Emergencies in Medical Practice

Emergencies in Medical Practice

Chief Advisor

Sukumar Mukherjee
MD FRCP (Lond) FRCP (Edinburgh) FICP FSMF
Honorary DSc (CU) Honorary D. Litt (Techno India University)
Head
Department of Medicine
Medical College
Kolkata, West Bengal, India

Editors

Om Tantia
MS FRCS (Eng) FACS FICS FAIS FMAS
Honorary Professor
Department of Surgery
Indian Medical Association (IMA)
Medical Director and Head
Department of Minimal Access and Bariatric Surgery
A Centre of Excellence (COE), Bariatric and Metabolic Surgery
ILS Hospitals
Kolkata, West Bengal, India

Ghanshyam Goyal
MBBS MD (Medicine)
Consultant Diabetologist and Director
Department of Diabetes and Metabolic Diseases
ILS Hospitals
Kolkata, West Bengal, India

Associate Editors

Tamonas Chaudhuri
MBBS MS FAIS FMAS FACS FACRSI (Hony)
Professor
Department of Surgery
Burdwan Medical College
Burdwan, West Bengal, India
Senior Consultant
Department of Minimal Access and Bariatric Surgery
ILS Hospitals
Kolkata, West Bengal, India

Gotam Pipara
MBBS MS (General Surgery) MCh (Urology,
Andrology and Renal Transplantation (St. John's – Bengaluru)
FRCS (Urology) (Edinburg)
Urology Consultant, Urologist,
and Andrologist
ILS Hospitals
Kolkata, West Bengal, India

Forewords

Pradeep Chowbey

Sukumar Mukherjee

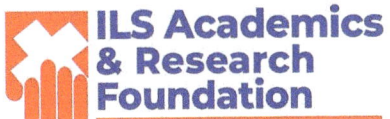

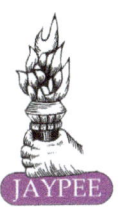

JAYPEE BROTHERS MEDICAL PUBLISHERS
The Health Sciences Publisher
New Delhi | London

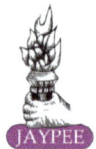

Jaypee Brothers Medical Publishers (P) Ltd

Headquarters

Jaypee Brothers Medical Publishers (P) Ltd
EMCA House, 23/23-B
Ansari Road, Daryaganj
New Delhi 110 002, India
Landline: +91-11-23272143, +91-11-23272703
+91-11-23282021, +91-11-23245672
Email: jaypee@jaypeebrothers.com

Corporate Office

Jaypee Brothers Medical Publishers (P) Ltd
4838/24, Ansari Road, Daryaganj
New Delhi 110 002, India
Phone: +91-11-43574357
Fax: +91-11-43574314
Email: jaypee@jaypeebrothers.com

Overseas Office

JP Medical Ltd
83 Victoria Street, London
SW1H 0HW (UK)
Phone: +44 20 3170 8910
Fax: +44 (0)20 3008 6180
Email: info@jpmedpub.com

Website: www.jaypeebrothers.com
Website: www.jaypeedigital.com

© 2023, Jaypee Brothers Medical Publishers

The views and opinions expressed in this book are solely those of the original contributor(s)/author(s) and do not necessarily represent those of editor(s) or publisher of the book.

All rights reserved. No part of this publication may be reproduced, stored or transmitted in any form or by any means, electronic, mechanical, photocopying, recording or otherwise, without the prior permission in writing of the publishers.

All brand names and product names used in this book are trade names, service marks, trademarks or registered trademarks of their respective owners. The publisher is not associated with any product or vendor mentioned in this book.

Medical knowledge and practice change constantly. This book is designed to provide accurate, authoritative information about the subject matter in question. However, readers are advised to check the most current information available on procedures included and check information from the manufacturer of each product to be administered, to verify the recommended dose, formula, method and duration of administration, adverse effects and contraindications. It is the responsibility of the practitioner to take all appropriate safety precautions. Neither the publisher nor the author(s)/editor(s) assume any liability for any injury and/or damage to persons or property arising from or related to use of material in this book.

This book is sold on the understanding that the publisher is not engaged in providing professional medical services. If such advice or services are required, the services of a competent medical professional should be sought.

Every effort has been made where necessary to contact holders of copyright to obtain permission to reproduce copyright material. If any have been inadvertently overlooked, the publisher will be pleased to make the necessary arrangements at the first opportunity.

Inquiries for bulk sales may be solicited at: jaypee@jaypeebrothers.com

Emergencies in Medical Practice

First Edition: **2023**

ISBN: 978-93-5696-122-7

Dedicated to

All the medical professionals who lost their lives while fighting the COVID-19 pandemic.

Section Editors

Ajoy Krishna Sarkar
MD (Medicine) MRCP (UK) FRCP (London)
Clinical Director
Department of Critical Care Unit
Peerless Hospital
Kolkata, West Bengal, India
Respiratory Emergencies

Anjan Lal Dutta MD DM FACC FCSI
Interventional Cardiologist and
Clinical Director
Department of Cardiology
Peerless Hospital
Kolkata, West Bengal, India
Past President
Cardiological Society of India
Cardiological Emergencies

Aruna Tantia MS FMAS FICOG Diploma in
Pelvic Endoscopy (Germany)
Director and Head, Department of
Obstetrics and Gynecology and Minimal
Invasive Gynecology, ILS Hospitals
Kolkata, West Bengal, India
Gynecological Emergencies

Arun Kumar Manglik
MD (Pediatrics) DNB (Pediatrics)
Pediatrician
Department of Pediatric Medicine
ILS Hospitals, Kolkata, West Bengal, India
Pediatric Emergencies

Dipashri Bhattacharya
MD (Anesthesiology) MNAMS FIAPM
Professor and Head
Department of Anesthesiology, Critical
Care and Pain
RG Kar Medical College
Kolkata, West Bengal, India
Director, Pain Clinic
COVID CCU In-Charge
Miscellaneous Emergencies-2

Ghanshyam Goyal MBBS MD (Medicine)
Consultant Diabetologist and Director
Department of Diabetes and Metabolic
Diseases, ILS Hospitals
Kolkata, West Bengal, India
Metabolic Emergencies

Goutam Gangopadhyay
MD DM (Neurology)
Ex-Professor and Senior Consultant
Neurologist
Department of Neurology
Bangur Institute of Neurosciences
and IPGME&R
Kolkata, West Bengal, India
Neurological Emergencies

Jayanta Mukherjee
MD (Medicine) DM (Gastroenterology)
Consultant Gastroenterologist
Department of Gastroenterology
ILS Hospitals
Kolkata, West Bengal, India
Gastrointestinal Emergencies

Jitendra Shah
MBBS Dip Ophthalmology FRCS (UK)
Consultant
Department of Ophthalmology
ILS Hospitals, Kolkata
New Alipore Eye Centre
Kolkata, West Bengal, India
Ophthalmological Emergencies

ML Saha
MBBS MS FAIS FMAS FALS
Professor and Head
Department of General Surgery
IPGME&R and SSKM Hospital
Kolkata, West Bengal, India
Miscellaneous Emergencies-1

Om Tantia
MS FRCS (Eng) FACS FICS FAIS FMAS
Honorary Professor
Department of Surgery
Indian Medical Association (IMA)
Medical Director and Head
Department of Minimal Access and
Bariatric Surgery
A Centre of Excellence (COE), Bariatric
and Metabolic Surgery
ILS Hospitals
Kolkata, West Bengal, India
Miscellaneous Emergencies-3

Pratim Sengupta
MD (Medicine) DM (Nephrology)
Consultant Nephrologist and Renal
Transplant Physician
Department of Nephrology
ILS Hospitals, Nephrocare India
Belle Vue Clinic
Kolkata, West Bengal, India
Nephrological Emergencies

Ramanuj Sinha MBBS DLO MS DNB FIAO
Professor
Department of ENT Medical College
Kolkata, West Bengal, India
ENT Emergencies

Sanjay Garg
MBBS MRCPsych (London) CCT (UK)
Head
Department of Psychiatry
Fortis Hospitals
Kolkata, West Bengal, India
Ex-Consultant
NHS Greater
Glasgow and Clyde
Glasgow, UK
Psychiatric Emergencies

Subhasish Deb MBBS FRCS
Consultant Orthopedic Surgeon
Department of Orthopedic
ILS Hospitals, Woodlands Hospital
AMRI Hospital
Kolkata, West Bengal, India
Trauma

Sukumar Mukherjee
MD FRCP (Lond) FRCP (Edinburgh) FICP FSMF
Honorary DSc (CU) Honorary D. Litt (Techno India
University)
Head
Department of Medicine
Medical College
Kolkata, West Bengal, India
Rheumatological Emergencies

Contributors

Abhraneel P Guha MBBS DNB (Medicine)
Registrar
Department of Medicine
Peerless Hospital
Kolkata, West Bengal, India

Adreesh Mukherjee
MD (Medicine) DM (Neurology)
Associate Professor
Department of Neurology
Bangur Institute of Neurosciences
and IPGME&R
Kolkata, West Bengal, India

Ajoy Krishna Sarkar
MD (Medicine) MRCP (UK) FRCP (London)
Clinical Director
Department of Critical Care Unit
Peerless Hospital
Kolkata, West Bengal, India

Arka Prava Chakraborty DM
Senior Resident
Department of Neuromedicine
Bangur Institute of Neurosciences
and IPGME&R
Kolkata, West Bengal, India

Arun Kumar Manglik
MD (Pediatrics) DNB (Pediatrics)
Pediatrician
Department of Pediatric Medicine
ILS Hospitals
Kolkata, West Bengal, India

Aruna Tantia
MS FMAS FICOG Diploma in Pelvic Endoscopy
(Germany)
Director and Head
Department of Obstetrics and
Gynecology and Minimal Invasive
Gynecology
ILS Hospitals
Kolkata, West Bengal, India

Avijit Das
MBBS MD (Tropical Medicine) FCCS (USA) MRCP (UK)
Consultant
Department of General Medicine
Peerless Hospital
Kolkata, West Bengal, India

Bhaswati Dasgupta Nath MRCP (UK)
Consultant
Department of Internal Medicine
Peerless Hospital and BK Roy Research
Center
Kolkata, West Bengal, India

Chintha Venkata Sriram DM (Neurology)
1st Year DM Resident
Bangur Institute of Neurosciences
and IPGME&R
Kolkata, West Bengal, India

Dayal Bandhu Majumdar MBBS DO
Senior Medical Officer
Department of Ophthalmology
Calcutta National Medical College
and Hospital
Kolkata, West Bengal, India
Technical Advisor, ICMR

Dipasri Bhattacharya
MD (Anesthesiology) MNAMS FIAPM
Professor and Head
Department of Anesthesiology, Critical
Care and Pain
RG Kar Medical College
Kolkata, West Bengal, India
Director, Pain Clinic, COVID CCU In-charge

Gautam Ghosh MD (Pediatrics) DNB (Pediatrics)
Pediatrician
Department of Pediatric Medicine
Park Clinics
Kolkata, West Bengal, India

Ghanshyam Goyal MBBS MD (Medicine)
Consultant Diabetologist and Director
Department of Diabetes and Metabolic
Diseases
ILS Hospitals
Kolkata, West Bengal, India

Goutam Gangopadhyay
MD DM (Neurology)
Ex-Professor and Senior Consultant
Neurologist
Department of Neurology
Bangur Institute of Neurosciences
and IPGME&R
Kolkata, West Bengal, India

Haseeb Hassan
MBBS MD (Medicine) DM (Neurology) Post-
doctoral Fellowship in Epilepsy
Neurologist/Consultant Epileptologist
Department of Neurology
Rabindranath Tagore International
Institute of Cardiac Sciences
Rabindranath Tagore Multispecialty Clinic
Narayana Superspecialty Hospital
AMRI Hospitals
Kolkata, West Bengal, India

Jasodhara Chaudhuri
MD (Pediatric Medicine) MRCPCH (UK) DM
(Neurology)
Pediatric Neurologist
Clinical Tutor
Department of Neurology
Bangur Institute of Neurosciences
and IPGME&R
Kolkata, West Bengal, India

Jayanta Mukherjee
MD (Medicine) DM (Gastroenterology)
Consultant Gastroenterologist
Department of Gastroenterology
ILS Hospitals
Kolkata, West Bengal, India

Jitendra Shah
MBBS Dip Ophthalmology FRCS (UK)
Consultant
Department of Ophthalmology
ILS Hospitals, Kolkata
New Alipore Eye Centre
Kolkata, West Bengal, India

Kallol K Dey
MBBS (Hons and Gold Medalist) MD (IPGMER Gold
Medal) MRCP (UK) FRCP (London)
Consultant Neurologist
Department of Neurology
CK Birla Group of Hospitals
Kolkata, West Bengal, India

Kamal Singh Chhajer
MBBS MS (General Surgery) MCh (Plastic Surgery)
Consultant General Surgeon
Plastic Surgeon
Calcutta Medical Research Institute and
ILS Hospitals
Kolkata, West Bengal, India

Contributors

Lopamudra Chowdhury
MBBS DA MD (Pharmacology)
Associate Professor and Head
Department of Pharmacology
Murshidabad Medical College
Murshidabad, West Bengal, India

Mihir Sirkar MD (Pediatrics)
Professor, In-Charge PICU
Department of Pediatrics
Medical College
Kolkata, West Bengal, India

Namrata Biswas MD (Anesthesia)
Senior Consultant
Department of Anesthesiology
ILS Hospitals, Columbia Asia, BIRTH Clinic
Neotia Hospital
Kolkata, West Bengal, India

Nandini Chatterjee
MBBS MD (Internal Medicine) FRCP (Glasgow) FICP
Professor
Department of Medicine
IPGME&R and SSKM Hospital
Kolkata, West Bengal, India
Editor, Journal of the Indian Medical
Association (JIMA)
Joint Secretary (Deans Place), API

Nitin Manglik
MD (Pediatrics) DCH (UK) MRCPCH (UK)
Pediatrician
Department of Pediatric Medicine
ILS Hospitals
Kolkata, West Bengal, India

Pankaj Kumar MS FACS
Associate Professor
Department of General Surgery
All India Institute of Medical Sciences
Bhubaneswar, Odisha, India

Pankaj Singhania MBBS MD
Senior Resident
Department of Endocrinology
Institute of Post Graduate Medical
Education and Research
Kolkata, West Bengal, India

Parthajit Das
MD FRCP (London) FRCP (Edinburgh) MRCP
(Rheumatology) MSC (Sports Medicine) CCST (UK)
Consultant Rheumatologist
Department of Rheumatology
Apollo Multispeciality Hospital, Kolkata
Assistant Professor
Department of Medicine
Ramakrishna Mission Seva Pratishthan
Kolkata, West Bengal, India

Piyas Gargari
MBBS MD DM (Endocrinology)
Senior Resident
Department of Endocrinology
Institute of Post Graduate Medical
Education and Research
Kolkata, West Bengal, India

Pradeep Singh
MBBS MRCP (UK) Fellowship in Intensive Care
Medicine
Acute Medicine Consultant, Recruitment
Lead
Department of Emergency Medicine
Princess Royal University Hospital
Orpington
King's College Hospital
NHS Foundation Trust
London, UK

Prakash Kumar Sasmal
MS (Gold Medal) FNB (Minimal Access Surgery)
FACS FACRSI FAIS FALS (Bariatric)
Additional Professor
Department of General Surgery
All India Institute of Medical Sciences
Bhubaneswar, Odisha, India

Pratik Biswas
MBBS MD (Pulmonary Medicine)
Consultant Pulmonologist
Department of Pulmonology
ILS Hospitals
Kolkata, West Bengal, India

Pratim Sengupta
MD (Medicine) DM (Nephrology)
Consultant Nephrologist and Renal
Transplant Physician
Department of Nephrology
ILS Hospitals, Nephrocare India
Belle Vue Clinic
Kolkata, West Bengal, India

Preethi Rubinath MS ENT
Senior Resident
Department of ENT
Medical College
Kolkata, West Bengal, India

Ramanuj Sinha MBBS DLO MS DNB FIAO
Professor
Department of ENT
Medical College
Kolkata, West Bengal, India

Rekha Basak Srivastava BAMS
Clinical Podiatrist and Clinical Research
Coordinator
Department of Diabetes and Metabolic
Diseases
ILS Hospitals
Kolkata, West Bengal, India

Rishika Pal MBBS
House Officer
Department of General Medicine
Peerless Hospitex Hospital and BK Roy
Research Centre
Kolkata, West Bengal, India

Saibal Moitra
MBBS MD (Chest Medicine) PhD FCCP MAMS
FRCP (Edinburgh)
Adjunct Professor and Senior Consultant
Division of Allergy and Immunology
Department of Respiratory Medicine
Apollo Multispeciality Hospital
Kolkata, West Bengal, India

Sanjay Garg
MBBS MRCPsych (London) CCT (UK)
Head
Department of Psychiatry
Fortis Hospitals
Kolkata, West Bengal, India
Ex-Consultant
NHS Greater Glasgow and Clyde
Glasgow, UK

Sanjay K Shah
MD MRCP CCST
Consultant Endocrinologist
Department of Endocrinology
Narayana Superspeciality Hospital
Howrah, West Bengal, India

Sanjukta Dey
DCH (Cal) DCH (UK) DNB MRCPCH (UK) FRCP (UK)
Dip Allergy (UK)
Clinical Director
Department of Pediatrics and
Neonatology
Peerless Hospital
Kolkata, West Bengal, India

Santanu K Tripathi
MBBS MD DM (Clinical Pharmacology)
Independent Clinical Pharmacologist and
Academic Dean
Professor and Head
Department of Pharmacology
Netaji Subhas Medical College and
Hospital
Patna, Bihar, India

Sarbajit Ray
MBBS MD (Internal Medicine)
Consultant
Department of Internal Medicine
ILS Hospitals, Kolkata
Assistant Professor
Department of Medicine
Medical College
Kolkata, West Bengal, India

Contributors

Saumitra Ray
MBBS MD FRCP FACC FESC FSCAI
Director
Department of Invasive Cardiology
MRI Hospitals (Dhakuria)
Kolkata, West Bengal, India

Shambo Samrat Samajdar
MBBS MD DM (Clinical Pharmacology) Fellowship in Respiratory and Critical Care (WBUHS) Fellow Allergy and Asthma Specialist Course (AAAAI) Dip Allergy Asthma Immunology (IAS) PG Dip Endo and Diabetes (RCP)
Consultant
Department of Medicine
Diabetes and Allergy-Asthma Specialty Clinic, Kolkata
Clinical Pharmacologist
Department of Medicine
School of Tropical Medicine
Kolkata, West Bengal, India

Shankha Shubhra Chaudhuri
MD (Internal Medicine) DM (Neurology)
Consultant
Department of Neurology
Eskag Sanjeevani Multispecialty Hospital
AMRI Hospitals
Kolkata, West Bengal, India

Shilanjan Roy MBBS MD DM (Cardiology)
Assistant Professor
Department of Cardiology
KPC Medical College
Kolkata, West Bengal, India

Sougata Sarkar
MBBS MD DM (Clinical Pharmacology)
Clinical Pharmacologist
Department of Medicine
School of Tropical Medicine
Kolkata, West Bengal, India

Souvik Dubey DM
Assistant Professor
Department of Neuromedicine
Bangur Institute of Neurosciences and IPGME&R
Kolkata, West Bengal, India

Srina Ray MBBS
Clinical Assistant
Department of Cardiology
Calcutta Cardiology Clinic
Kolkata, West Bengal, India

Subhasish Deb MBBS FRCS
Consultant Orthopedic Surgeon
Department of Orthopedic
ILS Hospitals, Woodlands Hospital
AMRI Hospital
Kolkata, West Bengal, India

Sujoy Ghosh
MBBS MD DM (Endocrinology)
Professor
Department of Endocrinology
Institute of Post Graduate Medical Education and Research
Kolkata, West Bengal, India

Sukumar Mukherjee
MD FRCP (Lond) FRCP (Edinburgh) FICP FSMF Honorary DSc (CU) Honorary D. Litt (Techno India University)
Head
Department of Medicine
Medical College
Kolkata, West Bengal, India

Sumanta Biswas MSc
Senior Research Associate
Department of Nephrology
Nephrocare India
Kolkata, West Bengal, India

Sunil Lhila MD DM (Cardiology)
Senior Interventional Cardiologist
Department of Cardiology
Rotary Narayana Nethralaya, Kolkata
Rabindranath Tagore International Institute of Cardiac Sciences
Kolkata, West Bengal, India

Sunipa Chatterjee MS FMAS FICMCH
Associate Consultant
Department of Obstetrics and Gynecology and Minimal Invasive Gynecology
ILS Hospitals
Kolkata, West Bengal, India

Tamoghna Banerjee
MBBS MRCP (UK)
Consultant
Department of Medicine
Peerless Hospitex Hospital
Kolkata, West Bengal, India

Tanya Panja MS DNB
Senior Resident
Department of ENT
Medical College
Kolkata, West Bengal, India

Titas Kar
MBBS MS (ENT) DNB (ENT) FEBORL-HNS (EU) DOHNS (UK)
ENT and Head Neck Surgeon
Department of ENT
Tamralipto Government Medical College
Tamluk, West Bengal, India

Usashi Biswas Bose MBBS
PG Trainee
Department of Diabetes and Metabolic Diseases
ILS Hospitals
Kolkata, West Bengal, India

Ushasi Mukherjee DGO DNB
Associate Consultant
Department of Obstetrics and Gynecology and Minimal Invasive Gynecology
ILS Hospitals
Kolkata, West Bengal, India

Vernon VS Bonarjee MD PhD FESC
Sr. Consultant
Department of Cardiology
Stavanger University Hospital
Stavanger, Norway

Vikas Prakash
DM (Hepatology) ILBS (Delhi)
Director
D'CosMedics Clinic
Kolkata, West Bengal, India

Vivek Shah MBBS
Medical Intern
Department of Endocrinology
Medical College
Kolkata, West Bengal, India

VK Mohun MD (Medicine)
Senior Registrar
Department of Nephrology
Nephrocare India
Kolkata, West Bengal, India

Foreword

I wish to congratulate, Dr Om Tantia on the publication of his Textbook on *Emergencies in Medical Practice*. It is rare in present times to have a textbook of repute that covers a wide range of medical specialties. This textbook is an admirable compilation of medical emergencies and their management across almost the entire spectrum of clinical medicine today. I cannot recollect any similar publication that deals in medical, surgical, neurological, gynecological, trauma, respiratory, poisoning and many other emergencies. Therein lies the immense value and scope of this textbook.

The specialty sections are written by eminent specialists with vast and long experience and expertise in their respective fields. Each chapter has been divided and written with subheadings to improve clarity and for ease of understanding. The style is lucid, reader-friendly with plenty of take home messages.

I am certain this publication will cater to a very wide audience. It should find pride of place in medical colleges and teaching hospital libraries for our younger colleagues in training. More importantly, I visualize this textbook to be a handy guide and a reference for practicing clinicians across several medical specialties.

The book will likely fill in a big gap that exists today on the subject. This is even more important today in the atmosphere of consumerism and litigation that has crept into the medical profession.

I wish Dr Om Tantia and his colleagues a long and productive professional career and hope that they will continue to contribute so generously to advance medical knowledge and expertise.

With warm regards,

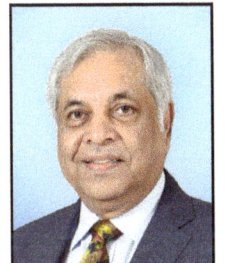

Pradeep Chowbey
MS MNAMS FRCS (London) FIMSA FAIS FICS FACS FIAGES FALS FAMS
Padma Shri awarded by the President of India
Chairman, Max Institute of Laparoscopic, Endoscopic and Bariatric Surgery, New Delhi
Chairman, Surgery and Allied Surgical Specialties, New Delhi, India
Honorary Laparoscopic Surgeon to the President of India
Honorary Laparoscopic Surgeon to Armed Forces Medical Services (AFMS)
Doctor of Science (Honoris Causa)
Surgeon to His Holiness Dalai Lama
President
International Federation for the Surgery of Obesity and Metabolic Disorders (IFSO) 2012–2013
Asia Pacific Chapter of IFSO (IFSO-APC) 2011–2013
Asia Pacific Metabolic and Bariatric Surgery Society (APMBSS) 2010–2012
Obesity and Metabolic Surgery Society of India (OSSI) 2006–2009
Founder President, Asia Pacific Hernia Society (APHS) 2004

Foreword

I feel privileged and enthused to write a Foreword for the book *"Emergencies in Medical Practice"*—an academic venture of Dr Om Tantia and Dr Ghanshyam Goyal, with the collaborative efforts of erudite and experienced clinicians.

Over the years, medical emergencies have taken a great stride with near-precision in various disciplines by the immense technological support and expertise. Basically, expectations of the patients are all time high. Bedside skill is still relevant toward success. In fact, emergency care has become a separate discipline with the broad classification of nontraumatic and traumatic care.

Medical emergencies by their own nature can occur at any time without warning and not necessarily in the usual clinical environment. It is, therefore, essential to be able to recognize the nature of the emergency as soon as it occurs and to have the knowledge, proficiency, and confidence to be able to undertake the appropriate remediable measures in opportune moment. The well-coordinated team of experts on multidirectional issues supported by technology has remained a benchmark in arriving at diagnosis for urgent care. The comprehensive book should be taken as a practical approach as provided by expert clinicians to yield a measurable success but individual variation should be duly respected.

This book edited by Dr Om Tantia, Dr Ghanshyam Goyal, and other senior specialists uniquely emphasizes on major disciplines of Internal Medicine in a logical way and to remain an eye-opener for emergency services supported by current scientific knowledge.

The additional scope of optimal care in other sections such as eye, ENT, pediatrics, psychiatry, burns, road-traffic accidents, drug interactions, etc., are of added value in diverse emergencies. Coverages of miscellaneous emergencies such as poisoning, drowning, etc., are welcome addition which is of immense value in rural settings.

I am optimistic all the physician, surgeons, and others would love it as an invaluable companion for evidence-based practice in emergency medicine.

I fervently wish Dr Tantia and Dr Goyal and their associates for their tireless efforts to bring out updated capsule of emergency care with grand success in time. Periodic revision is always welcome.

Best wishes and sincere regards.

Sukumar Mukherjee
MD FRCP (Lond) FRCP (Edinburgh) FICP FSMF
Honorary DSc (CU) Honorary D. Litt (Techno India University)
Head
Department of Medicine
Medical College
Kolkata, West Bengal, India

Preface

It gives us great pleasure to introduce this book on *Emergencies in Medical Practice*.

Medical emergencies usually deal with life-threatening situations and carry dire consequences. In these critical moments it is important for the clinician dealing with them to be equipped with the knowledge and correct guidelines regarding their management. Thus, clinicians dealing with emergency patients need to be a jack of all specialties. For example, a well-respected surgeon may be at wits end when faced with a cardiac emergency while traveling on a flight. Similarly, an endocrinologist may not know the correct protocol to be followed when treating a trauma patient. Similarly, treatment of snakebite is clouding by lots of myths. Our aim behind this book is to provide a comprehensive overview of all the common emergencies faced in clinical practice with evidence-based current guidelines. Each chapter deals with a specific emergency, has been written and reviewed by leading experts in their respective fields. The material is concise with salient points for emergencies at the end and has been backed by a number of illustrations to keep the reader engaged.

We hope that the book will serve as a useful tool for all clinicians, especially those who deal with emergencies in their routine practice.

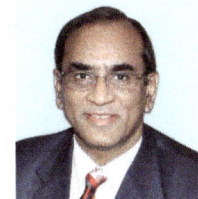

Om Tantia
MS FICS FAIS FMAS FACS FRCS (Eng) FALS (Bariatric) IAGES
Honorary Professor
Department of Surgery
Indian Medical Association (IMA)
Medical Director and Head
Department of Minimal Access and Bariatric Surgery
A Center of Excellence (COE), Bariatric and Metabolic Surgery
ILS Hospitals
Kolkata, West Bengal, India

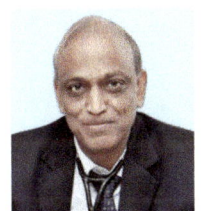

Ghanshyam Goyal
MBBS MD (Medicine)
Consultant Diabetologist and Director
Department of Diabetes and Metabolic Diseases
ILS Hospitals
Kolkata, West Bengal, India

Acknowledgments

It gives us great pleasure to acknowledge the efforts and contributions of the various persons involved in making this endeavor successful.

First and foremost, we would like to thank Professor Sukumar Mukherjee, who has inspired, guided, and supported us for creation of this book. We also thank him and Dr Pradeep Chowbey for their foreword.

All the contributors who have immense experience in their respective fields have shared their knowledge most passionately.

We would also like to acknowledge the efforts of Drs Tamonas Chaudhuri, Gotam Pipara, Aruna Tantia, Mridul Tantia, Shashi Khanna, Rajendar Rupavath, Pratik Biswas, Col. Shubhojeet Chatterjee, Ruchi Roumya Das, Abhinay Tibdewal, Abhishek Tiwari, Samiran Purkait, Rekha B Srivastava, and Usashi Biswas for sharing their valuable inputs and their constant support.

Staff and team at ILS Hospitals and ILS Academics, Kolkata, West Bengal, India deserve special acknowledgment for their unparalleled support and cooperation. Special credit must be given to Ms Kajari, our Clinical Research Assistant, who has relentlessly worked, coordinated, and compiled all the information and has been instrumental in completing this project. Our special thanks to Mr Subhranath Maitra for all the troubleshooting.

Finally, we also like to thank Shri Jitendar P Vij (Group Chairman), Mr Ankit Vij (Managing Director), Mr MS Mani (Group President), Ms Chetna Malhotra (Senior Director—Professional Publishing, Marketing and Business Development), Ms Pooja Bhandari (Production Head), Ms Suchita Gera (Development Editor), Mr Sabyasachi Hazra (Sr. Business Manager, Publishing) and the staff of M/s Jaypee Brothers Medical Publishers (P) Ltd, New Delhi, India.

Contents

Section 1   Cardiological Emergencies

Section Editor: Anjan Lal Dutta

1. **Cardiac Arrest and Cardiopulmonary Resuscitation** 3
   Pradeep Singh

2. **Approach to Syncope** 17
   Kallol K Dey

3. **Acute Coronary Syndrome: ST-elevation Myocardial Infarction** 29
   Sunil Lhila

4. **Acute Heart Failure** 34
   Vernon VS Bonarjee

5. **Cardiac Tamponade: Diagnosis and Management** 40
   Shilanjan Roy, Srina Ray, Saumitra Ray

Section 2   Respiratory Emergencies

Section Editor: Ajoy Krishna Sarkar

6. **Emergency Airway Management** 49
   Namrata Biswas

7. **Respiratory Failure** 57
   Tamoghna Banerjee

8. **Respiratory Emergencies** 61
   Ajoy Krishna Sarkar, Abhraneel P Guha, Sanjukta Dey, Pratik Biswas

9. **Massive Hemoptysis** 70
   Rishika Pal, Bhaswati Dasgupta Nath

10. **Acute Pulmonary Embolism** 77
    Avijit Das

11. **Acute Exacerbation of Asthma** 85
    Sanjukta Dey

Section 3   Neurological Emergencies

Section Editor: Goutam Gangopadhyay

12. **Approach to an Unconscious Patient** 95
    Chintha Venkata Sriram, Goutam Gangopadhyay

13. **Status Epilepticus** 104
    Haseeb Hassan

14. **Stroke** 111
    Shankha Shubhra Chaudhuri

15. **Acute Meningitis** 118
    Jasodhara Chaudhuri

16. **Acute Encephalitis** 123
    Arka Prava Chakraborty, Souvik Dubey

17. **Acute Migraine** 129
    Adreesh Mukherjee

Section 4: Gastrointestinal Emergencies

Section Editor: Jayanta Mukherjee

18. **Acute Abdomen: Approach** 137
    Jayanta Mukherjee

19. **Acute Gastrointestinal Hemorrhage: Approach** 142
    Jayanta Mukherjee

20. **Acute Pancreatitis: Approach** 146
    Jayanta Mukherjee

21. **Acute Hepatic Failure** 150
    Vikas Prakash

Section 5: Nephrological Emergencies

Section Editor: Pratim Sengupta

22. **Acute Renal Failure** 157
    Pratim Sengupta, VK Mohun, Sumanta Biswas

23. **Drugs and Kidney** 168
    Pratim Sengupta, VK Mohun, Sumanta Biswas

Section 6: Metabolic Emergencies

Section Editor: Ghanshyam Goyal

24. **Metabolic Emergencies (Electrolyte): Hyponatremia, Hypernatremia, Hypokalemia, and Hyperkalemia** 177
    Pankaj Singhania, Piyas Gargari, Sujoy Ghosh

25. **Metabolic-hyperglycemic Emergencies** 187
    Sanjay K Shah, Vivek Shah

26. **Endocrinal (Hypoglycemia)** 193
    Ghanshyam Goyal, Usashi Biswas Bose, Rekha Basak Srivastava

Section 7: Gynecological Emergencies

Section Editor: Aruna Tantia

27. **Gynecological Emergencies** 203
    Aruna Tantia, Sunipa Chatterjee, Ushasi Mukherjee

Section 8 — Trauma

Section Editor: *Subhasish Deb*

28. Road Traffic Accidents 215
    Subhasish Deb

29. Household Trauma 218
    Subhasish Deb

Section 9 — Psychiatric Emergencies

Section Editor: *Sanjay Garg*

30. Violence in Mental Health 223
    Sanjay Garg

Section 10 — Ophthalmological Emergencies

Section Editor: *Jitendra Shah*

31. Ophthalmic Emergencies 231
    Jitendra Shah

Section 11 — ENT Emergencies

Section Editor: *Ramanuj Sinha*

32. Emergencies in ENT 237
    Ramanuj Sinha, Titas Kar, Tanya Panja, Preethi Rubinath

    32.1 Foreign Bodies in ENT: A Nightmare for Patients and Doctors Alike! 237
        Ramanuj Sinha, Titas Kar

    32.2 Tracheostomy 240
        Ramanuj Sinha, Tanya Panja

    32.3 Otalgia 242
        Ramanuj Sinha, Preethi Rubinath

Section 12 — Pediatric Emergencies

Section Editor: *Arun Kumar Manglik*

33. Pediatric Emergencies 247
    Arun Kumar Manglik, Gautam Ghosh, Mihir Sirkar, Nitin Manglik

Section 13 — Rheumatological Emergencies

Section Editor: *Sukumar Mukherjee*

34. Emergencies in Rheumatological Practice 257
    Parthajit Das, Sukumar Mukherjee

Section 14: Miscellaneous Emergencies-1

Section Editor: ML Saha

35. **Burns** 267
    Kamal Singh Chhajer

36. **Postoperative Emergencies** 276
    Prakash K Sasmal, Pankaj Kumar

Section 15: Miscellaneous Emergencies-2

Section Editor: Dipashri Bhattacharya

37. **Code Blue and Crash Cart** 289
    Namrata Biswas

38. **Anesthetic Emergencies** 292
    Dipasri Bhattacharya

Section 16: Miscellaneous Emergencies-3

Section Editor: Om Tantia

39. **Unknown Poisoning** 305
    Nandini Chatterjee

40. **Snakebite: Initial Management, Myths, and Reality** 309
    Dayal Bandhu Majumdar

41. **Anaphylaxis** 316
    Shambo Samrat Samajdar, Sougata Sarkar, Saibal Moitra, Santanu K Tripathi

42. **Emergencies in Medical Practice: Common Drugs** 322
    Lopamudra Chowdhury

43. **Emergency Management of Drowning** 328
    Sarbajit Ray

Index .... *(Scan QR Code for detailed Index)*

SECTION 1

Cardiological Emergencies

Section Editor: *Anjan Lal Dutta*

1. **Cardiac Arrest and Cardiopulmonary Resuscitation**
   Pradeep Singh

2. **Approach to Syncope**
   Kallol K Dey

3. **Acute Coronary Syndrome: ST-elevation Myocardial Infarction**
   Sunil Lhila

4. **Acute Heart Failure**
   Vernon VS Bonarjee

5. **Cardiac Tamponade: Diagnosis and Management**
   Shilanjan Roy, Srina Ray, Saumitra Ray

CHAPTER 1: Cardiac Arrest and Cardiopulmonary Resuscitation

Pradeep Singh

INTRODUCTION

Countless numbers of people owe their lives to the quick application of cardiopulmonary resuscitation (CPR). The technique of coupling positive pressure ventilation and external cardiac compression was the result of the work of Peter Safar, who is also credited with the creation of one of the first intensive care units in the United States as well as one of the first paramedic emergency services. He is credited with multiple researches. CPR sciences are one of them which began in mid-20th century and gradually evolved to present state.[6]

Though this form important part of training in developed world but subcontinent dissemination of this science is still minimal. There could be various reason for the roadblock such as missing dedicated society funded by government at the level of state and center who will be responsible for research and sciences just like society of developed world namely American Heart Association (AHA), Resuscitation Council of UK, European Resuscitation Council and so on; missing protocolized clinical pathway of CPR sciences in healthcare institute private or government. Till date there is no concrete steps in this regard.

Few organization such as AHA have made entry to deliver these sciences in our country and that has been well accepted by private healthcare institute and by few government institutes. We believe these institute have workforce who were trained in developed country, and this could be the reason for acceptance in their workplace. Nevertheless, we are still far behind in terms of deliverance of care involving CPR sciences.

The world has gone through a very turmoil face of COVID-19 pandemic but few things which is understood during this phase is importance of infection control practices, triage, need of preparedness for disaster management, usefulness of CPR sciences, intensive care medicine, resource management, virtual consultation, paramedic support and need for integrated prehospital emergency medicine services such as ambulance service and on-going care.

This article is adaptation from updated guidelines of AHA, input from European Resuscitation Society and Resuscitation Council UK. It is an honest intent to simplify and bring the updated guidelines.

DATA FROM OTHER COUNTRIES WITH A STABILIZED EMERGENCY MEDICAL SYSTEM

The average overall survival to hospital discharge from 28,000 emergency medical services (EMS)-treated Out Hospital Cardiac Arrest (OHCA) in England is 8.6%, Holland 21.5%, Seattle 20%, and Norway 25%.

Countries with the highest rates of OHCA survival are those which have strengthened all four links in the chain of survival **(Fig. 1)**.

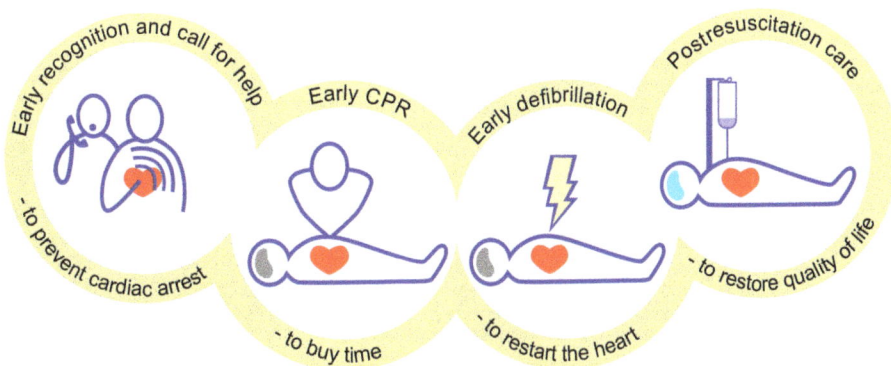

Fig. 1: Chain of survival.

Necessity: Bystander chest compression or knowledge of CPR can save life in out of hospital scenario. Victim could be anyone even your near or dear ones.

ADULT BASIC LIFE SUPPORT

Steps of CPR

Before you approach the person, who has collapsed, check your surroundings for danger.

1. Verify scene safety
2. Unresponsive (shake them gently), shout for nearby help, activate emergency response system via mobile device (if appropriate). Get automated external defibrillator (AED) and emergency equipment.
3. Look, listen and feel for signs of normal breathing or no normal or gasping breath (Look for the rise and fall of their chest normally) and check pulse simultaneously, is pulse felt definitely within 10 seconds?
4. Fetch an AED, if you can (difficult in Indian scenario but places such as airport have them). If someone is with you, ask them to fetch AED and bring it back.
5. Begin cycles of CPR 30 compressions and 2 breaths.
6. Start with high quality chest compressions if no pulse felt **(Fig. 2)**:
   - Interlock your fingers
   - Place your hands in the center of the chest on the line connecting nipples. Straighten your arms and position your shoulders directly over your hands.
   - Push down hard at least 5 cm up to 6 cm and then release twice per second (120/min) and do not stop.
   - Minimize interruption
   - Allow full chest recoil
7. Opening of the airway and giving breaths **(Figs. 3 to 5)**:
   - Position yourself at the patient's side so that the airway can be opened easily and breaths can be delivered to the patient.
   - If no trauma is involved, then head tilt-chin lift is performed following which mouth-to-mouth/mouth-to-mask breaths are delivered.
   - *Head tilt-chin lift:* Place one hand on the patient's forehead and push it your palm to tilt the head back simultaneously place the finger of other hand under bony part of lower jaw near the chin and lift the jaw to bring the chin forward.
   - *Mouth to mouth breathing:* After head tilt-chin lift, pinch the nose closed with your thumb and index finger of the hand on forehead then make an airtight seal with your lips around patient's mouth. Give 1 breath (blow for 1 second) and watch for chest rise as you give breath.
   - *Mouth to mask (barrier) breathing:* Position yourself at the patient's side. Place the mask, using nasal bridge as the guide. Place the thumb and index finger of the hand over the forehead along the border of the mask while place the thumb of the other hand along the lower margin of the mask. Now place the remaining fingers along the bony margin of the jaw and perform head tilt-chin lift. Give 1 breath (blow for 1 second) and watch for chest rise as you give breath.
8. If you have an AED, switch it on and follow the instructions.
   - An AED will tell you exactly what to do—just follow the prompt.
   - Common steps to use universal AED (Remember "PAAS")
     - P: *Power* on AED
     - A: *Attach* the right size pads. Make sure the area where the pad is applied is clean and dry.
     - A: *Analyze.* Let AED analyze the rhythm. Make sure no one is touching the patient.
     - S: *Shock.* AED advises you for the shock then keep all rescuer clear from the patient till shock is delivered. Continue CPR and follow above cycles after 2 minutes.

     Check for special situations.
9. *Continue CPR until:* The AED asks you to pause while it reanalyzes and gives another shock if needed, a trained medic arrives and tells you what to do or the person shows signs of life.

By developing the skills and confidence to follow these simple steps, you could be a lifesaver in an emergency. **Flowchart 1** shows an algorithm of adult basic life support.

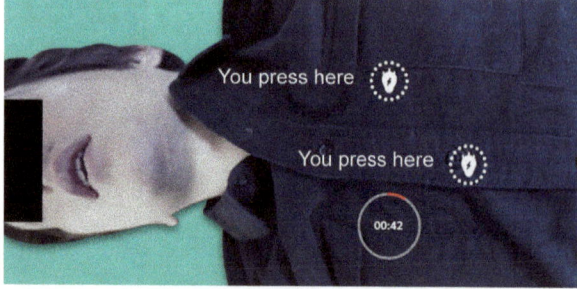 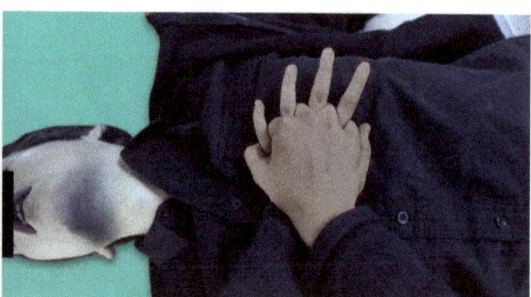

Fig. 2: Steps of cardiopulmonary resuscitation (CPR).
Source: Input taken from AHA updation and Resuscitation Council UK for nonprofitable and educational purpose.[1]

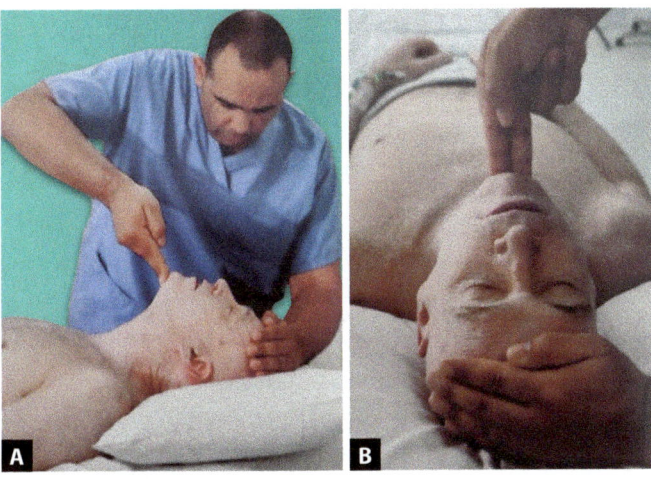

Figs. 3A and B: Head tilt-chin lift.
Source: Input taken from AHA updation and Resuscitation Council UK for nonprofitable and educational purpose.

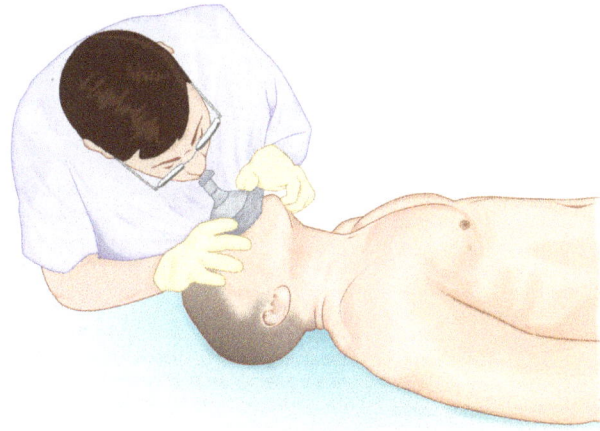

Fig. 5: Mouth to mask (barrier) breathing.
Source: Source: Input taken from AHA updation and Resuscitation Council UK for nonprofitable and educational purpose.

PREVENTION OF OUT-OF-HOSPITAL CARDIAC ARREST

Symptoms such as syncope (especially during exercise, while sitting or supine), palpitations, dizziness and sudden shortness of breath that are consistent with an arrhythmia should be investigated. Apparently healthy young adults who suffer sudden cardiac death (SCD) can also have signs and symptoms (e.g., syncope/presyncope, chest pain and palpitations) that should alert healthcare professionals to seek expert help to prevent cardiac arrest.

Young adults presenting with characteristic symptoms of arrhythmic syncope should have a specialist cardiology assessment, which should include an electrocardiogram (ECG) and in most cases echocardiography and an exercise test.

Systematic evaluation in a clinic specializing in the care of those at risk for SCD is recommended in family members of young victims of SCD or those with a known cardiac disorder resulting in an increased risk of SCD. Identification of individuals with inherited conditions and screening of family members can help prevent deaths in young people with inherited heart disorders.

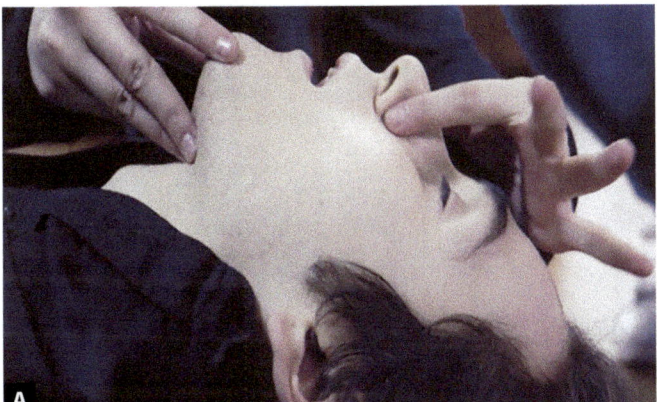
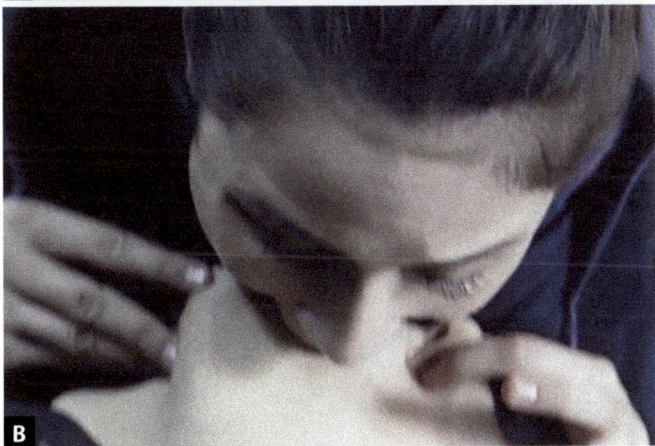

Figs. 4A and B: Mouth to mouth breathing.
Source: Input taken from AHA updation and Resuscitation Council UK for nonprofitable and educational purpose.

ADVANCE LIFE SUPPORT IN CARDIAC ARREST

It is also important to understand the cases which may undergo cardiac arrest. The various analysis of data as per European and UK Resuscitation Councils has led to new update in resus guidelines 2020. It highlights following ways of prevention of cardiac arrest in out-hospital and in-hospital patients.

PREVENTION OF IN-HOSPITAL CARDIAC ARREST

Shared decision making and advanced care planning which integrates resuscitation decisions with emergency care treatment plans to increase clarity of treatment goals and also prevent inadvertent deprivation of other indicated treatments, besides CPR. These plans should be recorded in a consistent manner.

Hospitals should use a track and trigger early warning score system for the early identification of patients who are critically ill or at risk of clinical deterioration.

Hospitals should train staff in the recognition, monitoring and immediate care of the acutely ill patient.

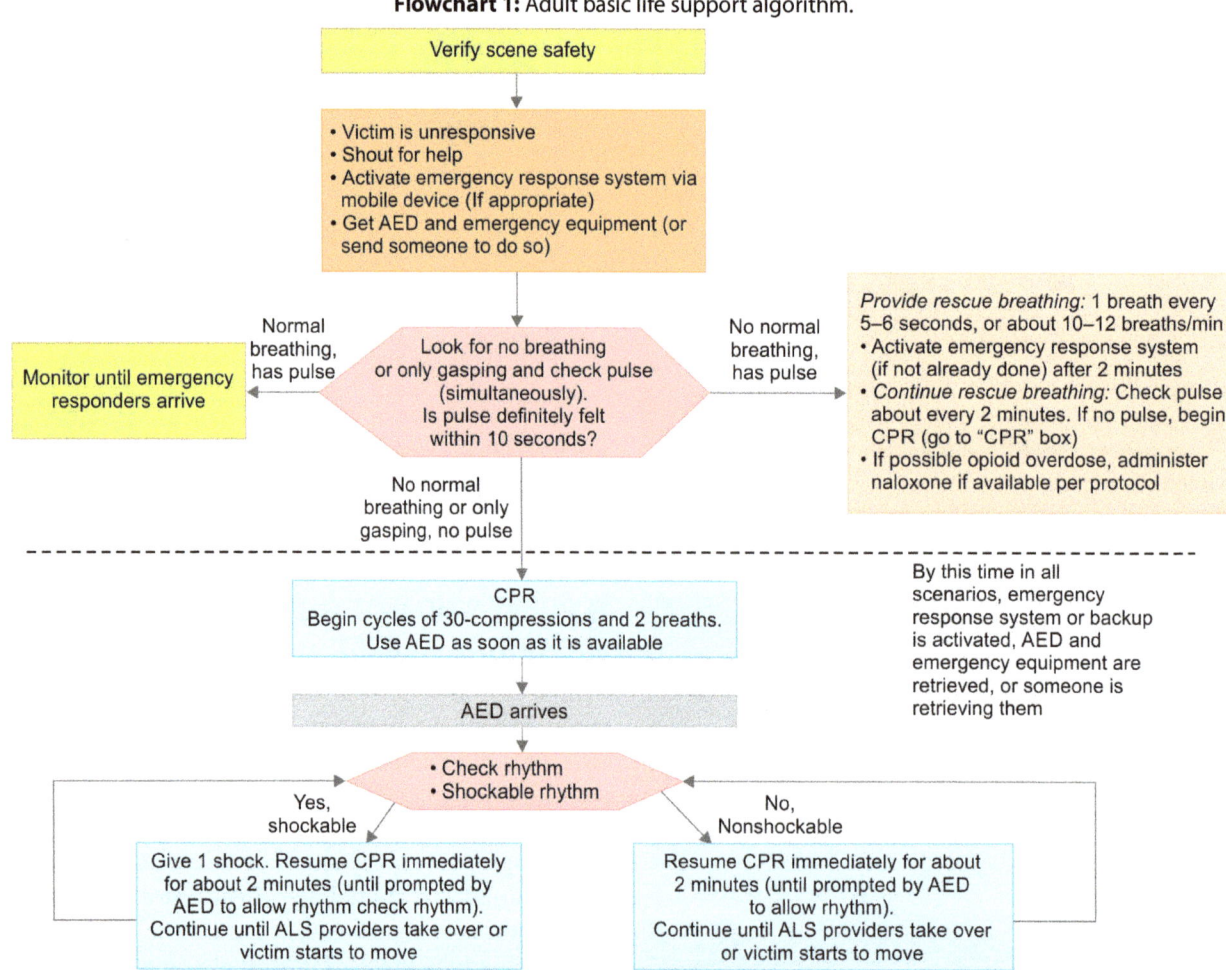

Flowchart 1: Adult basic life support algorithm.

(AED: automated external defibrillator; CPR: cardiopulmonary resuscitation)
Source: Input taken from AHA updation and Resuscitation Council UK for nonprofitable and educational purpose.

Hospitals should empower all staff to call for help when they identify a patient at risk of physiological deterioration. This includes calls based on clinical concern, rather than solely on vital signs.

Hospitals should have a clear policy for the clinical response to abnormal vital signs and critical illness. This may include a critical care outreach service and/or emergency team (e.g., medical emergency team, rapid response team).

Hospital staff should use structured communication tools to ensure effective handover of information.

Patients should receive care in a clinical area that has the appropriate staffing, skills, and facilities for their severity of illness.

Hospitals should review cardiac arrest events to identify opportunities for system improvement and share key learning points with hospital staff.

Next Step

Next step to resuscitation is advance life support. Which is self-explanatory as per **Flowchart 2**. Ideal way of training is through class and case based (online or offline) scenario to develop skills. Subsequently we have incorporated various different scenarios, modified intervention and prioritization needed for advance life support in opioid overdose, pregnancy, pediatric patient **(Flowchart 4 to 7)**.

The resuscitation protocols do not end with return of spontaneous circulation but need to be followed with therapeutic temperature monitoring and involvement of intervention as per adult postcardiac arrest care algorithm **(Flowchart 3)**.

IMPACT OF COVID-19 ON RESUSCITATION (BOX 1)

The resuscitation guidelines, which are usually updated in 5 years underwent an addition of new changes especially related to PPE use. The salient points are mentioned in subsequent **Flowcharts 4 to 7**.

CARDIAC ARREST SITUATIONS

Periarrest situation commonly leading to arrest situations, which are arrhythmias—tachycardia and bradycardia.

Flowchart 2: Adult advance cardiac arrest algorithm.[1]

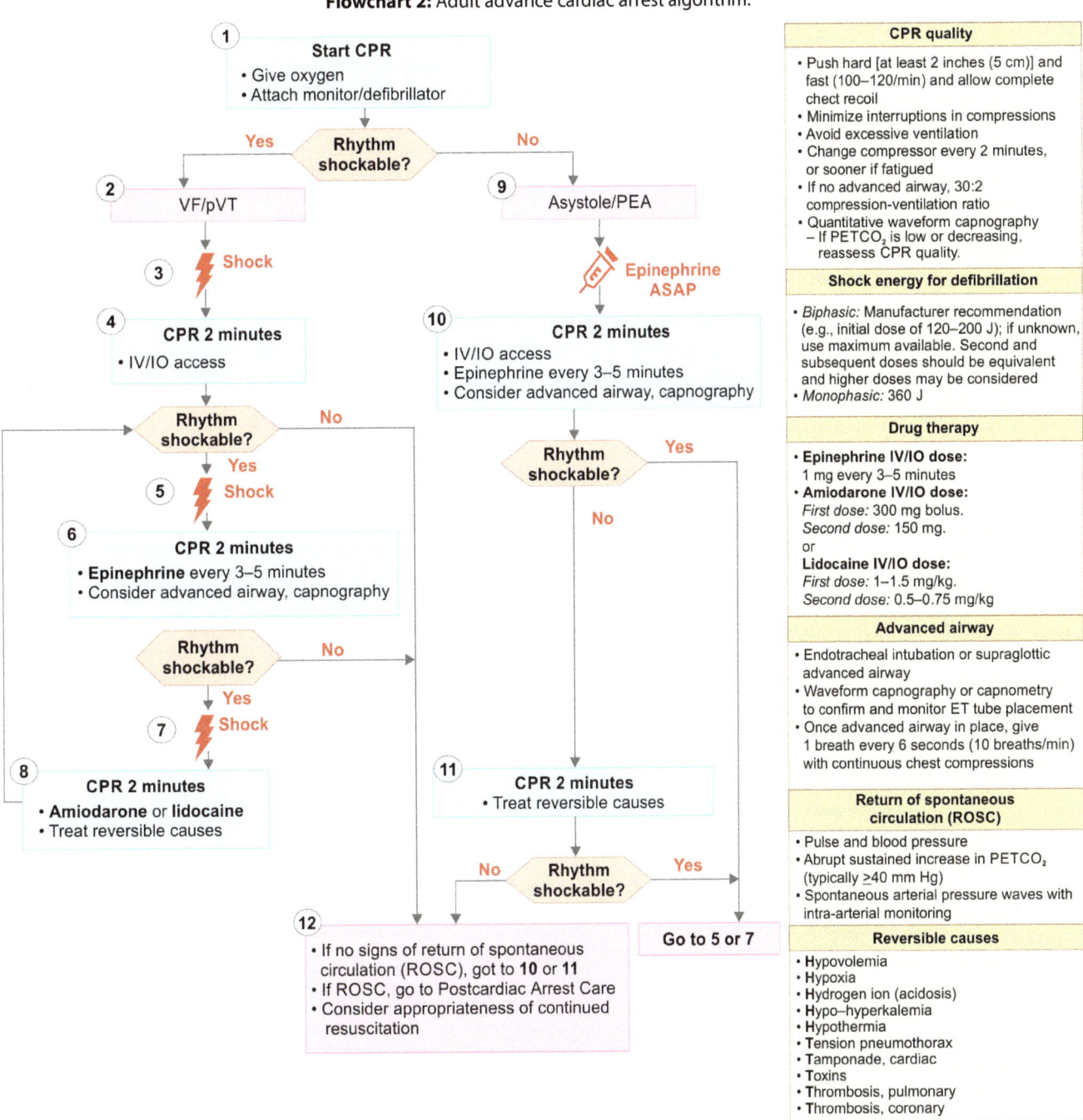

(CPR: cardiopulmonary resuscitation; IO: intraosseous; IV: intravenous; PEA: pulseless electrical activity; pVT: pulseless ventricular tachycardia; VF: ventricular fibrillation)
Source: Input taken from AHA updation and Resuscitation Council UK for nonprofitable and educational purpose.

Tachycardia: Salient Points

- Electrical cardioversion is the preferred treatment for tachyarrhythmia in the unstable patient displaying potentially life-threatening adverse signs.
- Conscious patients require anesthesia or sedation, before attempting synchronized cardioversion.
- To convert atrial or ventricular tachyarrhythmias, the shock must be synchronized to occur with the R wave of the ECG.
- *For atrial fibrillation:* An initial synchronized shock at maximum defibrillator output rather than an escalating approach is a reasonable strategy based on current data.
- *For atrial flutter and paroxysmal supraventricular tachycardia:* Give an initial shock of 70–120 J. Give subsequent shocks using stepwise increases in energy.
- *For ventricular tachycardia with a pulse:* Use energy levels of 120–150 J for the initial shock. Consider stepwise increases if the first shock fails to achieve sinus rhythm.

Flowchart 3: Adult postcardiac arrest care algorithm.[1]

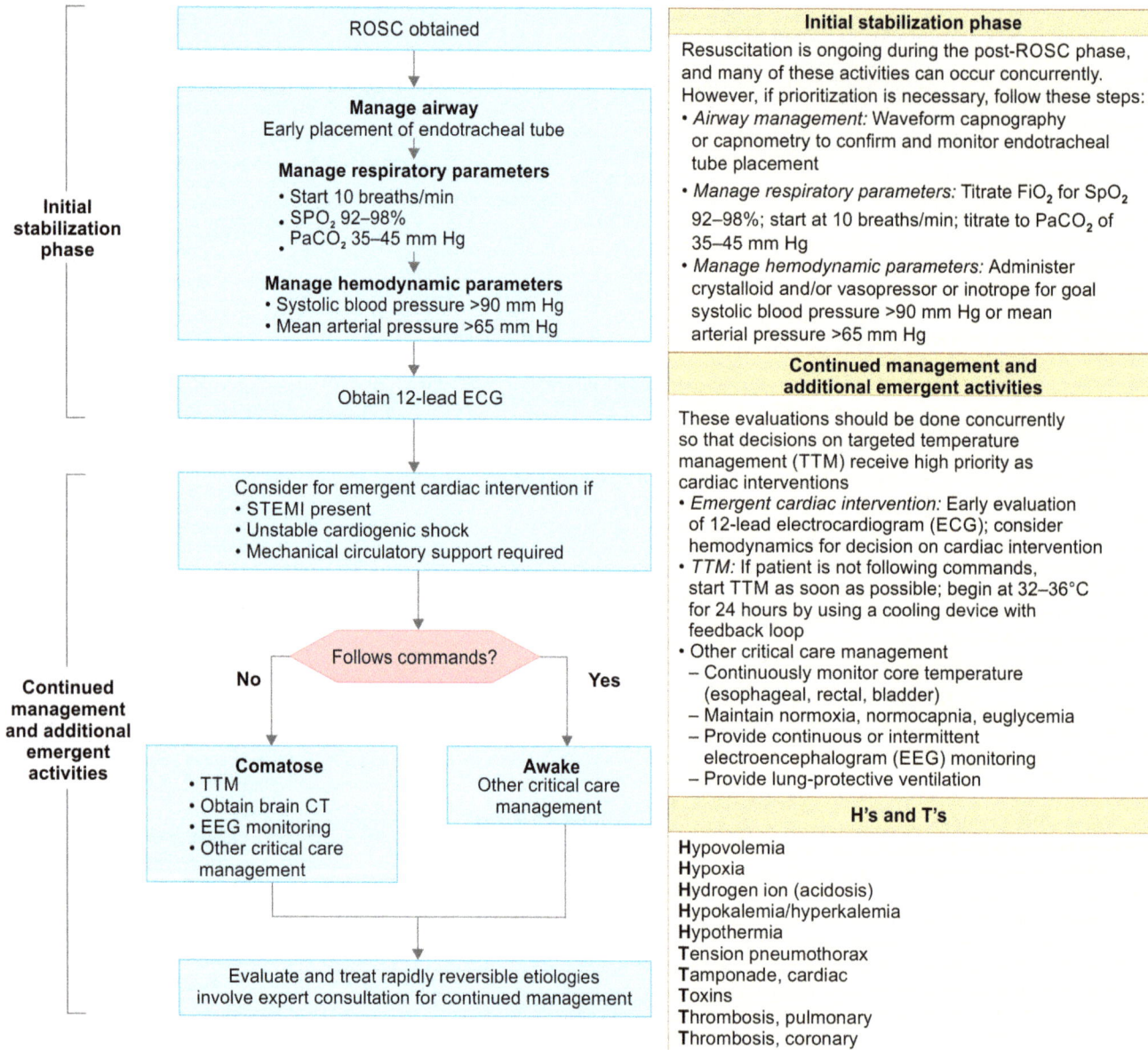

(ROSC: return of spontaneous circulation; STEMI: ST-elevation myocardial infarction elevation)
Source: Input taken from AHA updation and Resuscitation Council UK for non-profitable and educational purpose

---

BOX 1: Resuscitation of adult COVID-19 patients in acute hospital settings.

- Recognize cardiac arrest. Look for the absence of signs of life and normal breathing. Feel for a carotid pulse if trained to do so. Do not listen or feel for breathing by placing your ear and cheek close to the patient's mouth. When calling cardiac arrest code
- If wearing level 2 PPE (surgical mask, gloves, apron and eye protection) and a defibrillator is readily available, defibrillate shockable rhythms rapidly prior to starting chest compressions. The early restoration of circulation may prevent the need for further resuscitation measures. Local guidance must be followed about equipment entering the area
- Full aerosal generating procedure (AGP) personal protective equipment (PPE) (disposable gloves, fluid resistant gown/suit, filtering face piece respirator and eye protection) must be worn by all members of the resuscitation/emergency team before entering the room. Sets of AGP PPE must be readily available where resuscitation equipment is being locally stored. No chest compressions or airway procedures such as those detailed below should be undertaken without full AGP PPE. Once suitably clothed, start compression-only CPR and monitor the patient's cardiac arrest rhythm as soon as possible. Do not do mouth-to-mouth ventilation or use a pocket mask. If the patient is already receiving supplemental oxygen therapy using a face mask, leave the mask on the patient's face during chest compressions as this may limit aerosol spread. If not in situ, but one is readily available, put a simple oxygen mask on the patient's face. Restrict the number of staff in the room (if a single room). Allocate a gatekeeper to do this

Contd...

Contd...

- Airway interventions (e.g., supraglottic airway (SGA) insertion or tracheal intubation) must be carried out by experienced individuals. Individuals should use only the airway skills (e.g., bag-mask ventilation) for which they have received training. For many HCWs this will mean two-person bag-mask techniques with the use of an oropharyngeal airway. Tracheal intubation or SGA insertion must only be attempted by individuals who are experienced and competent in this procedure. Use a viral filter between the self-inflating bag and airway (mask, SGO or tracheal tube). Liaise with your anesthetic department about the use of filters
- Identify and treat any reversible causes (e.g., severe hypoxemia) before considering stopping CPR. Discussion should be maintained throughout the resuscitation event and early planning of the postresuscitation phase undertaken. Contact senior help and gain advice from critical care partners as part of the planning
- Dispose of, or clean, all equipment used during CPR following the manufacturer's recommendations and local guidelines. Any work surfaces used for airway/resuscitation equipment will also need to be cleaned according to local guidelines. Specifically, ensure equipment used in airway interventions (e.g., laryngoscopes, face masks) is not left lying on the patient's pillow, but is instead placed in a tray. Do not leave the Yankauer sucker placed under the patient's pillow; instead, put the contaminated end of the Yankauer inside a disposable glove
- Remove PPE safely to avoid self-contamination and dispose of clinical waste bags as per local guidelines. Hand hygiene has an important role in decreasing transmission. Thoroughly wash hands with soap and water; alternatively, alcohol hand rub is also effective
- Postresuscitation debrief is important and should be planned

Source: Input taken from Resuscitation Council UK for nonprofitable and educational purpose.

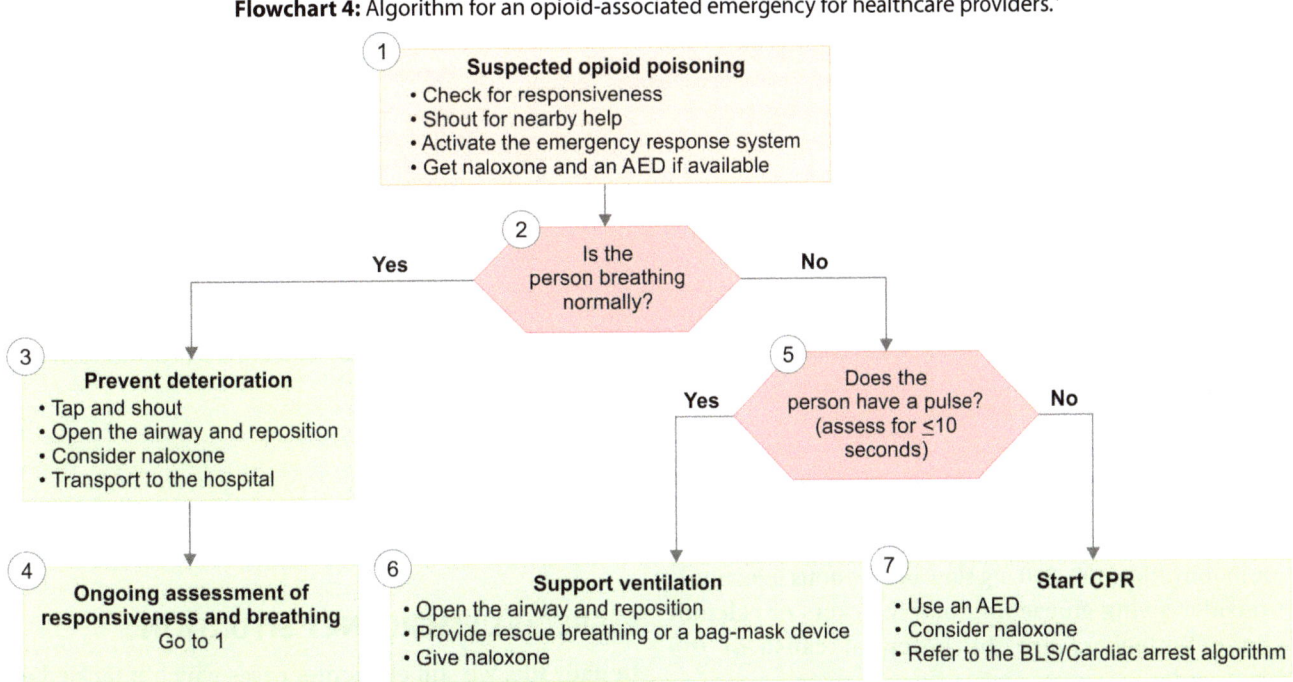

Flowchart 4: Algorithm for an opioid-associated emergency for healthcare providers.[1]

(AED: automated external defibrillator; BLS: basic life support; CPR: cardiopulmonary resuscitation)
Source: Input taken from AHA updation and Resuscitation Council UK for nonprofitable and educational purpose.

- If cardioversion fails to restore sinus rhythm and the patient remains unstable, give amiodarone 300 mg intravenously over 10–20 minutes (or procainamide 10–15 mg/kg over 20 minutes) and reattempt electrical cardioversion. The loading dose of amiodarone can be followed by an infusion of 900 mg over 24 hours.
- If the patient with tachycardia is stable (no life-threatening adverse signs or symptoms) and is not deteriorating, pharmacological treatment may be possible.
- Consider amiodarone for acute heart rate control in AF patients with hemodynamic instability and severely reduced left ventricular ejection fraction (LVEF). For patients with LVEF <40% consider the smallest dose of beta-blocker to achieve a heart rate <110/min. Add digoxin if necessary.

Bradycardia: Salient Points

- If bradycardia is accompanied by life-threatening adverse signs, give atropine 500 µg IV (IO) and, if necessary, repeat every 3–5 minutes to a total of 3 mg.
- If treatment with atropine is ineffective, consider second line drugs. These include isoprenaline (5 µg/min starting dose), and adrenaline (2–10 µg/min).

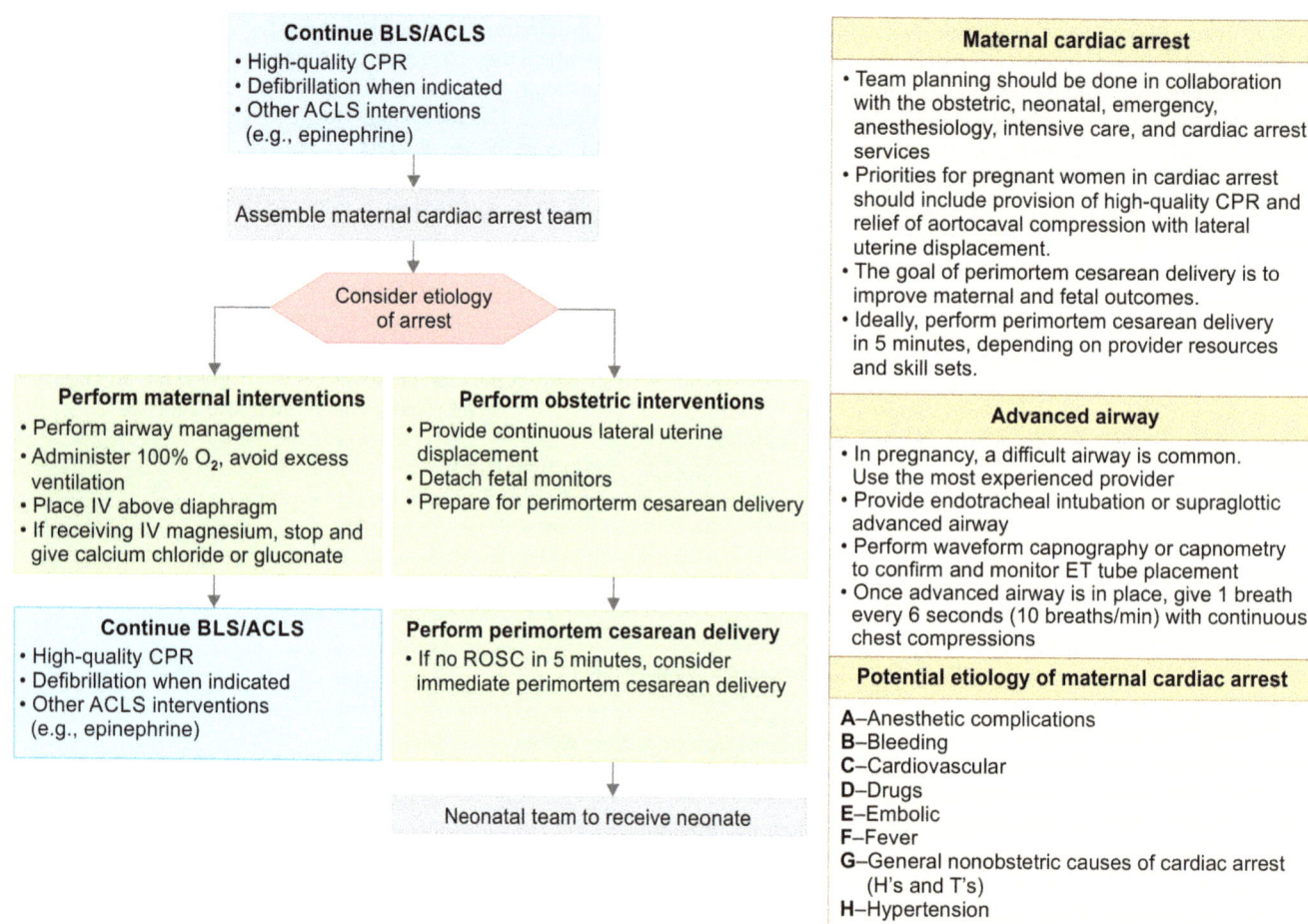

Flowchart 5: Cardiac arrest in pregnancy in-hospital ACLS algorithm.[1]

(ACLS: advanced cardiac life support; BLS: basic life support; CPR: cardiopulmonary resuscitation; ET: endotracheal; ROSC: return of spontaneous circulation)
Source: American Heart Association, 2020.

- For bradycardia caused by inferior myocardial infarction, cardiac transplant or spinal cord injury, consider giving aminophylline (100–200 mg slow intravenous injection).
- Consider giving glucagon if beta-blockers or calcium channel blockers are the potential cause of the bradycardia.
- Do not give atropine to patients with cardiac transplants—it can cause a high-degree AV block or even sinus arrest—use aminophylline.
- Consider pacing in patients who are unstable, with symptomatic bradycardia refractory to drug therapies.
- If transcutaneous pacing is ineffective, consider transvenous pacing. Whenever a diagnosis of asystole is made, check the ECG carefully for the presence of P waves because unlike true asystole, this is more likely to respond to cardiac pacing.
- If atropine is ineffective and transcutaneous pacing is not immediately available, fist pacing can be attempted while waiting for pacing equipment.

Flowcharts 8 and 9 show how to deal with adult tachycardia with pulse and adult bradycardia. It is based on Resuscitation Council UK guidelines but also include input from AHA updates.

■ SPECIAL EMERGENCY SITUATION

In daily life, we still encounter cases which if tackled early on then cardiac arrest can be avoided. Choking leading to airway obstruction is such a case.

There have been few changes made recently and those are back slaps on adult patient followed by Heimlich maneuver.

Steps to handle a choking or foreign body airway obstruction is discussed here and shown in **Figures 6A and B**.

Choking: Foreign Body Airway Obstruction

- Foreign body airway obstruction: Suspect choking if someone is suddenly unable to speak or talk, particularly if eating.
- Encourage the person to cough.

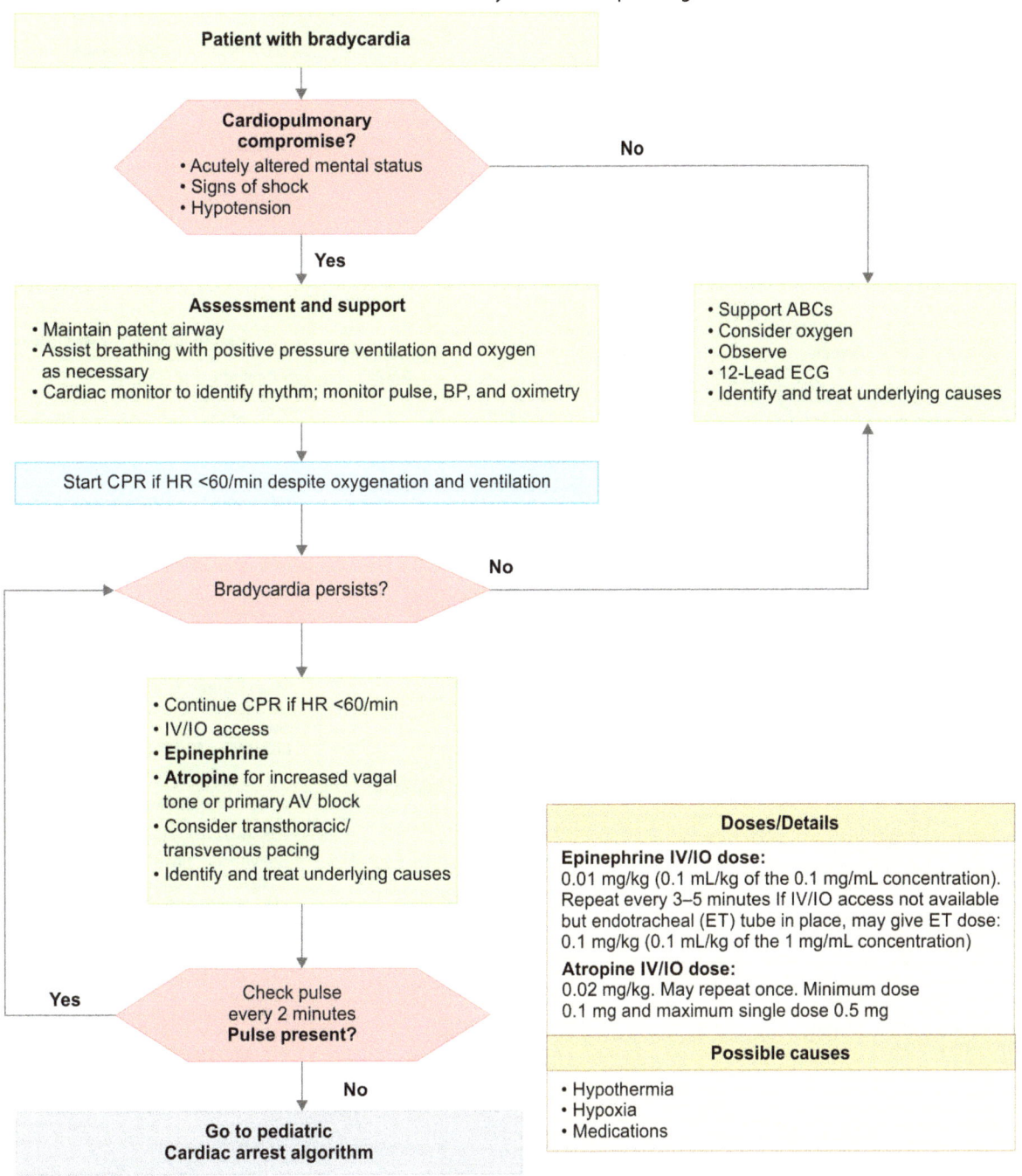

Flowchart 6: Pediatric bradycardia with a pulse algorithm.[1]

(ABC: airway, breathing, and circulation; CPR: cardiopulmonary resuscitation; ECG: electrocardiogram; HR: heart rate)
Source: Input taken from AHA updation and Resuscitation Council UK for nonprofitable and educational purpose.

- If the cough becomes ineffective, give up to five back blows, lean the person forward. Apply blows between the shoulder blades using the heel of one hand **(Fig. 6A)**.

If back blows are ineffective, give up to five abdominal thrusts: Stand behind the person and put both your arms around the upper part of their abdomen. Lean the person forward. Clench your fist and place it between the umbilicus (navel) and the ribcage. Grasp your fist with the other hand and pull sharply inward and upward **(Fig. 6B)**.

If choking has not been relieved after five abdominal thrusts, continue alternating five back blows with five abdominal thrusts until it is relieved, or the person becomes unresponsive. If the person becomes unresponsive, start CPR.

Recovery Position for Adults and Children

This needs a mention. As less vigilant ward or out-hospital scenarios where we get patient in unconscious state can be easily managed in this position and avoid potential dangers such as aspiration and airway obstruction.

Flowchart 7: Pediatric cardiac arrest algorithm.[1]

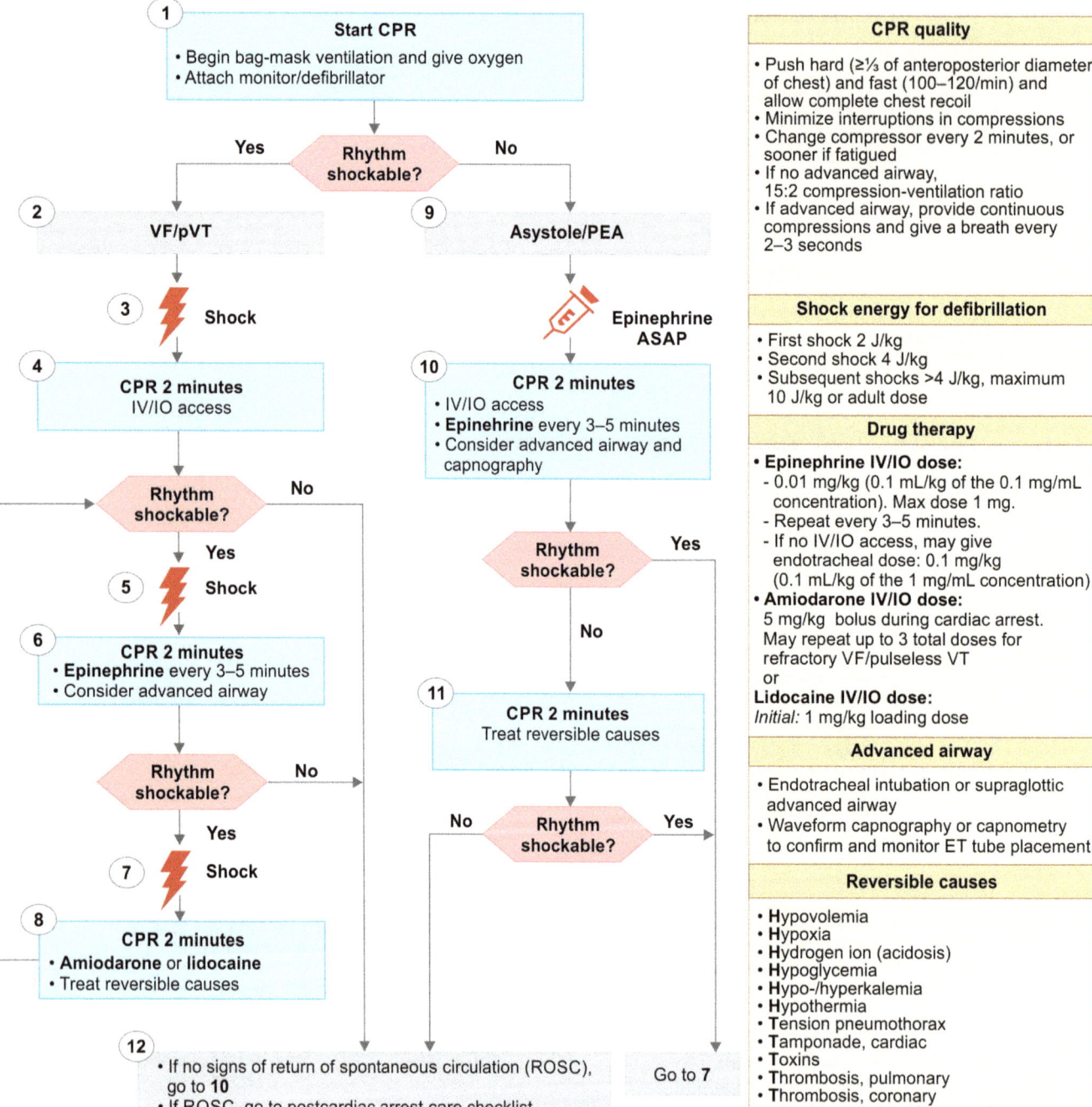

(CPR: cardiopulmonary resuscitation; IO: intraosseous; IV: intravenous; PEA: pulseless electrical activity; pVT: pulseless ventricular tachycardia; VF: ventricular fibrillation)
Source: Input taken from AHA updation and Resuscitation Council UK for nonprofitable and educational purpose.

Recovery position for adults and children with a decreased level of responsiveness due to medical illness or nonphysical trauma, who do not meet the criteria for the initiation of rescue breathing or chest compressions (CPR).

It is recommended that they can be placed into a lateral, side-lying recovery position. Overall, there is little evidence to suggest an optimal recovery position, but resuscitation councils recommend the following sequence of actions **(Fig. 7)**:

- Kneel beside the person and make sure that both legs are straight.
- Place the arm nearest to you out at right angles to the body with the hand palm uppermost.
- Bring the far arm across the chest and hold the back of the hand against the person's cheek nearest to you.
- With your other hand, grasp the far leg just above the knee and pull it up, keeping the foot on the ground.

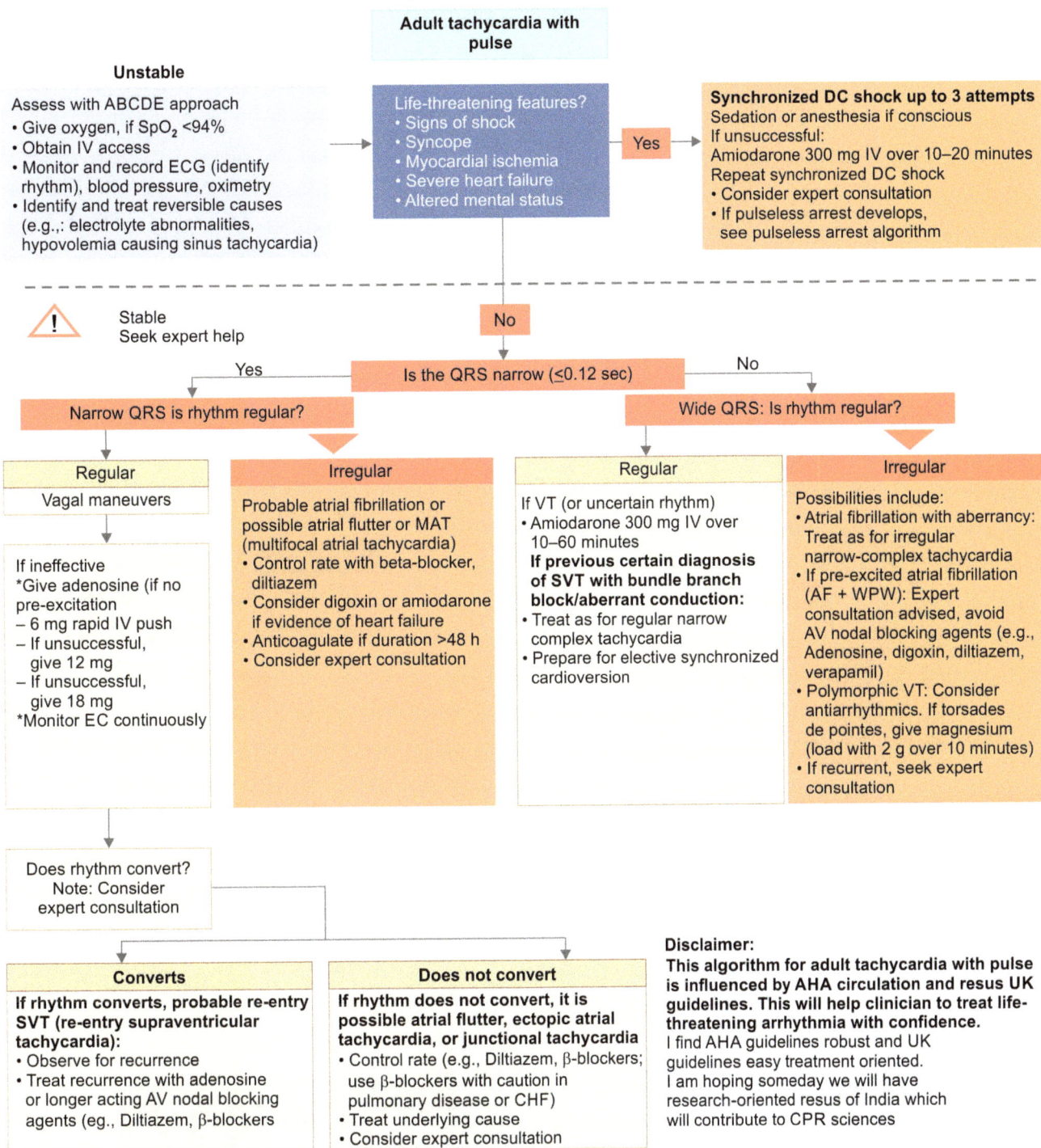

Flowchart 8: Algorithm to treat adult tachycardia with pulse.

(ABCDE: airway, breathing, circulation, disability, and exposure; CHF: congestive heart failure; SVT: supraventricular tachycardia)

- Keeping the hand pressed against the cheek, pull on the far leg to roll the person towards you onto their side. Adjust the upper leg so that both the hip and knee are bent at right angles.
- Tilt the head back to make sure the airway remains open. Adjust the hand under the cheek, if necessary, to keep the head tilted and facing downward to allow liquid material to drain from the mouth.

Check regularly for normal breathing. Only leave the person unattended if absolutely necessary, e.g., to attend to other people. It is important to stress the importance of maintaining a close check on all unresponsive individuals until the EMS arrives to ensure that their breathing remains normal. In certain situations, such as resuscitation-related agonal respirations or trauma, it may not be appropriate to move the individual into a recovery position.

Flowchart 9: Algorithm to treat adult bradycardia.

```
Assess with ABCDE approach
           ↓
Give oxygen if appropriate and obtain IV access
           ↓
Monitor ECG, BP, SpO₂, record 12-lead ECG
           ↓
Identify and treat reversible causes
e.g., electrolyte abnormalities
           ↓
• Life-threatening features?
• Signs of shock
• Syncope
• Myocardial ischemia
• Severe heart failure
• Altered mental status
```

Yes → Atropine 500 mcg IV → Satisfactory response?
- Yes → Risk of asystole?
- No → Interim measures:
  - Atropine 500 mcg IV repeat to maximum of 3 mg
  - Adrenaline 2–10 mcg min-1 IV
  - Alternative drugs* or
  - Transcutaneous pacing
  → Seek expert help → Arrange transvenous pacing

No → Risk of asystole?
- Recent asystole
- Mobitz II AV block
- Complete heart block with broad QRS
- Ventricular pause >3s

Risk of asystole? Yes → Interim measures (above)
Risk of asystole? No → Observe

AHA
**Alternatives include
• Dopamine 2–10 mcg/Kg min-1 IV
• Adrenaline 2–10 mcg min-1 IV

Resus UK
**Alternatives include
• Aminophylline
• Dopamine
• Isoprenaline 5 mcg min-1 IV
• Glucagon (if beta-blocker or calcium channel blocker overdose)
• Glycopyrrolate can be used instead of atropine

(ABCDE: airway, breathing, circulation, disability, and exposure)

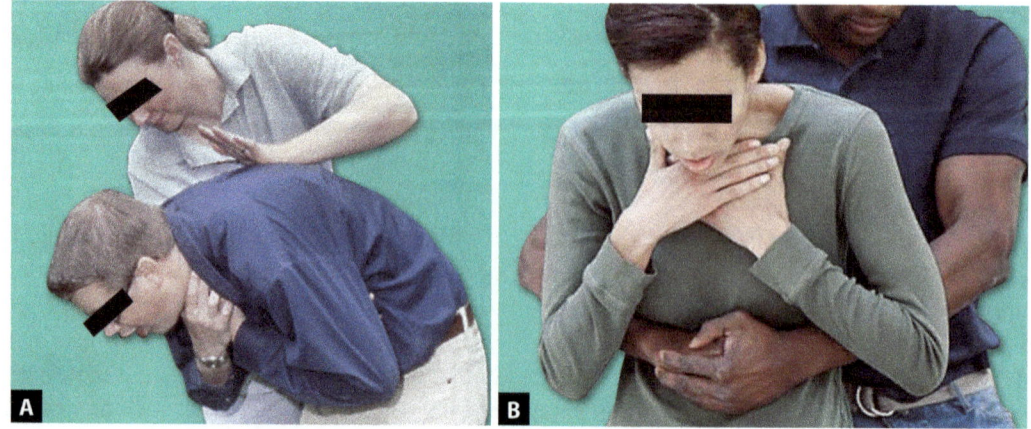

Figs. 6 A and B: Combined techniques to treat foreign body airway obstruction.
Source: Input taken from Resuscitation Council UK for nonprofitable and educational purpose.

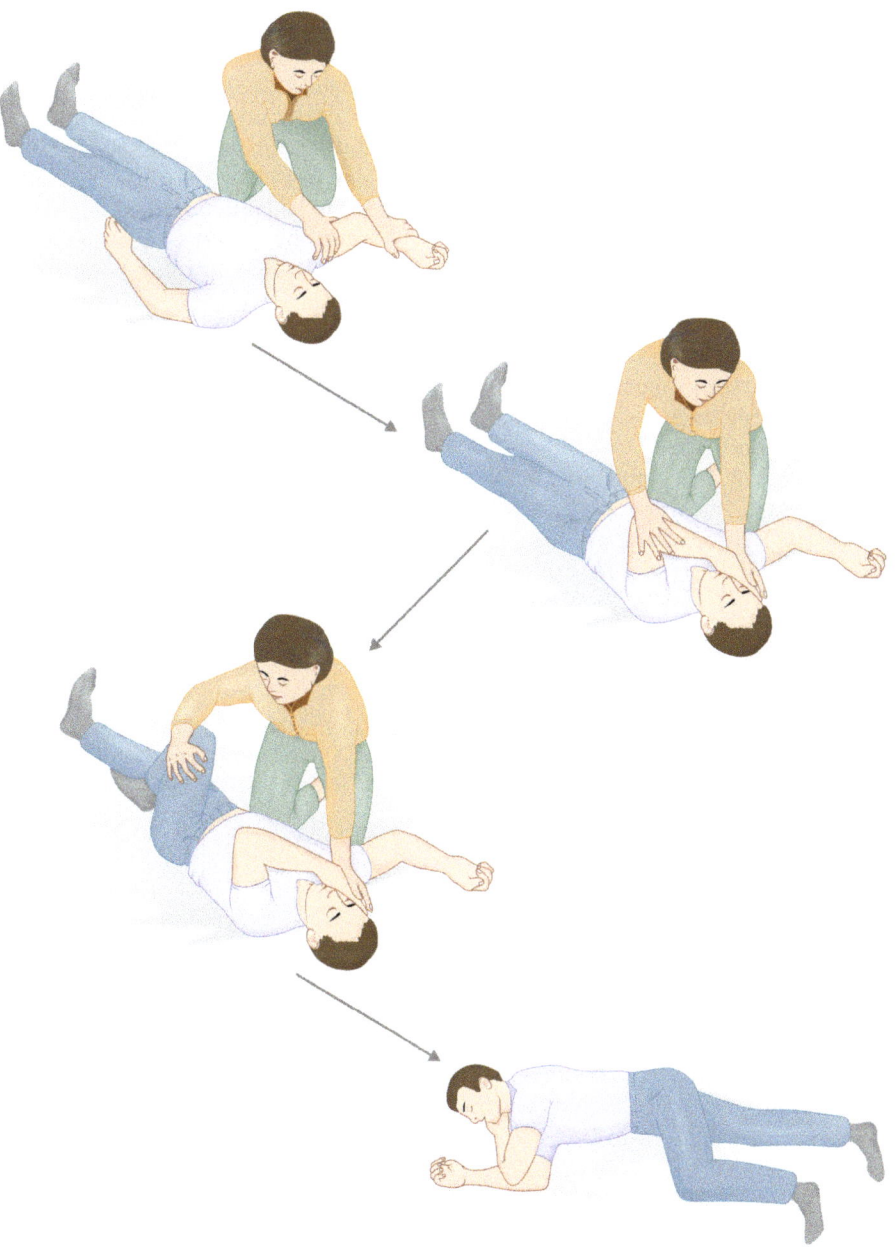

Fig. 7: How to move a person into the recovery position.

CONCLUSION

- Cardiopulmonary resuscitation sciences, which started in 1950s and developed to this extent, is still minimal in our country though initiatives are taken to educate masses, but we are still in stone age if we compare education of CPR.
- There are number of deaths in hospital and out hospital due to lack of knowledge of CPR as it is still not mandatory in medical school to teach CPR.
- There is no integration of healthcare institute in India to collaborate data, which can add on to research and analysis for CPR evolution.
- There is no *resuscitation body* at state level or central level in India such as AHA, Resuscitation Council UK, European Resuscitation Council, Australian Resuscitation Council which can look into this.
- Cardiopulmonary resuscitation adaptions are done majorly from AHA education which can be good for USA but research at Indian level may yield a different result.
- Cardiopulmonary resuscitation education is still a discouragement for medics as it comes at a cost.
- Gray areas such as patient wishes, patient not fit for CPR are not incorporated. There is no legal or government support to investigate this.
- Considering all above points CPR use and education is institute- and individual-centric till date.
- We have tried to incorporate AHA and Resuscitation Council UK input to familiarize all with CPR knowledge and easy way to administer clinical care.

> **Take Home Messages**
> - The more we spread the knowledge the more we save lives.
> - More importantly, if all clinical and nonclinical people can decide and influence law makers to constitute a *resuscitation body* which can begin with CPR research and teaching, that would be ideal.

■ REFERENCES

1. American Heart Association. Highlights of the 2020 American Heart Association's Guidelines for CPR and ECC.pdf. [online] Available from: https://cpr.heart.org/-/media/cpr-files/cpr-guidelines-files/highlights/hghlghts_2020_ecc_guidelines_english.pdf. [Last Accessed January 2023].
2. European Resuscitation Council. ERC Guidelines. [online] Available from: cprguidelines.eu. [Last Accessed January 2023].
3. Resuscitation Council (UK). Statements and resources on COVID-19 (Coronavirus): CPR and Resuscitation. [online] Available from: https://www.resus.org.uk/sites/default/files/2020-06/Resuscitation%20Council%20UK%20Statement%20on%20COVID-19%20in%20relation%20to%20CPR%20and%20resuscitation%20in%20first%20aid%20and%20community%20settings13052020.pdf. [Last Accessed January 2023].
4. Resuscitation Council (UK). e-Lifesaver. [online] Available from: https://www.resus.org.uk/public-resource/how-we-save-lives/lifesaver-learning/e-lifesaver. [Last Accessed January 2023].
5. Johns Hopkins Medicine. A Father of CPR. [online] Available from: https://www.hopkinsmedicine.org/news/publications/hopkins_medicine_magazine/class_notes/winter-2016/a-father-of-cpr#:~:text=James%20Jude%20pioneered%20external%20cardiac%20massage.&text=Tens%20of%20thousands%20of%20people,He%20was%2087. [Last Accessed January 2023].
6. Acierno LJ, Worrell LT. Peter Safar: father of modern cardiopulmonary resuscitation. Clin Cardiol. 2007;30(1):52-4.

CHAPTER 2

Approach to Syncope

Kallol K Dey

■ INTRODUCTION

*"I faint, I perish with my love! I grow
Frail as a cloud whose pale
Under the evening's ever-changing glow:
I die like mist upon the gale,
And like a wave under the calm I fail"*

—Percy Bysshe Shelley[1]

The poet perfectly captures the essence of syncope and its associated autonomic symptoms.

The word *syncope* is derived from the post-classical Latin *sincopis* (accusative *sincopin*) meaning sudden loss of strength or consciousness.[2] The word is in use in English since 1400. In Greek, the word *Synkope* means cutting short.

The relationship between the heart and brain has been known to the mankind since the time of Galen of Pergamon (129 AD–c200).[3] A Persian physician Ibn Sina (ca980-1037) known as Avicenna was the first to describe carotid hypersensitivity.[4] In the late 18th and 19th centuries, various authors, e.g., Denis Diderot, Jane Austen, Charles Dickens, Gustave Flaubert, George Eliot, Fyodor Dostoevsky—portrayed vasovagal syncope in their work. One such graphic description is from Diderot (173-1784) a French philosopher, art critic and writer:

"I moved towards the superior with my arms held out in supplication and my body leaning backwards, swooning. I fell, but it was not a heavy fall. In such fainting fits when one's strength abandons one, the limbs seem to give way and as it were fold up unawares; nature, unable to hold up, seems to try to collapse gently. I lost consciousness and the sense of feeling, and merely heard confused and distant voices buzzing round me; whether it was real speech or a singing in my ears, I could make out nothing but this continual buzzing".[5]

Although syncope is far more common in real life than epilepsy, in classical paintings syncope is far rarer and is usually depicted as a reaction to high drama and emotion.[6,7] The best and most common depictions of syncope in classical art show Mary, mother of Jesus, fainting at the Cross. The finest example is "The Deposition" by Rogier van der Weyden (c. 1435–40)—the oil painting is kept at the Museo del Prado, Madrid, Spain. Octavia was having a syncope in Jean-Joseph Thaillasson's 'Virgil reading the Aeneid to Augustus and Octavia (c. 1787) at the National Gallery, London. Marguerite Gerard's "Bad News" (1804) in Musee de Louvre, Paris portrayed a mother's response on hearing the news of her son's death while an attendant tries to awake her senses by smelling salt. When men faint in paintings, there is usually a medically serious, often life-threatening cause. Benjamin West's "The Death of Nelson" in Walker Art gallery, Liverpool and "The Death of the Earl of Chatham" at the Kimbell Art Museum, Texas are prime examples of men fainting.[7-9]

■ SYNCOPE—A DEFINITION

To put things in perspective, let us first define transient loss of consciousness (TLOC). Transient loss of consciousness is defined as a short-lived loss of consciousness with spontaneous recovery.[5] Syncope is defined as TLOC due to cerebral hypoperfusion characterized by loss of muscle tone followed by spontaneous recovery.[5]

The 2018 Task Force for the Diagnosis and Management of Syncope of the European Society of Cardiology noted that low blood pressure and global cerebral hypoperfusion are the central final common pathway of syncope. Loss of consciousness will be produced by a sudden cessation of cerebral blood flow for as short as 6–8 seconds, or a systolic blood pressure of 50–60 mm Hg at the heart level (corresponding to 30–45 mm Hg at the brain level in the upright position).[10]

There are four items to consider as a checklist:
1. Amnesia-gap in memory
2. Not responsive to speech or touch
3. Abnormal motor control
   a. Always tendency to fall
   b. Flaccid or stiff, movements or still
4. Short-few minutes.

There are conditions when the above criteria are not met. However, in these group of conditions there is apparent LOC:
- Abnormal motor control/fall

- Not responsive
- Amnesia.

Examples of the above would be falls without LOC, transient ischemic attack (TIA), stroke, altered consciousness but no falls (for example, focal epilepsy).[11] Loss of consciousness due to hypoglycemia and intoxication is for a longer duration. TLOC may be categorized into not traumatic and traumatic (concussion) **(Flowchart 1)**. Nontraumatic causes include:
- Syncope
- Tonic-clonic seizure
- Psychogenic:
  - Psychogenic nonepileptic seizures (PNES)
  - Psychogenic pseudosyncope (PPS)
  - Rare causes.

Syncope is often misdiagnosed as epilepsy. A systematic review of 27 studies showed that the diagnosis is wring in 1,249 out of 6,912 cases (mean 18%, range 2–71%).[12] The main reasons of misdiagnosis are:
- False interpretation of EEG[13]
- Inadequate history[13]
- No knowledge of other conditions.[14]

Presyncope and near syncope are terms used to describe a state that resembles the prodrome of syncope which is not followed by loss of consciousness although the mechanisms involved are the same as in syncope is not entirely clear.

■ CLASSIFICATION OF SYNCOPE

Syncope may be classified as reflex (neurally mediated), secondary to orthostatic hypotension, and cardiovascular[11,15] **(Box 1)**.

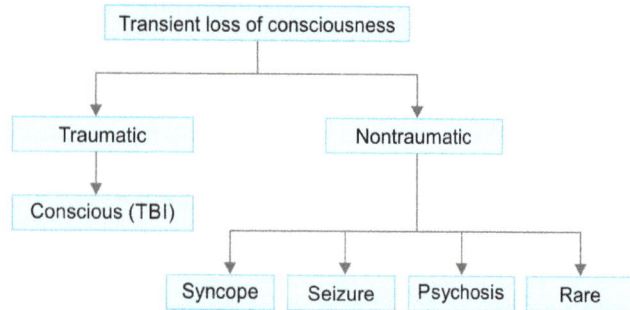

Flowchart 1: Transient loss of consciousness.

Reflex Syncope

Reflex syncope (also known as autonomic mediated syncope, neurocardiogenic syncope, neurally mediated syncope) encompasses a heterogeneous group of disorders mediated by cardiovascular reflexes that are inappropriately triggered, producing vasodilation or bradycardia, with a consequent fall in both blood pressure and cerebral perfusion without preexisting orthostatic hypotension. Blood pressure falls because of sympathetic withdrawal and heart rate falls because of increased vagal activity. The effects are more likely when upright. There are typically no abnormalities between the attacks.

Reflex syncope can be classified as vasovagal, situational, carotid sinus, and atypical. Vasovagal syncopes are the most common reflex syncopes and include the common faint; they are often triggered by emotional distress, fear, pain, and instrumentation (e.g., needle). Atypical vasovagal syncope may be associated with a short or absent prodrome and amnesia for loss of consciousness, thus, increasing the possibility of misdiagnosis with nonsyncopal falls.[16]

Glossopharyngeal neuralgia is an uncommon cause of reflex syncope. Situational syncopes are triggered by specific circumstances such as coughing/sneezing, swallowing, defecation, visceral pain, micturition (or immediately postmicturition), postexercise, postprandial, trumpet-blowing (trumpet blower's syncope), exposure to heat and weightlifting.

Orthostatic Hypotension

Definition: A BP fall of 20 mm Hg systolic or 10 mm Hg diastolic on rising from the supine, to sitting, standing or during a 60-degree tilt test. **Box 2** summarizes the variety of conditions causing orthostatic hypotension. Syncope due to orthostatic hypotension may result from primary autonomic failure (e.g., pure autonomic failure, multisystem atrophy, Parkinson disease, Lewy body dementia), secondary autonomic failure (e.g., alcoholism, diabetes mellitus, spinal cord injury), drugs (e.g., alcohol, vasodilators, alpha-blockers, beta-blockers, diuretics, phenothiazines, antidepressants), and volume depletion (e.g., dehydration, hemorrhage,

---

BOX 1: Classification of syncope.

- *Neurally-mediated/reflex syncope/autonomic mediated syncope/ neurocardiogenic syncope (17–22%):*
  - Vasovagal (14%)
  - Situational
  - Carotid sinus hypersensitivity
- *Orthostatic hypotension (11%)*
- *Cardiovascular syncope (17%):*
  - Arrhythmia (14%)
  - Structural
- *Unknown (39%)*

Source: Figures from Kapoor (1983).[17]

BOX 2: Common causes of orthostatic hypotension.

Neurogenic:
- Multiple system atrophy
- Parkinson's disease
- Dementia with Lewy bodies
- Pure autonomic failures
- Peripheral or autonomic neuropathies

Non-neurogenic:
- Hypovolemia (acute blood loss, dehydration)
- Medication use
- Adrenal insufficiency
- Reduced cardiac output (aortic stenosis, cardiomyopathy)

> **BOX 3:** Symptoms resulting from orthostatic hypotension and impaired perfusion.
>
> - *Cerebral hypoperfusion:*
>   - Dizziness
>   - Visual disturbances
>   - Blurred—tunnel
>   - Scotoma
>   - Greying out—blacking out
>   - Color defects
>   - Syncope
>   - Cognitive deficits
> - *Muscle hypoperfusion:*
>   - Paracervical and suboccipital (coat-hanger) ache
>   - Lower back/buttock ache
> - *Subclavian steal-like syndrome*
> - *Renal hypoperfusion:*
>   - Oliguria
> - *Spinal cord hypoperfusion*
> - *Nonspecific:*
>   - Weakness, lethargy, fatigue
>   - Falls

> **BOX 4:** Factors influencing orthostatic hypotension.
>
> - Speed of positional change
> - Time of day (worse in the morning)
> - Prolonged recumbency
> - Warm environment (hot weather, central heating, hot bath)
> - Raising intrathoracic pressure—micturition, defecation or coughing
> - Food and alcohol ingestion
> - Water ingestion
> - Physical exertion
> - Physical maneuvers and positions (bending forward, abdominal compression, leg crossing, squatting, activating calf muscle pump)
> - Drugs with vasoactive properties (including dopaminergic agents)

diarrhea, vomiting). **Box 3** sets out to summarize the various symptoms due to orthostatic hypotension and impaired cerebral perfusion. Hypotension may vary, syncope can occur instantly. Occasionally, a hypoxic seizure can follow cerebral hypoperfusion.

There are several factors which influence the development of orthostatic hypotension **(Box 4)**.

In neurogenic orthostatic hypotension, plasma noradrenaline levels do not rise when upright unlike normally. Hypoperfusion of the organs above the heart such as the brain causes malaise, nausea, dizziness, and the visual disturbances that often precede syncope.

Cardiovascular Syncope

Cardiovascular syncope may result from two causes: (1) arrythmia-like bradycardia (e.g., sinus node dysfunction including bradycardia/tachycardia syndrome, atrioventricular conduction system disease, and implanted device malfunction), tachycardia (supraventricular or ventricular) and structural heart disease (e.g., aortic stenosis, acute myocardial ischemia or infarction, hypertrophic cardiomyopathy, atrial myxoma, pericardial tamponade); and (2) cardiopulmonary conditions and disorders of the great vessels, (e.g., pulmonary embolism, acute aortic dissection, and pulmonary hypertension). The cardiac subtype is also likely to yield the highest rate of electrocardiographic abnormality. A cardiac cause of syncope is an independent predictor of sudden death, and mortality rates are higher in patients with cardiac syncope compared with those of noncardiac or unknown origin.[17]

Syncope in Paced Patients

The most common cause of syncope in paced patients is cardiovascular autonomic dysfunction.[18] In a study of 39 paced patients with syncope, orthostatic hypotension (41%) and vasovagal syncope (31%) were the most common diagnoses—there was no case of pacemaker dysfunction. Predictors of syncope recurrence and fall-related injury after pacemaker implantation include treated hypertension, renal failure, and atrial fibrillation (AF).[18]

■ EPIDEMIOLOGY OF SYNCOPE

Syncope is a prevalent disorder, accounting for 3–5% of emergency department visits and 1–3% of hospital admissions. Overall, neurological causes make up 40% of syncope cases.[19] Syncope due to orthostatic hypotension represents approximately 1/10th cases in the general population and up to one-fourth of cases presenting to accident and emergency. Pulmonary emboli represent a common cause of syncope in the hospitalized patients for syncope. Approximately one-third of syncope remains unexplained.

A large international multicenter study looked at syncope in people aged 40 or more presenting to the emergency department with a syncope in the preceding 12 hours.[20] The incidence of recurrent syncope was 20% within the first 24 months. The risk factors for recurrence are cardiac syncope and syncope of unknown cause. Occurrence of more than three previous episodes of syncope was the only predictor identified for recurrent syncope. Recurrent syncope carried an increased risk for death (HR 1.87) and major cardiovascular events (HR 2.69) over 24 months of follow up.

Syncope or presyncope in patients hospitalized with COVID-19 is uncommon and is infrequently associated with a serious underlying pathology (e.g., cardiac etiology) or adverse outcomes compared to those who do not present with these symptoms.[21] In another series of 35 cases associated with SARS-CoV-2 onset, affected patients had significantly lower heart rates compared to 68 SARS-CoV-2-positive patients who did not have syncope.[22]

In children with "syncope", the most common causes are neurocardiogenic (vasovagal, 63%), "pseudosyncope" (13%), cardiac (10%), neurologic (10%), and indeterminate (3%).[23]

PATHOPHYSIOLOGY OF SYNCOPE

The human body has an ability to maintain a stable blood pressure in the face of forces that constantly shift and redistribute the circulating blood volume. Even a simple change in posture such as standing up can result in a relatively "empty" ventricle due to shift of blood from the thorax to the abdomen and lower limbs. The shift in blood volume can markedly reduce the cardiac output. The decreased output is sensed by arterial baroreceptors in the carotid sinus and aortic arch. These receptors transmit signals to the nervous system and result in reflex-increased sympathetic output.[24] In addition, the vascular system responds locally by vasoconstriction restricting blood supply to nonvital organs such as skin, muscles, and adipose tissue. Clinically, the response is manifested by increase in the heart rate by 10–15 beats and a gradual diastolic pressure increase of about 10 mm Hg. In autonomic mediated syncope or neurally-mediated syncope there is "hypersensitivity" of the autonomic nervous system in response to various stimuli, most notably orthostatic stress. **Flowchart 2** presents the sequence of events schematically.[24]

CLINICAL MANIFESTATIONS OF SYNCOPE

It is important to recognize the progression of symptoms so that a clinician can identify the reported features to reach an accurate diagnosis of syncope. **Box 5** summarizes the events in abrupt syncope with acute standstill of perfusion of the brain and retina along with those in gradual onset syncope with autonomic activation and symptoms of hypoperfusion.[25]

A videometric study of syncope by Lempert and colleagues made video of 56 volunteers who induced syncope by squatting and hyperventilation, followed by Valsalva (the Mess Trick).[26] They demonstrated the range of features that can be associated with syncope—in particular multifocal jerks, head turns and other brief motor movements—and transformed the clinical assessment of patients with blackouts as many of these were previously supposed to be highly specific for seizures. This study should prevent many patients with syncope being misdiagnosed as having had a seizure.

DIAGNOSTIC EVALUATION OF SYNCOPE

In the evaluation of syncope, history, physical examination, and electrocardiogram (ECG) have the greatest utility.

History remains the cornerstone in the diagnosis of syncope and its further evaluation. A checklist approach may be helpful. There are six historical clues one should try to elicit when faced with a patient presenting with transient loss of consciousness.[11] The clues are as follows:

1. Triggers
2. Features at the onset
3. Features during the attack
4. Other aspects
5. State after the attack
6. Antecedent disorders.

One clinically useful pointer to make a correct diagnosis is trigger. Syncope is often triggered, epilepsy rarely. The triggers also differ in the two groups. The usual triggers for epilepsy are flashing lights, various cognitive tasks, while those for the syncope are pain, fear, standing (vasovagal), exercise, supine (cardiac), fever, water in face, alarm clock, etc.

BOX 5: Sequence of symptoms and signs in the prodromal phase of syncope.

Abrupt syncope with acute standstill of perfusion of the brain and retina.
- After approximately 6 seconds: Darkened vision (black out), staring, "freeze"
- 7–13 s: Fixation in the midline or upward turning of the eyes, loss of muscle tone, loss of consciousness
- After approximately 14 s muscle jerks
- Gradual onset syncope with autonomic activation and symptoms of hypoperfusion

Autonomic activation
- Sweating
- Facial pallor
- Nausea
- Pupillary dilatation
- Palpitations
- Yawning
- Hyperventilation

Symptoms of hypoperfusion
- *Brain:* Light-headedness, unclear thinking
- *Retina:* Blurred vision, loss of peripheral and color vision (gray out, darkened vision (black out)
- *Shoulders:* Coat hanger pain
- Angina pectoris
- Hypotensive TIA

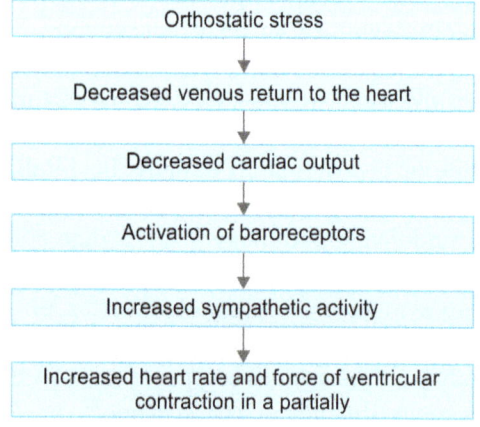

Flowchart 2: Steps of development of syncope.

Contrary to popular teaching, certain historical features do not help us in distinguishing syncope from seizure **(Table 1)**: incontinence, opening of eyes, presence of jerks, fatigue, and sleep.

These features may be present in both the conditions. For example, if the bladder is full during the event the patient may experience incontinence even with a syncope.

Serum prolactin level does not help distinguish a syncope from a seizure.[27]

There are three clinical features that are helpful in distinguishing syncope from seizure: jerks, location of tongue bite and timeline of recovery **(Table 2)**.

One useful rule to remember to distinguish a seizure from a syncope is the "10-20 rule". In syncope the jerks are irregular, 0–10 in number and was noted in 66% of cases (31/47). In tonic-clonic seizure the jerks are rhythmic, 20–191 jerks and noted in 100% of cases studied. (48/48).[28]

It is often difficult to differentiate syncope from psychogenic events: psychogenic nonepileptic syndrome (PNES) and psychogenic pseudosyncope (PPS). **Table 3** lists the features are useful in making a correct diagnosis.

In PPS the patient is flaccid, motionless, and eyes are closed.[29] It is useful to have an event captured on a video on mobile phones. Compared with vasovagal syncope, eye closure during the event, long periods of apparent TLOC, and high HR and BP are highly specific for PPS.

Physical examination should include blood pressure measurement in each arm, orthostatic blood pressure measurement (three sets of pulse and blood pressure: after supine for 5 minutes, on standing, and after standing for 3 minutes), neck auscultation, cardiac examination, examination of the extremities for swelling, and examination of cranial nerves and motor function.[30]

It is important to use the diaphragm of the stethoscope because it detects the higher frequency sounds of arterial bruits rather better than the bell. Ask the patient to breathe in and hold their breath. Listen over an area beginning from just behind the upper end of the thyroid cartilage to just below the angle of the jaw, in other words over the line of the common carotid artery leading up to the bifurcation into the internal and external carotid arteries.[31] Apply only sufficient pressure to ensure the diaphragm rests squarely on the skin. Excessive pressure can compress the underlying artery enough to cause a bruit even when the artery is normal.

Orthostatic hypertension is defined as a sustained fall in systolic blood pressure of at least 20 mm Hg (at least 30 mm Hg in those with supine hypertension), or diastolic blood pressure of 10 mm Hg, or a decrease in systolic blood pressure to <90 mm Hg within 3 minutes of standing or head-up tilt to at least 60 degrees on tilt table testing. Delayed orthostatic hypotension is similar to orthostatic hypotension but it occurs after 3 minutes and may occur up to 45 minutes after standing.[32] Tilt table testing is particularly helpful to evaluate patients for delayed orthostatic hypotension.

Orthostatic Intolerance with Posturally Induced Tachycardia

Orthostatic intolerance without hypotension but with a substantial rise in heart rate is known as orthostatic intolerance with posturally-induced tachycardia (PoTS). This tends to affect women younger than 50. Dizziness on postural change or modest exertion, presyncope and syncope may occur without generalized autonomic features. Associations include joint hypermobility (Ehlers-Danlos III), chronic fatigue, mitral valve prolapse and hyperventilation.[33]

Diagnostic Testing: ECG, Echo, Tilt Table Testing

If there is a cardiac history, abnormal ECG suggesting structural heart disease (see later), abnormal findings suggesting cardiac disease on physical examination, history of arrhythmia or evidence on the ECG then proceed to cardiac investigations before engaging on carotid sinus massage (CSM) and tilt table testing.

The clinical examination along with electrocardiography, as part of multivariable scores, can accurately identify patients with and without cardiac syncope.[34] According to the EGSYS Rule, there are positive and negative predictors that carry different weights for cardiac syncope and 2-year mortality: (1) palpitations before syncope (4 points);

TABLE 1: Features not helpful in distinction between seizure and syncope.

Features	Syncope	Seizure
Incontinence	Yes	Yes
Eye open	Yes	Yes
Presence of jerks	Yes	Yes
Fatigue, Sleep	Yes	Yes

TABLE 2: Helpful features: syncope versus seizure.

Features	Seizure	Syncope
Jerks	1 minute <20	Few seconds <10
Tongue bite	Side of tongue	Rare (if so, tip)
Recovery	Minutes, Confusion (No imprinting)	Secondary No confusion

TABLE 3: Somatic or psychogenic.

Somatic syncope/seizure	Psychogenic PNES/PPS	
Eyes	Open	Closed
Frequency	<1 per week	Up to >1 per day
Duration	About a minute	1–45 minute

(PNES: psychogenic nonepileptic syndrome; PPS: psychogenic pseudosyncope)

(2) abnormal ECG or heart disease (3 points); (3) syncope during effort (3 points); (4) syncope while supine (2 points); (5) autonomic prodrome with nausea/vomiting (-1 point); and (6) the presence of predisposing or precipitating factors (e.g., warm crowded place, prolonged standing, fear, pain, intense emotion) (-1 point).[35] An EGSYS score of <3 is associated with lower likelihood of cardiac syncope: the probability of cardiac syncope is 2% with a total score of <3, 13% with a score of 3, 33% with a score of 4, and 77% with a score of >4.[35]

Clinical predictors of cardiac syncope include the following, based on systematic reviews:[34,36] (1) age at first syncope of at least 35 years; (2) history of atrial fibrillation or flutter; (3) known severe structural heart disease; and (4) cyanosis witnessed during the episode. Negative predicators of cardiac syncope include the following: (1) age at first syncope younger than 35 years; (2) certain prodromal symptoms prior to syncope, including mood change, preoccupation with details, feeling cold, or headache; (3) mood changes after syncope; and (4) inability to remember behavior prior to syncope.

Electrocardiogram Abnormalities Suggesting a Cardiac Cause of Syncope[37,38]

The Task Force for the Diagnosis and Management of Syncope of the European Society of Cardiology has identified specific ECG findings suggestive of an arrhythmic basis for syncope, which were modified somewhat from 2009 to 2018: (1) bifascicular block (i.e., left or right bundle branch block combined with left anterior or left posterior fascicular block); (2) other intraventricular conduction abnormalities with QRS duration of at least 0.12 seconds; (3) Mobitz I second-degree atrioventricular block and first degree AV block with a markedly prolonged PR interval; (4) asymptomatic inappropriate sinus bradycardia (40–50 bpm) or slow atrial fibrillation (40–50 bpm) in the absence of negative chronotropic medications or athletic physical training; (5) nonsustained ventricular tachycardia; (6) pre-excited QRS complexes; (7) long (>460 ms) or short (<340 ms) QT intervals; (8) early repolarization; (9) a right bundle branch block pattern with ST elevation in leads V1 to V3 (Brugada syndrome); (10) negative T waves in the right precordial leads (epsilon waves) suggestive of arrhythmogenic right-ventricular cardiomyopathy; and (11) left ventricular hypertrophy suggesting hypertrophic cardiomyopathy.[10,15]

Arrhythmic syncope is considered highly probable when the ECG shows any of the features listed in **Box 6**. **Box 7** enumerates the examples of structural heart diseases where cardiovascular syncope is likely.

Cardiac ischemia-related syncope is confirmed when syncope presents with evidence of acute myocardial ischemia (with or without myocardial infarction). Syncope

> **BOX 6:** ECG findings in arrhythmic syncope.
> - Arrhythmic syncope is considered highly probable when the ECG shows any of the following:
>   - Persistent sinus bradycardia or slow atrial fibrillation of <40 bpm or repetitive sinoatrial block or pauses of at least 3 seconds
>   - Mobitz II seconds or third-degree atrioventricular block
>   - Alternating right and left bundle branch block
>   - Ventricular tachycardia or rapid paroxysmal supraventricular tachycardia
>   - Episodes of polymorphic ventricular tachycardia with either a long or short QT interval
>   - Malfunction of a pacemaker or implanted cardiac defibrillator with resulting cardiac pauses

> **BOX 7:** Example of heart disease in which cardiopulmonary syncope is likely to occur.
> - Cardiomyopathy with episodes of overt heart failure
> - Systolic dysfunction (Ejection fraction <40%)
> - Ischemic cardiomyopathy following an acute myocardial infarction
> - Right ventricular dysplasia
> - Hypertrophic cardiomyopathy
> - Congenital heart disease
> - Cardiac tumors
> - Outflow tract obstruction
> - Pulmonary embolism, aortic dissection

due to structural cardiopulmonary disorders is highly probable when syncope presents in patients with any of the following: prolapsing atrial myxoma, left atrial ball thrombus, severe aortic stenosis, pulmonary embolus, or acute aortic dissection.

Pulmonary embolus as a cause of syncope should be suspected in patients with elevated troponin levels or a dilated right ventricle on echocardiogram.[39]

Echocardiography

The yield of echocardiography in the setting of sorting out syncope is low. Echocardiography should be performed if there is previously known heart disease, data suggestive of structural heart disease or syncope due to cardiovascular cause. Patients presenting with syncope aged >60 years with ECG abnormality and elevated brain natriuretic peptide should get an echocardiogram.

Two-dimensional and Doppler echocardiography during exercise in the standing, sitting, or semi-supine position is useful to detect provocable left ventricular outflow tract obstruction in patients with hypertrophic cardiomyopathy, a history of syncope, and a resting or provoked peak instantaneous left ventricular outflow tract gradient of <50 mm Hg.

Holter Monitoring

True yield is low as compared to the cost per diagnosis. Although Holter monitoring may rarely reveal transient bradyarrhythmias or tachyarrhythmias in patients with syncope, symptoms do not recur during monitoring in most patients.

Event Recorders

External event recorders are applied by the patient when symptoms occur. They can be useful for evaluation of palpitations but not for syncope. External loop recorders have a higher diagnostic yield than Holter monitoring and can be useful for patients with relatively frequent syncope and those with recurrent unexplained syncope.

Pacemaker or Defibrillator Interrogation

This is useful only in patients with syncope after a recent device implantation.

Electrophysiological Testing

The testing to determine the threshold for induction of atrial and ventricular dysrhythmias may be diagnostic and help decide on the radiofrequency ablation or implantation of a permanent automated implanted defibrillator.

Neurological Investigations

Electroencephalography (EEG) in unselected patients is of little diagnostic value. There is a danger of wring interpretation of false-positives on EEG and misdiagnosis of epilepsy, especially in children. EEG is useful if there is diagnostic uncertainty between syncope and seizure. EEG during a syncopal spell shows initial slowing followed by generalized large amplitude delta activity, and absence of epileptiform discharges despite clinical convulsion.[40]

The telemetry with prolonged EEG recording is useful in elucidating ictal bradycardia and asystole.[41]

Neuroimaging such as CT and MRI may be helpful in select population but not recommended as a routine testing.

Autonomic Testing

In most centers, evaluation of patients presenting with syncope includes noninvasive cardiovascular monitoring to identify abnormalities in the parasympathetic and sympathetic nervous systems.[32]

- The most widely used test of cardiac parasympathetic function is heart rate variability, besides heart rate responses to a Valsalva maneuver and to standing.
- The common tests of sympathetic adrenergic function include the blood pressure response to postural change with tilt table testing and active standing, as well as the blood pressure response to a Valsalva maneuver. In addition to these four tests, the Ewing protocol also includes the blood pressure response to sustained hand grip, reflecting sympathetic function;[11] however this is not commonly performed in the clinical laboratory setting.
- Autonomic testing can help in the diagnosis of orthostatic hypotension, neurally mediated syncope, postural tachycardia syndrome and delayed orthostatic hypotension.

Quantitative sweat testing has been used to assess differences in sudomotor sympathetic activity in relation to the type of reflex syncope.[42] They found that in the cardioinhibitory type, sweating started in 7–9 patients after syncope, whereas in vasodepressor type, sweating started in 11 of 12 patients before syncope. In mixed type, sweating started before syncope in 20 patients and after syncope in 10 patients. They also noted that the onset of sweating correlated significantly with the onset of syncope symptoms.

Carotid Sinus Massage

Carotid sinus massage may be diagnostic, and traditional recommendations suggest that it should generally be performed in patients over age 40 with syncope of unknown etiology after initial evaluation is completed.

The procedure is contraindicated in stroke or TIA in previous 3 months unless carotid artery disease is excluded by means of carotid dopplers and presence of carotid bruits.

The test is considered positive if symptoms are reproduced during or immediately after the massage in the presence of asystole longer than 3 s and/or a fall in systolic blood pressure of 50 mm Hg or more. A positive response is diagnostic of the cause of syncope in the absence of any other competing diagnosis.

Head-up Tilt Testing

It was first introduced into clinical practice by Kenny et al. in 1986 and remains a pivotal modality for the investigation of syncope in appropriate patients.[43]

Tilt table testing can sometimes be useful in correcting misdiagnoses of epilepsy in those with convulsive syncope and in identifying rare cases of ictal asystole. Tilt table testing can also help establish a diagnosis of pseudosyncope by the constellation of apparent loss of consciousness with loss of motor control, normal blood pressure, heart rate, and electroencephalography.[15]

Indications for Tilt Table Testing

Class 1 (full consensus): In cases of unexplained single syncopal episodes in high-risk settings (e.g., occurrence of, or potential risk for, physical injury or with occupational implications), or recurrent episodes in the absence of organic heart disease, or, in the presence of organic heart disease, after cardiac causes of syncope have been excluded.

When it will be of clinical value to demonstrate susceptibility to neurally-mediated syncope to the patient.

Class 2 (no full consensus): When an understanding of the hemodynamic pattern in syncope may alter the therapeutic approach.

- For differentiating syncope with jerking movements from epilepsy
- For evaluating patients with recurrent unexplained falls
- For assessing recurrent presyncope or dizziness.

Class 3 (may be harmful): A single episode without injury and not in a high-risk setting.

The standard protocol used for tilt table test (TTT) in most institutions is the one based on the 2004 protocol by Brignole et al. The test is performed in a quiet room that is equipped with a resuscitation trolley. The patient lies supine on a Tilt couch (Akron Streamline, Arjo Huntleigh Ltd., Gloucester, UK).[8,44] The continuous heart rate and blood pressure recording is done by Finapres® or Portapres® system.

The test begins with a pre-tilt supine position with the patient laying still for 5–20 min and then at a tilt of 60° for approximately 20 min. If there has not been any change, a CSM is performed at this time. The patient is then brought back to the supine position and is maintained for another 20 min, following which another CSM is performed. During the test, the patient is monitored with the Task force 3040i Monitor (CN systems, Graz, Austria). The endpoints are either induction of syncope or completion of planned test.

While proceeding with the TTT it is mandatory to obtain an informed consent and explain the risk of complications: Stroke or TIA (mild 1:100, moderate or severe 1:1,000–1:10,000), arrhythmia especially AF, syncope, VT and palpitations with isoproterenol, headache with glyceryl trinitrate (GTN).

If carotid bruit is present, the procedure is abandoned and a carotid Doppler is arranged.

Supine Carotid Sinus Massage

- Allow patient to lie flat for 5 minutes (usually coincides with preparation time, if IV cannulation is performed extend to 20 min, usually only done for IV isoproterenol provoked tilt test), ask patient to report any symptoms they may have during the procedures.
- Find point of maximum carotid pulsation with index finger, start on right side.
- Apply firm pressure moving finger slightly up and down in longitudinal direction for 5 seconds whilst ECG is recorded continuously and BP drop is observed on Finapres®. Record baseline and minimal BP and pulse rate.
- Repeat on opposite side after 1–2 min rest. Allow BP/pulse to come back to baseline levels (1–2 min) before proceeding to the following:

Erect Carotid Sinus Massage

- Tilt table to 60 degrees
- Perform same task as under supine CSM
- Record baseline and post CSM BP and heart rate
- If clinical syncope occurs immediately lower tilt table to supine position.

Tilt Table Test, Passive Phase (20 minutes)

- Allow patient to rest for at least 5 minutes supine. If there was vasomotor instability on CSM testing (but no syncope) then allow patient to lie supine for 20 minutes, leave all equipment in place.
- Record baseline supine BP and HR using sphygmomanometer and Finapres® readings (they may differ)
- Place Patient in 60-degree head up position
- Record immediate BP and HR from Finapres®
- Record 2-minute BP and HR post start of head up tilt
- Record BP and HR using Finapres® and sphygmomanometer ever 1–3 minutes or when clinically indicated up until 20 minutes have elapsed. Proceed to provoked Tilt table test, patient remains in upright position.

Tilt table test findings: In patients without structural heart disease, tilt testing can be considered diagnostic, and no further tests need to be performed when spontaneous syncope is reproduced. In patients with structural heart disease, arrhythmias or other cardiac causes should be excluded prior to considering positive tilt test results as evidence suggesting neurally-mediated syncope. The clinical meaning of abnormal responses other than induction of syncope may be unclear at times.

It is crucial to recognize that seizure-like activities are commonly precipitated by head-up tilt table testing.[45]

In this study of head-up tilt testing for suspected vasovagal syncope, 47 of 71 patients (66%) showed seizure-like activities at the time of syncope during head-up tilt testing: 14 with eyeball deviation but without abnormal limb movements, and 33 with eyeball deviation and abnormal limb movements (e.g., myoclonic or tonic-clonic activities).[45]

Classification of positive response on TTT[19]

Type 1: Mixed—heart rate falls at the time of syncope but the ventricular rate does not fall to <40 beats/min or falls to <40 beats/min for <10 s with or without asystole of <3 s. Blood pressure falls before the heart rate falls.

Type 2A: Cardioinhibition without asystole. Heart rate falls to a ventricular rate <40 beats/min for >10 s but asystole of >3 s does not occur. Blood pressure falls before the heart rate falls.

Type 2B: Cardioinhibition with asystole. Asystole occurs for >3 s. Blood pressure fall coincides with or occurs before the heart rate fall.

Type 3: Vasodepressor. Heart rate does not fall >10% from its peak at the time of syncope.

- *Exception 1:* Chronotropic incompetence. No heart rate rises during the tilt testing (i.e., <10% from the pretilt rate).

- *Exception 2:* Excessive heart rate rise. An excessive heart rate rises both at the onset of the upright position and throughout its duration before syncope (i.e., >130 beats/min).

DIFFERENTIAL DIAGNOSIS OF SYNCOPE

It is crucial to make an accurate diagnosis of syncope as many patients with transient loss of consciousness have been misdiagnosed to have epilepsy or other conditions and have been given inappropriate treatment for decades imposing undue restrictions on employment, driving and life in general.

Seizure remains the most common differential diagnosis of syncope. **Table 4** highlights the important points on history and physical examination to help distinguish between the two.[46]

If the patient is unable to recall events just moments prior to postural collapse, syncope may still be the correct diagnosis, but one must consider seizure. The presence of postictal confusion and reports of convulsion from observers would support a diagnosis of seizure, but one must be careful not to misattribute the myoclonus of convulsive syncope to an epileptic convulsion. The 10–20 rule discussed earlier would be useful in this regard.

- Diagnosis of reflex syncope is supported by a long history of recurrent syncope (with onset before the age of 40 years); evidence of typical triggers; occurrence in crowded or hot places; occurrence during a meal; occurrence with head rotation or when pressure is placed on the carotid sinus from tumors, shaving, or tight collars; or evidence of autonomic activation prior to syncope, absent of heart disease.
- A prodrome duration of 5 seconds or less suggests arrhythmic syncope, whereas a prodrome duration of >10 seconds in the absence of structural heart disease suggests reflex syncope.
- Vasovagal syncope is diagnosed if syncope is precipitated by emotional or orthostatic stress and is associated with a typical prodrome.
- Situational syncope is diagnosed if it occurs during or immediately after specific triggers such as coughing/sneezing, swallowing, defecation, visceral pain, micturition, exertion, or after eating.
- Orthostatic hypotension is the likely basis for syncope if syncope and presyncope are present during standing, absent while lying, and less severe or absent while sitting.

Diagnosis of syncope due to orthostatic hypotension is supported by the following: (1) an appropriate triggering situation; (2) a temporal association with starting or changing dosage of medications known to cause orthostatic hypotension; and (3) a history of autonomic neuropathy or parkinsonism.

Diagnosis of cardiovascular syncope is supported by the presence of structural heart disease, a family history of unexplained sudden death or channelopathy, occurrence during exertion or while supine, occurrence of syncope following palpitations, and specific ECG findings suggesting arrhythmic syncope.

Migraine with brainstem aura (formerly known as "basilar-type migraine," "basilar migraine", "basilar artery migraine", or "Bickerstaff migraine") may be confused with a syncope. Because the involvement of the basilar artery is unlikely, the term migraine with brainstem aura is preferred. The associated symptoms clearly originate from

TABLE 4: Distinguishing syncope from a seizure.

	Before spell	
	Seizure	**Syncope**
• Trigger (position, emotion, Valsalva)	• Common	• Rare
• Sweating and nausea	• Common	• Rare
• Aura (e.g., déjà vu, smell) or unilateral symptoms	• Rare	• Common
	During spell (from Eyewitness)	
	Seizure	**Syncope**
• Pallor • Cyanosis • Duration of LOC • Movements	• Common • Rare • <20 seconds • A few clonic or myoclonic jerks; brief tonic posturing (few seconds); duration <15 seconds; always begin after LOC	• Rare • Common • >60 seconds • Prolonged tonic phase, transitioning to rhythmic clonic phase; duration >1 minute • May begin at onset of LOC • Before; Unilateral jerking (partial seizure)
Automatisms	Occasional	Common (in complex partial and secondarily generalized seizures)

the brainstem and are not ischemic in etiology. According to the International Classification of Headache Disorders. 3rd Edition (ICHD-3), the diagnosis is based on the findings of full reversible speech or language, sensory, or visual auras that are not accompanied by retinal or motors symptoms. There must be at least two of the following "brainstem" symptoms present: dysarthria, vertigo, tinnitus, hypacusis, diplopia, ataxia not attributable to sensory deficit, and decreased level consciousness (Glasgow Coma Scale ≤13). By definition, the aura symptoms spread over 5 or more minutes, last from 5 to 60 minutes, and may be followed by a headache within 1 hour. Some authors have proposed requiring three rather than the current criteria of two brainstem aura symptoms for diagnosis, while setting a more stringent criterion of combining hearing loss and tinnitus into a single auditory feature, criterion B ("hearing loss and/or tinnitus").[47,48]

Metabolic causes of transient loss of consciousness may include hypoglycemia and hypoxemia, but the mechanism of loss of consciousness is not a decrease in global cerebral perfusion, and the alteration in consciousness is rarely of sudden onset and offset.

Unlike syncope, episodes of pseudosyncope (or psychogenic nonsyncopal collapse) are not associated with compromised cerebral circulation.[49] Pseudosyncope is usually a manifestation of conversion disorder and, as such, shares many features with pseudoseizure. Psychiatric disease and age of >45 years are risk factors for pseudosyncope. Some patients may have a combination of tilt-induced vasovagal syncope and psychogenic pseudosyncope:[50] such individuals are more likely to have a high attack frequency (including multiple attacks in a single day), delayed recovery following apparent transient loss of consciousness, episodes without prodromes, lacking or atypical triggers, eye closure and especially forced eye closure with attempted passive eye-opening by the examiner (the eyes are typically not closed during epileptic seizures and syncope), apparent loss of consciousness lasting longer than 1 minute (affected patient may lie on the floor for 15 minutes or longer), and tearfulness associated with fainting. It is important to note that physical injury does not exclude pseudosyncope.

A perhaps underrecognized cause of episodic loss of consciousness is the ictal bradycardia syndrome, which occurs when epileptic discharges profoundly disrupt normal cardiac rhythm, resulting in cardiogenic syncope during the ictal event.[41] The ictal bradycardia syndrome should be considered in patients with unusual or refractory episodes of syncope, or in patients with a history suggestive of both epilepsy and syncope. It suggests seizure onset in temporal lobe, and is more commonly diagnosed in males. Diagnosis may be aided by ambulatory EEG/ECG monitoring. Cardiac pacemaker implantation along with antiepileptic drug therapy may be necessary to minimize the possibility of death.[41]

Characteristics considered to be typical of ictal asystole (focal, left temporal seizures appearing on grounds of a long-lasting, intractable epilepsy) seem only partially legitimate. Another study suggests that in new-onset IA, female gender and a preexisting heart condition could serve as predispositions in an otherwise benign epilepsy. They speculate that in late-onset IA, male-predominant changes in neuronal networks in chronic, intractable epilepsy and an accompanying autonomic dysregulation serve as facilitating factors.[51]

■ FUTURE DIRECTIONS

Setting up of a Rapid Access Blackout or Faint/Falls Clinic or TIA/Syncope Clinic would be an effective strategy to sort out syncope at the first point of contact at the hospital, especially the emergency department.[52] Syncope is a common presentation to Emergency Departments (EDs). Estimates on the frequency of visits (0.6–1.7%) and subsequent rates of hospitalizations (12–85%) vary according to country. For those deemed intermediate risk, access to specialist assessment and related testing may occur in a syncope unit in the emergency department—this is a cost-effective solution to the problem.

Twin studies, highly focused genome-wide association studies, and gene duplicate studies all suggest genetic association of the vasovagal syncope, although the specific genes, pathways, and proteins are unknown. A recent large, candidate gene study of kindreds with high, multigenerational prevalence of the vasovagal syncope identified three genes that associate with vasovagal syncope.[53] The best evidence to date is for central signaling genes involving serotonin and dopamine.

Take Home Messages

- Syncope is a frequently encountered clinical condition but it is often misdiagnosed.
- One must be precise in using the term *syncope* only for the patients where TLOC is due to cerebral hypoperfusion. TLOC and syncope should not be used interchangeably. Syncope is a subset of TLOC.
- Overdiagnosis of epilepsy is common in clinical practice. Care must be exercised in making a positive diagnosis of epilepsy.
- A neurologist must be prepared to undiagnose the transient loss consciousness with a wrong diagnostic label of epilepsy with a clear and detailed explanation to the patient and relatives.
- History remains the cornerstone of diagnosis. One must be ready to spend time asking the right questions (six key questions–*see* **Box 8**) and get as much information as possible from the eyewitness.
- It is important to understand that various motor phenomena, jerks, eye boll rolling may happen in syncope. Presence of those clinical features do not make the patient epileptic.
- Remember that 40% of patients with syncope do not have a clear-cut explanation at presentation. It is crucial to keep them under follow-up.

BOX 8: Suspected syncope: Six key questions to ask.
1. Triggers
2. At the onset
3. During the aback
4. Other aspects
5. After the attack
6. Antecedent disorders

- Rational use of tilt table testing is to be encouraged.
- Autonomic testing is often underutilized in sorting out TLOC.
- Rather than having a tick-box approach to syncope with a battery of tests, it is vital to order tests with a clear expectation and rationale.
- A separate area in the emergency dealing with TLOC would be useful to streamline the patients with suspected syncope avoiding needless testing and misdiagnosing the condition. Setting up a TIA/syncope clinic by a neurologist is a significant way forward.

REFERENCES

1. Poetry.com. I Faint, I Perish With My Love! (Shelley, PB). [online] Available from: https://www.poetry.com/poem/29134/i-faint%2C-i-perish-with-my-love%21. [Last Accessed January, 2023].
2. Oxford University Press (OED). (2022). Syncope. [online] Available from: https://www.oed.com/viewdictionaryentry/Entry/196418. [Last Accessed January, 2023].
3. Nahm F, Freeman R. Syncope and the history of nervous influences on the heart. Arch Neurol 2003;60(2):282-7.
4. Shoja MM, Tubbs RS, Loukas M, Khalili M, Alakbarli F, Cohen-Gadol AA. Vasovagal syncope in the Canon of Avicenna: the first mention of carotid artery hypersensitivity. Int J Cardiol, 2009;134(3):297-301.
5. Diderot D. The Nun. London: Penguin Books; 1974.
6. Smith P. Fainting in classical art. Int Rev Neurobiol. 2006;74: 79-88.
7. Smith PEM. (2005). Fainting painting. Pract Neurol. 2005;5(6): 366-9.
8. Brignole M, Alboni P, Benditt DG, Bergfeldt L, Blanc JJ, Bloch Thomsen PE, et al. Guidelines on management (diagnosis and treatment) of syncope—update 2004. Europace. 2004;6(6): 467-537.
9. Thijs RD, Wieling W, Kaufmann H, van Dijk G. Defining and classifying syncope. Clin Auton Res. 2004;14(Suppl 1):4-8.
10. Brignole M, Moya A, de Lange FJ, Deharo JC, Elliott PM, Fanciulli A, et al. 2018 ESC Guidelines for the diagnosis and management of syncope. Eur Heart J. 2018;39(21): 1883-948.
11. Brignole M, Moya A, de Lange FJ, Deharo JC, Elliott PM, Fanciulli A, et al. Practical Instructions for the 2018 ESC Guidelines for the diagnosis and management of syncope. Eur Heart J. 2018;39(21):e43-e80.
12. Xu Y, Nguyen D, Mohamed A, Carcel C, Li Q, Kutlubaev MA, et al. Frequency of a false positive diagnosis of epilepsy: a systematic review of observational studies. Seizure. 2016; 41:167-74.
13. Oto MM. The misdiagnosis of epilepsy: appraising risks and managing uncertainty. Seizure. 2017;44:143-6.
14. Chitre M. Pitfalls in the diagnosis and misdiagnosis of epilepsy. Paediatr Child Health. 2013;23(6):237-42.
15. Task Force for the Diagnosis and Management of Syncope; European Society of Cardiology (ESC); European Heart Rhythm Association (EHRA); Heart Failure Association (HFA); Heart Rhythm Society (HRS), Moya A, Sutton R, Ammirati F, Blanc JJ, Brignole M, Dahm JB, et al. Guidelines for the diagnosis and management of syncope (version 2009). Eur Heart J. 2009;30(21):2631-71.
16. Kenny RA, McNicholas T. (2016). The management of vasovagal syncope. QJM. 2016;109(12):767-73.
17. Kapoor WN, Karpf M, Wieand S, Peterson JR, Levey GS. A prospective evaluation and follow-up of patients with syncope. N Engl J Med. 1983;309(4):197-204.
18. Yasa E, Ricci F, Holm H, Persson T, Melander O, Sutton R, et al. Cardiovascular Autonomic Dysfunction Is the Most Common Cause of Syncope in Paced Patients. Front Cardiovasc Med. 2019;6:154.
19. Brignole M, Menozzi C, Del Rosso A, Costa S, Gaggioli G, Bottoni N, et al. New classification of haemodynamics of vasovagal syncope: beyond the VASIS classification. Analysis of the pre-syncopal phase of the tilt test without and with nitroglycerin challenge. Vasovagal Syncope International Study. Europace. 2000;2(1):66-76.
20. Zimmermann T, du Fay de Lavallaz J, Nestelberger T, Gualandro DM, Strebel I, Badertscher P, et al. Incidence, characteristics, determinants, and prognostic impact of recurrent syncope. Europace. 2020;22(12):1885-95.
21. Oates CP, Turagam MK, Musikantow D, Chu E, Shivamurthy P, Lampert J, et al.Syncope and presyncope in patients with COVID-19. Pacing Clin Electrophysiol. 2020;43(10):1139-48.
22. Canetta C, Accordino S, Buscarini E, Benelli G, La Piana G, Scartabellati A, et al. Syncope at SARS-CoV-2 onset. Auton Neurosci. 2020;229:102734.
23. Mohanty S, Kumar CPR, Kaku SM. Clinico-Etiological Profile of Pediatric Syncope: a Single Center Experience. Indian Pediatr. 2021;58(2):134-7.
24. Zaqqa M, Massumi A. Neurally mediated syncope. Tex Heart Inst J. 2000;27(3):268-72.
25. Wieling W, Thijs RD, van Dijk N, Wilde AA, Benditt DG, van Dijk JG. (2009). Symptoms and signs of syncope: a review of the link between physiology and clinical clues. Brain. 2009;132(Pt 10):2630-42.
26. Lempert T, Bauer M, Schmidt D. Syncope: a videometric analysis of 56 episodes of transient cerebral hypoxia. Ann Neurol. 1994;36(2):233-7.
27. Chen DK, So YT, Fisher RS; Therapeutics and Technology Assessment Subcommittee of the American Academy of Neurology. Use of serum prolactin in diagnosing epileptic seizures: report of the Therapeutics and Technology Assessment Subcommittee of the American Academy of Neurology. Neurology. 2005;65(5):668-75.
28. Shmuely S, Bauer PR, van Zwet EW, van Dijk JG, Thijs RD. Differentiating motor phenomena in tilt-induced syncope and convulsive seizures. Neurology. 2018;90(15):e1339-e1346.
29. Tannemaat MR, van Niekerk J, Reijntjes RH, Thijs RD, Sutton R, van Dijk JG. The semiology of tilt-induced psychogenic pseudosyncope. Neurology. 2013;81(8):752-8.

30. MedLink®. (2022). Syncope (Lanska JD). [online] Available from: https://www.medlink.com/articles/syncope. [Last Accessed January, 2023].
31. Sandercock PAG, Kavvadia E. (2002). The Carotid Bruit. Pract Neurol. 2002;2(4):221-4.
32. Jones PK, Gibbons CH. Autonomic function testing: an important diagnostic test for patients with syncope. Pract Neurol, 2015;15(5):346-51.
33. Charles C. Neurology-A Clinical Handbook. London: Wiley Publishing Co.; 2022.
34. Albassam OT, Redelmeier RJ, Shadowitz S, Husain AM, Simel D, Etchells EE. Did This Patient Have Cardiac Syncope?: The Rational Clinical Examination Systematic Review. JAMA. 2019;321(24):2448-57.
35. Del Rosso A, Ungar A, Maggi R, Giada F, Petix NR, De Santo T, et al. Clinical predictors of cardiac syncope at initial evaluation in patients referred urgently to a general hospital: the EGSYS score. Heart. 2008;94(12):1620-6.
36. Malik V, Gallagher C, Linz D, Elliott AD, Emami M, Kadhim K, et al. Atrial fibrillation is associated with syncope and falls in older adults: a systematic review and meta-analysis. Mayo Clin Proc. 2020;95(4):676-87.
37. Dovgalyuk J, Holstege C, Mattu A, Brady WJ. The electrocardiogram in the patient with syncope. Am J Emerg Med. 2007;25(6):688-701.
38. Marine JE. ECG Features that suggest a potentially life-threatening arrhythmia as the cause for syncope. J Electrocardiol. 2013;46(6):561-8.
39. Ammar H, Ohri C, Hajouli S, Kulkarni S, Tefera E, Fouda R, et al. Prevalence and Predictors of Pulmonary Embolism in Hospitalized Patients with Syncope. South Med J. 2019; 112(8):421-7.
40. Brenner RP. Electroencephalography in syncope. J Clin Neurophysiol. 1997;14(3):197-209.
41. Reeves AL, Nollet KE, Klass DW, Sharbrough FW, So EL. The ictal bradycardia syndrome. Epilepsia. 1996;37(10):983-7.
42. Struhal W, Mišmaš A, Kirchmayr M, Bartl S, Javor A, Vosko MR, et al. Onset of sweating depends on the type of reflex syncope. Auton Neurosci. 2014;184:73-6.
43. Kenny RA, Ingram A, Bayliss J, Sutton R. Head-up tilt: a useful test for investigating unexplained syncope. Lancet. 1986;1(8494):1352-5.
44. Sandhu KS, Khan P, Panting J, Nadar S. Tilt-table test: its role in modern practice. Clin Med (Lond). 2013;13(3), 227-32.
45. Joo BE, Koo DL, Yim HR, Park J, Seo DW, Kim JS. Seizure-like activities in patients with head-up tilt test-induced syncope. Medicine (Baltimore). 2018;97(51):e13602.
46. Rowland LP, Pedley TA. Syncope, Seizures and their Mimics. In: Rowland LP, Pedley TA (Eds). Merritt's Neurology. Philadelphia: Lippincott Williams and Wilkins; 2010.
47. Lempert T, Seemungal BM. How to define migraine with brainstem aura. Brain. 2020;143(5):e35.
48. Yamani N, Chalmer MA, Olesen J. Migraine with brainstem aura: defining the core syndrome. Brain, 2019;142(12): 3868-75.
49. Heyer GL, Harve RA, Islam MP. Comparison of specific fainting characteristics between youth with tilt-induced psychogenic nonsyncopal collapse versus reflex syncope. Am J Cardiol. 2017;119(7):1116-20.
50. Blad H, Lamberts RJ, van Dijk GJ, Thijs RD. Tilt-induced vasovagal syncope and psychogenic pseudosyncope: overlapping clinical entities. Neurology. 2015;85(23): 2006-10.
51. Tényi D, Gyimesi C, Kupó P, Horváth R, Bóné B, Barsi P, et al. Ictal asystole: a systematic review. Epilepsia. 2017;58(3): 356-62.
52. Sandhu RK, Sheldon RS. Syncope in the Emergency Department. Front Cardiovasc Med. 2019;6:180.
53. Sheldon RS, Sandhu RK. The Search for the Genes of Vasovagal Syncope. Front Cardiovasc Med. 2019;6:175.

CHAPTER 3

Acute Coronary Syndrome: ST-elevation Myocardial Infarction

Sunil Lhila

INTRODUCTION

Cardiovascular (CV) emergencies are certain life-threatening conditions, which if not recognized promptly and managed immediately can lead to unseen morbidity and mortality.

A few CV emergencies are:
- Acute coronary syndrome (ACS)
- Sudden cardiac death (SCD) and malignant cardiac arrhythmias
- Hypertensive crisis and aortic dissection
- acute pulmonary edema
- Acute pulmonary embolism
- Cardiac tamponade
- Tension pneumothorax.

We will limit the scope of this chapter to ACS with special reference to ST-elevation myocardial infarction (STEMI) in cardiac emergencies.

EPIDEMIOLOGY

Cardiovascular disease (CVD) kills about 7.5 million people every year which tantamount to one-third of total deaths worldwide. Two million out of this 7.5 million die due to ACS and its complications.

Incidence of ACS increase with age. Below the age of 60 years, ACS occurs 3–4 times more often in males; however, after the age of 75 years, women are the majority of patients.[1] It is commonly believed that breast cancer is the most common killer in women. The fact is 1 in 3 women die due to CVD whereas the mortality due to breast cancer is 1 in 31 globally. The Indian scenario is no better. CVD is not just the most common killer, the accelerated build-up of fat deposits (plaque) that starts in the arteries at an early age makes the situation more dismal. This happens a decade earlier in Indian population compared to western counterparts.

Acute coronary syndrome occurs as a result of sudden reduced blood flow into the heart muscle. It ranges from unstable angina (UA) where there is no heart muscle loss to acute myocardial infarction (AMI) where there is definite death of heart muscles. AMI are classified as non-ST-elevation myocardial infarction (NSTEMI) to STEMI. Early recognition of the condition followed by definitive treatment helps not only in preventing permanent loss of heart muscle but also reduces mortality.[2]

PATHOPHYSIOLOGY

Fat deposits in the wall of arteries (plaque) results in narrowing of the lumen of arteries and compromises the blood flow to the heart muscles. Once there is fissure or rupture of these plaques, there is a sudden thrombus formation on this plaque, which occludes the artery subtotally or totally, resulting in NSTEMI or STEMI respectively. The thrombus formation is platelet rich and occludes the artery incompletely in NSTEMI (white thrombus). It is red in nature in STEMI due to presence of fibrin along with platelets and erythrocytes (red thrombus). Thus, thrombolytic therapy (TT) which primarily dissolves fibrin rich clot works only in STEMI and has no role in NSTEMI where it is contraindicated. Occasionally, ACS results from nonthrombotic occlusion of the coronary arteries (CA). This happens due to prolonged and complete coronary artery spasm. Such condition is known as myocardial infarction of non-obstructive coronary artery (MINOCA).[3]

RISK FACTORS

Risk factors can be classified as modifiable and nonmodifiable.

Modifiable Risk Factors
- Hypertension
- Diabetes
- High blood cholesterol
- Smoking
- Obesity
- Sedentary lifestyle.

Nonmodifiable Risk Factors
- Age
- Family history of ischemic heart disease
- Ethnicity.

SYMPTOMS

- *Chest Pain:* Crushing, tightness or burning in chest that radiates to both arms, neck, jaws, upper abdomen at times
- Nausea and vomiting
- Excessive sweating (diaphoresis)
- Shortness of breath (dyspnea)
- Dizziness or fainting.

Chest pain is the most common symptom but may be absent in diabetic, women and elderly subjects (silent heart attack).[4]

One should seek immediate medical help if any of these symptoms occur and are not relieved within half an hour.

MANAGEMENT

Rapid identification of patients with ACS reporting in emergency room (ER) with chest pain is of paramount importance as aggressive and time sensitive strategy of revascularization is the cornerstone of ACS management.

Initial Assessment of the Patient with a TIMI Risk

Thrombolysis in myocardial infarction (TIMI) Risk Calculator is preferable to assess patients risk along with few tests **(Table 1)**.

INVESTIGATIONS

Electrocardiogram

Electrocardiogram (ECG) is the gold standard and first test to be performed for the diagnosis of ACS. It should be performed within 10 minutes of first medical contact (FMC).

In 10% of patients ECG can be normal with ongoing chest pain. In such cases, subsequent serial ECGs are recommended. Right sided chest leads, posterior chest leads and continuous ST-segment monitoring may be helpful in certain patients. Normal ECG even after 12 hours of ongoing chest pain, usually has a high negative predictive value for ACS.[5]

Newly developed left bundle branch block (LBBB) or a diagnosis of ischemic changes in patients with pacing rhythm and having symptoms of ACS possess a diagnostic and therapeutic challenge to clinician. Several ECG scoring systems has been suggested in rapidly identifying individual with LBBB and STEMI equivalent. One such is Sgarbossa criteria which is used along with cardiac biomarkers to clinch the diagnosis.

Sgarbossa Criteria (Fig. 1)[6]

- Concordant ST elevation >1 mm *in leads with a positive QRS complex (score 5)*
- Concordant ST depression >1 mm *in V1–V3 (score 3)*
- Excessively discordant ST elevation >5 mm *in leads with a –ve QRS complex (score 2).*

These criteria are specific, but not sensitive (36%) for myocardial infarction. A total score of ≥3 is reported to have a specificity of 90% for diagnosing myocardial infarction.

ST-segment elevation in aVR along with ST depression of 1 mm or more in 8 or more surface leads suggests left main coronary artery obstruction, particularly if the patient presents with hemodynamic compromise.

Localizing the ischemic areas and the associated complications is reasonably possible by ECG in STEMI **(Table 2)**.[7]

Cardiac Biomarkers

Cardiac high sensitivity troponins (HsTn): Both Trop I (TnI) and Trop T (TnT) are the most sensitive and specific tools in providing both diagnostic and prognostic information of patients. They are found to be raised within 4–6 hours of onset of chest pain. These enzymes are released in the blood if there is heart muscle damage.

In certain conditions, there could be false elevation of troponin. They are chronic kidney disease (CKD), blood clot in the lungs and congestive heart failure (CCF)

Measurement of creatine kinase (CK)-MB, the isoenzyme specific to heart muscle is another biomarker which is used

TABLE 1: Risk score using the TIMI Risk Calculator.

Inclusion criteria	Scoring system	
	TIMI score	Risk
Thrombolysis in myocardial infarction (TIMI) risk score (1 point for each item) • Age (>65 years) • More than 3 coronary risk factors • Prior angiographic coronary obstruction • ST-segment deviation • More than 2 angina events within 24 hours • Use of aspirin within 7 days • Elevated cardiac markers	0–2	Low
	3–4	Intermediate
	5–7	High
	TIMI risk score is a very useful tool to stratify the risk in UA/NSTEMI patients. This allows the clinician to categorize the patients into high, intermediate or low risk. A 7-point TIMI risk score must be publicized for the practice and should be provided to as many hospital emergency rooms as possible	

(TIMI: thrombolysis in myocardial infarction; NSTEMI: non-ST segment elevated myocardial infarction; UA: unstable angina)

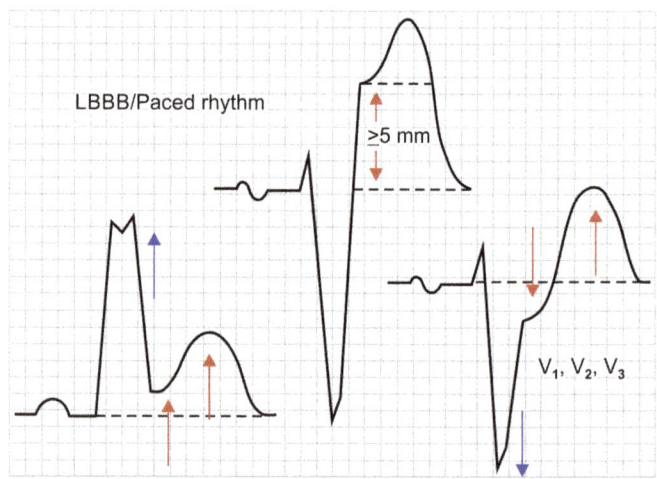

Fig. 1: Sgarbossa criteria.

TABLE 2: ECG lead changes due to injury or infarct with coronary artery, anatomic area of damage, and associated complications.

Leads with ECG	Injury/Infarct-related artery	Area of damage	Associated complications
V_1–V_2	LCA: LAD-septal branch	Septum, His bundle, bundle branches	Infranodal block and BBBs
V_3–V_4	LCA: LAD-diagonal branch	Anterior wall LV	LV dysfunction, CHF, BBBs, complete heart block, PVCs
V_5–V_6 plus I and aVL	LCA: Circumflex branch	High lateral wall LV	LV dysfunction, AV nodal block in some
II, III, aVF	RCA: Posterior descending branch	Inferior wall LV, posterior wall LV	Hypotension, sensitivity to nitroglycerin and morphine sulfate
V_4R (II, III, aVF)	RCA: proximal branches	RV, inferior wall LV, posterior wall LV	Hypotension, supranodal and AV-nodal blocks, arterial fibrillation/flutter, PACs, adverse medical reactions
V_1 through V_4 (marked depression)	Either LCA-circumflex or RCA-posterior descending branch	Posterior wall LV	LV dysfunction

(AV; atrioventricular; BBBs: bundle branch blocks; CHF: congestive heart failure; ECG: echocardiograpm; LAD: left anterior descending; LCA: left coronary artery; LV: left ventricular; RCA: right coronary artery; PVCs; premature ventricular contractions)

to diagnose heart attack. It was the principal biomarker for heart muscle injury till troponin supplemented it.[8]

Echocardiogram

Echocardiography is an inexpensive noninvasive test, which, if available, should be done at earliest in ER only. Appearance of regional wall motion abnormalities (RWMA) in ACS is the first sign to appear and can be easily picked by echocardiogram. In fact, absence of RWMA during active chest pain is highly reliable sign of nonischemic origin. It is an important tool in diagnosing acute mechanical complications of ACS such as acute mitral valve regurgitation, ventricular or myocardial free wall rupture and papillary muscle rupture. All of these mechanical complications, once diagnosed, require urgent surgical interventions to prevent mortality.[9]

■ TREATMENT

Once diagnosis of STEMI is confirmed, the patients should immediately receive dual antiplatelet therapy (DAPT).[10]

Tablet Aspirin 325 mg to be chewed along with Tablet Clopidogrel 300–600 mg or Tablet Ticagrelor 180 mg. Different trials have shown that 600/150 mg for 1 week of Clopidogrel results in better platelet inhibition that 300/75 mg daily. Tablet Prasugrel should not be given in ER and can only be used in cardiac catheterization laboratory once primary angioplasty is definitely planned. Tablet Atorvastatin 80 mg should be given along with the antiplatelet.

Beta blockers should be used if not contraindicated. Nitroglycerin can be used sublingual or intravenous if blood pressures are high. It should be avoided in patients with right ventricular (RV) MI.

Routine oxygen inhalation if SpO_2 >94 should be discouraged.[11]

Revascularization

Early revascularization is the treatment of choice in ACS. Prompt restoration of blood flow in the occluded artery is of prime importance in saving the heart muscle from getting damaged permanently as "time is muscle". Minimizing heart muscle loss is the most important factor in defining both short term and long-term outcomes regardless of the method of revascularization. It could be achieved by pharmacological means with thrombolytic therapy (TT), mechanical means by primary percutaneous coronary intervention (PCI) or a combination of both TT followed by PCI known as pharmacoinvasive therapy.

Thrombolytic Therapy

Thrombolytics are the clot buster medicines which dissolve clots responsible for blockage of the artery. Currently, the commercially available thrombolytic agents are:
- Streptokinase (STK)
- Alteplase (tPA)
- Tenecteplase (TNK-tPA)
- Reteplase (R-tPA)
- Urokinase.

Thrombolytic therapy is contraindicated in NSTEMI as there is a platelet rich plaque. Before administering TT, clinician should always fill in a check list in ER to avoid contraindications and complications.[12]

Contraindications to Thrombolytic Therapies

Absolute contraindications:
- Previous intracranial hemorrhage (ICH) or stroke of unknown origin at anytime
- Ischemic stroke in preceding 6 months
- Known malignant intracranial neoplasm or AV malformation (AVM)
- Aortic dissection
- Known bleeding diathesis (excluding menses)
- Gastrointestinal bleeding within past month
- Recent major trauma/surgery/head injury within past month
- Noncompressible punctures in past 24 hours (liver biopsy, lumbar puncture).

Relative contraindications:
- Transient ischemic attack in preceding 6 months

- Severe uncontrolled hypertension on presentation (SBP >180 mm Hg or DBP >110 mm Hg)
- On oral anticoagulants
- Active peptic ulcer
- Pregnancy or within 1st week of postpartum
- Advanced liver disease
- Infective endocarditis
- Traumatic or prolonged (>10 minutes) cardiopulmonary resuscitation (CPR).

Thrombolytic therapy should be administered to patients with STEMI if primary PCI is not feasible within 120 minutes from first medical contact (FMC). It should be given within 30 minutes (door to needle time). Once administered, the patient should be transferred immediately to a PCI capable center so that they can undergo rescue PCI immediately in case of a failed thrombolysis. In case of a successful thrombolysis, patient undergoes a planned PCI within the next 24 hours as a pharmacoinvasive procedure.[13]

Prehospital thrombolysis, if indicated, appears to be safe and feasible. This needs to be administered by some skilled personnel. It could change the outcome dramatically. Agents such as TNK-tPA or reteplase are relatively safe and recommended for prehospital usage.[14]

If presentation is <3 hours and there is no delay to an invasive strategy, there is no preference for either strategy **(Table 3)**.

Primary Percutaneous Coronary Intervention

Primary PCI is the treatment of choice for STEMI. It is the preferred treatment modality over TT.[15]

It has survival benefits over TT in the following conditions:
- Acute cardiogenic shock
- Age >75 years
- High risk populations with hemodynamic instability, malignant arrhythmia, and survivors of aborted sudden cardiac death.

Primary PCI performed by radial route has significant lower morbidity and mortality over femoral route.[16]

Stenting with a drug eluting stent is preferred over plain balloon angioplasty.[17]

Routine use of thrombosuction devices should be avoided and should be limited to patients with slow flow or no flow.[18]

At present, opening of infarct related artery (IRA) in multivessel coronary artery disease and STEMI during primary PCI followed by complete revascularization within next 6 weeks appears to be reasonably safe and noninferior to complete revascularization. However, in patients with cardiogenic shock, revascularization with primary PCI, and complete revascularization if multivessel disease is present, are the preferred treatments.[19]

Delayed routine primary PCI in asymptomatic patients can be done up to 48 hours of FMC. Beyond 48 hours, opening of IRA is contraindicated.[20]

TABLE 3: Feasibility of prehospital initiation of thrombolytic therapy.

Fibrinolysis is preferred if—	An invasive strategy is preferred if—

• Duration of onset of symptoms <12 hours and primary PCI is not possible within 120 minutes of FMC
• Invasive strategy is not an option
  – Catheterization laboratory occupied/not available
  – Vascular access difficulties
  – Lack of access to a skilled PCI laboratory
	• Skilled PCI laboratory available with door-to-wire time of <120 minutes of FMC
	• High risk from STEMI
	  – Cardiogenic shock
	  – Killip class is ≥3
	  – Ongoing chest pain >12 hours of duration
	  – Malignant arrhythmias

(FMC: first medical contact; PCI: percutaneous coronary intervention; STEMI: ST-elevation myocardial infarction)

SECONDARY PREVENTION AND HEART HEALTHY LIFESTYLE

Patients who survive the first event of ACS should follow a heart healthy lifestyle to lead a normal or near normal life and mitigate the chances of a second event. A second event occurs in 25% of patients within first 3 years of the first event.

A heart healthy lifestyle includes:
- Quit smoking
- Eat heart healthy diet and watch body weight
- Be active and undertake rehabilitation exercise program under supervision
- Check blood cholesterol levels from time to time. Keep low-density lipoprotein (LDL) cholesterol levels <55 mg/dL with high intensity statin therapy indefinitely
- Take DAPT preferably with Aspirin and Ticagrelor or Prasugrel for at least 1 year and subsequently, if required
- Control blood pressure and blood sugar levels
- Manage stress by yoga, etc.
- Moderate alcohol intake
- Visit your physician routinely and do not omit medications without the physician's advise.

CONCLUSION

Tremendous progress has been made in reducing fatality from ACS, yet many deaths occur as people fail to recognize the signs early and do not seek timely medical advice. Early diagnosis of ACS by healthcare providers with skilled, efficient, and coordinated out of hospital care and in ER care subsequently improves survival significantly.

Take Home Messages

- Although the rate of mortality associated with STEMI are decreasing, it is still the single most common cause of death worldwide. The in-hospital mortality rates of unselected patients with STEMI varies between 4 and 12%.
- Women tend to receive reperfusion therapy and other evidence-based treatments less frequently and/or delayed compared to men. Women and men receive equal benefit from a reperfusion and other STEMI-related therapies, and so both genders must be managed equally.

- Getting a prehospital ECG in STEMI expedites the treatment and leads to timely angiography and PCI. Patient transfer to the PCI center should bypass the emergency department.
- STEMI patients should undergo a primary PCI strategy unless the anticipated absolute time from STEMI diagnosis to PCI-mediated reperfusion is >120 min, when TT should be initiated immediately.
- Following TT, patient should be shifted to PCI capable center immediately for subsequent rescue angioplasty or pharmacoinvasive angioplasty.
- Patients with STEMI postresuscitation following cardiac arrest should undergo a primary PCI
- Routine radial access and routine DES implant is the standard of care during primary PCI. Routine thrombus aspiration is contraindicated.
- Treatment of non-IRA should be considered before hospital discharge. In cardiogenic shock, non-IRA PCI should be considered during the index procedure.
- DAPT are the cornerstones of the pharmacological approach in the acute phase of STEMI. Following loading dose of aspirin and clopidogrel/ticagrelor/prasugrel, maintenance therapy with DAPT should be continued for 1 year.
- After reperfusion therapy, patients should be monitored for at least 24 h. Early ambulation and early discharge are the best options in uncomplicated patients.
- Noninvasive imaging such as echocardiography is very important for the acute and long-term management of STEMI patients.
- A sizeable proportion of STEMI patients do not present significant coronary artery stenosis on urgent angiography. This is defined as MINOCA. It is important to perform additional diagnostic tests in these patients to identify the etiology.

REFERENCES

1. Writing Group Members, Mozaffarian D, Benjamin EJ, Go AS, Arnett DK, Blaha MJ, Cushman M, et al. Heart Disease and Stroke Statistics-2016 Update: A Report From the American Heart Association. Circulation. 2016;133(4):e38-360.
2. Switaj TL, Christensen SR, Brewer DM. Acute coronary syndrome: current treatment. Am Fam Physician. 2017; 95(4):232-40.
3. Abdu FA, Mohammed AQ, Liu L, Xu Y, Che W. Myocardial Infarction with Nonobstructive Coronary Arteries (MINOCA): a review of the current position. cardiology. 2020;145(9): 543-52.
4. de Torbal A, Boersma E, Kors JA, van Herpen G, Deckers JW, van der Kuip DA, et al. Incidence of recognized and unrecognized myocardial infarction in men and women aged 55 and older: the Rotterdam Study. Eur Heart J. 2006;27(6):729-36.
5. Diercks DB, Peacock WF, Hiestand BC, Chen AY, Pollack CV Jr, Kirk JD, et al. Frequency and consequences of recording an electrocardiogram >10 minutes after arrival in an emergency room in non-ST-segment elevation acute coronary syndromes (from the CRUSADE Initiative). Am J Cardiol. 2006;97(4): 437-42.
6. Sgarbossa EB, Pinski SL, Barbagelata A, Underwood DA, Gates KB, Topol EJ, et al. Electrocardiographic diagnosis of evolving acute myocardial infarction in the presence of left bundle-branch block. GUSTO-1 (Global Utilization of Streptokinase and Tissue Plasminogen Activator for Occluded Coronary Arteries) Investigators. N Engl J Med. 1996;334(8):481-7.
7. Rokos IC, Farkouh ME, Reiffel J, Dressler O, Mehran R, Stone GW. Correlation between index electrocardiographic patterns and pre-intervention angiographic findings: insights from the HORIZONS-AMI trial. Catheter Cardiovasc Interv. 2012;79(7):1092-8.
8. Chacko S, Haseeb S, Glover BM, Wallbridge D, Harper A. The role of biomarkers in the diagnosis and risk stratification of acute coronary syndrome. Future Sci OA. 2018; 4(1):FSO251.
9. Greaves SC. Role of echocardiography in acute coronary syndromes. Heart. 2002;88(4): 419-25.
10. Kubica J, Adamski P, Ostrowska M, Sikora J, Kubica JM, Sroka WD, et al. Morphine delays and attenuates ticagrelor exposure and action in patients with myocardial infarction: the randomized, double-blind, placebo-controlled IMPRESSION trial. Eur Heart J. 2016;37(3):245-52.
11. Stub D, Smith K, Bernard S, Nehme Z, Stephenson M, Bray JE, et al. Air versus oxygen in ST segment-elevation myocardial infarction. Circulation. 2015;131(24):2143-50.
12. Fibrinolytic Therapy Trialists' (FTT) Collaborative Group. Indications for fibrinolytic therapy in suspected acute myocardial infarction: collaborative overview of early mortality and major morbidity results from all randomised trials of more than 1000 patients. Lancet. 1994;343(8893):311-22.
13. Le May MR, Wells GA, Labinaz M, Davies RF, Turek M, Leddy D, et al. Combined angioplasty and pharmacological intervention versus thrombolysis alone in acute myocardial infarction (CAPITAL AMI study). J Am Coll Cardiol. 2005; 46(3):417-24.
14. Huber K, De Caterina R, Kristensen SD, Verheugt FW, Montalescot G, Maestro LB, et al. Prehospital reperfusion therapy: a strategy to improve therapeutic outcome in patients with ST-elevation myocardial infarction. Eur Heart J. 2005;26(19):2063-74.
15. Dalby M, Bouzamondo A, Lechat P, Montalescot G. Transfer for primary angioplasty versus immediate thrombolysis in acute myocardial infarction: a meta-analysis. Circulation. 2003;108(15):1809-14.
16. Romagnoli E, Biondi-Zoccai G, Sciahbasi A, Politi L, Rigattieri S, Pendenza G, et al. Radial versus femoral randomized investigation in ST-segment elevation acute coronary syndrome: the RIFLE-STEACS (Radial Versus Femoral Randomized Investigation in ST-Elevation Acute Coronary Syndrome) study. J Am Coll Cardiol. 2012;60(24):2481-9.
17. Nordmann AJ, Hengstler P, Harr T, Young J, Bucher HC. Clinical outcomes of primary stenting versus balloon angioplasty in patients with myocardial infarction: a meta-analysis of randomized controlled trials. Am J Med. 2004;116(4):253-62
18. Jolly SS, Cairns JA, Yusuf S, Meeks B, Pogue J, Rokoss MJ, TOTAL Investigators, et al. Randomized trial of primary PCI with or without routine manual thrombectomy. N Engl J Med. 2015;372(15):1389-98.
19. Hannan EL, Samadashvili Z, Walford G, Holmes DR Jr, Jacobs AK, Stamato NJ, et al. Culprit vessel percutaneous coronary intervention versus multivessel and staged percutaneous coronary intervention for ST-segment elevation myocardial infarction patients with multivessel disease. JACC Cardiovasc Interv. 2010;3(1):22-31.
20. Ioannidis JP, Katritsis DG. Percutaneous coronary intervention for late reperfusion after myocardial infarction in stable patients. Am Heart J. 2007;154(6):1065-71.

CHAPTER 4

Acute Heart Failure

Vernon VS Bonarjee

■ DEFINITION

Heart failure (HF) is a clinical syndrome with symptoms of breathlessness, fatigue and swelling of the lower extremities, accompanied by clinical signs of pulmonary congestion, elevated Jugular venous pressure, and peripheral edema. It is caused by a structural and/or a functional abnormality of the heart resulting in elevated intracardiac pressures and/or inadequate cardiac output at rest or during exercise.[1]

Acute HF (AHF) is most often due to acute decompensated chronic HF (ADCHF), where the onset of severe symptoms forces the patient to seek urgent medical attention. It can also be de novo acute HF (DNHF) due to sudden cardiac dysfunction.[2] Patients with acute HF need urgent evaluation and treatment, and often require hospitalization or consultation at an emergency department.[3]

■ PREVALENCE

Acute HF is a phase of the chronic HF syndrome. AHF does not exist over time, but either has a fatal outcome, recovers or moves into the chronic phase. In the US, 6.4 million currently have HF with 1 million new cases a year.[4] Prevalence and incidence increase with age with a 5-year mortality of 65%.[5] There are no systematic survey data from India, but a conservative estimate of the prevalence of HF in India is 1.3–2.4 million, with an annual incidence up to 1.8 million.[6] AHF also has a high in-hospital mortality. A study showed in-hospital mortality of 12.7%, the highest being 62.7% in patients with cardiogenic shock (CS).[7]

■ EARLY DIAGNOSIS

Acute HF is a medical emergency and time to diagnosis and treatment is crucial. Patients are breathless, presenting with pulmonary congestion. They may have stable blood pressure (BP) and cardiac output (CO), termed wet and warm, but may be hypotensive with low CO, termed wet and cold. In cardiogenic shock there is circulatory collapse. A history of cardiac disease or objective findings of cardiac dysfunction will support the diagnosis. Initial diagnosis may not be difficult in ADCHF and treatment may be initiated without further diagnostic considerations. However, in DNHF a more extensive diagnostic process to investigate the underlying cardiac pathology is required to determine appropriate treatment.

■ DIFFERENTIAL DIAGNOSIS

Many noncardiogenic causes of dyspnea can mimic AHF.
- Acute respiratory distress syndrome (ARDS) may occur in some severe clinical conditions such as septicemia and severe pancreatitis which may cause inflammation and noncardiogenic pulmonary edema.[8]
- *Pneumonia:* Bacterial or viral
- Chronic obstructive pulmonary disease with exacerbation
- Pulmonary embolism
- Pneumothorax
- Diffuse parenchymal lung disease and interstitial pulmonary fibrosis
- Neurogenic pulmonary edema, a relatively rare form of pulmonary edema may occur in central nervous system insults such subarachnoidal hemorrhage, cerebral hemorrhage, and traumatic brain injury
- Acute kidney disease may cause acute fluid overload, acidosis, and hyperkalemia, mimicking AHF
- Acute heart failure may be the presenting symptom of an acute myocardial infarction.

■ APPROACH TO THE PROBLEM

Acute decompensated HF and DNHF are actually two entities with a similar clinical presentation. Acute coronary syndrome, valvular dysfunction, hypertensive heart disease, viral myocarditis and toxic insults are usual in DNHF resulting mainly in acute systolic dysfunction. ADCHF is more common and is often due to infections, poor treatment compliance, inadequate medication, excessive sodium intake, alcohol, and drug abuse, resulting in fluid overload and redistribution. Maladaptive neurohumoral activation is often seen.[9,10]

Initial Evaluation

The first task in suspected AHF is to evaluate cardiopulmonary status. In addition to pulmonary rales on auscultation one needs to look at respiratory rate, ability or inability to lie flat, degree of hypoxia (oxygen saturation), and effort of breathing to assess the severity of the problem. Blood pressure must be measured and heart rate and rhythm must be noted. Look for signs of hypoperfusion and check mental status, peripheral edema, and jugular venous distension.

There are four clinical presentations of AHF[1] **(Table 1)** that may guide treatment. This initial evaluation should give an idea of the severity of the condition and determine the approach to further treatment.[3]

■ LABORATORY ASSESSMENT

In case of acute decompensated HF, it is important to identify the precipitating factor. In case of de novo AHF it is important to diagnose the cause. **Table 2** presents the main tests that should be done in AHF patients. **Table 3** presents the blood tests that should be taken.

■ ROLE OF BIOMARKERS

There are numerous biomarkers that can be measured in relation to HF. Some may be elevated in response to myocardial stretch such as natriuretic peptides, others such as troponins may reflect myocardial injury. Level of neurohormone activation as well as biomarkers for inflammation and fibrosis can be measured.[13] Numerous studies have shown a relationship between these biomarkers and heart failure, also as markers of prognosis.[14] However, many of the biomarkers may be elevated due to other conditions and are not specific for heart failure. Not all are readily available for clinical use. The biomarkers most relevant for HF are discussed here.

Natriuretic Peptides

Brain natriuretic peptide (BNP) and NT-proBNP act as the gold standard in HF. BNP is predominantly released from the ventricles in response to volume expansion and overload. The biologically inactive segment of its prohormone, NT-proBNP is the preferred biomarker. NT-proBNP is highly sensitive and specific for the diagnosis of AHF. NT-proBNP level <300 pg/mL can rule out AHF, with a negative predictive value of 99%.[15] Another advantage is that—the novel class of drugs angiotensin receptor-neprilysin inhibitors (ARNi) that are used to treat HF increase the level of BNP but does not affect NT-proBNP concentrations. Numerous studies have shown that BNP and NT-proBNP are independent predictors of mortality in AHF.[16] Fall in NT-proBNP following treatment is also associated with improved prognosis.[17]

Bedside kits are available for rapid analysis of BNP in the emergency room and can be helpful to distinguish AHF from other causes of dyspnea.[18] Other available natriuretic peptides are atrial natriuretic peptide (ANP), NT-proANP and a novel marker MR-proANP.[19]

Troponins

Troponins are the part of the regulatory complex of myocyte thin filaments.[20] Cardiac troponin (cTn) isoform T and I are distinct from their skeletal muscle counterparts and highly specific and sensitive assays exist to detect them in the circulation. They are released from injured myocardium and are the primary biomarker for the detection of myocardial necrosis and acute myocardial infarction (MI).

TABLE 1: Clinical presentations in acute heart failure.

	Onset	Key features	Hemodynamics	Primary treatment*
Acute decompensated heart failure	Gradual over days	Sodium and water retention	High LVEDP normal or low SBP	Diuretics and inotropes/vasopressors
Acute pulmonary edema	Rapid	Hypertension, valvular HD, diastolic LV dysfunction	High LVEDP. Normal or high SBP	Diuretics. Vasodilators
Isolated right ventricular failure	Rapid or gradual	Right ventricular dysfunction or precapillary pulmonary hypertension	Elevated central venous pressure with jugular distension. Hypotension due to low LV filling. Pulmonary congestion may be absent	• Treat cause such as RV infarction or pulmonary emboli. Diuretics for peripheral congestion • Vasopressors if hypotension
Cardiogenic shock	Rapid or gradual	Dominated by severe cardiac dysfunction, pulmonary congestion, hypotension and systemic hypoperfusion	Elevated LVEDP, low SBP and low CO	• Treat cause if possible • Inotropes, vasopressor agents and diuretics • Mechanical circulatory support

(CO: cardiac output; HD: heart disease; LVEDP: left ventricular end diastolic pressure; SBP: systolic blood pressure)
*In all cases adequate ventilatory support is essential. This includes noninvasive positive pressure ventilation (NIV) or intubation if necessary.

TABLE 2: Examinations recommended in acute heart failure.

Test	Time Point	Evaluation	Consequence
ECG	On admission. Prehospital if possible	• Identify acute MI or ischemia as cause. • Identify arrythmia • Identify cardiac hypertrophy, dyssynchrony or old MI (Q-waves)	• Decide treatment such as primary PCI or early angiography • Need to treat arrhythmia • Identify cause of HF such as old MI, conduction defects
Chest X-ray	On admission	Quantify pulmonary congestion. Help in the differential diagnoses such as pneumonic infiltration, pulmonary fibrosis, pneumothorax, pleural effusion, etc	• Evaluate degree of pulmonary congestion • Identify other causes of acute dyspnea
Lung ultrasound[11,12]	On admission if available	Evaluate degree of pulmonary congestion	Identify pulmonary congestion in the emergency room
Echocardiography	Early after admission in ADHF. During hospital stay in ADCHF	Study LV and RV function. Evaluate valve function. Identify other cardiac pathology such as septal or papillary rupture, pericardial fluid. Measure pulmonary pressure if there is TI	• Identify cause or the precipitating factor for AHF • Guide treatment
Coronary angiography	• On admission if STEMI. 2–24 hours after admission in NSTEMI • Otherwise during hospital stay or after discharge if necessary to find cause. If low risk for coronary disease on can do CT coronary angiography	Identify acute coronary occlusion/stenosis. Identify ischemic cardiomyopathy as a cause	Revascularization if needed in STEMI and in ischemic cardiomyopathy
Right heart catheterization	Indicated only in cardiogenic shock patients	Measure cardiac filling pressures and cardiac output	Guide treatment strategies

(ADCHF: acute decompensated acute heart failure; ADHF: acute de novo heart failure; ECG: electrocardiogram; MI: myocardial infarction; PCI: percutaneous coronary intervention; STEMI: ST-elevation MI; NSTEMI: non-ST elevation MI; TI: tricuspid insufficiency)

A small amount (<10%) of cTn exists free in the cytosol of cardiomyocytes and may be released without myocyte necrosis. Elevated levels may be detected in conditions such as HF,[21] kidney disease, severe infection, and cerebral injury.

Measuring cTn is useful in AHF first of all to confirm or exclude myocardial infarction as the cause or precipitating factor for AHF, but also, as an important prognostic indicator.

In AHF an elevated cTn level has been repeatedly shown to correlate with increased short- and long-term mortality and readmission rates.[22]

■ PREHOSPITAL CARE

Monitoring

Prehospital management of AHF is critical and time to treatment is important.[3] Patients with AHF need emergency care and should be to be monitored until admission. The clinical picture can change markedly within a short period. Noninvasive examination, including pulse oximetry, Blood pressure (BP), heart rate and respiratory rate should be measured. A continuous ECG monitoring should be instituted when available. An intravenous line should be put in as soon as possible. Emergency units should have dedicated protocols for AHF treatment.[23]

Treatment

Oxygen therapy should be given only to hypoxemic patients (oxygen saturation is <90%) as it may causes vasoconstriction and a reduction in cardiac output in HF.[24] Oxygen therapy may also suppress ventilation and increase hypercapnia in patients with COPD.[1]

Noninvasive positive pressure ventilation (NIV) improves respiration in patients with respiratory distress (respiratory rate >25 breaths/min, SpO$_2$ <90%) and should be started as soon as possible. A meta-analysis has shown that NIV may improves dyspnea, reduces the need for intubation and reduce mortality, compared with traditional oxygen therapy, especially if AHF is due to ischemia.[25]

Intravenous diuretics are the cornerstone of AHF treatment.[1,11] They decrease fluid overload and congestion by increasing renal excretion of salt and water. Loop diuretics are preferred due to their rapid onset of action and efficacy. 20–40 mg of furosemide should be given IV.

TABLE 3: Recommended blood tests in acute heart failure.

	Time Point	Reason
NT-proBNP	On admission and before discharge	To confirm or exclude HF on admission. As a prognostic marker
BNP using bed side kit	On admission if available	To confirm or exclude HF on admission
Hemoglobin	On admission	To detect anemia as a precipitating factor
White blood cell count	On admission and later if necessary	To confirm or exclude infection
Cardiac troponins	On admission and 1–3 hours after	To diagnose myocardial infarction or injury. As a prognostic marker
Serum electrolytes	On admission and later if necessary	Reveal electrolyte disorder, especially in ADCHF with prior diuretics
D-dimer	On admission	To diagnose thromboembolism and pulmonary emboli
Serum creatinine	On admission and later if necessary	To detect renal disorder as a precipitating factor
TSH	During hospital stay	To detect hypo- or hyperthyroidism as a cause of HF
Arterial blood gas	On admission in severe cases	Evaluate respiratory function
Serum lactate	On admission in severe cases	To detect lactacidosis and evaluate perfusion status

(ADCHF: Acute Decompensated Chronic Heart Failure; BNP: Brain Natriuretic Peptide; NT-proANP: N terminal pro brain natriuretic peptide, it is the biomarker of choice but others are commercially available; TSH: thyroid-stimulating hormone)

Most patients with AHF have normal or high blood pressure at presentation and may benefit from vasodilator therapy in addition to diuretics. If systolic BP (SBP) is ≥110 mm Hg, IV nitroglycerin may be started. Alternatively, sublingual nitrates may be considered.[3] There are however, few clinical trials to support this.[26] Prehospital vasodilators are not recommended if there is aortic stenosis or low cardiac output.

Opiates such as morphine relieve dyspnea and anxiety. They may be used as sedative agents but are associated with increased adverse outcomes, and are only recommended in case of severe pain or anxiety.

Additional treatment with vasopressors, inotropes, digoxin, and intubation may be needed, but is only possible out of hospital if adequate expertise and monitoring are available.

Prehospital treatment should aim to stabilize the patient. Unless there is a rapid symptomatic recovery, patients need to be admitted to the nearest hospital with necessary facilities. Initial prehospital treatment should not delay hospital admission.

OUTCOME ASSESSMENT

It is important to do a cardiopulmonary assessment on admission and perform necessary diagnostic tests as mentioned. A cause of AHF such as acute MI, tachy- or bradyarrhythmia must be treated as necessary.

Diuresis should be monitored and repeated dose of loop diuretics must be given if there is <100 mL urine/hour. Augmented effect may be seen if combined with thiazide diuretics. In case of diuretic resistance or renal failure renal replacement therapy may be necessary.

If SBP is >110 mm hg a vasodilator such as IV nitroglycerin or sodium nitroprusside should be started. In low output cases with SBP <90 mm Hg and systemic hypoperfusion one may need inotropic drugs such as dopamine or dobutamine. Intravenous levosimendan, an inotrope with vasodilator properties may provide rapid and durable symptomatic relief in patients with ADHF.[27] Initial hypotension may be avoided by omitting the loading dose and starting with an infusion rate of 0.1 μg/kg/min for 24 hours.

Vasopressors may be necessary in severe hypotension to increase perfusion to vital organs. Norepinephrine is preferred. Inotropes and vasopressors must be administered under proper monitoring capabilities with invasive arterial pressure measurements. There should be proper treatment protocols and treatment should be as short as possible as the drugs may actually increase mortality.

Ventilatory support is of utmost importance. If NIV is not sufficient intubation and respirator treatment may be necessary, especially in pulmonary edema.

Cardiogenic shock, which is the most severe form for AHF needs immediate treatment in an emergency unit with adequate facilities. The cause, which may be myocardial infarction or a mechanical complication needs to be identified and treated. All the abovementioned treatments may be necessary but here one may also need additional mechanical circulatory support (MCS) such as intra-aortic balloon pump, Impella pump or extracorporeal membrane oxygenation. Randomized controlled trials on MCS do not support the routine use of such treatment in cardiogenic shock.[1] However, in selected cases MCS may potentially translate into improved survival.[28]

Acute RV failure is uncommon and may be due to RV infarction or massive pulmonary embolism that needs specific treatment.

Clinical response to initial treatment is an important indicator of outcome. Subjective improvement, no hypotension, resting heart rate <100, adequate urine output and oxygen saturation >95% in room air are signs of a favorable outcome.

Early follow-up should include daily weight assessment to follow fluid balance. Renal function and electrolytes should be monitored. Invasive hemodynamic monitoring is only indicated in patients with cardiogenic shock. Predischarge NT-proBNP and a fall in its concentration is a good prognostic indicator.[29]

Evidence-based foundational oral treatment for HF must be initiated as soon as the patient is stable. This includes angiotensin-converting enzyme inhibitors (ACE-I)/angiotensin receptor blockers (ARB), beta-blockers, mineralocorticoid receptor antagonists, diuretics and sodium-glucose cotransporter-2 (SGLT-2) inhibitors. ACE-I/ARBs may be replaced by the ARNi valsartan/sacubitril. Most patients have comorbidities such as diabetes mellitus, renal failure, chronic pulmonary disease, etc. Proper care of comorbidities is important. Early follow-up in a dedicated HF clinic may prevent readmission and improve long-term prognosis.

CONCLUSION

Acute heart failure is a medical emergency with poor outcome if not treated properly. It is most often due to acute decompensation of chronic heart failure but may be de novo due to sudden cardiac dysfunction. Time is important and treatment should be initiated prehospital with rapid transfer to a hospital with necessary facilities. Adequate ventilatory support and IV loop diuretics are the primary treatment, together with a vasodilator such as IV nitroglycerin if BP is adequate. In-hospital treatment depends on the cause and primary clinical presentation. Biomarkers such as NT-proBNP and cardiac troponins are particularly useful in the diagnostic process and determining prognosis.

Take Home Messages

- Patients with respiratory distress need urgent attention. With pulmonary congestion, especially in patients with known HF one should start immediate treatment. Measure BP, check pulse and oxygen saturation, put in IV lead and give first dose of loop diuretics such as furosemide 20–40 mg. If no IV lead, one can give first dose intramuscular.
- Give oxygen if available if saturation is below 90%. Secure breathing and start noninvasive positive pressure ventilation in patients who need support.
- If systolic BP is >110 mm Hg in patients without aortic stenosis on can give 0.5 mg nitroglycerin sublingual.
- Check patient status and transfer patient to hospital. Initial in-hospital action is to do a cardiopulmonary status including ECG and chest X-ray. Do tests as mentioned. One can do a bedside BNP measurement to confirm HF. Try to ascertain the cause of AHF and treat according to clinical presentation. Ventilation and decongestion with diuretics is most important. Circulatory support with inotropes and vasopressors may be needed but should be given as short time as possible. Mechanical circulatory support may be given in advanced cardiogenic shock, but the effect on long-term prognosis is, at the best, marginal. Proper long-term follow-up with guideline-based treatment is essential for good prognosis.

REFERENCES

1. McDonagh TA, Metra M, Adamo M, Gardner RS, Baumbach A, Böhm M; ESC Scientific Document Group, et al. 2021 ESC Guidelines for the diagnosis and treatment of acute and chronic heart failure. Eur Heart J. 2021;42(36):3599-726.
2. Mosterd A, Hoes AW. Clinical epidemiology of heart failure. Heart. 2007;93(9):1137-46.
3. Mebazaa A, Yilmaz MB, Levy P, Ponikowski P, Peacock WF, Laribi S, et al. Recommendations on pre-hospital and early hospital management of acute heart failure: a consensus paper from the Heart Failure Association of the European Society of Cardiology, the European Society of Emergency Medicine and the Society of Academic Emergency Medicine. Eur J Heart Fail. 2015;17(6):544-58.
4. Savarese G, Lund LH. Global Public Health Burden of Heart Failure. Card Fail Rev. 2017;3(1):7-11.
5. Bleumink GS, Knetsch AM, Sturkenboom MC, Straus SM, Hofman A, Deckers JW, et al. Quantifying the heart failure epidemic: prevalence, incidence rate, lifetime risk and prognosis of heart failure The Rotterdam Study. Eur Heart J. 2004;25(18):1614-9.
6. Huffman MD, Prabhakaran D. Heart failure: epidemiology and prevention in India. Natl Med J India. 2010;23(5):283-8.
7. Spinar J, Parenica J, Vitovec J, Widimsky P, Linhart A, Fedorco M, et al. Baseline characteristics and hospital mortality in the Acute Heart Failure Database (AHEAD) Main registry. Crit Care. 2011;15(6):R291.
8. Pierrakos C, Karanikolas M, Scolletta S, Karamouzos V, Velissaris D. Acute respiratory distress syndrome: pathophysiology and therapeutic options. J Clin Med Res. 2012;4(1):7-16.
9. Pranata R, Tondas AE, Yonas E, Vania R, Yamin M, Chandra A, et al. Differences in clinical characteristics and outcome of de novo heart failure compared to acutely decompensated chronic heart failure - systematic review and meta-analysis. Acta Cardiol. 2021;76(4):410-20.
10. Raffaello WM, Henrina J, Huang I, Lim MA, Suciadi LP, Siswanto BB, et al. Clinical characteristics of de novo heart failure and acute decompensated chronic heart failure: are they distinctive phenotypes that contribute to different outcomes? Card Fail Rev. 2021;7:e02.
11. Palazzuoli A, Evangelista I, Beltrami M, Pirrotta F, Tavera MC, Gennari L et al. Clinical, Laboratory and Lung Ultrasound Assessment of Congestion in Patients with Acute Heart Failure. J Clin Med. 2022;11(6):1642.
12. Platz E, Campbell RT, Claggett B, Lewis EF, Groarke JD, Docherty KF, et al. Lung Ultrasound in Acute Heart Failure: Prevalence of Pulmonary Congestion and Short- and Long-Term Outcomes. JACC Heart Fail. 2019;7(10):849-58.
13. Sarhene M, Wang Y, Wei J. Biomarkers in heart failure: the past, current and future. Heart Fail Rev. 2019;24:867-903.
14. Lassus J, Gayat E, Mueller C, Peacock WF, Spinar J, Harjola VP, GREAT-Network, et al. Incremental value of biomarkers to clinical variables for mortality prediction in acutely decompensated heart failure: the Multinational Observational Cohort on Acute Heart Failure (MOCA) study. Int J Cardiol. 2013;168(3):2186-94.
15. Januzzi JL Jr, Camargo CA, Anwaruddin S, Baggish AL, Chen AA, Krauser DG, et al. The NT-proBNP investigation of dyspnea in the emergency department (PRIDE) study. Am J Cardiol. 2005;95(8):948-54.

16. Santaguida PL, Don-Wauchope AC, Oremus M. BNP and NT-proBNP as prognostic markers in persons with acute decompensated heart failure: a systematic review. Heart Fail Rev. 2014;19:453-70.
17. Zile MR, Claggett BL, Prescott MF, McMurray JJ, Packer M, Rouleau JL, et al. Prognostic Implications of Changes in N-Terminal Pro-B-Type Natriuretic Peptide in Patients with Heart Failure. J Am Coll Cardiol. 2016;68(22):2425-36.
18. Maisel AS, Krishnaswamy P, Nowak RM, McCord J, Hollander JE, Duc P, Breathing Not Properly Multinational Study Investigators, et al. Rapid measurement of B-type natriuretic peptide in the emergency diagnosis of heart failure. N Engl J Med. 2002;347(3):161-7.
19. Idzikowska K, Zielińska M. Midregional pro-atrial natriuretic peptide, an important member of the natriuretic peptide family: potential role in diagnosis and prognosis of cardiovascular disease. J Int Med Res. 2018;46(8):3017-29.
20. Parmacek MS, Solaro RJ. Biology of the troponin complex in cardiac myocytes. Prog Cardiovasc Dis. 2004;47(3):159-76.
21. Wettersten N, Maisel A. Role of Cardiac Troponin Levels in Acute Heart Failure. Card Fail Rev. 2015;1(2):102-6.
22. Peacock WF 4th, De Marco T, Fonarow GC, Diercks D, Wynne J, Apple FS, Wu AH; ADHERE Investigators. Cardiac troponin and outcome in acute heart failure. N Engl J Med. 2008;358(20):2117-26.
23. Harjola P, Miró Ò, Martín-Sánchez FJ, Escalada X, Freund Y, Penaloza A, EMS-AHF Study Group, et al. Pre-hospital management protocols and perceived difficulty in diagnosing acute heart failure. ESC Heart Fail. 2020;7(1):289-96.
24. Park JH, Balmain S, Berry C, Morton JJ, McMurray JJ. Potentially detrimental cardiovascular effects of oxygen in patients with chronic left ventricular systolic dysfunction. Heart. 2010;96(7):533-8.
25. Weng CL, Zhao YT, Liu QH, Fu CJ, Sun F, Ma YL, et al. Meta-analysis: noninvasive ventilation in acute cardiogenic pulmonary edema. Ann Intern Med. 2010;152(9):590-600.
26. Wakai A, McCabe A, Kidney R, Brooks SC, Seupaul RA, Diercks DB, et al. Nitrates for acute heart failure syndromes. Cochrane Database Syst Rev. 2013;8:CD005151.
27. Packer M, Colucci W, Fisher L, Massie BM, Teerlink JR, Young J, REVIVE Heart Failure Study Group, et al. Effect of levosimendan on the short-term clinical course of patients with acutely decompensated heart failure. JACC Heart Fail. 2013;1(2):103-11.
28. Tehrani BN, Truesdell AG, Psotka MA, Rosner C, Singh R, Sinha SS, et al. A Standardized and Comprehensive Approach to the Management of Cardiogenic Shock. JACC Heart Fail. 2020;8(11):879-91.
29. Cohen-Solal A, Logeart D, Huang B, Cai D, Nieminen MS, Mebazaa A. Lowered B-type natriuretic peptide in response to levosimendan or dobutamine treatment is associated with improved survival in patients with severe acutely decompensated heart failure. J Am Coll Cardiol. 2009;53(25):2343-8.

Cardiac Tamponade: Diagnosis and Management

Shilanjan Roy, Srina Ray, Saumitra Ray

INTRODUCTION

The normal pericardium is a fibroelastic sac containing a thin layer of fluid that surrounds the heart. When larger amounts of fluid accumulate (pericardial effusion) or when the pericardium becomes scarred and inelastic, one of three pericardial compressive syndromes may occur:

1. *Cardiac tamponade:* It may be acute or subacute and is characterized by the accumulation of fluid in pericardial space causing pressure in cardiac chambers.
2. *Constrictive pericarditis:* It is a chronic process of scarring and loss of elasticity of the pericardial sac thereby impeding normal relaxation of cardiac chambers.
3. *Effusive-constrictive pericarditis:* It is characterized by presence of fluid in pericardial space with underlying constrictive physiology due to inelasticity of pericardium, can be associated with tamponade.

PHYSIOLOGY

In cardiac tamponade, the primary abnormality is compression of all cardiac chambers due to increased pericardial pressure.[1] Once the pericardium reaches its highest limit of elasticity due to accumulated fluid, the cardiac chambers competes with the intrapericardial fluid as the intrapericardial volume is more or less fixed. As tamponade progresses, the cardiac chambers become compressed and smaller. Diastolic compliance of chambers is also reduced.

Consequences as a result from this constrained cardiac filling are:

- *Progressive changes in systemic venous return:* Venous return in heart follows a bimodal pattern, peaking during ventricular systole and early diastole. The effusion produces compression in all four chambers throughout the cardiac cycle, and as cardiac tamponade becomes more severe, venous return is progressively reduced, the cardiac chambers collapses and cardiac output and blood pressure (BP) falls resulting in shock.
- *Respiratory variation in venous return:* Inspiratory decline in thoracic pressure is transmitted through the pericardium to the right sided cardiac chambers and the pulmonary vasculature. As a result, systemic venous return to the right heart increases with inspiration, venous return to the left heart from the pulmonary veins reduces with inspiration.

In cardiac tamponade, the fluid in pericardium prevents the transmission of negative intrathoracic pressure and free wall from expanding. The distension of the right ventricle during inspiration along with relative underfilling of the left ventricle causes the septum to bulge to the left, reducing left ventricular cavity size, and compliance. It further contributes to decreased filling of the left ventricle during inspiration. This hemodynamic interaction is known as "ventricular interaction" or "ventricular interdependence".

These changes start occurring once pericardial pressure becomes substantially higher than ventricular end-diastolic pressures (**Figs. 1A and B**).

- An acute collection, even if it is as small as 50–100 mL can rapidly lead to cardiac tamponade in a stiff pericardium.
- In comparison, chronic slow accumulation of a pericardial effusion (e.g., due to renal failure or malignancy) allows a much higher amount of collection due to gradual increase in pericardial compliance before tamponade develops.

ETIOLOGY

Infectious

- *Viral:* Human immunodeficiency virus, echovirus, coxsackievirus, adenovirus, and Epstein-Barr virus (EBV).
- *Bacterial: Mycobacterium tuberculosis* (4–5%), *Coxiella burnetii*, other rare causes such as pneumococcus, meningococcus, gonococcus, *Staphylococcus*, and *Leptospira*.
- Fungal and parasitic infections are rare and usually seen in immunocompromised host.

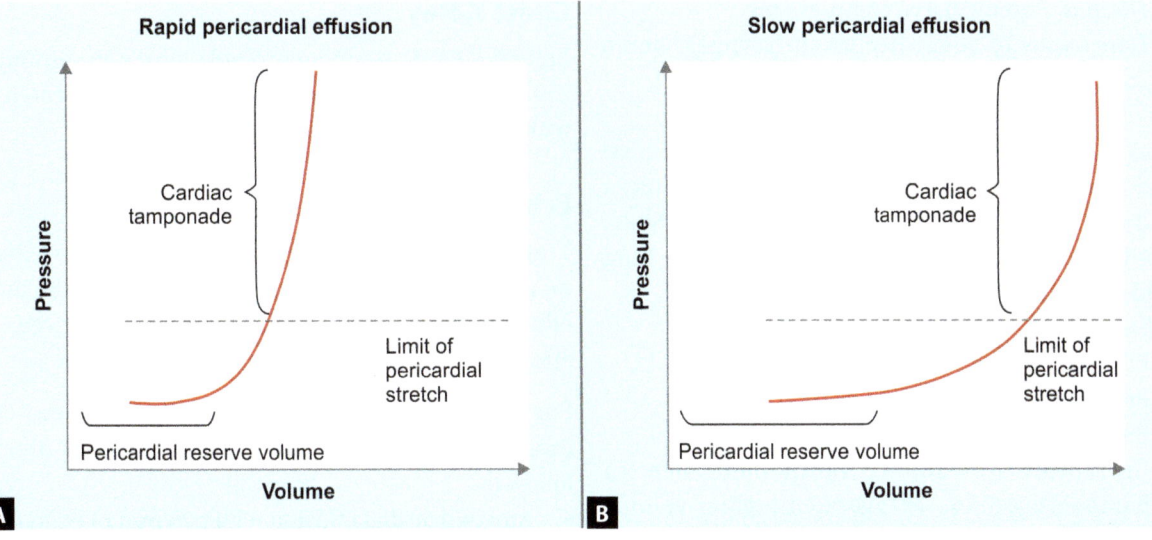

Figs. 1A and B: Pressure/volume curve of the pericardium with fast accumulating pericardial fluid leading to cardiac tamponade with a smaller volume (A) compared with the slowly accumulating pericardial fluid reaching cardiac tamponade only after larger volumes (B).

Noninfectious

- *Autoimmune/inflammatory:* Systemic lupus erythematosus (SLE), rheumatoid arthritis, Sjögren syndrome, systemic vasculitis, Behçet syndrome and sarcoidosis.
- *Pericardial injury syndromes:* Postacute myocardial infarction (AMI), postpericardiotomy, and post-traumatic.
- *Iatrogenic:* Radiation induced, postcardiac interventional procedure like atrial fibrillation (AF) ablation, balloon mitral valvotomy (BMV), percutaneous coronary intervention (PCI), and left atrial appendage (LAA) closure.
- *Neoplastic:* Primary tumors and pericardial mesothelioma.
- *Secondary metastatic:* Lung or breast carcinoma, lymphoma, and melanoma.
- *Metabolic:* Uremia, metabolic, and amyloidosis.
- *Drugs and toxins:* Procainamide, hydralazine, and immunosuppressive therapies.

■ CLINICAL PRESENTATION

The presentation of patients with cardiac tamponade primarily depends upon the time over which pericardial fluid accumulates and the clinical scenario:

- *Acute cardiac tamponade* can occur within minutes, due to trauma, myocardial rupture, as a complication of an invasive diagnostic, or therapeutic procedure.

    Patient usually presents with cardiogenic shock that requires urgent reduction in pericardial pressure by pericardiocentesis. Low BP, tachycardia, and narrow pulse pressure are common clinical presentations due to the decline in cardiac output. Patients can also present with various types of arrhythmias including pulseless electrical activity. Patients in cardiogenic shock will have cold extremities, peripheral cyanosis, and decreased urine output.
- *Subacute cardiac tamponade* characterized by fluid collection over days to weeks before developing tamponade and can be associated with neoplastic, uremic, or tubercular pericarditis. Symptoms include exertional dyspnea, chest heaviness, edema, and fatigability. The physical examination in subacute severe cardiac tamponade may reveal hypotension with a low volume/thready pulse. However, patients with preexisting hypertension may remain hypertensive.
- *Regional cardiac tamponade* occurs when a loculated/septated effusion or localized hematoma compresses any specific cardiac chamber.
- *Low pressure cardiac tamponade:* Patients having severe hypovolemia because of traumatic hemorrhage, hemodialysis or ultrafiltration, or overdiuresis at presentation may have low pressure cardiac tamponade in which the intracardiac and pericardial diastolic pressures are only 6–12 mm Hg.[1] A fluid challenge with a rapid infusion of 1 L of normal saline in the catheterization laboratory will unmask typical cardiac tamponade hemodynamics.

■ PHYSICAL FINDINGS

Depending upon the type and severity of cardiac tamponade clinical presentation can be varied:

- *Symptoms:*
  - Dull aching pain in chest
  - Dyspnea on exertion
  - Other nonspecific symptoms secondary to fluid collection are:
    - *Dysphagia:* Esophageal compression

- *Hiccups:* Phrenic nerve compression
- *Hoarseness of voice:* Recurrent laryngeal nerve compression
- Signs:
  - *Beck's triad* namely low BP, dilated neck veins, and muffled heart sounds are present in only a minority of cases of acute cardiac tamponade. Sinus tachycardia is the rule. Tachypnea with clear lung fields is typical.
  - *Other signs include:*
    - Elevated JVP
    - Prominent "x" descent
    - Blunted/absent "y" descent
    - In rapidly developing tamponade like in hemopericardium, exaggerated jugular venous pulsation is seen without distension as there is no time for compensatory mechanisms to develop.
  - *Pulsus paradoxus:*
    - Pulsus paradoxus is an exaggerated fall in systolic BP during inspiratory phase of normal respiration, while the diastolic pressure usually remains unchanged. This occurs because of the phenomenon of ventricular interdependence already described earlier.
    - The assessment of pulsus paradoxus should always be performed during normal quiet respiration because deep inspiration may result in false-positive findings.[2]
    - Pulsus paradoxus is not specific for cardiac tamponade. It can also be seen in severe obstructive airway disease, obstructive sleep apnea, massive pulmonary embolism, severe hypovolemic shock, right ventricular myocardial infarction, bilateral pleural effusion, tension pneumothorax, restrictive cardiomyopathy, and extrinsic cardiac compression.[3]
  - *Ewart's sign:* Dullness to percussion and bronchial breathing below the left scapular angle.

DIAGNOSIS AND WORKUP

Electrocardiogram
- The most common electrocardiogram (ECG) finding in large pericardial effusion is low voltage complex.
- Electrical alternans is a marker of massive effusion because of the swinging of heart along both axes.[4]
- Combined P and QRS waves alternans is specific for pericardial tamponade.
- Different stages of pericarditis can present with diffuse ST elevation with concavity upward with depression of PR segment.
- T wave alternans.
- Electromechanical dissociation in agonal phase.

Chest X-Ray
Enlarged cardiac silhouette (only after a minimum of 200–250 mL of fluid is accumulated), sharply demarcated margins with decreased pulmonary vascularity.

Echocardiography
Transthoracic echocardiography (TTE) is the diagnostic modality of choice to diagnose and quantify the amount of effusion. However, it cannot differentiate between various etiologies of effusion.[5]

For circumferential pericardial effusions, the common quantitative measurements in Echo Doppler are as follows:
- Any pericardial effusion with ≥20 mm of echo free space is considered as large, usually corresponding to a fluid volume >500 mL.
- The echocardiographic findings of tamponade include:
  - Diastolic collapse of right atrium (a sensitive sign with >80% specificity)[6]
  - Early diastolic collapse of right ventricle (this usually requires higher pressure difference between the intrapericardial space and cardiac chambers than right atrial collapse, thereby making this sign more specific albeit with a lesser sensitivity)[7]
  - Exaggerated respiratory variation of tricuspid and mitral valves inflow velocities in Doppler (a decrease in transmitral E wave amplitude by >25% during inspiration is highly suggestive of cardiac tamponade. Tricuspid inflow variation in PW Doppler is more exaggerated (up to 40–60% in tamponade) than mitral and aortic flow velocities at least in initial phase of tamponade.
  - Plethoric inferior vena cava (IVC), i.e., engorged and noncollapsible IVC (which can also mimic as constrictive physiology), and rarely left atrial diastolic collapse which can be seen only in 25 % of tamponade cases but is a highly specific sign.[8]

Both right atrial and right ventricular collapses are subject to current perfusion state. Right ventricular hypertrophy such as that in pulmonary hypertension can delay right ventricular collapse until significant intrapericardial pressure is existent.

Computed Tomography/Magnetic Resonance Imaging
- High resolution computed tomography (CT) scan is an excellent modality for visualization of the amount, distribution, and nature of the accumulated fluid in the pericardium.

- Magnetic resonance imaging (MRI) may be used in selected cases of chronic effusion for detection of loculated collections and pericardial thickening.
- However, the clinical utility of CT and MRI is restricted because echocardiography itself provides us with most of diagnostic information with high degree of accuracy in bedside.
- CT/MRI also has potential safety concerns in acutely ill patients and none of the modality has role in acute tamponade.
- The utility of nonechocardiographic diagnostic modalities is restricted to only doubtful, complicated, and atypical presentations mainly to find out the etiology.[9]

Invasive Hemodynamics

Role of right heart catheterization (RHC) is very limited in the era of advanced echo Doppler technology. It is not necessary in patients where clinical and echocardiographic findings are consistent with tamponade and, in fact, may delay the definitive treatment.[10]

Right heart catheterization can only be beneficial in borderline cases where there is uncertainty regarding tamponade physiology and help in exact quantification of the early/subtle hemodynamic compromise.

Right atrial pressure tracing shows:
- Prominent "x" descent
- Absent/blunted "y" descent
- Equalization of end diastolic pressure
- Alterations in systolic ejection period.

■ MANAGEMENT

Overview of Treatment

- Definitive treatment of cardiac tamponade is achieved by removal of the pericardial fluid thereby relieving the elevated intrapericardial pressure and improving hemodynamic status.
- Supportive care with fluid resuscitation and/or inotropic support may be of temporary benefit but should not be considered a substitute for drainage of the effusion.
- The decision to drain a pericardial effusion with suspected cardiac tamponade should be focused clinical assessment, echocardiographic findings, and the risk of the procedure.
- Cardiac tamponade causing overt hemodynamic compromise requires urgent pericardiocentesis, *and it produces a rapid and dramatic improvement in cardiac and systemic hemodynamics.*
- Early cardiac tamponade with no/minimal evidence of hemodynamic compromise may be managed with serial echocardiographic studies (every 1–3 days), avoiding of volume depletion, and treatment of the underlying cause of the pericardial effusion.
- In inflammatory effusions associated with "early" cardiac tamponade (e.g., idiopathic pericardial effusion/pericarditis, connective tissue disease, etc.) may resolve with anti-inflammatory therapy [e.g., nonsteroidal anti-inflammatory drugs (NSAIDs) and colchicine].

Choosing Percutaneous or Surgical Drainage

Both percutaneous drainage (i.e., pericardiocentesis) and surgical drainage of a pericardial effusion are highly effective at removal of fluid and relief of symptoms associated with hemodynamic compromise.

- Catheter pericardiocentesis is the treatment of choice in most patients, according to the 2015 European Society of Cardiology (ESC) guidelines on pericardial disease.
- An indwelling pigtail catheter is generally left in the pericardial space until fluid return is <25 mL/day, while a more extended drainage period is frequently preferred in neoplastic effusions.
- Catheter pericardiocentesis under real-time echo guidance, permits the operator to select the best site and angle for puncture, much easier and less expensive than surgery, and facilitates more precise assessment of hemodynamics and diagnosis of effusive constrictive pericarditis.

Surgical drainage has the advantages of:
- Allowing pericardial biopsies to be taken for exact etiological diagnosis.
- Pericardiectomy can be performed if needed.
- Direct surgical visualization of pericardium may be helpful in case of fluid reaccumulating after catheter drainage, loculated effusions, when biopsy is needed, or the patient has a coagulopathy.
- However, surgical drainage requires general anesthesia, which may worsen hemodynamic compromise if percutaneous needle drainage is not performed first to reduce the severity of the cardiac tamponade.

The echocardiography-guided approach is also preferred in hemodynamically unstable patients because of its ability to be performed more rapidly, whereas an open surgical approach might be preferred for traumatic cases, purulent pericarditis, or with recurrent malignant pericardial effusions which may require pericardiectomy also.

There are several specific settings, however, in which there is a clear preference for one of these procedures.
- *Effusion characteristics:* With effusions that are small, organized, and/or loculated, needle aspiration should generally be avoided unless a highly skilled operator well versed in echocardiographically-guided percutaneous techniques is available.
- On the other hand, large, free-flowing effusions can usually be drained safely and effectively using a percutaneous approach.

- *Acuity:* An exception to the rule regarding the size of an effusion is acute cardiac tamponade complicating a cardiac procedure (e.g., percutaneous coronary intervention, invasive electrophysiology study or ablation) where anticoagulation has been given.

    In this setting, the effusion is often small, but pericardial pressure rises very quickly, resulting in hemodynamic compromise and the need for urgent fluid removal. Pericardiocentesis is technically more challenging, with more associated risk, if there is <1 cm of effusion. However, most skilled interventional cardiologists or electrophysiologists can safely tap the effusion, especially with echocardiographic guidance

- *Aortic dissection or myocardial rupture:* In suspected aortic dissection or myocardial rupture causing tamponade, needle drainage should not be attempted as relief of cardiac tamponade may lead to further bleeding and pericardial collection. Emergent surgical intervention is the therapy of choice in such cases.

Relative Contraindications to Pericardial Fluid Drainage

While pericardiocentesis can be safely performed in most patients, there are situations in which the procedure may need to be postponed.

- *Severe pulmonary hypertension:* Here the pericardial effusion may be preventing significant dilatation of the right ventricle, which may be crucial to supporting the right ventricle. Drainage of the pericardial fluid may lead to loss of this support of the right ventricle, causing worsening of right ventricular function and more severe tricuspid regurgitation.
- *Bleeding diathesis/coagulopathy:* The relative risks and benefits of pericardiocentesis should be cautiously weighted if a bleeding diathesis or coagulopathy is present. In addition, the subcostal approach should be avoided in the setting of a coagulopathy as bleeding from liver injury can be life threatening.

In most cases, however, the potential benefits for a patient with significant hemodynamic compromise related to cardiac tamponade will outweigh the risks associated with the procedure.

Evaluation of the Removed Fluid

While pericardial fluid drainage in the setting of cardiac tamponade is done primarily for its therapeutic benefit, the procedure may also be diagnostic, particularly in patients with an uncertain etiology for the effusion.

Monitoring Postprocedure

Monitoring for at least 24–48 hours following either percutaneous or surgical drainage of a pericardial effusion is recommended.

Serial assessment with two-dimensional and Doppler echocardiography prior to discharge from the hospital is required to confirm adequate fluid removal and to detect any possible recurrence of fluid accumulation.

In general, a follow-up echo should be performed within 1–2 weeks after discharge and additional follow-up study in 2–6 months depending on the etiology of the effusion, recurrence of symptoms, etc.

Complications of Fluid Removal

Pericardiocentesis performed electively under controlled conditions is generally safe and effective. The incidence of major complications in experienced hands is 1.2–1.6%.

- Rarely, pericardiocentesis to relieve cardiac tamponade is complicated by acute left ventricular failure with pulmonary edema.
- Acute dilation of the right ventricle following pericardiocentesis is also rare.

Volume Repletion

Patients with cardiac tamponade may require volume expansion with agents such as blood, plasma, dextran, or saline but only as a temporary measure until therapeutic pericardial fluid drainage can be performed. Systolic BP <100 mm Hg was predictive of a favorable response to volume expansion.

Therapies to Avoid

In general, treatment with inotropes and positive pressure ventilation should be avoided whenever possible, due to the possibility of worsening hemodynamics in patients with cardiac tamponade.

Take Home Messages

- Cardiac tamponade is a type of cardiogenic shock and a medical emergency.
- Cardiac tamponade may occur in various conditions that affect the pericardium, including acute and subacute pericarditis, malignancies, tuberculosis, chronic renal failure, thyroid disease, autoimmune disease, etc.
- TTE is the most important tool for diagnosis, grading, during drainage, and for follow-up.
- Clinicians should be able to quickly diagnose cardiac tamponade, particularly in cases without large pericardial effusion where it may be challenging, and correlate the clinical features with the echocardiographic findings.
- The drainage of cardiac tamponade is lifesaving.

REFERENCES

1. Spodick DH. Acute cardiac tamponade. N Engl J Med. 2003; 349:684-90.
2. Diaz-Arocutipa C, Saucedo-Chinchay J, Imazio M. Pericarditis in patients with COVID-19: a systematic review. J Cardiovasc Med (Hagerstown). 2021;22:693-700.

3. Beck CS. Two cardiac compression triads. JAMA. 1935;104: 714-16.
4. Spodick DH. Images in Cardiology. Truly Total Electric Alternation of the Heart. Clin Cardiol. 1998;21(6):427-8.
5. Manning WJ. Pericardial disease. In: Goldman L, Ausiello D (Eds). Cecil Medicine, 23rd edition: Philadelphia: Saunders/Elsevier; 2008. pp. 548-52.
6. Gillam LD, Guyer DE, Gibson TC, King ME, Marshall JE, Weyman AE. Hydrodynamic compression of the right atrium: a new echocardiographic sign of cardiac tamponade. Circulation. 1983;68:294-301.
7. Traylor JJ, Chan K, Wong I, Roxas JN, Chandraratna PA. Large pleural effusions producing signs of cardiac tamponade resolved by thoracentesis. Am J Cardiol. 2002;89:106-8.
8. Reydel B, Spodick DH. Frequency and Significance of Chamber Collapses during Cardiac Tamponade. Am Heart J. 1990;119(5):1160-3.
9. Verhaert D, Gabriel RS, Johnston D, Lytle BW, Desai M, Klein AL. The Role of Multimodality Imaging in the Management of Pericardial Disease. Circ Cardiovasc Imaging. 2010; 3(3):333-43.
10. Meltser H, Kalaria VG. Cardiac Tamponade. Catheter Cardiovasc Interv. 2005;64(2):245-55.

SECTION 2

Respiratory Emergencies

Section Editor: Ajoy Krishna Sarkar

6. **Emergency Airway Management**
   Namrata Biswas

7. **Respiratory Failure**
   Tamoghna Banerjee

8. **Respiratory Emergencies**
   Ajoy Krishna Sarkar, Abhraneel P Guha, Sanjukta Dey, Pratik Biswas

9. **Massive Hemoptysis**
   Rishika Pal, Bhaswati Dasgupta Nath

10. **Acute Pulmonary Embolism**
    Avijit Das

11. **Acute Exacerbation of Asthma**
    Sanjukta Dey

CHAPTER 6

Emergency Airway Management

Namrata Biswas

INTRODUCTION

Airway management is an essential skill and requires a team approach. But in an emergency, an expert airway provider or a supporting team is not available. The unfamiliar complicated instruments or the international algorithms with many intermediate steps and arrows provide confusion and stress to the clinician present. So a practical simple step guideline is required to manage the patient efficiently and safely. A protocol that takes into account that the initial management can be done by an operator with basic skills and rudimentary equipment is more suitable in the initial phase of an emergency.

Success or failure of airway management is often due to complex factors especially in an emergency. The availability of trained personnel, adjunct airway devices, equipment for tracheal intubation, monitoring of lung ventilation, and oxygenation are key factors that prevent brain damage or death. Any flaw in airway management may lead to grave morbidity or mortality.

For treatment of patients in cardiac and respiratory distress, a common acronym *CAB-D* (circulation, airway, breathing, defibrillate) is used to assess the patient.[1]

In a situation where a patient is lying on the ground:
The rescuer needs to ensure the *safety of the scenario* for the resuscitator and the patient. Shift patient to a safe site away from danger before the attempting any resuscitation.[2]

Assess responsiveness: Tap on the shoulders and speak to the person on the ground asking if he/she is ok. Verify the chest and abdomen for movement and respiration. Assess if the person is gasping.

If the person is unresponsive:
- If there is only one rescuer then as a first step, emergency response team to be called and bring an automatic external defibrillator (AED) to the patient.
- If there are two rescuers or more then someone near should call the emergency
- response team and bring the AED.

Find a hard flat surface and place the patient on it in a supine position. Check for a carotid pulse on either one side of the neck with the tip of the fingers for 5–10 seconds (do not test for more than 10 seconds) **(Fig. 1)**.

If carotid artery pulsations are felt, start with airway management:
- Give 10 rescue breaths/minute (one breath every 6 seconds)
- Every 2 minutes you have to recheck for the artery pulsations.

If carotid pulsations are absent then:
Begin cardiopulmonary resuscitation *(CPR) for 5 cycles* (lasts a total of 2 minutes).

Chest compressions should be started immediately **(Figs. 2A and B)**:
- A total of 100–120 compressions/minute have to be given. Count loudly while doing it. Approximately 30 compressions every 15–18 seconds.
- Identify the midline of the person's sternum, and place your palms one over the other between the patient's nipples and on the lower 1/3 of the patient's sternum.

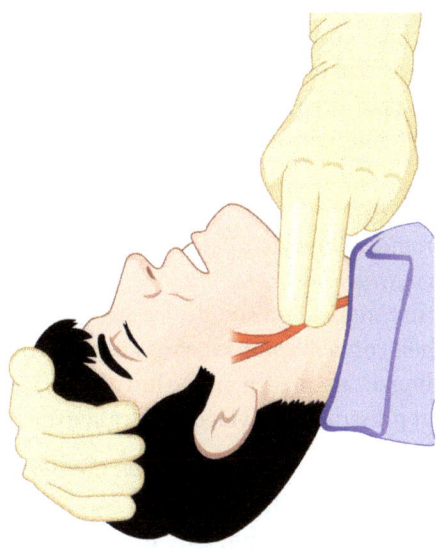

Fig. 1: Palpation of pulsations of carotid artery.

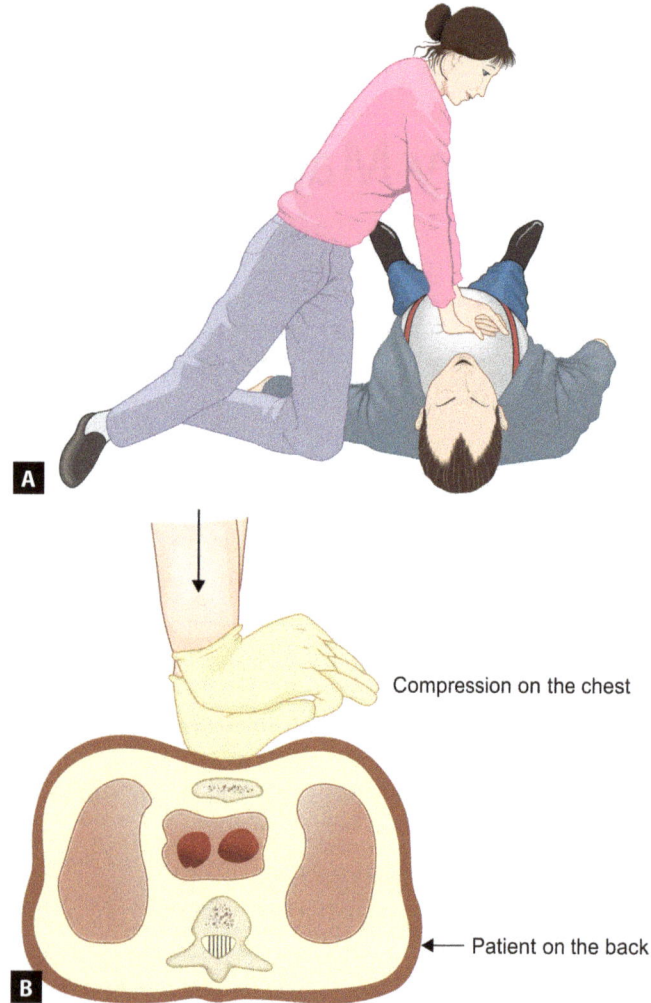

Figs. 2A and B: The proper position for the chest compressions.

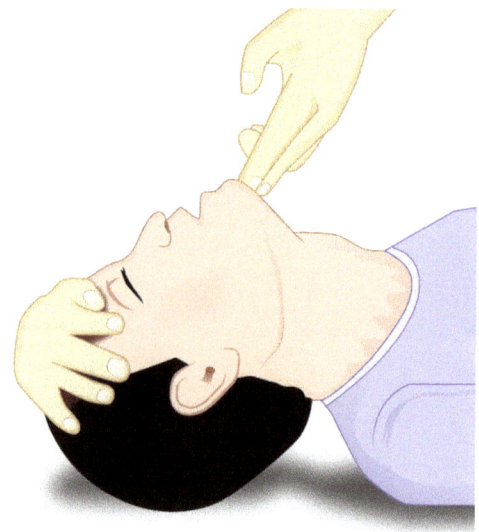

Fig. 3: The head tilt-chin lift maneuver.

- Lock your elbows.
- Give pressure to a depth of 2–2.4 inches (5–6 cm) or more using two arms on the person's chest.
- Compressions should be fast and hard.
- Allow for full recoil of the chest between each compression.

Thirty chest compressions of the chest and then two rescue breaths comprise of one cycle of adult CPR.

If two trained rescuers are present then every five cycles of CPR switch rolls between compressor and rescue breather.

■ AIRWAY

When a provider finds an adult who has collapsed or in an unwitnessed drowning or trauma:
A Jaw-Thrust maneuver should be used to maintain the airway (when cervical spine injury is suspected):
- Three fingers are placed on the lower rami of the jaw.
- Anterior pressure is provided to advance the jaw forward.

When there is a witnessed collapse then there is no reason to assume a cervical spine injury:
The proper Head Tilt-Chin Lift maneuver is shown in **Figure 3**.

Tilt the head backwards by applying pressure with your palm on the patient's forehead and use two fingers of your other hand to pull the chin forward and cephalic.

■ BREATHING

Scan the patient's abdomen and chest for any abnormal jerky breathing or gasping.

If the patient is breathing smoothly, adequately, and regularly then

Continue to assess the patient, put the patient in the recovery position and maintain the patent airway as described above.

The recovery position is used to maintain a patent airway in the unconscious person.
- Place the patient close to a true lateral position with the head dependent to allow fluid to drain.
- Assure the position is stable.
- Avoid pressure on the chest that could impair breathing.
- Position the patient in such a way that it allows turning them onto their back easily.
- Take precautions to stabilize the neck in case of cervical spine injury.

Continue to assess and maintain access of the airway.

Avoid the recovery position if it will sustain injury to the patient.

Recovery Position (Lateral Recumbent or ¾ Prone Position) (Fig. 4)

If the patient is not breathing or gasping or has inadequate breathing:
- Check for carotid pulsations, if present then:
- Start immediately with the rescue breaths. *If you suspect that there is a foreign body obstruction*
- Perform abdominal thrusts.

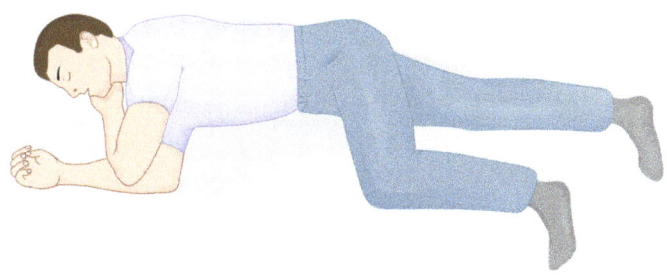

Fig. 4: Maintaining recovery position.

■ MANAGING PATIENTS WHO ARE CHOKING

The patient has both hands wrapped around the base of their throat is the universal sign of choking. With complete airway obstruction, the child is unable to cry, speak, or provide any sounds of respiration. The patient may be weak, confused or cyanotic.

Partial airway obstruction may result in stridor or a high-pitched audible noise during respiration. Partial airway obstruction may allow for a productive cough or allow the patient to speak.
- Do not attempt the Heimlich maneuver.

Complete airway obstruction:
- (One provider) immediately call the emergency response team.
- (One provider) Attempt Heimlich maneuver
- (Two providers) Send someone to call the emergency response team while attempting the Heimlich maneuver.[3]

Heimlich Maneuver (Fig. 5)
- Stand directly behind the child/adult.
- Place both of your arms around the patient's waist.
- Make a fist with one hand and grab the fist with the opposite hand.
- Position the thumb end of the fisted hand immediately above the patient's naval
- (ample distance away from the xiphoid process).
- Perform fast upward and inward diaphragmatic abdominal thrusts.
- Continue abdominal thrusts until the obstruction is removed.

If the patient becomes unconscious:
- Initiate CPR.
- Before attempting rescue breaths during normal CPR, assess the airway, removing any visually present obstruction.
- Do not use a blind finger sweep in an attempt to remove an obstruction.

■ CHOKING: INFANT <1 YEAR OLD
Infant Choking

The initial steps of assessment and response are the same as in adults only the position of the infant is different **(Fig. 6)**.

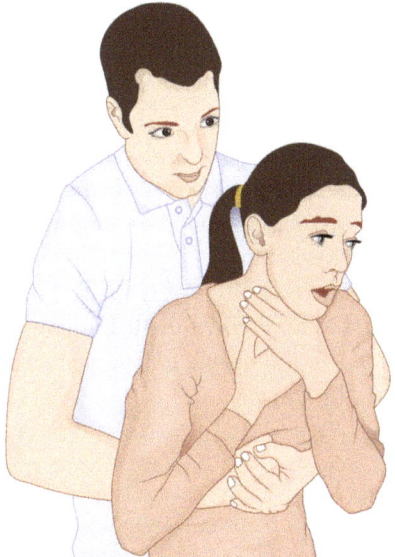

Fig. 5: Heimlich maneuver.

- Lay the infant's face and torso down on the forearm (prone) with the chest being supported by your palm and their head and neck by your fingers.
- Tilt the infant's body at a 30° angle, head downward (Trendelenburg).
- Use your thigh or another object for support.

Interventional Back Blows
Provide five rapid forceful blows using a flat palm on the infant's back between the two scapulae.

Reposition the Patient
Rotate the infant face up (supine), and head downward (Trendelenburg) by switching the infant to the opposite arm.

Interventional Chest Thrusts
- Place your two fingers on the center of the infant's sternum immediately below the nipple line.
- Provide five rapid compressions, with thrusts equaling 1/3 to 1/2 the total depth of the chest.
- Continue cycling back and forth between interventional back blows and chest thrusts until the obstruction is removed or until consciousness is lost.

If the infant becomes unconscious:
- Initiate CPR.
- Before attempting rescue breaths during normal CPR, assess the airway, removing any visually present obstruction.
- Do not use a blind finger sweep in an attempt to remove an obstruction.

■ EMERGENCY AIRWAY MANAGEMENT IN DROWNING

Avoid head down positioning or abdominal thrusts as they delay ventilation and increase vomiting, which increases the risk of aspiration and mortality. Heimlich maneuver is no longer recommended for drowning.[4]

If there is history of unobserved loss of consciousness think C-spine precautions, intoxication, arterial gas embolism (AGE)—if history and circumstances suggest it (e.g., scuba diver surfacing unconscious or with neuro complaint)[4] If AGE is suspected, begin notification of hyperbaric chamber team.

Consider gastric decompression as many drowning patients swallow water before inhaling and between 60–80% will vomit at some point during recovery or resuscitation.

Keep the victim warm.

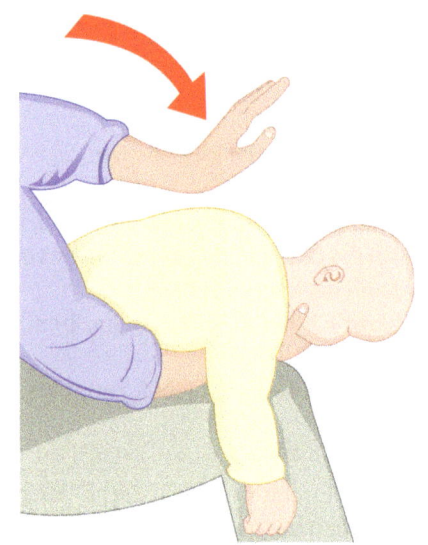

Fig. 6: Infant positioning for removing choking.

EMERGENCY TRAUMA AIRWAY MANAGEMENT

Managing airway in trauma patients is challenging and requires a different protocol. Hemodynamic instability, cervical immobility, direct airway trauma, oropharyngeal bleeding, and risk of aspiration all complicate airway management.[5] Calling for help is the most important first step. Sniffing position of the head in whom it can be undertaken safely (exclude spine injury), bougies and supraglottic airways improve the success rate of quick airway management. Rapid sequence intubation (RSI) is preferred to prevent aspiration.

Rapid sequence intubation involves administering a sedating agent and a neuromuscular block to facilitate endotracheal intubation.

- Preoxygenate the patient—3 minutes with >15l/minute O_2
- Position—ear to sternal notch or rapid airway management position (RAMP) if obese.
- Suction, paralysis and sedation, cricoid pressure, and bougie.
- Monitoring—$ETCO_2$, SpO_2, ECG, NIBP
- The most experienced medical personnel to intubate.
- Maximum two attempts in 2 minutes, reoxygenate if SpO_2 <92% and call for the anesthesiologist **(Flowchart 1)**.

Patients die or suffer brain death from failure to ventilate and oxygenate, rather than failure to intubate. So it is imperative to identify and manage difficult ventilation first to prevent brain damage.

Flowchart 1: Airway management in trauma patient in an emergency.

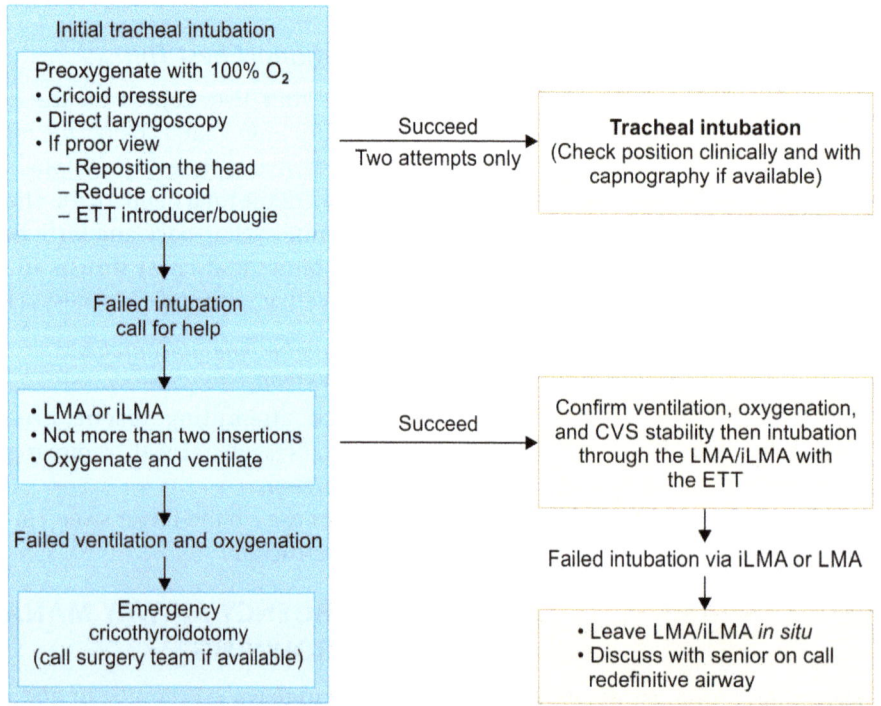

(CVS: cardiovascular system; LMA: laryngeal mask airway).

Techniques for Difficult Ventilation

- Proper positioning and call for help **(Fig. 7)**
- Oral and nasopharyngeal airways
- Laryngeal mask airway
- Esophageal tracheal Combitube
- Intratracheal jet stylet
- Invasive airway access.

Obstruction at different levels in the respiratory tract requires different measures.

Pharynx because of tongue fall back or deceased tone: Two components of the triple airway maneuver, mouth opening, and the jaw thrust are accomplished with the oral airway. The third, head extension, is occasionally necessary to free the base of the tongue from the posterior pharyngeal wall.

Oropharyngeal airway: The airway is placed over the tongue once the mouth is opened. The easiest technique is to insert it after depressing the tongue with a blade. Another method is to insert the tube with the convexity caudad and then rotate it **(Fig. 8)**.

Nasopharyngeal tubes: These are better tolerated by patients who are not in coma and have active gag reflexes **(Fig. 9)**. The tube is advanced until maximal airflow is heard. Insertion of a nasopharyngeal airway is also useful in patients with seizures, trismus, or cervical spine injuries. In addition, a nasogastric tube can be passed through a nasopharyngeal tube to prevent intracranial placement in patients with cribriform plate fractures.[6]

Supraglottic obstruction: The laryngeal mask airway (LMA) is inserted blindly into the oropharynx **(Fig. 10)**. It is easy to insert and very useful in patients with difficult airway to ventilate and prevent aspiration.[7]

Esophageal Tracheal Combitube

This plastic twin-lumen has one lumen resembling an esophageal obturator airway (EOA) and the other an ET tube **(Fig. 11)**. The Combitube has a proximal pharyngeal sealing balloon (100–140 mL air) that functionally replaces the EOA mask. The distal balloon holds 15–20 mL of air. Potential advantages of the pharyngeal cuff (Combitube) over an oral cuff (PTLA) include a fairly consistent inflation volume to achieve a seal and less dental trauma to the cuff.[2]

Glottic or subglottic obstruction: Tracheal tube or cricothyrotomy or tracheostomy **(Fig. 12)**.

■ TECHNIQUES FOR DIFFICULT INTUBATION[8]

- Laryngoscopy with a blade of a different size.
- Awake intubation with video laryngoscope or fiberoptic laryngoscope.
- Using an Intubating stylet or tube changer like a Cook catheter or an angled soft bougie.
- Use appropriately sized LMA which can act as an intubating conduit.
- Use a light wand to guide the tube and the trachea and larynx.

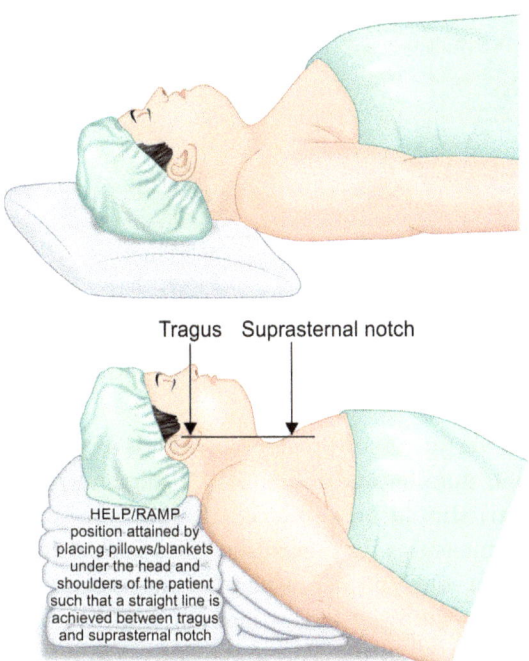

Fig. 7: Rapid airway management position (RAMP).

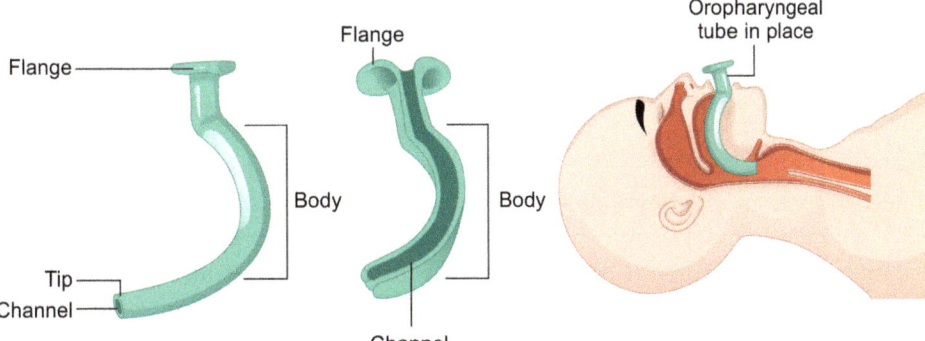

Fig. 8: Oropharyngeal airway.

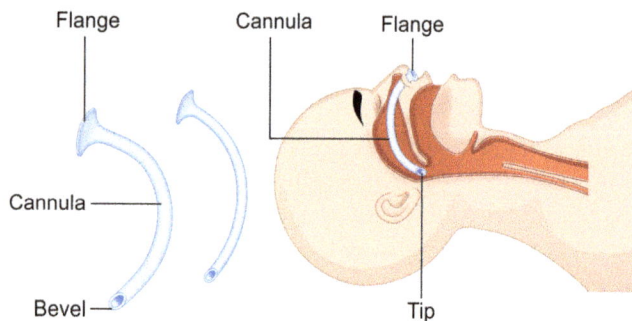

Fig. 9: Nasopharyngeal airway.

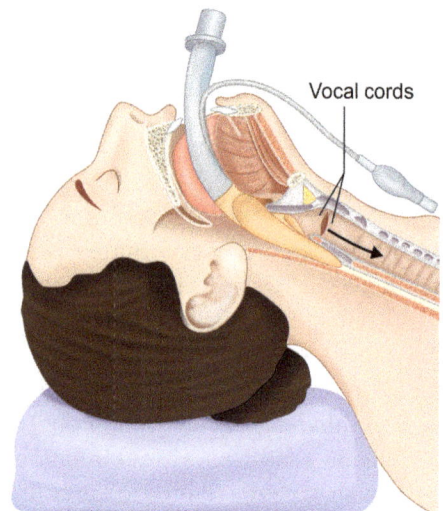

Fig. 10: Placement of laryngeal mask airway.

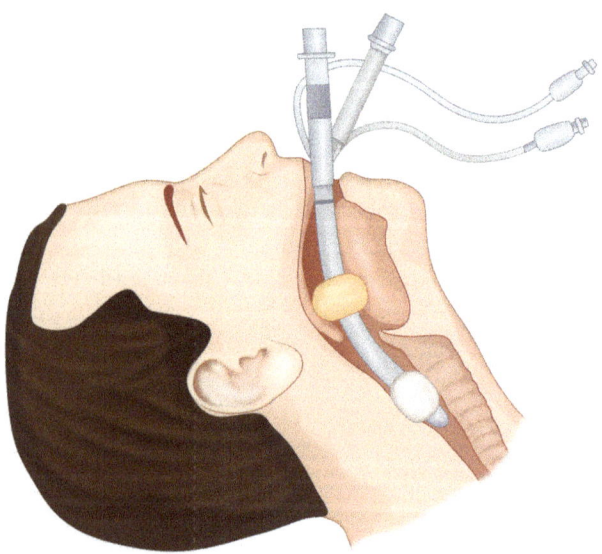

Fig. 11: Combitube placement.

- Retrograde intubation
- Surgical airway access such as cricothyroidotomy or tracheostomy.

A randomized controlled trial comparing *a video laryngoscope combined with a flexible bronchoscope reported a greater first attempt success rate with the combination technique than with a video laryngoscope alone.*[9]

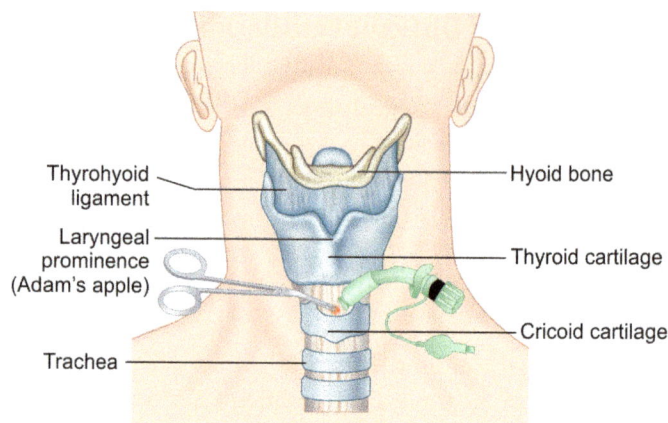

Fig. 12: Cricothyrotomy.

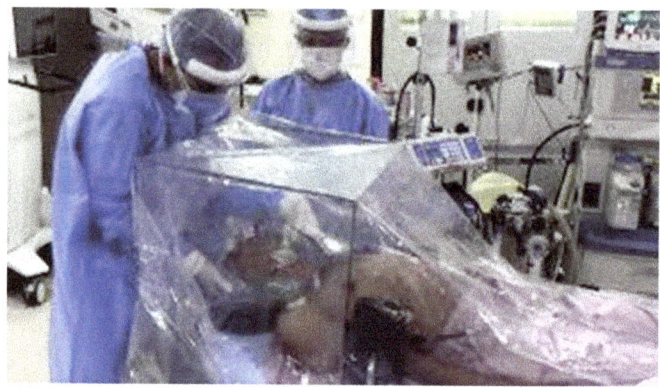

Fig. 13: Protection in COVID times.

SAFETY OF THE EXPERIENCED AIRWAY OPERATOR

While training the rescue providers, methods of proper hand sanitization, donning and doffing of PPE (personal protective equipment) should be emphasized. These are the most important measures for preventing cross-contamination.[10] After the procedure, proper disposal of pieces of equipment and PPE kits, followed by subsequent sterilization plays an important part in preventing the spread of infection.[11] A non-permeable barrier between the patient and the trained rescuer is absolutely necessary for the safety of the person performing the procedure **(Fig. 13 and Flowchart 2)**.

There should be proper and thorough training on the mannequins of all the personnel involved in the management of airway of the patients in a hospital.

Managing both the anticipated and unanticipated difficult airway successfully and safely requires technical expertise. When and how to intervene are equally important decisions for a successful outcome. Airway management in an emergency rarely starts with the placement of an endotracheal tube but begins as soon as patient contact is made. Securing an intravenous access, starting the fluid resuscitation, and giving oxygen are lifesaving. These bridging interventions allow for the safe execution of more

CHAPTER 6: Emergency Airway Management

Flowchart 2: Management of airway during COVID.

Management of unanticipated difficult tracheal intubation in adults during the COVID-19 pandemic

Call For Help

STEP 1: Laryngoscopy and tracheal intubation

Unable to intubate during first attempt at direct/videolaryngoscopy
- Continue nasal oxygen using O_2 flow at 5 L/min
- Maximum two more attempts **preferably with a videolaryngoscope** repeat attempts only if $SpO_2 \geq 95\%$)
- **Gentle mask ventilation between attempts (if $SpO_2 <95\%$) with two-person technique and optimal mask fit***
- Optimise position, use external laryngeal manipulation, release cricoid pressure, use bougie/stylet if required
- Consider changing device/technique/operator between attempts
- Maintain depth of anesthesia and **optimal neuromuscular blockade**

→ **Succeed** → Confirm tracheal intubation using capnography

Failed Intubation ↓ *If necessary, resume gentle mask ventilation** (with optimal mask fit) with 100% O_2)

Step 2: Insert SAD to maintain oxygenation

- Continue nasal oxygen using O_2 flow at 5 L/min
- Use second generation SAD
- Maximum two attempts (only if $SpO_2 \geq 95\%$)
- **Gentle mask ventilation between attempts (if $SpO_2 <95\%$) with two-hand two-person technique and optimal mask fit***
- Consider changing size or type of SAD
- Maintain depth of anesthesia and optimal neuromuscular blockade

→ **Succeed** → Consider one of the following options:
- **Preferably** wake up the patient
- Continue anesthesia using the SAD only if considered safe for the patient, keeping in mind the risk of aerosolisation
- Tracheostomy and tracheal intubation through SAD are not preferred

Failed ventilation through SAD ↓

Step 3: Rescue face mask ventilation

- **Continue nasal oxygen using O_2 flow at 5 L/min**
- Ensure neuromuscular blockade
- Final attempt at gentle mask ventilation* using optimal technique

→ **Succeed** → Wake up the patient

Complete ventilation failure ↓   **Call for additional help**

Step 4: Emergency cricothyroidotomy

- Continue nasal oxygen using O_2 flow at 5L/min and efforts at rescue mask ventilation
- Perform surgical cricothyroidotomy with optimal neuromuscular blockade

Post-procedure plan
- Ensure proper disposal of single use items and disinfection of reusable items as per the institutional policy
- Supervised doffing of PPE with proper disposal, followed by hand hygiene
- Further airway manamement plan
- Treat airway oedema if suspected
- Monitor for complications
- Counselling and documentation
- Debriefing

This flowchart should be used in conjuction with the text
SAD = Supraglottic airway device O_2 = Oxygen
PPE = Personal protective equipment SpO_2 = Pxygen saturation

Bold underlined text represents modifications in AIDAA algorithm.

*A viral filter should be present between the mask and the breathing circuit and the patient's face should be covered with a transparent plastic sheet or a customised intubation box during mask ventilation

Source: Patwa A, Shah A, Garg R, Divatia JV, Kundra P, Doctor JR, et al. All India difficult airway association (AIDAA) consensus guideline for airway management in the operating room during the COVID-19 pandemic. Indian J. Anaesth 2020;S107-15

definitive procedures later on in the management of the patient. Then, securing the airway will have the best chance of making a positive difference in patient outcomes.

CONCLUSION

A successful airway management, specially a difficult one in unknown areas, needs an interprofessional team approach. The charts and the algorithms helps provide a comprehensive pathway for everyone to follow. Simulation labs for training of the personnels will help reduce the mortality and morbidity of the patient. Regular review of recent guidelines, educating and training of the airway management team will go a long way to save lives in the critical moment.

Take Home Messages

- A *call for help* is the first step in any resuscitation procedure.
- The gold standard is to remember that the patient *dies because of failure to ventilate and not because of failure to intubate. So ensure oxygenation and ventilation.*
- When a difficult airway is anticipated it is safer to *perform awake intubation especially when difficult ventilation is also anticipated.*
- There is permanent brain damage after 4 minutes without oxygen and death can occur as soon as 4–6 minutes later, so *be aware of the passage of time.*

REFERENCES

1. Garg R, Ahmed SM, Kapoor MC, Rao SC, Mishra BB, Kalandoor MV, et al. Comprehensive cardiopulmonary life support (CCLS) for cardiopulmonary resuscitation by trained paramedics and medics inside the hospital. Indian J Anaesth. 2017;61(11):883-94.
2. Handley AJ. Basic life support. Br J Anaesth. 1997;79(2):151-8.
3. Netter FH. The Heimlich Maneuver. [produced by Ciba Pharmaceutical Co., Medical Education Division]. Summit, NJ: The Division; 1979.
4. Parenteau M, Stockinger Z, Hughes S, Hickey B, Mucciarone J, Manganello C, et al. Drowning management. Military Med. 2018;183(suppl_2):172-9.
5. Dupanovic M, Fox H, Kovac A. Management of the airway in trauma. Curr Opin Anesthesiol. 2010;23(2):276-82.
6. Atanelov Z, Aina T, Amin B, Rebstock SE. Nasopharyngeal airway. In: StatPearls [Internet]. Treasure Island (FL): StatPearls Publishing; 2022.
7. Garg R, Ahmed SM, Kapoor MC, Mishra BB, Rao SC, Kalandoor MV, et al. Basic cardiopulmonary life support (BCLS) for cardiopulmonary resuscitation by trained paramedics and medics outside the hospital. Indian J Anaesth. 2017;61(11):874-82.
8. Auerbach PS, Cushing TA, Harris NS. Auerbach's Wilderness Medicine. In: Drowning and Submersion Injuries (Chapter 69); 7th edition, 2017. ISBN: 978-0-323-35942-9.
9. Grigonytė M, Kraujelytė A, Januškevičiūtė E, Šėmys G, Bružytė-Narkienė G, Kriukelytė O, et al. Current recommendations for airway management techniques in COVID-19 patients without respiratory failure undergoing general anaesthesia: a nonsystematic literature review. Acta Med Litu. 2021;28(1):19-30.
10. Myatra SN, Shah A, Kundra P, Patwa A, Ramkumar V, Divatia JV, et al. All India Difficult Airway Association 2016 guidelines for the management of unanticipated difficult tracheal intubation in adults. Indian J Anaesth. 2016;60(12):885-98.
11. Quintard H, Higgs A, Lyons G, Pottecher J. Critical airway management in the intensive care unit: homogeneity in practice?. Br J Anaesth. 2019; 122:533-6.

CHAPTER 7

Respiratory Failure

Tamoghna Banerjee

■ DEFINITION

Respiratory failure is primarily a defect in either oxygenation, leading to low oxygen content in blood (or hypoxemia), or ventilation, leading to carbon dioxide trapping (or hypercapnia) and respiratory acidosis. The former one is also known as type one respiratory failure while the latter one is called type two respiratory failure.

■ INTRODUCTION

Respiratory failure is a fairly common medical emergency, the signs of which can be picked up just by staring at the patient. Therefore, it takes little effort to acknowledge that junior and middle grade doctors working in accident and emergency/acute medicine medical on-call must have a thorough foundation on the principles of respiratory failure. To this end, this chapter will take the reader through to defining respiratory failure and understanding the epidemiology of respiratory failure and its importance in the era of emerging respiratory infectious diseases. Also, there will be a discussion on how to anticipate an impending respiratory failure, navigate through the various causes and finally settle on an initial management plan. Moreover, there is a brief discussion on the basics of noninvasive ventilation and the predictors of outcome in respiratory failure.

■ PREVALENCE

A serial cross-sectional study conducted between 2002 and 2017 primarily in the US showed that the incidence of all-cause respiratory failure nearly doubled in this period, while the hospital mortality rate more than halved from 28 to 12%. Institution of assisted ventilation (both invasive and noninvasive) modestly reduced in-hospital mortality ranging between 20 and 40%. The epidemiology of respiratory failure and the statistical analysis of outcomes with assisted ventilation are of utmost importance now, more than ever, thanks to the emergence of respiratory viral infections, notably the novel coronavirus. Studies are underway that are evaluating emerging as well as existing management protocols in respiratory failure and whether they yield similar results with coronavirus disease-2019 (COVID-19) cases.

■ EARLY DIAGNOSIS

The key to the diagnosis of an impending respiratory failure (either type) is a brief history and swift clinical examination which is then followed up with blood gases and other targeted investigations. An individual would usually present with respiratory distress, typically not able to complete sentences when providing a history and that is when you pick up the distress and start working toward management hand in hand with history taking and a physical examination. Almost all medical emergencies begin with securing the airways and circulation. Respiratory distress and impending respiratory failure is not an exception. Poor breathing effort with a low respiratory rate in a patient is a sign of respiratory fatigue and should be considered for assisted ventilation in consultation with a senior colleague. Note that in a case of bronchial asthma with an acute exacerbation, partial pressure of carbon dioxide (pCO_2) level in the normal range is actually a sign of impending respiratory arrest and escalation of management should be immediately discussed with your respiratory team involving senior colleagues. This happens due to fatigue of the muscles of respiration leading to gradual build-up of carbon dioxide which then rises from an initially low level due to hyperventilation to a normal range and further up **(Fig. 1)**.

A careful physical examination can reveal a great deal about a patient. A typical individual presenting with an exacerbation of chronic obstructive airway disease, may appear flushed [facial flushing would be due to secondary polycythemia caused by chronic hypoxia in a case of chronic obstructive pulmonary disease (COPD)] and breathing with lips pursed. A look at the hands might reveal some form of clubbing along with tar staining of fingers (if he is a chronic smoker). Presence of fever or an acute confusional state may hint toward an underlying pneumonia. However, never forget to evaluate other potential causes of confusion, i.e., dyselectrolytemia. A patient with chronic heart failure

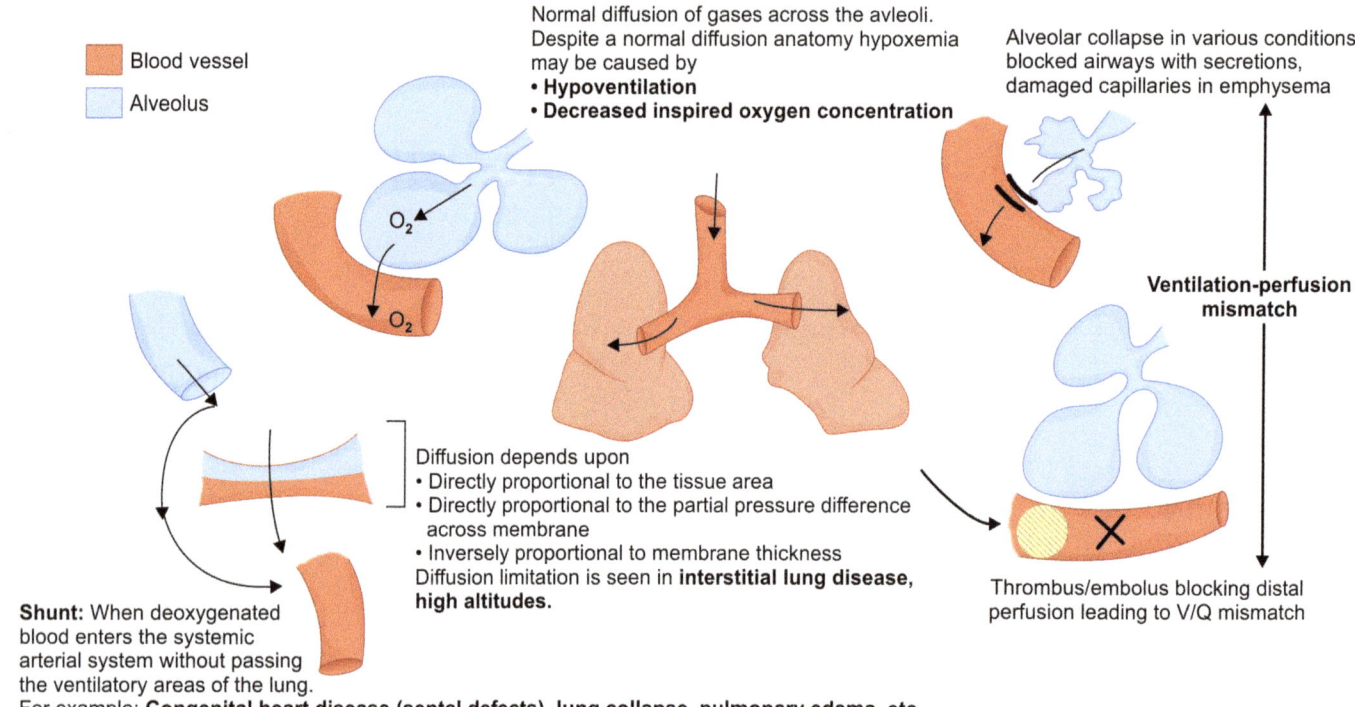

Fig. 1: Schematic diagram showing various causes of hypoxemia.

often present with respiratory distress alongside dependent edema and a jugulovenous distension. Presence of a distended jugular venous pressure (JVP) only means there is an ongoing right heart failure, which could either be due to a coexistent left heart failure or cor pulmonale (right heart failure due to a respiratory cause) or, albeit rarely, otherwise. Chest auscultation can reveal a myriad of sounds, from normal vesicular breath sounds in a case of pulmonary embolism, to a distressing wheezing to even a silent chest in life-threatening asthma. The physical examination must be quick and should go along with data gathering so that the decision making process is undertaken within an appropriate time.

LABORATORY ASSESSMENT: FIRST 48 HOURS THROUGH 96 HOURS (FLOWCHART 1)

The initial clues to the type and severity of respiratory distress/failure come from the blood gases or "arterial blood gas (ABG)". In a case of hypoxemic failure (or type I respiratory failure), the primary aim is correction of this hypoxemia by treating the underlying pathology alongside working on the airway, breathing, and circulations (ABCs). Here the ABG would typically show a low partial pressure of arterial oxygen (pAO_2) in association with low saturation levels. Hypoxemia typically resets the respiratory rate to a higher limit which explains the drop in pCO_2 level in ABG. Thereafter the line of investigation is dictated by the possible list of diagnoses in the given scenario.

A chest X-ray may be done to know any worsening of a previously existing lung infection to exclude a pneumothorax

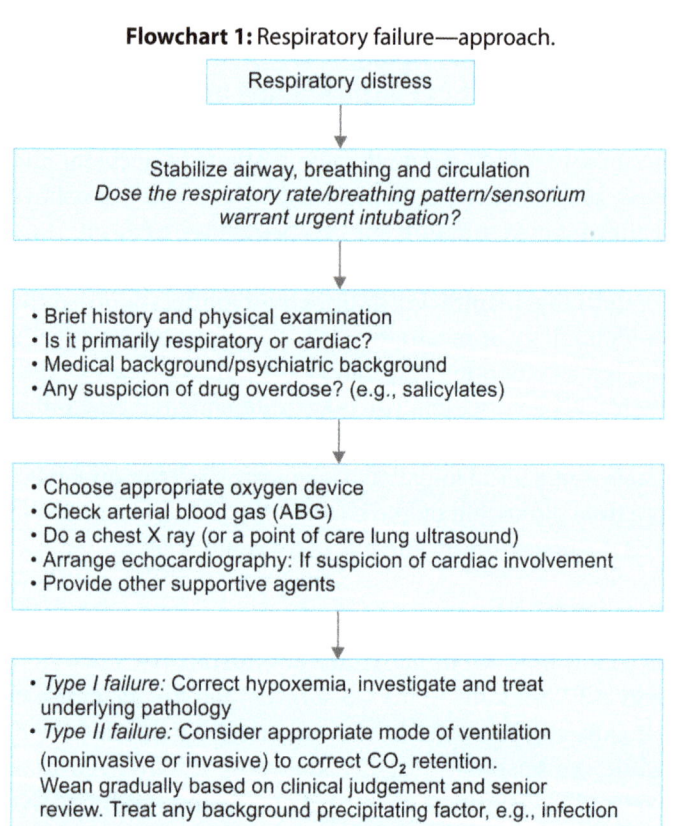

Flowchart 1: Respiratory failure—approach.

or to look for signs of acute respiratory distress syndrome (ARDS) in a patient admitted with any severe systemic illness, e.g., pancreatitis. It should be noted that in the event of a pulmonary embolism leading to respiratory failure the chest X-ray would be unremarkable. In that case, a patient should ideally undergo a two-level Wells' scoring followed by scanning of leg veins and D-dimer testing and consideration of anticoagulation.[1] Although rare, a 12-lead electrocardiogram (ECG) may show the classical S1Q3T3 pattern. It must be borne in mind that a suspected pulmonary embolism in pregnancy shall be investigated with a ventilation-perfusion scan, if required, instead of CT pulmonary angiography.

In an acute exacerbation of COPD, the initial line of investigations remains more or less similar. CO_2 retention would be observed alongside hypoxemia in type II or ventilatory failure. Increased CO_2 concentration in the blood leads to increased H^+ concentration (rate of forward reaction exceeds that of backward reaction due to lowering of gradient between arterial bicarbonate and arterial carbon dioxide) which lowers the pH of the blood.[2]

$$CO_2 + H_2O \longleftrightarrow HCO_3^- + H^+$$

To exclude an acute decompensated heart failure, which presents in the same way as any respiratory decompensation leading to respiratory failure, an N-terminal pro B-type natriuretic peptide (NT-proBNP) level must be sought along with arranging for an echocardiography. In the event the NT-proBNP level is found to be raised, the patient should be screened for any coexistent sepsis, chronic kidney disease, or pulmonary hypertension as in these conditions the biomarker has been observed to be falsely elevated thereby confounding the diagnosis of heart failure.

In case there is a suspicion of drug overdose leading to respiratory failure, urinary and blood samples should be collected at the very first instance and properly stored for toxicology screening. Certain blood parameters may be checked to corroborate the clinical suspicion and have an in-depth review of all the organ systems during the period of ongoing illness. This is a brief summary of how you may navigate through the initial stages of evaluation and management of respiratory failure. Assessment of severity and response to initial management dictates the prognosis as well as predicts in-hospital morbidity.

Once you tide over the acute emergency and the patient has stabilized, further evaluation is based on disease categorization and targeted therapy (if any) followed by institution of measures that prevent or reduce recurrences.

NONINVASIVE VENTILATION IN RESPIRATORY FAILURE

As outlined in the section under prevalence, noninvasive ventilation (NIV) has essentially become one of the central pillars in management of respiratory failure. It is the most preferred method of ventilation when a patient is conscious, and therefore not at risk of aspiration, able to generate his own respiratory rhythm, has an intact airway, and an unaltered facial anatomy. **Table 1** highlights the key situations in which invasive ventilation is preferred over NIV. There are two types of positive pressure ventilation (PPV), continuous positive airway pressure (CPAP), and bi-level positive airway pressure (BiPAP). Unlike CPAP, in BiPAP, the pressure can be customized during inspiration and expiration separately.

Noninvasive ventilation works by reducing the workload of respiratory muscles, generating a positive intrathoracic pressure which leads to decreased left ventricular (LV) afterload (decreased LV afterload potentially augments LV ejection fraction, thereby relieving any features of heart failure and reduces dyspnea). Being a noninvasive process, it has a direct positive impact on nosocomial infections and therefore better mortality data compared to intubation and mechanical ventilation.

In hypoxemic or type I respiratory failure, NIV acts by reducing the respiratory muscle overactivity and consequent fatigue, along with treating hypoxemia. This in turn prevents the vicious circle of refractory hypoxemia leading to hyperventilation, respiratory fatigue, CO_2 retention, and ultimately, respiratory arrest **(Fig. 2)**.

TABLE 1: Situations where noninvasive ventilation (NIV) is contraindicated.

Situation	Explanation
Altered mental status/encephalopathy/hemodynamic instability	Airway protection compromised/risk of aspiration/depressed brainstem response
Acute severe upper gastrointestinal (GI) bleeding	Risk of aspiration and consequent respiratory arrest
Airway secretions	Risk of aspiration, inability to protect airways
Polytrauma/road traffic accident	Facial anatomy altered and hence the interface cannot be fixed properly, inability to protect airways/depressed brainstem response
Upper airway obstruction	Inability to protect airways

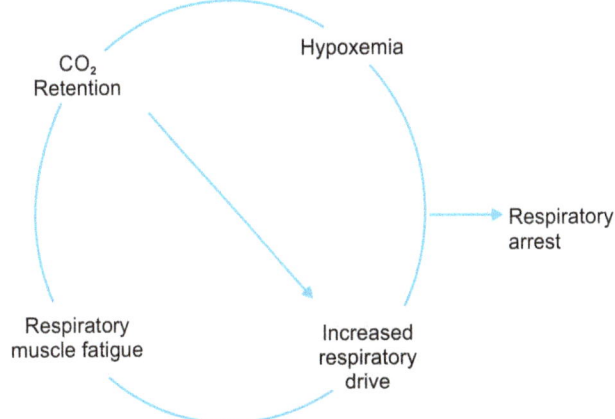

Fig. 2: A schematic diagram that shows how a refractory hypoxemic acute respiratory failure may cause a vicious circle that may ultimately lead to respiratory arrest, if left untreated.

> **BOX 1:** Prerequisites for noninvasive ventilation (NIV), as part of good medical practice.
>
> - *Prerequisites for NIV*
>   - Ensure you have a baseline arterial blood gas (ABG)
>   - Ensure you have evaluated for all reversible causes of respiratory failure (e.g., pneumothorax)
>   - Ensure you have an agreed upon plan in case of NIV failure
>
> *Source:* Adapted from BTS/ICS guidelines.

In hypercapnic or type II respiratory failure, the idea is to deliver a fair amount of tidal volume against the least work of breathing, so as to maintain adequate alveolar ventilation, which is the primary defect in this type of respiratory failure. This in turn reverse hypoxia and related hypercapnia and acidosis. Persistent acidosis with a pH falling between 7.25 and 7.35 in combination with pCO_2 6.5 kPa or higher despite initial medical management warrants institution of NIV.[3] In an adult with an acute exacerbation of COPD, NIV can be safely initiated with an inspiratory positive airway pressure (IPAP) of 15, gradually increased as per response, and an expiratory positive airway pressure (EPAP) ranging between 5 and 8.[4] An even higher degree of acidosis should be considered for invasive mechanical ventilation. Mechanics of invasive ventilation falls beyond the scope of this chapter. **Box 1** summarizes the necessary practice points before initiation of NIV.

> **Take Home Messages**
>
> - Outcome in respiratory failure really depends on the severity at presentation, whether the patient required intensive care on admission and any associated organ-system involvement besides the lungs.

- Studies have consistently shown favorable outcomes[5] in those developing respiratory failure from an acute exacerbation of COPD compared with those due to any other etiology.
- Prognosis and outcome is commonly assessed with scoring systems such as quick sequential organ failure assessment (qSOFA) [in the emergency department (ED), because it is quick and easy, saves time], SOFA (in the intensive care), National Early Warning Score (NEWS), and others.
- Generally speaking, cessation of smoking in individuals with COPD, early diagnosis of an impending respiratory failure, institution of NIV at an appropriate time, shorter intensive care unit (ICU) stay, and lesser number of organ-system involvement are associated with a better prognosis.

REFERENCES

1. National Institute for Health and Care Excellence. Venous thromboembolic diseases: diagnosis, management and thrombophilia testing. London: National Institute for Health and Care Excellence (NICE); 2020.
2. Patel S, Sharma S. Respiratory Acidosis. Treasure Island (FL): StatPearls Publishing; 2022.
3. National Institute for Health and Care Excellence. Chronic obstructive pulmonary disease in adults. London: National Institute for Health and Care Excellence (NICE); 2011.
4. Davidson AC, Banham S, Elliott M, Kennedy D, Gelder C, Glossop A, et al. BTS/ICS guideline for the ventilatory management of acute hypercapnic respiratory failure in adults. Thorax. 2016;71 Suppl 2:ii1-35.
5. Gillespie DJ, Marsh HM, Divertie MB, Meadows JA 3rd. Clinical outcome of respiratory failure in patients requiring prolonged (greater than 24 hours) mechanical ventilation. Chest. 1986;90(3):364-9.

CHAPTER 8

Respiratory Emergencies

Ajoy Krishna Sarkar, Abhraneel P Guha, Sanjukta Dey, Pratik Biswas

■ INTRODUCTION

Respiratory emergencies are quite common in emergency room (ER). The early identification and management of these patients are critical, as early identification affects morbidity and mortality. Facilities that are not capable of dealing with advanced respiratory care should be able to refer to the higher health facility. Pulmonary symptoms and signs usually occur when lung is unable to meet the metabolic demand of the body leading to inadequate tissue oxygenation and carbon dioxide homeostasis. In this chapter we will be discussing common respiratory emergencies in brief.

■ ACUTE EXACERBATION OF CHRONIC OBSTRUCTIVE PULMONARY DISEASE[1]

An exacerbation of chronic obstructive pulmonary disease (COPD) is defined as an acute worsening of respiratory symptoms that result in additional therapy. As exacerbations of COPD leads to disease progression and most of the time readmission, they negatively impact health status of COPD patients.

It comprises of complex events where there is marked airway inflammation, profuse mucus production, and increase in gas trapping. All of these lead to increase in dyspnea which is the main symptom of an exacerbation. Increase in cough, wheeze, increase in volume of sputum or purulence of sputum are other symptoms seen in exacerbation of COPD.

While dealing with patient of exacerbation of COPD, other clinical conditions which worsens respiratory symptoms in COPD such as pneumonia, pneumothorax, pleural effusion, pulmonary embolism (PE), pulmonary edema, and arrhythmia should be considered before diagnosis of a COPD exacerbation is made.

Exacerbations are classified as:
- Mild (treated with short-acting bronchodilators only, SABDs)
- Moderate (treated with SABDs plus antibiotics and/or oral corticosteroids)
- Severe (patient requires hospitalization or visits the ER). Severe exacerbations may also be associated with acute respiratory failure.

Indication of Hospitalization
- Symptoms such as increased breathlessness, tachypnea, drop in oxygen saturation (SpO_2), if the patient gets drowsy or confused.
- Occurrence of new signs such as edema, cyanosis, etc.
- Failure to respond to initial management
- Coexisting comorbidities such as congestive heart failure, etc.
- Lack of support at home.

Management of Exacerbations
- History taking and physical examination to assess severity, arterial blood gas analysis and chest X-ray
- Administer oxygen (*no over oxygenation*, target SpO_2 being 88–92%)
- Short-acting inhaled beta-2-agonists (SABA), with or without short-acting anticholinergics (SAMAs), are recommended bronchodilators to treat exacerbation of COPD (either increase dose and/or frequency or both). The patients should be put on long-acting bronchodilators when they become stable. (To use spacers or air-driven nebulizers as appropriate depending on the patient.)
- Systemic corticosteroids (oral route preferred) improves forced expiratory volume in 1 second (FEV1-lung function), oxygenation, and shorten recovery time and hospital duration. Recommended duration is of about 5–7 days.
- Since methylxanthines have increased side effects profile, they are not recommended.
- Noninvasive mechanical ventilator (NIV) should be first mode of ventilation used in COPD patients with acute respiratory failure who have no absolute contraindication because it improves gas exchange, reduced work of breathing and the need for intubation, decreases hospitalization duration, and improved survival.

- To monitor fluid balance.
- Thromboembolism prophylaxis is an important consideration—either with subcutaneous heparin or low molecular weight heparin.
- Coexisting conditions should be addressed like congestive heart failure, arrhythmias, pulmonary embolism, etc.

Indications for Noninvasive Mechanical Ventilation

- Respiratory acidosis ($PaCO_2$ >45 mm Hg and arterial pH ≤7.35)
- Severe breathlessness with clinical signs of respiratory muscle fatigue, increased work of breathing (e.g., accessory muscles working, paradoxical movement of the abdomen, or retraction of intercostal spaces), or both
- Persistent desaturation despite oxygen therapy.

Indications of Invasive Mechanical Ventilation

- Noninvasive ventilation failure
- Life-threatening hypoxemia in patients unable to tolerate NIV
- Patients who have decrease in level of consciousness or psychomotor agitation which are inadequately controlled by sedation
- In order to protect airway such as in massive aspiration or persistent vomiting or not able to remove excessive respiratory secretions
- Severe hemodynamic instability without response to fluids and vasoactive drugs
- Severe life-threatening arrhythmias
- Postcardiac arrest or postrespiratory arrest.

ACUTE EXACERBATION OF ASTHMA[2]

Exacerbations of asthma are episodes in which there is progressive increase in symptoms of dyspnea, wheezing, cough or chest tightness, and also associated with progressive decrease in lung function, which ultimately requires a change in treatment. They may have been previously diagnosed with asthma or may even present for the first time.

There are certain triggers which can lead to exacerbation: allergen exposure like pollen grains, respiratory viral infections, seasonal changes, food allergy, outdoor pollution, poor adherence to inhaled steroid for asthma, etc.

Certain conditions which increase risk of asthma-related death are:
- History of near-fatal asthma which eventually required intubation and mechanical ventilation
- Emergency care visit for asthma or hospitalization in the past year
- Recently stopped or currently using oral corticosteroids (a marker of event severity)
- Not currently using inhaled corticosteroids (ICS) or poor adherence
- Overuse of SABAs
- History of psychosocial problems or psychiatric disease
- Food allergy in patient with asthma
- Other comorbidities such as diabetes and arrhythmia

Management Guidelines

In the acute setting, measurement like peak expiratory flow (PEF) or FEV1 which shows decline as compared to previous values of the patient or the predicted values are more reliable indicators of the severity of the exacerbation than symptoms. The more sensitive marker for onset of exacerbation is frequency of symptoms than PEF **(Table 1)**.

- Increase frequency of ICS-formoterol/SABA as reliever [either pressurized metered dose inhaler (pMDI) with spacer or nebulizer]. For mild-to-moderate exacerbations, repeated administration of inhaled SABA

TABLE 1: Severity assessment.

At primary care	Patient presents with acute or subacute asthma exacerbation
Assess the patient	• Is it asthma? • Factors for asthma-related death? • Severity of exacerbation? (Consider worst feature)

Mild or moderate	Severe	Life-threatening
Talks in phrases, prefers sitting to lying, not agitated	Talks in words, sits hunched forward, agitated	Drowsy and confused
Respiratory rate 20–30 breaths per minute	Respiratory rate >30 breaths per minute	Silent chest
Accessory muscles not used	Accessory muscles in use	
Pulse rate 100–120 beats per minute	Pulse rate >120 beats per minute	
SpO_2 room air 90–95%	SpO_2 room air <90%	
PEF >50% predicted or best	PEF ≤50% predicted or best	
Start treatment • SABA 4–10 puffs by pMDI + Spacer, repeat every 20 minutes for 1 hour • *Prednisolone:* Adults 40–50 mg • *Controlled oxygen:* Target SpO_2 93–95%	• Transfer to acute care facility • *While waiting:* Give SABA, ipratropium bromide, O_2, systemic corticosteroid	

(PEF: peak expiratory flow; pMDI: pressurized metered dose inhaler; SABA: short-acting inhaled beta-2-agonist; SpO_2: oxygen saturation)

like salbutamol (4–10 puffs every 20 minutes for the first hour). After the first hour, the dose of SABA varies from 4–10 puffs every 3–4 hours to 6–10 puffs every 1–2 hours or more often. If there is a good response to initial treatment, no additional SABA is needed. (PEF > 60–80% of predicted or personal best for 3–4 hours)
- Quadruple ICS dose during exacerbation which the patient was on. Based on product information, the maximum recommended dose of ICS-formoterol in a single day is a total of 48 μg formoterol for beclomethasone-formoterol and 72 μg formoterol for budesonide-formoterol.
- Treatment with ipratropium bromide in addition to SABA was associated with fewer hospitalization for adults and children with moderate-severe exacerbation.
- Add oral corticosteroids for severe exacerbations (PEF or FEV1 <60% personal best or predicted) or patient not responding to treatment over 48 hours or exacerbation developed while patient was taking oral corticosteroid or the patient has a history of previous exacerbations requiring oral corticosteroids. Once started, morning dosing is preferable. For adults, prednisolone 40–50 mg/day usually for 5–7 days is needed. Tapering is not required if oral corticosteroids are prescribed for <2 weeks.
- Controlled oxygen-target SpO_2 93–95% (no excess oxygen for the fear of development of hypercapnia).
- Routine antibiotics not recommended unless there is strong evidence of infection.
- Intramuscular (IM) epinephrine is indicated in addition to standard therapy for acute asthma associated with anaphylaxis and angioedema.
- Aminophylline and theophylline should not be used in view of poor efficacy and safety profile.
- Sedatives must be avoided.
- Limited role of leukotriene receptor antagonists in exacerbation.
- Evidence of NIV in asthma is weak. If required, patient should be intubated and ventilated.

PNEUMOTHORAX[3]

- The term "pneumothorax" refers to presence of air in the pleural cavity.
- **Secondary spontaneous pneumothorax (SSP)** is the pneumothorax with diseased underlying lung and **Primary Spontaneous Pneumothorax (PSP)** is without underlying diseased lung. SSP has higher morbidity and mortality compared to PSP.
- It is important to stop smoking in order to prevent recurrence of pneumothorax.
- Symptom like breathlessness is more in SSP, even with small pneumothorax radiologically. **Breathlessness is the most important criteria to decide treatment modality than size**. Severe sign and symptoms may be indicative of tension pneumothorax.
- Rather than expiratory films, erect chest X-ray in inspiration is recommended for diagnosis.
- CT scanning is the investigation recommended for uncertain or complex cases. CT scanning also helps in accurate calculation of the size of the pneumothorax.
- In order to define the size of pneumothorax, the interpleural distance is measured at the level of hilum. **A cut off of 2 cm is used to differentiate large from small pneumothorax.** The size of the pneumothorax determines the rate of resolution and is a relative indication for active intervention.
  - Supportive treatment in the form of oxygen supplementation is also given.
  - Chest drains are given to the patient who fails initial management as mentioned in the **Flowchart 1** or tension or bilateral pneumothorax.
  - Unless there were technical difficulties while performing needle aspiration, it should not be repeated.
  - For pneumothorax, small-bore (<14 F) chest drain insertion is recommended rather than large bore.
  - **Most patients of SSP will require the insertion of a small-bore chest drain.** All patients especially SSP will require early referral to a chest physician.
  - Those who have a persistent air leak should be referred to a thoracic surgeon at 48 hours.

Flowchart 1 shows approach to pneumothorax.

PLEURAL EFFUSION[4]

Pleural effusion is defined as presence of fluid in the pleural cavity. The possibility of pleural effusion should always be kept in mind whenever an abnormal chest X-ray is seen. Increased densities, especially at the lower zone on the chest X-ray, are frequently attributed to parenchymal infiltrates, but is actually pleural fluid. If this costophrenic angle is blunted, the patient should be ideally be evaluated with ultrasound to see whether free pleural fluid is present or not. **Flowchart 2** provides a guide to the approach to a patient with an undiagnosed pleural effusion. In presence of confirmed pleural effusion, the aspirant should be subjected to cytology, biochemical analysis and culture sensitivity. This gives a clue to clinch the diagnosis **(Flowcharts 3 and 4)**.

PNEUMONIA[5]

It is defined as lung inflammation caused by bacterial or viral infection and is diagnosed by presence of infiltrate in lung parenchyma on chest X-ray. Once the diagnosis of pneumonia is made clinicoradiologically, the most important decision for managing pneumonia is the decision regarding site of care, as pneumonia can present in a very mild to life-threatening form with significant mortality.

Flowchart 1: Approach to pneumothorax.

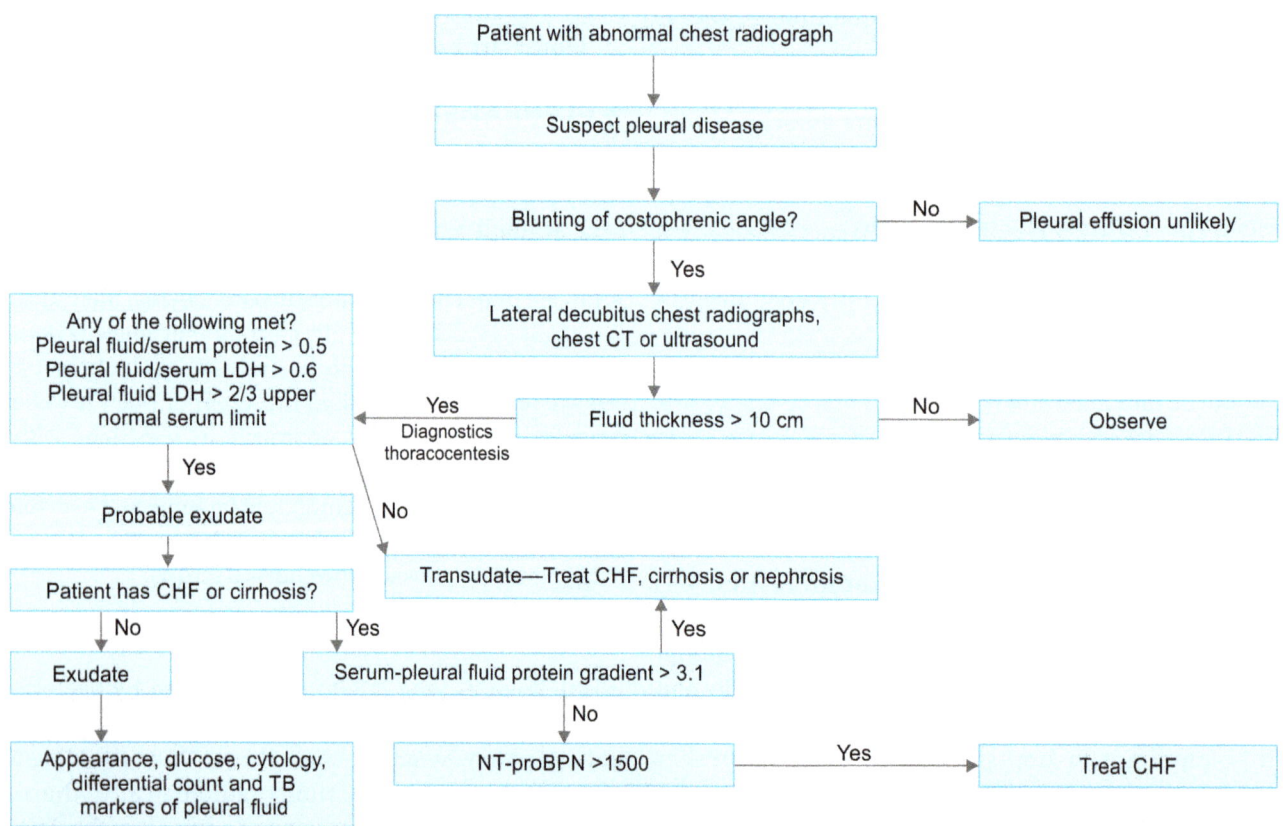

(CXR: chest X-ray; OPD: outpatient department)

Flowchart 2: Approach to undiagnosed pleural effusion.

(CHF: congestive heart failure; LDH: lactate dehydrogenase; NT-proBNP: N-terminal pro-B-type natriuretic peptide; TB: tuberculosis)

Flowchart 3: Appearance of the aspirant and its analysis (biochemical, cytological, and culture) clinches the diagnosis and guide the management.

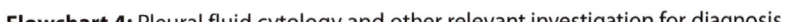

Flowchart 4: Pleural fluid cytology and other relevant investigation for diagnosis.

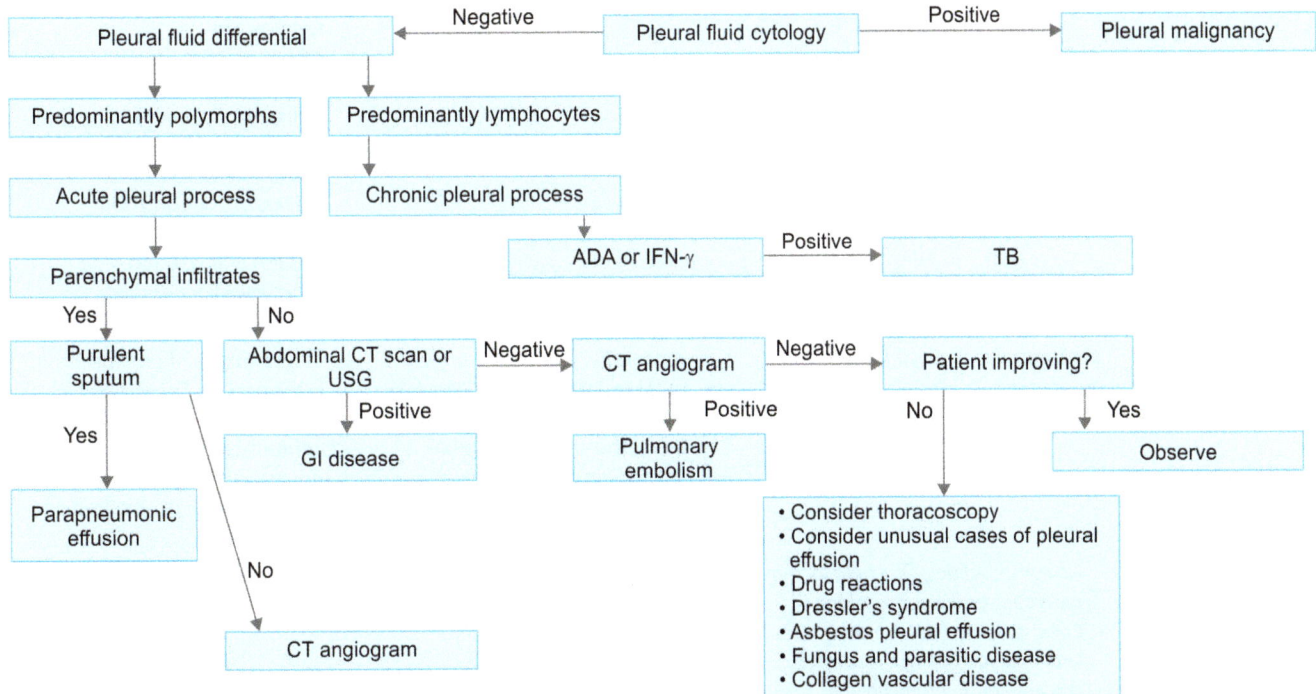

(ADA: adenosine deaminase; CT: computed tomography; GI: gastrointestinal; IFN-γ: interferon-γ; TB: tuberculosis USG: ultrasonography)

- CURB 65 is the most common and simpler to remember and easy to apply in day to day practice. CURB65 uses variables:
  - Confusion
  - Urea >20 mg/dL
  - Respiratory rate >30 breaths/minute
  - Blood pressure (systolic blood pressure <90 mm Hg or diastolic blood pressure <60 mm Hg)
  - Age >65 years

  Each of the variable is allotted one point to get the score. For score 0–1 it is recommended to manage patient as outpatient, for score of 2 to manage as inpatient, and 3 or more in intensive care unit (ICU).
- The next step is the decision regarding initiation of appropriate empirical antibiotic as soon as the diagnosis is made.
- Early initiation leads to decrease in mortality, complications, and also decreases the duration of illness. Studies have shown that clinical and radiological picture may be suggestive of the pathogen but is not a good predictor.
- The most appropriate empirical antibiotics for the patients being managed in outpatient department (OPD) basis might be a beta-lactam plus macrolide in the outpatient setting and an intravenous (IV) beta-lactam plus a respiratory fluoroquinolone in the indoor setting **(Table 2)**.
- All the indoor and ICU patients should be monitored for their vitals regularly (pulse, blood pressure, respiratory rate, temperature, oxygen saturation SpO_2, and mental status).
- Supportive management includes oxygen to maintain a $pO_2 > 60$ mm Hg or SpO_2 above 94%, IV fluid, deep venous thrombosis (DVT) prophylaxis if bedridden, nutritional support, and ventilatory support.
- NIV or continuous positive airway pressure (CPAP) should only be tried in ICU setting with facilities for intubation and invasive ventilation.

TABLE 2: Antibiotic regimens.

	Outpatient	Inpatient (non-ICU)	Inpatient (ICU)
IDSA/ATS consensus guidelines (2007)	• Healthy with no use of antimicrobials in the previous 3 months: *Macrolides or doxycycline* • Comorbidities including chronic heart, lung, liver or renal disease; diabetes; alcoholism; malignancy; immunosuppressed state; use of antimicrobials in the previous 3 or in areas with high rate of infection with high level macrolide-resistant *Streptococcus pneumoniae*: *A respiratory fluoroquinolone* or *A beta lactam plus a macrolide*	*A respiratory fluoroquinolone* or *A beta lactam plus a macrolide*	• *A beta lactam* (cefotaxime, ceftriaxone or ampicillin sulbactam) *plus azithromycin/ a respiratory fluoroquinolone* • If pseudomonas is suspected: *An antipneumococcal, antipseudomonal beta lactam* (piperacillin-tazobactam, cefepime, meropenem or imipenem) *plus ciprofloxacin or levofloxacin* or *Above beta lactam plus aminoglycoside and azithromycin* or *Above beta lactam plus aminoglycoside and anti-pneumococcal fluoroquinolones* • If MRSA is suspected: Add *vancomycin or linezolid*
BTS guidelines (October 2009)	*Amoxicillin 500–1000 mg thrice a day or clarithromycin/erythromycin or doxycycline*	• If oral therapy possible: *Amoxicillin plus clarithromycin or Doxycycline or Levofloxacin or Moxifloxacin* • If oral therapy not possible: *IV amoxicillin or benzylpenicillin plus clarithromycin or IV levofloxacin*	*Co-amoxiclav plus clarithromycin* (*plus levofloxacin* if *Legionella* is suspected) or *Cefuroxime/cefotaxime/ceftriaxone plus clarithromycin* (*plus levofloxacin* if *Legionella* is suspected) or *Benzylpenicillin plus levofloxacin/ciprofloxacin*
PGIMER, Chandigarh guidelines (2006)	• *No comorbidities:* Oral beta lactam or macrolide or fluoroquinolone • *Coexisting medical comorbidities:* Oral beta lactam plus macrolide/doxycycline/fluoroquinolone	*Oral/IV beta lactam plus macrolide/respiratory fluoroquinolone*	*IV beta lactam plus macrolide/respiratory fluoroquinolone*

(ATS: American Thoracic Society; BTS: British Thoracic Society; ICU: intensive care unit; IDSA: Infectious Diseases Society of America; IV: intravenous; MRSA: Methicillin-resistant *Staphylococcus aureus*; PGIMER: Postgraduate Institute of Medical Education and Research)

- Hospitalized patients generally require antibiotics for 7–10 days, but may be prolonged for 14–21 days depending on response.
- Radiologically, response lags behind clinical response and need not be repeated if the patient shows adequate response clinically. It needs to be repeated only if the patient deteriorates, inadequate response, or is a case of nonresolving pneumonia.
- There are certain factors which help in predicting the etiology and hence in deciding treatment options:
  - Comorbidities such as COPD, asthma, and diabetes
  - Alcoholic/smoker
  - Structural lung disease
  - Severity of illness
  - In the background of human immunodeficiency virus (HIV) infection
  - IV drug abuser
  - During an epidemic or pandemic like influenza or coronavirus disease-2019 (COVID-19)
  - Travel history
  - Background situation when the pneumonia occurs, like after a binge of alcohol (also other conditions predisposing to aspiration)
  - Resident in nursing home
  - Local prevalent resistance pattern
  - Chronic or recurrent antibiotic abuse
- *Streptococcus pneumoniae* is the most common organism in all settings and drug-resistant *Streptococcus pneumoniae* are being identified with increasing frequency.

PULMONARY EMBOLISM[6]

Pulmonary embolism occurs due to disruption of flow of blood in pulmonary artery or its branches caused by a thrombus originating from somewhere else. Spectrum of Pulmonary embolism and DVT together is known as venous thromboembolism which is third most common acute cardiovascular event after acute myocardial infarction and stroke. Pulmonary embolism although is a common clinical condition has a varied presentation, thus require multidisciplinary approach in order to make diagnosis in time to improve outcome. **Flowcharts 5 to 7** illustrate the brief approach to pulmonary embolism.

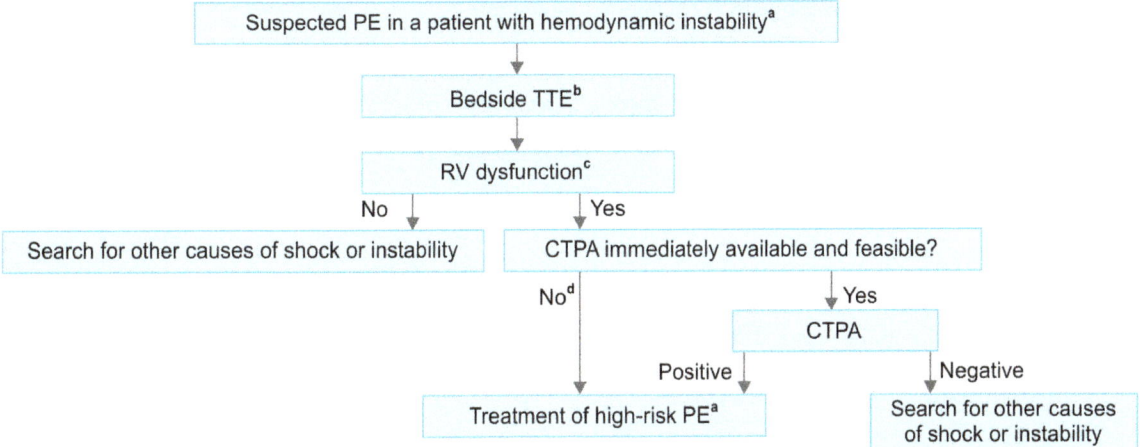

Flowchart 5: Approach to pulmonary embolism in patients with hemodynamic instability.

[a]Definition of hemodynamic instability, which delineates acute high-risk pulmonary embolism (one of the following clinical manifestations at presentation)

Cardiac arrest	Obstructive shock	Persistent hypotension
Need for CPR	Systolic BP < 90 mm Hg or vassopressors required to achieve a BP ≥ 90 mm Hg despite adequate filling status And End-organ hypoperfusion (altered mental status; cold, clammy skin; oliguria/anuria increased serum lactate)	Systolic BP < 90 mm Hg or systolic BP drop ≥ 40 mm Hg, lasting longer than 15 minutes and not caused by new onset arrhythmia, hypovolemia, or sepsis

[b]Ancillary bedside imaging tests may include TOE, which may detect emboli in the pulmonary artery and its main branches; and bilateral venous CUS, which may confirm DVT and thus VTE.
[c]In the emergency situation of suspected high-risk PE, this refers mainly to a RV/LV diameter ratio >1.0
[d]Includes the cases in which the patient's condition is so critical that it only allows bedside diagnostic tests. In such cases, echocardiographic findings of RV dysfunction confirm high-risk PE and emergency reperfusion therapy is recommended

(BP: blood pressure; CPR: cardiopulmonary resuscitation; CTPA: computed tomography pulmonary angiogram; CUS: compression ultrasonography; DVT: deep venous thrombosis; LV: left ventricular; PE: pulmonary embolism; RV: right ventricular; TOE: transesophageal echocardiogram; TTE: transesophageal echocardiography; VTE: venous thromboembolism)

Flowchart 6: Approach to pulmonary embolism in hemodynamically stable patient.

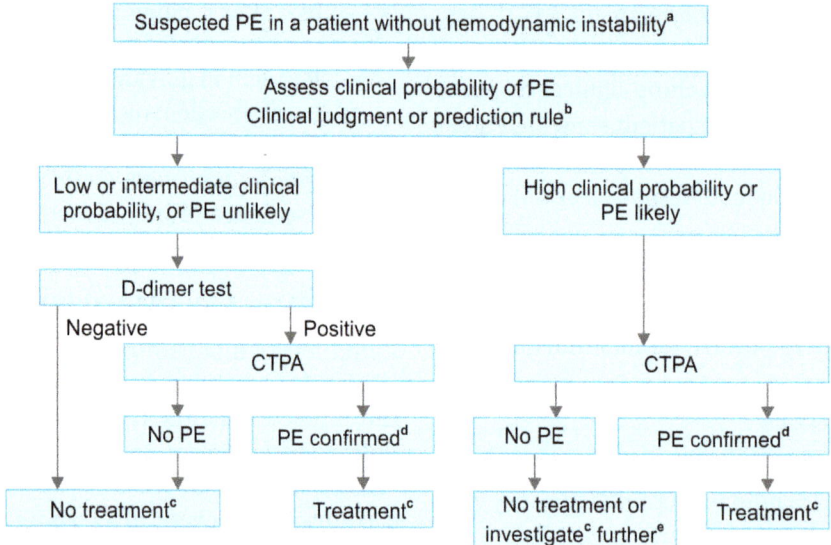

[a] Definition of hemodynamic instability mentioned in previous chart
[b] When using a moderately sensitive assay, D-dimer measurement should be restricted to patients with low clinical probability or a PE-unlikely classification, while highly sensitive assays may also be used in patients with intermediate clinical probability of PE due to a higher sensitivity and negative predictive value. Note that plasma D-dimer measurement is of limited use in suspected PE occurring in hospitalized patients.
[c] Treatment refers to anticoagulation treatment for PE.
[d] CTPA is considered diagnostic of PE if it shows PE at the segmental or more proximal level.
[e] In case of a negative CTPA in patients with high clinical probability, investigation by further imaging tests may be considered before withholding PE-specific treatment.
(CTPA: computed tomography pulmonary angiogram; PE: pulmonary embolism)

Flowchart 7: Management protocol of pulmonary embolism.

(CTPA: computed tomography pulmonary angiogram; PE: pulmonary embolism; RV: right ventricular; TTE: transthoracic echocardiography)

▪ THROMBOLYTIC REGIMENS

See **Table 3**.

TABLE 3: Thrombolytic regimens.

Molecule	Regimen	Contraindications to fibrinolysis
rtPA	100 mg over 2 hours 0.6 mg/kg over 15 minutes (maximum dose 50 mg)	*Absolute* • History of hemorrhagic stroke or stroke of unknown origin • Ischemic stroke in previous 6 months • Central nervous system neoplasm • Major trauma, surgery or head injury in previous 3 weeks • Bleeding diathesis • Active bleeding
Streptokinase	250000 IU as a loading dose over 30 minutes, followed by IU/h over 12–24 h *Accelerated regimen:* 1.5 million over 2 h	
Urokinase	4400 IU/kg as a loading dose over 10 minutes, followed by 4400 IU/kg over 12-24 h Accelerated regimen: 3 million IU over 2 h	*Relative* • Transient ischemic attack in previous 6 months • Oral anticoagulation • Pregnancy or first postpartum week • Noncompressible puncture sites • Traumatic resuscitation • Refractory hypertension (systolic BP >180 mm Hg) • Advanced liver disease • Infective endocarditis • Active peptic ulcer

(BP: blood pressure; rtPA: recombinant tissue plasminogen activator)

TABLE 4: Low-molecular-weight heparin and Fondaparinux (subcutaneous).

	Dosage	Interval
Enoxaparin	1.0 mg/kg	Every 12 hours
Dalteparin	• 100 IU/kg • 200 IU/kg	• Every 12 hours • Once daily
Fondaparinux	• 5 mg (body weight < 50 kg) • 7.5 mg (body weight 50–100 kg) • 10 mg (body weight >100 kg)	Once daily

LOW-MOLECULAR WEIGHT HEPARIN AND FONDAPARINUX (SUBCUTANEOUS)

See **Table 4**.

CONCLUSION

Dyspnea can be caused by different conditions and the cause can be sometimes difficult to determine. The origin of respiratory disease could be either in airways, lung parenchyma, pleural space or even in thoracic vasculature. Proper history taking and clinical examination forms the cornerstone of management, because stabilising the patient in the ER is the priority rather than finding the actual cause then and there. Then based on the clinical findings, relevant investigations especially imaging, are carried out to confirm the diagnosis. A few of the common emergencies in respiratory medicine have been covered above and their management has been described as per the latest guidelines.

Take Home Messages

- SABA with or without SAMA, systemic corticosteroid, oxygen, and NIV are used to treat acute exacerbation of COPD.
- Compared to exacerbation of COPD where NIV trial is indicated, evidence of NIV is weak in severe or life-threatening asthma where the patient needs to be intubated.
- Breathlessness forms the most important criteria to decide about the treatment rather than the size of pneumothorax.
- Bilateral pneumothorax, hemodynamically unstable, SSP >2cm or breathlessness requires chest drainage.
- Basic biochemical analysis of pleural fluid helps in classifying pleural fluid into exudate or transudate (as per Light's criteria).
- Bed sound ultrasonography is more sensitive than X-ray for evaluation of pleural effusion.
- CURB 65 scoring is commonly used to decide the site of care in pneumonia.
- Early initiation, appropriate antibiotic in appropriate dosage and for appropriate duration affects the outcome in case of pneumonia.
- Possibility of PE is suspected in patients presenting with breathlessness, chest pain, syncope or even hemoptysis in appropriate background.
- D-DIMER followed by CTPA to be done for evaluation of PE.

REFERENCES

1. Global Initiative for Chronic Obstructive Lung Disease. Gold 2022. https://goldcopd.org/
2. Global Initiative for Asthma. GINA 2022. https://goldcopd.org/
3. MacDuff A, Arnold A, Harvey J; BTS Pleural Disease Guideline Group. Management of spontaneous pneumothorax: British Thoracic Society pleural disease guideline 2010. Thorax. 2010; 65 Suppl 2:ii18-31.
4. Light RW. Pleural Disease, 6th edition. Philadelphia: Lippincott Williams & Wilkins; 2013.
5. Guleria R, Kumar J. Management of community acquired pneumonia. J Assoc Physicians India. 2012;60 (Suppl):21-4.
6. Konstantinides SV, Meyer G, Becattini C, Bueno H, Geersing G-J, Harjola V-P, et al. 2019 ESC Guidelines for the diagnosis and management of acute pulmonary embolism developed in collaboration with the European Respiratory Society (ERS). Eur Heart J. 2020;41(4):543-603.

CHAPTER 9

Massive Hemoptysis

Rishika Pal, Bhaswati Dasgupta Nath

■ DEFINITION

Hemoptysis is defined as expectoration of blood from the pulmonary parenchyma or tracheobronchial tree below the level of glottis.

Greek word "haima", meaning blood and "'ptysis" meaning spitting. Hemoptysis can range from blood streaking of sputum to the presence of frank blood in the absence of any accompanying sputum.[1]

The lungs have dual bloody supply, namely the bronchial and pulmonary circulation, respectively. Most of the massive hemoptysis incidentally arises from the bronchial circulation, which being a high-pressure system and which facilitates neovascularization of tumors and/or dilated airways in bronchiectasis or cavitary lesions, precludes the possibility of cessation of bleeding by simple measures.

From accumulated data and systematic reviews, it has been observed that 4.8–14% of patients presenting with hemoptysis tend to have massive hemoptysis,[2] which, however remains debatable considering the heterogeneity of studied populations. Amongst various etiologies, tuberculosis, bronchiectasis, lung abscesses and mycetomas remain consistent as culprits of massive hemoptysis.[3]

Massive hemoptysis sometimes involves both circulatory and respiratory system leading to death by asphyxiation or exsanguation.[4,5] Massive hemoptysis is a common emergency complaint, but only 1–5% of cases are massive or life threatening. In these cases, the mortality rate approaches nearly 50–100%, if prompt intervention is not executed.[6] In 90% of cases, it arises from the high-pressure bronchial circulation. In another 5% of cases, it arises from causes related to the aorta, such as ruptured aneurysm or aortobronchial fistulae, or from nonbronchial systemic circulation pertaining to intercostal arteries, coronary arteries, thoracic arteries and/or phrenic arteries, while in the rest 5% of cases, it arises from the pulmonary vessels.[7,8]

There are a multitude of patterns of bronchiolar arteriolar anatomy according to literature. The most common of them being a single intercostal trunk on the right giving rise to the right bronchial arteries and a single left bronchial artery in 30.5%. The second most common pattern being an intercostal trunk on the right yielding the right bronchial artery and a second common trunk from which right and left bronchial arteries arise (25%); In 12.5% of cases, a right intercostal trunk giving rise to a bronchial artery and two bronchial arteries on the left.[9]

Massive hemoptysis in cystic fibrosis is reported to have annual incidence of 0.9–4.1%.[10,11]

Massive hemoptysis categorically has been stated as either >400 mL in 24 hours or >150 mL in a single episode,[12] that is potentially acutely life threatening usually results due to bleeding from a bronchial artery in 90% of cases, most commonly due to bronchiectasis, tuberculosis, bronchogenic carcinoma and fungal infections.

■ ETIOLOGY

Studies by Rao[13] in 1960, suggested that tuberculosis had remained the most common cause of hemoptysis in India. The scenario still remains the same today. On the contrary nontubercular causes such as malignancy, bronchiectasis and pneumonia remains more common causes of hemoptysis in developed countries.

The various causes of hemoptysis are illustrated is **Table 1**.

- *Pulmonary tuberculosis:* It is the leading cause, wherever the disease is endemic.[15] Here, the cause of bleeding is usually bronchiolar ulceration with necrosis of adjacent blood vessels or rupture of a Rasmussen's aneurysm (**Fig. 1**).[16] In the latter, weakening of pulmonary arterial wall is accountable for the same with a prevalence of 5%[17] and it must be taken into consideration wherever cavitary tuberculosis is suspected or diagnosed.
- *Bronchiectasis:* Chronic airway inflammation mediated by neutrophils, T-lymphocytes and cytokines causing tortuosity and permanent dilatation of the bronchial tree, owing to release of elastase and collagenase.
- *Fungal infections:* These are more prevalent among immunocompromised individuals or those with preexisting cavitary lung disease. Among these, the most

TABLE 1: Etiology of hemoptysis.	
Causes	**Examples**
Infections	Mycobacteria, mycetomas, lung abscess (*Klebsiella, Pseudomonas, Streptococcus, Actinomyces*), Bacterial endocarditis, paragonimiasis, hydatid cyst
Neoplastic	• Bronchogenic carcinoma • Endobronchial tumors (carcinoid, adenoid cystic carcinoma) • Pulmonary metastases • Sarcoma
Pulmonary causes	• Bronchiectasis (including cystic fibrosis) • Chronic bronchitis • Alveolar hemorrhage and underlying causes • Diffuse alveolar damage
Hematology	• Coagulopathy, platelet disorders • Thrombotic thrombocytopenic purpura
Trauma	• Catheter-induced PA rupture • Blunt or penetrating chest injury • Transtracheal procedures • Iatrogenic secondary to interventional pulmonology procedures • Bronchoscopic biopsy
Vascular	• Pulmonary and bronchial arterial aneurysms • Pulmonary infarct (embolism) • Pulmonary hypertension • Congenital cardiac or pulmonary malformations • Airway-vascular fistulae, arteriovenous malformations, Mitral stenosis • Left-ventricular failure • Pulmonary veno-occlusive disease
Drugs and toxins	• Penicillamine • Solvents • Crack cocaine • Trimellitic anhydride • Bevacizumab • Isocyanates • Nitrofurantoin
Vasculitis/ Collagen vascular diseases	• Granulomatosis with polyangiitis • Goodpasture's syndrome • Behçet's disease • Systemic lupus erythematosus • Essential mixed cryoglobulinemia • Henoch-Schonlein purpura • Mixed connective tissue disease • Progressive systemic sclerosis • Rheumatoid arthritis • Systemic necrotizing vasculitis • Immune complex associated glomerulonephritis • Pauci-immune glomerulonephritis
Miscellaneous	• Cryptogenic • Endometriosis • Lymphangioleiomyomatosis • Broncholithiasis, foreign body aspiration • Lung transplantation • Tuberous sclerosis • Idiopathic pulmonary hemosiderosis, catamenial • Hemoptysis (pulmonary endometriosis)[10,14]

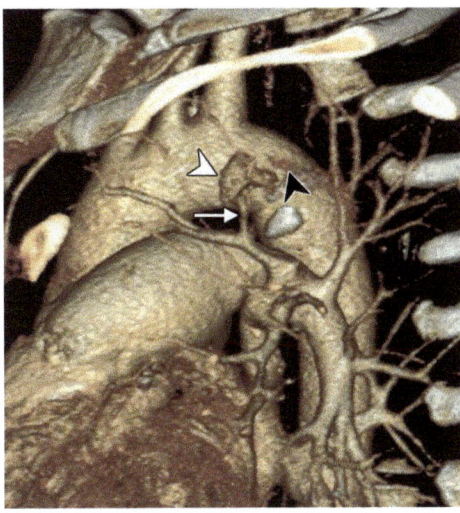

Fig. 1: A Rasmussen's aneurysm (white arrowhead) originating from a small pulmonary artery branch (arrow) over the left upper lobe. Adjacent contrast medium extravasations (black arrowhead) indicate rupture of the aneurysm.

common cause is an aspergilloma.[18] Other offending causes include histoplasmosis and blastomycosis.
- *Bronchogenic carcinoma:* This is common with large and centrally located tumors, especially squamous cell carcinoma. In the setting of malignancy, myriad pathological factors play a role in influencing the volume and rate of bleeding, such as neovascularization in and relative to neoplasm, exfoliation of tumor surface, tumor necrosis, erosion of airways into surrounding vascular structures.
- *Immunologic lung diseases:* Goodpasture syndrome, Wegener's granulomatosis, systemic lupus erythematous (SLE), lupus pneumonitis, and microscopic polyangiitis.

APPROACH TO THE PROBLEM (FLOWCHART 1)
- Identify whether it is true hemoptysis
- Identify the severity of hemoptysis
- History and examinations
- Diagnostic investigations
- Appropriate management.[1,10,14]

Identifying True Hemoptysis
It should be below the vocal cords and persists as blood-tinged sputum. There should be a history of cardiopulmonary disease. Chest X-ray will reveal abnormal lung parenchymal lesion.

Identifying the Severity of Hemoptysis
- *Mild:* >100 mL blood loss per day
- *Moderate:* 100-150 mL blood loss per day
- *Severe:* Up to 200 mL blood loss per day
- *Massive:* >500 mL blood loss per day or >150 mL per hour or 100 mL blood loss per day for >3 days.

History and Examination

Hemoptysis is the presenting symptoms for many different diseases.

History

- Acute onset of fever, cough, bloody sputum is suggestive of bronchitis or pneumonia. Productive cough is suggestive of bronchiectasis.
- Fever, nights sweats, history of travel from endemic region are suggestive of tuberculosis
- Dyspnea and pleuritic chest pain are suggestive of pulmonary embolism.
- Chronic weight loss, change in cough and extensive use of tobacco is suggestive of bronchogenic carcinoma.
- Minor hemoptysis with dyspnea is suggestive of mitral stenosis or alveolar hemorrhage diseases.
- Hemoptysis, hematuria with renal insufficiency suggests Goodpasture syndrome
- *Drug history:* Patients taking antiplatelets and/or anticoagulants have a higher preponderance to bleed. Ernst et al. in his study showed that 89% of patients taking clopidogrel and 100% of those taking both clopidogrel and aspirin respectively yielded higher rates of mild, moderate, and severe hemoptysis.[19]

Examination

- Start with checking the airway, breathing and circulation of the patient. Keep monitoring the vital signs side by side.
- Tachypnea is indicative or respiratory compromise with hypoxemia.
- Hypotension seen in massive hemoptysis.
- Cardiac examination reveals valvular heart diseases (diastolic murmur of mitral stenosis).
- Nasal and oral cavities should be examined properly to exclude out any extrapulmonary source of bleeding (pseudohemoptysis).

Diagnostic Investigations

- *Chest X-ray (PA and lateral view):* 20–30% patients with hemoptysis usually have normal chest X-rays. Abnormalities may include preexisting chronic lung diseases or infiltration resulting from pulmonary hemorrhage rather than identifying the cause for bleeding.
- *Arterial blood gas*
- *Complete blood count:* To rule out any thrombocytopenia and for evaluation of anemia/microcytosis (for any chronic blood loss or malignancy)
- *Coagulation profile:* To find out patients with history of coagulopathy or current use of anticoagulants.
- *Urea and electrolytes:* For the assessment of underlying kidney function.
- Electrocardiogram
- Urine analysis
- Bronchoscopy
- *Sputum* (fungal culture, Gram stain, acid fast bacilli smear, and cytology): If infective etiology is suspected.
- *High resolution computerized tomography (HRCT):* To find out any additional information/evidence which is not detected in the chest X-ray.
- *Nasal endoscopy, biopsy, CT or MRI* is indicated if the source of bleeding is from the upper airway for example nasal polyps, laryngeal carcinoma or pharyngeal tumor.
- *Other imaging:* Ventilation perfusion scan is an alternative procedure of CT in those selected patients with suspected pulmonary embolism.
- *Pulmonary or bronchial angiography:* It is useful if bleeding is ongoing and no source is found by other means.[1,10,14]

Appropriate Management (Flowchart 1)

Airway

The most lethal sequelae of hemoptysis is hypoxia due to ventilation-perfusion match which occurs due to small airways and alveoli getting flooded with blood. In such cases oxygen saturation is to be maintained at >94% by administering supplemental oxygen. In life-threatening hemoptysis, the airway has to be secured by large diameter (8 mm or larger) endotracheal tube (ETT) to allow for bronchoscopy if required, without jeopardizing the ventilation and oxygenation. In case of persisting bleeding and if the bleeding side can be localized, then ETT is advanced in the main stem bronchus of nonbleeding side, so as to improve the ventilation. It has been seen that the right main stem bronchus is easier to enter than the left bronchus.

Double lumen ETT, containing two small working channels, provides single lung ventilation and facilitates isolation of the bleeding side. However, these can get obstructed with clots and is hence not an effective tool for clot retraction.

Breathing

In patients with a known lateralizing source of bleeding, a mitigating "lung down" approach can be employed, where the patient is positioned with the bleeding lung in the dependent position. This will promote and protect the unaffected lung and thus will improve the oxygenation.

Circulation

Hemodynamic instability occurs due to massive hemorrhage, hence following measures can be taken:

- To secure an IV channel with a large bore cannula and crystalloids can be administered.
- Blood transfusion may be considered in patients with massive hemoptysis

Flowchart 1: Algorithm for management of massive hemoptysis.

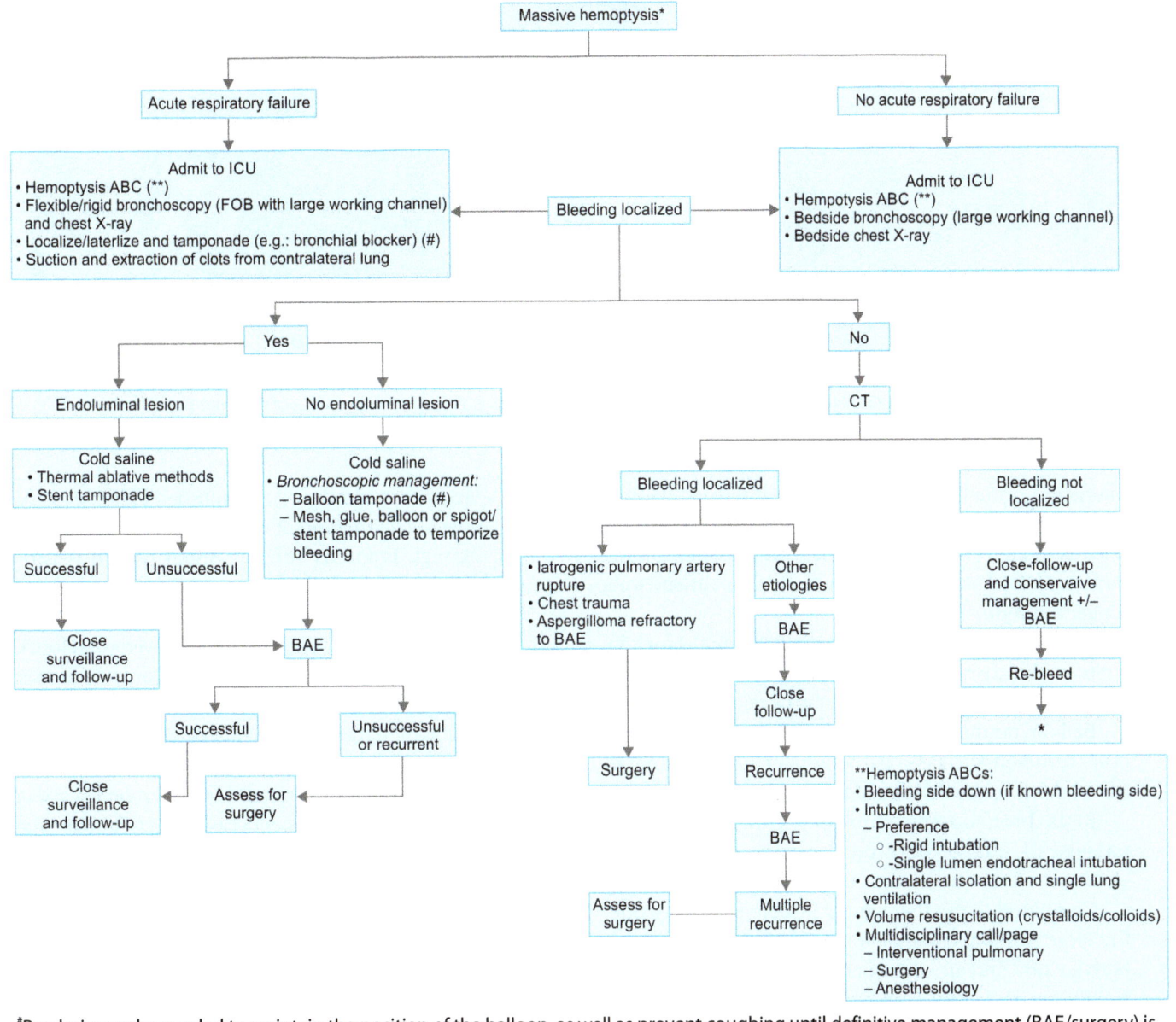

#Paralysis may be needed to maintain the position of the balloon, as well as prevent coughing until definitive management (BAE/surgery) is carried out
*Starting from the top of the diagram
**See ABC hemoptysis. BAE: bronchial artery embolization

- Any coagulopathy if present should be corrected
- Injection tranexamic acid 1 g intravenous bolus can be administered followed by oral tranexamic acid 500 mg 8 hourly.

Antibiotics

In case of mild hemoptysis due to bronchitis or bronchiectasis, the administration of antibiotics should be considered, if there is any evidence of bacterial infection.

Bronchoscopy

Early bronchoscopy should be performed at bedside, which will facilitate direct visualization of the central airway thus allowing therapeutic intervention. These include injection of vasoactive agents, balloon and topical hemostatic tamponade and thermocoagulation.

- *Bronchial blocking techniques:* Bronchial blocking techniques are deployed in order to localize the bleeding site and prevent aspiration and contamination of the unaffected lung, thereby facilitating continued ventilation to the same. Moreover, it provides sufficient time to undertake therapeutic intervention.

A bronchial blocker is a long flexible catheter of length 65–78 cm (4.5–9F) inserted through the endotracheal tube into the bleeding lung under Bronchoscopic guidance. They are usually placed in the

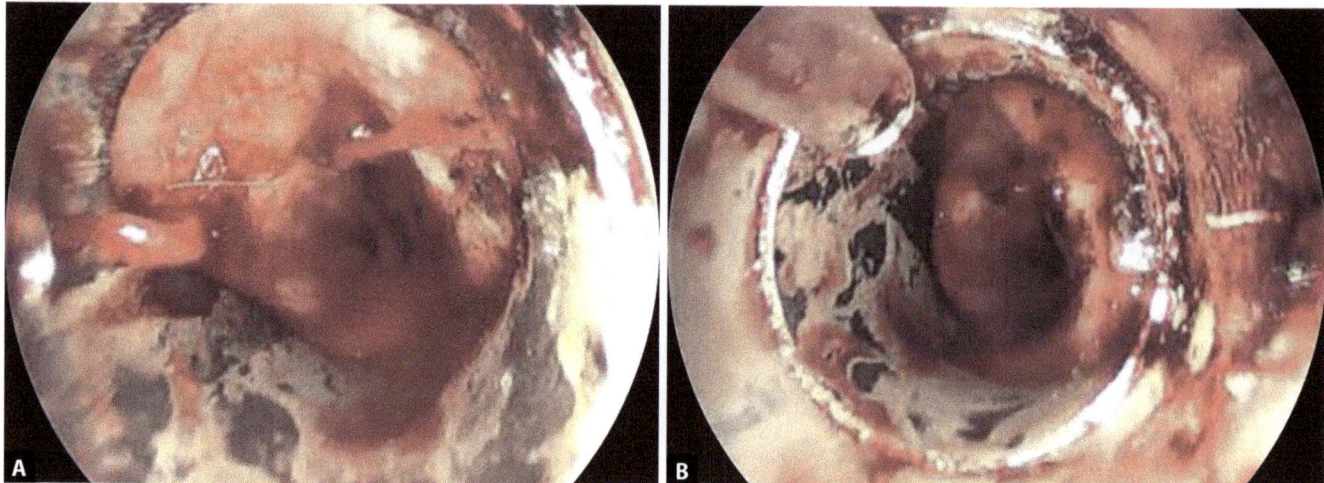

Figs. 2A and B: (A) Submucosal tumor infiltration of bronchus intermedius isolated from the bevel of the rigid bronchoscope; (B) Simultaneous argon plasma coagulation therapy and suction of blood for airway clearance.

mainstem bronchus or the bronchus intermedius. It is a temporizing measure often in the first 48–72 hours, as it leads to atelectasis, pneumonia, compression trauma and necrosis of bronchial wall mucosa if kept in-situ for a longer duration.[20]

Several commercially available bronchial blockers such as Arndt blocker, Cohen Flexitip blocker, Fuji Uniblocker, and the EZ Blocker may be used.[21]

Balloon tamponade can also be achieved by means of other catheters such as Fogarty catheter inserted through the working channel of flexible bronchoscope.[22]

Rigid bronchoscopy provides a large lumen for passage of a large bore rigid suction which allows clearance of obstructive clots under direct visualization.

Compared to the therapeutic flexible bronchoscope, the large working channel of a rigid bronchoscope aids both suction and airway visualization simultaneously by facilitating passage of a rigid suction catheter, a small soft suction catheter and a flexible bronchoscope for both suction and airway visualization, simultaneously.

- Bronchoscopic interventions for control of bleeding
  - *Endobronchial medical therapy*
    - Ice cold saline irrigation[11]
    - Epinephrine and norepinephrine
    - *Antidiuretic hormone (ADH)-derivatives:* Terlipressin, Ornipressin
    - Bronchoscopic-guided topical hemostatic tamponade therapy using oxidized regenerated cellulose.
  - *Thermal ablative methods*
    - LASER Therapy: Nd:YAG (Neodymium yttrium aluminum garnet): The energy from laser beam is absorbed by tissues and converted to heat, thereby producing local effects by photocoagulation, vaporization and necrosis, respectively **(Figs. 2A and B)**[23,24]
    - Electrocauterization: Accomplished either by using noncontact method of conducting electrical energy through inert gas such as Argon (Argon Plasma photocoagulation) (Morice et al.)[25] or by using contact method of conducting electrical energy (electrocautery).[26] The tissue then converts the electrical energy to heat resulting in coagulation and necrosis.
  - *Endobronchial stents:* Silicone stents, with or without adjunctive endobronchial management modalities, are primarily being used for control of hemoptysis arising due to malignancies, especially when bronchial artery embolization fails. Number of case reports have proven the efficacy of this management strategy to be worthwhile in managing hemoptysis **(Figs. 3A and B).**[19,27]
  - *Brachytherapy and extrathoracic radiotherapy:* Brachytherapy was pioneered in the management of neoplasms, in 1920s, whereby a radioactive emitting substance, mounted on wire, used to be introduced via fiberoptic bronchoscope upto the proximity of the tumor, after adequate debulking, in order to accomplish the same. Although it was found to be efficacious in alleviating mild hemoptysis, its role in massive ones is limited.

In the past few decades, extrathoracic radiotherapy has shown to have moderate effect on hemoptysis, but substantially being palliative. Presently, its utility is guarded considering the recent day advancements.

CT Chest

In hemodynamically stable patients, HRCT chest will give valuable information to localize the site of bleeding and thereby guiding bronchial artery embolization (BAE), if required. Bronchial artery embolization was first described by Remy et al., in 1974. Spinal cord ischemia results from embolization of anterior spinal arteries, which is considered to be the most feared complication of BAE.

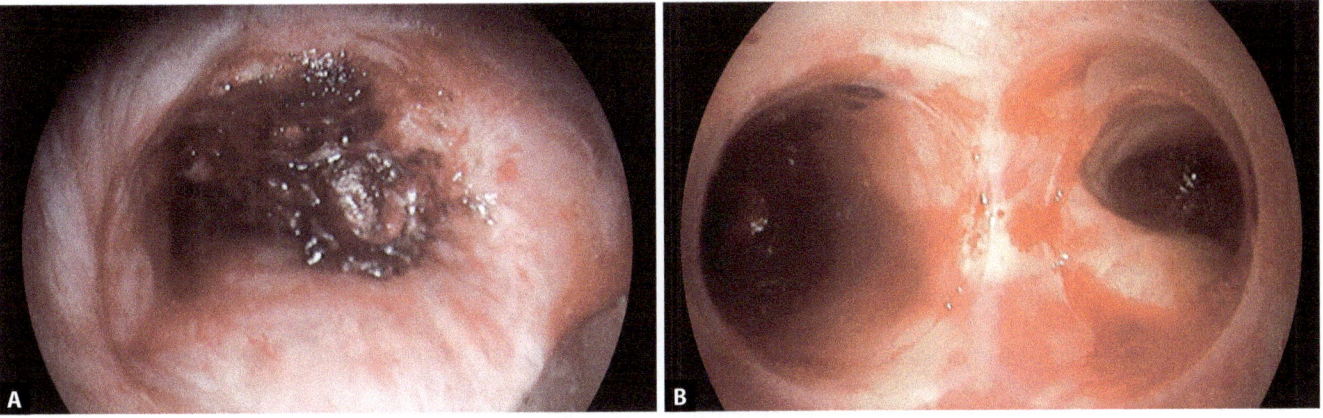

Figs. 3A and B: (A) Endobronchial bleeding tumor; (B) Tamponade effect obtained after stent placement following laser therapy and debulking.

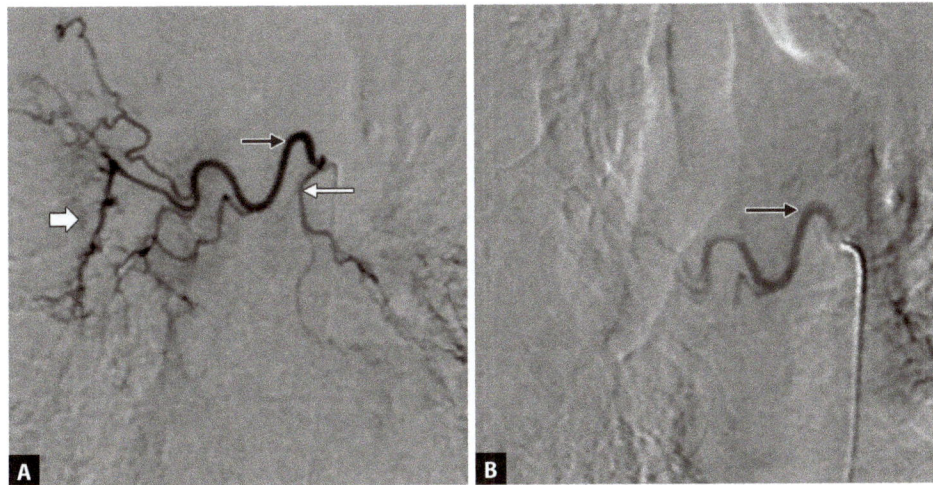

Figs 4A and B: (A) Pre-embolization digital subtraction angiographic (DSA) image showing selective catheterization of common bronchial artery with hypertrophied right bronchial artery *(black arrow)* and left bronchial artery *(white arrow)* with parenchymal blush *(white block arrow)*; (B) Postembolization DSA image showing contrast stasis in right bronchial artery *(black arrow) with* obliterated left bronchial artery and no residual parenchymal blush suggestive of successful embolization.

Interventional Angiography

For those patients who are unable to tolerate bronchoscopy or surgery, bronchial artery embolization is the first line of therapy. Massive bleeding due to tuberculosis and bronchiectasis respond well to it. Complications may arise from non-target embolization, either to the esophagus resulting in dysphagia or to the spinal arteries resulting in transverse myelitis. Rare complications include dissection and arterial perforation.[1,11,28]

Bronchial Artery Embolization

The two most common indications of this in controlling hemoptysis are due to pulmonary tuberculosis and post tuberculosis sequelae such as fibrosis, aspergillosis and bronchiectasis.

Initially transfemoral arteriogram is performed followed by embolotherapy using any one of the following agents: gelatin sponge, polyvinyl alcohol (PVA) particles, microspheres, liquid embolic agents such as n-butyl-2-cyanoacrylate, and metallic coil.

Success rates of BAE in neoplasm related hemoptysis ranges from 60 to 90%.[29] Semi and Shimono evaluated results of a novel technique using chemotherapeutic agents such as cisplatin and fluorouracil, to infiltrate the feeding vessels of a neoplasm followed by embolization with gelatin sponge particles, whereby success rates reached 90% in alleviating hemoptysis **(Figs. 4A and B)**.[30,31]

■ CONCLUSION

The diagnostic evaluation of patients with life-threatening hemoptysis remains focused on the localization of the leading site and underlying cause, which can be performed quickly with CT imaging in patients who have adequate oxygenation, ventilation, and are hemodynamically stable. Bronchoscopy remains invaluable for patients needing airway control and those in whom CT imaging cannot localize the bleeding site. The more widespread availability of bronchial artery embolization has led to a shift in the management of life-threatening hemoptysis.

> **Take Home Messages**
> - Try to establish that this is true hemoptysis and nothing else
> - Identify the severity of hemoptysis.
> - Detailed history taking and clinical examination might help to identify the cause.
> - Appropriate investigations are essential to find out the site as well as the nature of lesions.
> - Management includes basic resuscitation of patient, correction of blood loss, control of bleeding by applying modern technology and finally treatment of the cause of hemoptysis.

REFERENCES

1. Wilkinson IB, Raine T, Wiles K, Goodhart A, Hall C, O'Neil H. Oxford handbook of clinical medicine tenth edition. New York: Oxford University Press Inc.; 2017. pp. 48-9.
2. Hirshberg B, Biran I, Glazer M, Kramer MR. Hemoptysis: etiology, evaluation, and outcome in a tertiary referral hospital. Chest. 1997;112(2):440-4.
3. Dweik RA, Stoller JK. Role of bronchoscopy in massive hemoptysis. Clin Chest Med. 1999;20(1):89-105.
4. Yoon W, Kim JK, Kim YH, Chung TW, Kang HK. Bronchial and nonbronchial systemic artery embolization for life-threatening hemoptysis: a comprehensive review. Radiographics. 2002;22(6):1395-409.
5. Jean-Baptiste E. Clinical assessment and management of massive hemoptysis. Critical care medicine. 2000;28(5):1642-7.
6. Najarian KE, Morris CS. Arterial embolization in the chest. Journal of thoracic imaging. 1998;13(2):93-104.
7. Remy J, Remy-Jardin M, Voisin C. Endovascular management of bronchial bleeding. Lung biology in health and disease. 1992;57:667-723.
8. Sakr L, Dutau H. Massive hemoptysis: an update on the role of bronchoscopy in diagnosis and management. Respiration. 2010;80(1):38-58.
9. Uflacker R, Kaemmerer A, Picon PD, Rizzon CF, Neves CM, Oliveira ES, et al. Bronchial artery embolization in the management of hemoptysis: technical aspects and long-term results. Radiology. 1985;157(3):637-44.
10. Cham G, Dilley S. Hemoptysis. In: George PC, Kelly AM, Brown A, Little M. Textbook of Adult Emergency Medicine, 4th edition. New York: Elsevier; 2015. p. 324.
11. Radchenko C, Alraiyes AH, Shojaee S. A systematic approach to the management of massive hemoptysis. J Thorac Dis. 2017;9(Suppl 10):S1069-S1086.
12. Kritek P, Fanta C. Cough and Hemoptysis. In: Longo DL, Kasper DL, Larry JJ, Fauci AS, Hauser SL (Eds). Harrison's Principles of Internal Medicine, 18th edition. New York: The McGraw's Hill Companies; 2012. pp. 282.
13. Rao PU. Hemoptysis as a symptom in a chest clinic. Indian J Chest Dis. 1960;2(219):8.
14. Devnani T, Holthaus C, Aggarwal P, Levine MD, Gilmore WS. The Washington Manual of Emergency Medicine South Asian edition. New York: Wolters Kluwer publication; 2021. pp. 503.
15. Ozgül MA, Turna A, Yildiz P, Ertan E, Chairman S, Yilmaz V. Risk factors and recurrence patterns in 203 patients with hemoptysis. Tuberk Toraks. 2006;54(3):243-8.
16. Shih SY, Tsai IC, Chang YT, Tsan YT, Hu SY. Fatal hemoptysis caused by a ruptured Rasmussen's aneurysm. Thorax. 2011;66(6):553-4.
17. Khalil A, Parrot A, Nedelcu C, Fartoukh M, Marsault C, Carette MF. Severe hemoptysis of pulmonary arterial origin: signs and role of multidetector row CT angiography. Chest. 2008;133(1):212-9.
18. Cahill BC, Ingbar DH. Massive hemoptysis: assessment and management. Clinics in chest medicine. 1994;15(1):147-68.
19. Ernst A, Eberhardt R, Wahidi M, Becker HD, Herth FJ. Effect of routine clopidogrel use on bleeding complications after transbronchial biopsy in humans. Chest. 2006;129(3):734-7.
20. Alraiyes AH, Alraies MC, Machuzak MS. Q: Does massive hemoptysis always merit diagnostic bronchoscopy? Cleveland Clin J Med. 2014;81(11):662-4.
21. Hiebert CA. Balloon catheter control of life-threatening hemoptysis. Chest. 1974;66(3):308-9.
22. Solomonov A, Fruchter O, Zuckerman T, Brenner B, Yigla M. Pulmonary hemorrhage: a novel mode of therapy. Respiratory medicine. 2009;103(8):1196-200.
23. Kvale PA, Eichenhorn MS, Radke JR, Miks V. YAG laser photoresection of lesions obstructing the central airways. Chest. 1985;87(3):283-8.
24. Gershman E, Guthrie R, Swiatek K, Shojaee S. Management of hemoptysis in patients with lung cancer. Ann Translat Med. 2019;7(15):9.
25. Morice RC, Ece T, Ece F, Keus L. Endobronchial argon plasma coagulation for treatment of hemoptysis and neoplastic airway obstruction. Chest. 2001;119(3):781-7.
26. Sheski FD, Mathur PN. Cryotherapy, electrocautery, and brachytherapy. Clinics in chest medicine. 1999;20(1):123-38.
27. Barisione E, Genova C, Grosso M, Pasquali M, Blanco A, Felletti R, et al. Palliative treatment of life-threatening hemoptysis with silicone stent insertion in advanced lung cancer. Monaldi Arch Chest Dis. 2017;87(1).
28. Gagnon S, Quigley N, Dutau H, Delage A, Fortin M. Approach to Hemoptysis in the Modern Era. Canadian Resp J. 2017:1565030.
29. Fruchter O, Schneer S, Rusanov V, Belenky A, Kramer MR. Bronchial artery embolization for massive hemoptysis: long-term follow-up. Asian Cardiovasc Thorac Ann. 2015;23(1):55-60.
30. Seki A, Shimono C. Transarterial chemoembolization for management of hemoptysis: initial experience in advanced primary lung cancer patients. Japanese J Radiol. 2017;35(9):495-504.
31. Panda A, Bhalla AS, Goyal A. Bronchial artery embolization in hemoptysis: a systematic review. Diagnostic and Interventional Radiology. 2017;23(4):307.

CHAPTER 10

Acute Pulmonary Embolism

Avijit Das

DEFINITION

Pulmonary embolism (PE) also known as "the Great Masquerader"[1] refers to obstruction of the pulmonary artery or one of its branches by material (e.g., thrombus, tumor, air or fat) that originated elsewhere in the body.[2] The thrombus usually originates in the deep venous system of the lower extremities but also from pelvic, renal, upper extremity veins, or the right heart chambers.[3] It may lead to severe PE that may lead to right ventricular failure.[4] Pulmonary embolism is categorized as hemodynamically stable or unstable. It is further classified as follows:

- *Massive PE (5–10%):* This is a hemodynamically unstable condition is characterized by extensive thrombosis affecting at least half of the pulmonary vasculature. Dyspnea, syncope, hypotension and cyanosis are the hallmarks of massive PE.
- *Submassive or intermediate risk PE (20–25%):* RV strain pattern present, patient hemodynamically stable.
- *Low risk PE (65–75%):* RV strain pattern absent, patient hemodynamically stable with excellent prognosis.

PREVALENCE

Indian Perspective

Though the exact epidemiology of PE in India is largely unknown, an autopsy study showed the overall incidence of PE in patients admitted in medical wards of tertiary care center in North India to be 15.9%, mainly affecting the younger population <50 years of age. The incidence of significant PE contributing to the death of the patients was 12.6%.[5] The prevailing notion that the incidence of VTE in Asians is less than that in the Western population has been disproved by recent studies. The incidence of postoperative DVT in Indian patients undergoing major lower limb surgery is as high (43.2% and 60% patients in the groups with and without prophylaxis, respectively) as seen in the Western world.[6] In a meta-analysis that included seven studies have shown that the pooled prevalence of PE in unexplained AE-COPD was 16.1% [95% confidence interval (CI) 8.3–25.8%].[7]

Worldwide Perspective

The annual incidence of PE is <120 per lakh population.[8] PE ranks third in the list of cardiovascular disease after coronary artery disease and embolic cardiovascular accident[9] males suffers most from PE compared to females.[10]

EARLY DIAGNOSIS, LABORATORY ASSESSMENT, ROLE OF BIOMARKERS AND APPROACH TO THE PROBLEM

It is very difficult to diagnose PE early as because of its varied clinical presentation. Unexplained breathlessness, chest pain, and cough are the most common symptoms of PE, while fever, tachycardia, abnormal pulmonary signs and peripheral vascular collapse are the most common physical findings.[11] Distal PE give rise to pleuritic chest pain while central or proximal PE simulates like angina pain.[12-14] For most patients with suspected PE we usually divide it into high risk and intermediate risk or low risk groups. For high-risk group, urgent echocardiography or computerized tomography pulmonary angiography (CTPA) done; and for the latter group PE is likely or not is assessed by WELLS criteria, if PE is unlikely D-dimer assay done, if it is negative an alternative diagnosis is considered and if it is positive CTPA/VQ (ventilation-perfusion scan) performed or to be treated pending imaging if >1 hour as in case of PE likely.

WELLS criteria: 3 points each for clinical symptoms of DVT and other diagnosis less likely than PE, 1.5 points each for immobilization for 3 or more days or surgery in last 4 weeks, heart beats >100/min and past history of DVT, 1 point for hemoptysis and malignancy. Points >4 is considered PE likely and points ≤4 is considered PE unlikely.

The revised version of Geneva clinical prediction for PE is given in **Table 1**.

TABLE 1: The revised Geneva clinical prediction rule for pulmonary embolism.		
	Clinical decision rule points	
Items	**Original version**	**Simplified version**
Previous PE or DVT	3	1
Heart rate		
• 75–94 b.p.m.	3	1
• ≥95 b.p.m.	5	2
Surgery or fracture within the past month	2	1
Hemoptysis	2	1
Active cancer	2	1
Unilateral lower-limb pain	3	1
Pain on lower-limb deep venous palpation and unilateral oedema	4	1
Age >65 years	1	1
Clinical probability		
Three-level score		
• Low	0–3	0–1
• Intermediate	4–10	2–4
• High	11	>5
Two-level score		
• PE-unlikely	0–5	0–2
• PE-likely	≥6	≥3

Role of Echocardiography in Early Diagnosis of Pulmonary Embolism

Echocardiographic examination is not mandatory but more than one-fourth of patients with PE have right ventricular dilatation which is considered to be an important risk measuring parameter of the disease.[17] McConnell's sign (reduced contraction of right ventricular fee wall in comparison to RV apical movement in echocardiography) and sign of 60/60 (blood flow rate at right ventricular outflow tract measured as acceleration time <60 ms with gradient at tricuspid valve during peak systolic period <60 mm Hg) together is suggestive of PE.[18] and justifies emergency reperfusion treatment for PE.

Important Biomarkers

D-dimer

As we know D-dimer is elevated in several clinical condition other than PE so a normal D-dimer excludes PE hence cannot confirm PE, ELISA method is 95% sensitive however specificity above 80 years age steadily goes down to 10%.[19] D-dimer testing on spot can be applied in remote areas but is less sensitive and less negative predictive values as compared to laboratory testing.[20,21]

Others

The more of right ventricular dysfunction the more is myocardial stretch because of pressure overload as a result of which blood levels of B type natriuretic (BNP) peptide and N terminal pro BNP are elevated as also troponin levels in severe PE.[22,23]

Computed Tomographic Pulmonary Angiography (CTPA)

Computed tomographic pulmonary angiography (CTPA) being noninvasive with perfect visualization of subsegmental pulmonary vessels and at the same time its similar diagnostic accuracy to that of pulmonary angiography (variable and operator dependent), it replaced the later which was once a decade old gold standard diagnostic modality of PE.[24,25] For high risk or intermediate group positive predictive value is high compared to low likelihood group -96% versus 58%.[26] It is contraindicated in iodinated contrast allergy and renal impairment patient. A multicentric prospective cohort study in 457 patients showed RV enlargement is an important prognostic marker of PE which is detected by CTPA along with other indicators of RV enlargement.[27] Ultrasound Doppler is recommended for those who are not candidates of CTPA as in pregnant women but the same is not applicable for non-pregnant patient where it gives 90% negative result.[28]

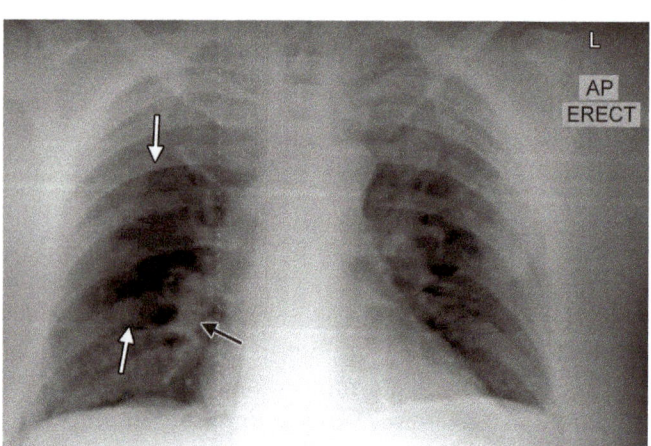

Fig. 1: Pulmonary embolism: Hamptons sign (hump-like opacity in peripheral lung—white arrows) and Watermarks signs (black arrow).

Diagnostic Workup

Diagnostic work starts with routine blood tests, arterial blood gas (ABG) analysis, ECG, chest X-ray, and echocardiography in general. CO_2 wash out with wide $PO_2(A-a)$ is noted in ABG. ECG findings are although nonspecific.[15] The most common ECG findings in PE is sinus tachycardia, S1Q3T3 is typical of PE. Both Hamptons sign (hump-like opacity in peripheral lung) and Watermarks signs (shown in below chest ray) for distal oligemia are specific although rare in PE **(Fig. 1)**.[16] In figure below the hyperlucency secondary to oligaemia is watermark sign.

Lung Scintigraphy

Among selected group of patients namely pregnant, with history of contrast anaphylaxis and severe renal failure V/Q scan remains the test of choice and they are subdivided into normal scan that is PE excluded, high probability scan and nondiagnostic scan.[29,30] Not to give anticoagulation therapy in a normal test result is practiced as safe strategy is depicted in multiple studies.[31]

Compression Ultrasonography

Compression ultrasonography (CUS) has successfully picked up DVT in 30-50% patients with PE as its specificity and sensitivity both >90% and has replaced lower limb venography.[32,33]

Differential Diagnosis of Pulmonary Embolism

- Pneumonia
- Asthma, chronic obstructive pulmonary disease (COPD)
- Congestive cardiac failure
- Pericarditis
- *Pleurisy:* Viral syndrome, costochondritis, musculoskeletal discomfort
- Rib fracture
- Pneumothorax
- Acute coronary syndrome
- Anxiety.

Approach to a Patient with Acute Pulmonary Embolism (Flowcharts 1 and 2)

The primary steps are supportive measures like administration of supplemental O_2 in patients with SaO_2 <90% and also high flow O_2 via high flow nasal cannula if required[34,35] and in cases of extreme clinical instability one may require invasive or noninvasive mechanical ventilation (NIV). Intubation is done only when patients cannot cope up with NIV. According to feasibility NIV or high flow oxygenation is preferred. During intubation, anesthetic medication causes hypotension hence should be used with caution or better avoided. In high-risk patients like circulatory collapse or cardiac arrest venoarterial extracorporeal membrane oxygenation (VA-ECMO) should be applied. Intravenous fluid with normal saline around halt to 1 liter is recommended cautiously as large volumes should be avoided. If perfusion fails to respond with normal saline vasopressor is administered (norepinephrine 0.2-1 mg/kg/min; dobutamine 2-20 mg/kg/min), however too much vasoconstriction may lead to tissue ischemia.

Empiric anticoagulation should be started with low risk of bleeding in a patient with high clinical suspicion for PE without any delay. However, if these patients are unstable systemic thrombolytic therapy rather than empiric anticoagulation/no therapy is suggested. Low molecular weight heparin or fondaparinux is recommended over UFH when used in intermediate or low risk patients.[36-39] Among oral anticoagulants NOACs (apixaban, dabigatran, edoxaban, or rivaroxaban), a NOAC is recommended in preference to a VKA.[40-44] When patients are treated with a VKA, overlapping with parenteral anticoagulation is recommended until an INR of 2.5 (range 2.0-3.0) is reached.[45,46] NOACs are not recommended in pregnant or lactating mother, antiphospholipid antibody syndrome and in patients with CKD.

Rescue thrombolytic therapy with streptokinase 250,000 IU as loading dose in 30 min followed by 100,000 IU over 12-24 hours or rtPA 0.6 mg/kg over 15 minutes is applied in patients who are hemodynamically unstable with anticoagulation therapy.[47] Other alternatives in these patients are percutaneous catheter directed treatment or surgical embolectomy. IVC filter deployed in recurrent PE and in absolute contraindication to anticoagulants.

■ OUTCOME ASSESSMENT (TABLE 2 AND BOX 1)

Original and simplified pulmonary embolism severity index **(Table 2)**.

■ COMPLICATIONS

- Right heart failure
- Cardiogenic shock
- Recurrent thromboembolism
- Chronic thromboembolic pulmonary hypertension.

■ CONCLUSIONS AND AUTHOR'S PERSPECTIVE

Pulmonary embolism is a common clinical problem with varied manifestations ranging from benign to fatal. In view of complexities in diagnosis, approach and therapies, collaborative multidisciplinary approach is helpful.

Clinical

Sudden onset respiratory distress, tachycardia, tachypnea, and hypotension in a patient with absence of another reasonable clinical explanation, and in the presence of major risk factor should arouse the clinical suspicion of PE. All the patients with possible PE should have clinical probability assessed and documented. An alternative clinical explanation should always be considered at presentation and sought when PE is excluded. Once PE is suspected, a determination of pretest probability using either the WELLS or Geneva scores may be used.

Diagnosis

D-dimer value adjusted according to age or clinical probability is preferred over fixed cut-off values. Blood D-dimer assay should only be considered following

Flowchart 1: Treatment algorithm for hemodynamically stable patients with suspected pulmonary embolism (PE).

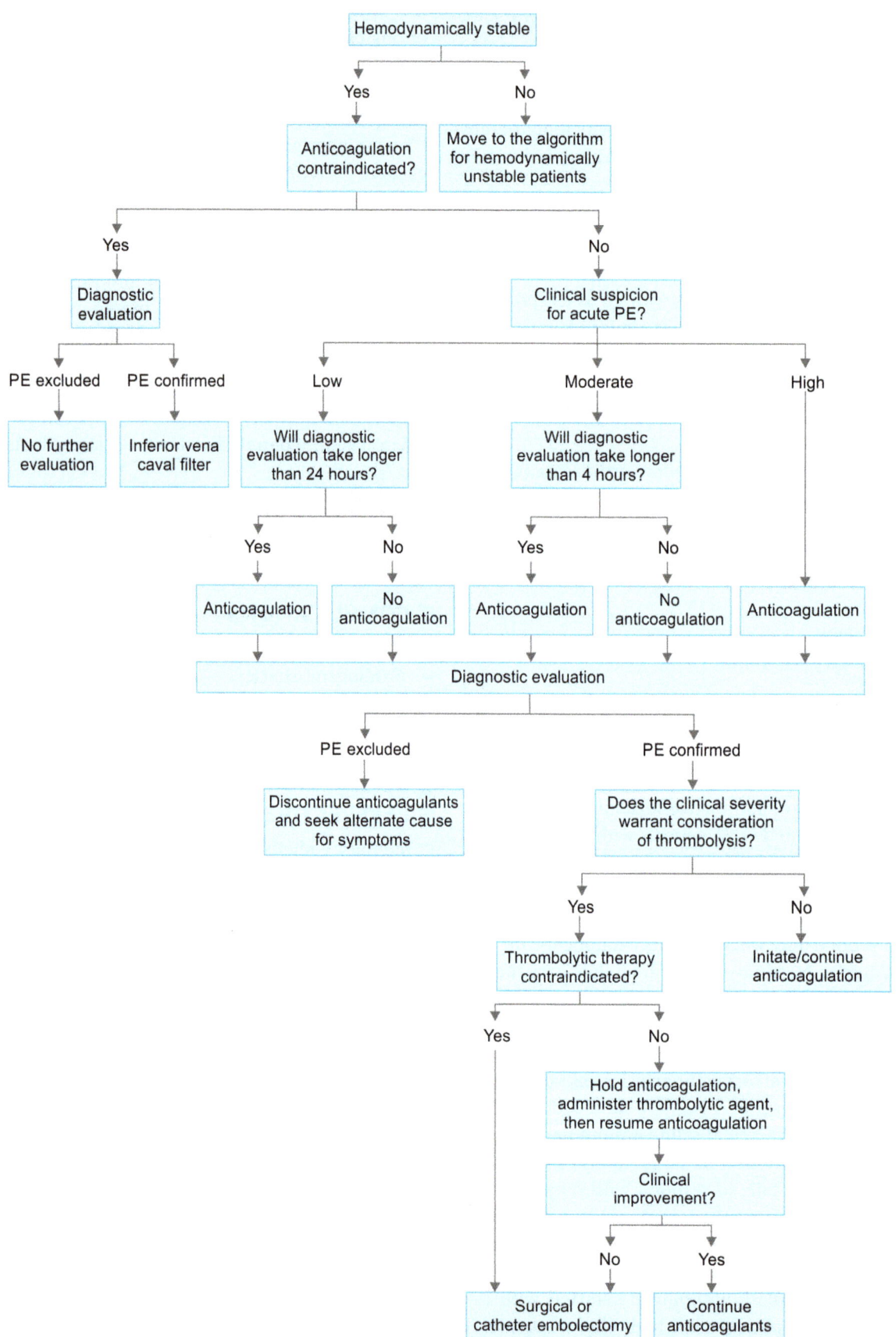

Flowchart 2: Treatment algorithm for hemodynamically unstable patients with suspected pulmonary embolism (PE).

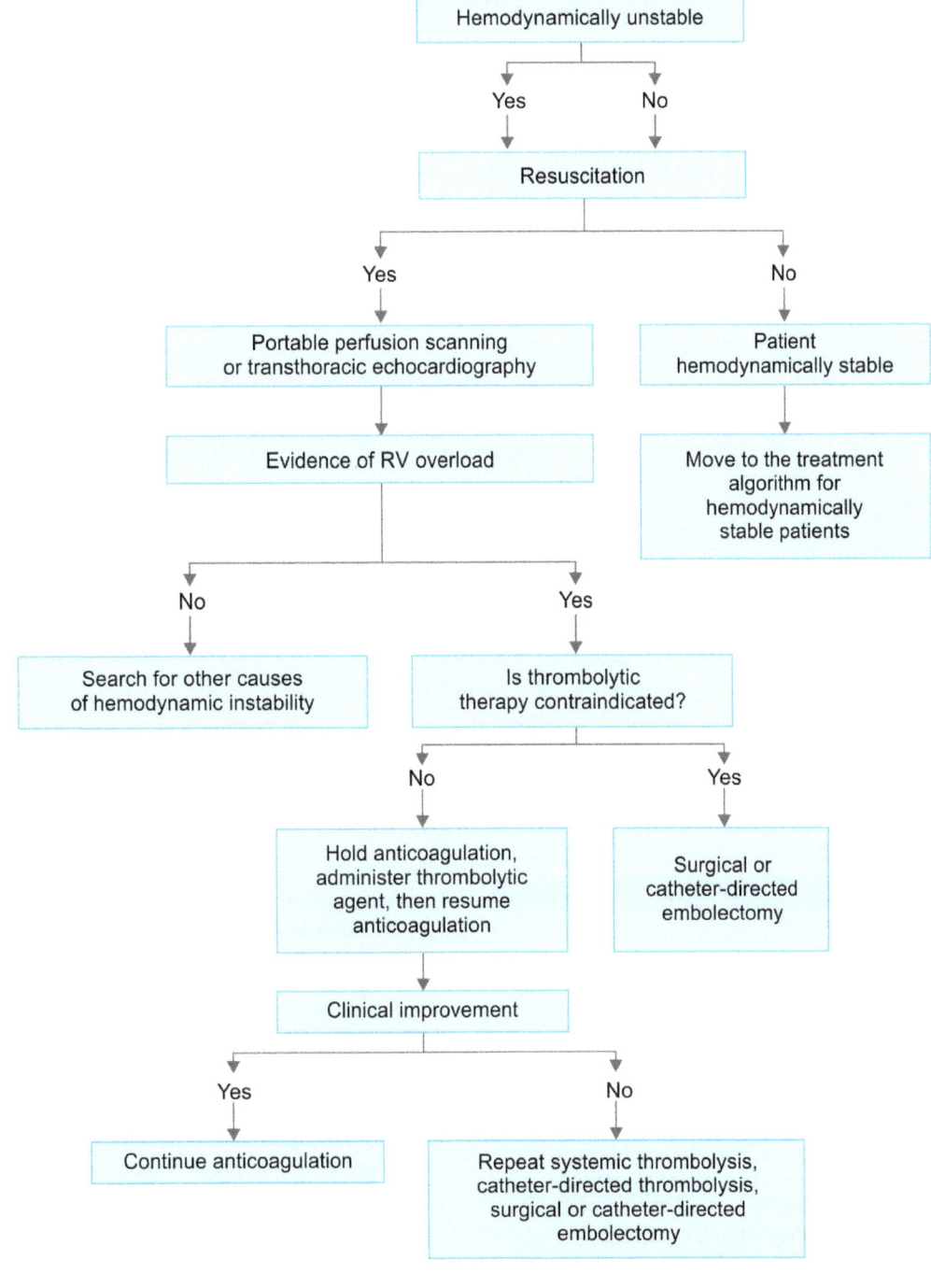

assessment of clinical probability. Even for low PEPSI or 0 PEPSI, RV status should be assessed along with biomarkers. For patients with intermediate or high pretest probability or a positive D-dimer, CTPA is indicated. For low clinical probability or PE unlikely group CTPA may be normal. Patients with a good quality negative CTPA do not require further investigation or treatment for PE.

Treatment

Initial approach should aim at stabilizing the patient with respiratory and hemodynamic support. In first half an hour cautious volume replacement in a patient with hypotension is crucial in one hand and on other hand volume overload my worsen RV function so concurrent use of vasopressor is suggested.[48] NOAC replaced VKA as anticoagulants and in cancer patients edoxaban and rivaroxaban is preferred over LMWH except in gastrointestinal cancer with PE. Thrombolysis is recommended for pregnant patients as NOAC is contraindicated in them. In hemodynamically unstable patient ECMO with surgical embolectomy or catheter directed treatment may be lifesaving. Clinical follow up done after 3–6 months of acute PE.

TABLE 2: Original and simplified Pulmonary Embolism Severity Index.

Parameter	Original version	Simplified version
Age	Age in year's	1 point (if age >80 years)
Male sex	+10 points	—
Cancer	+30 points	1 point
Chronic heart failure	+10 points	1 point
Chronic pulmonary disease	+10 points	1 point
Pulse rate ≥110 b.p.m.	+20 points	1 point
Systolic BP <100 mm Hg	+30 points	1 point
Respiratory rate >30 breaths per min	+20 points	—
Temperature <36°C	+20 points	—
Altered mental status	+60 points	—
Arterial oxyhaemoglobin saturation <90%	+20 points	1 point
Risk strata[a]		
	• Class I: ≤65 points very low 30 day mortality risk (0–1.6%) • Class II: ≤66–85 points low mortality risk (1.7–3.5%)	0 points = 30 day mortality risk 1.0% (95% CI 0.0–2.1%)
	• Class III: 86–105 points moderate mortality risk (3.2–7.1%) • Class IV: 106–125 points high mortality risk (4.0-11.4%) • Class V: >125 points very high mortality risk (10.0–24.5%)	≥1point(s) = 30 day mortality risk 10.9% (95% CI 8.5–13.2%)

(b.p.m.: beat per minute; BP: blood pressure; CI: confidence interval)
[a]Based on the sum of points.

BOX 1: Recommendations for prognostic assessment.

Recommendations
- Initial risk stratification of suspected or confirmed PE, based on the presence of hemodyonamic instability, is recommended to Identify patients at high risk of early mortality
- In patients without hemodynamic instability, further stratification of patients with acute PE into intermediate- and low-risk categories is recommended
- In patients without hemodynamic instability, use of clinical prediction rules integrating PE severity and comorbidity preferably the PESI or sPESI, should beconsidered for risk assessment in the acute phase of PE
- Assessment of the RV by imaging methods or laboratory biomarkers should be considered, even in the presence of a low PESI or a negative sPeSI
- In patients without hemodynamic instability, use of validated scores combining clinical, imaging, and laboratory PE-related prognostic factors may be considered to further stratify the severity of the acute PE episode

(PE: pulmonary embolism; PESI: pulmonary embolism severity index; RV: right ventricle; sPESI: simplified pulmonary embolism severity index)

Take Home Messages

- High clinical suspicion of PE despite its overlapping clinical features with other cardiac and pulmonary diseases from a clinician view point is needed in daily clinical practice that will help in early diagnosis and also categorizing them as low, intermediate and high risk groups.
- Subsequent checking of D-dimer and using other radiological techniques especially CTPA for early detection of PE is very important during golden hours of presentation.
- Treatment is supportive and definitive. Supportive treatment includes oxygen therapy, IV-fluids, vasopressors if needed besides NIV/IV support. Empiric anticoagulation with LMWH and NOAC is recommended. Thrombolytic therapy is for hemodynamically unstable patients following resuscitation.
- Decision for IVC filter placement should be judicious as IVC filter itself is a source of PE and will invite inadvertent events of recurrent PE.
- All patients with unprovoked PE should receive at least 3 months of anticoagulation (As per American college of clinical pharmacy guidelines). Risk benefit ratio should be assessed for extended therapy at the end of 3 months. Hence follow-up after 3 months of acute PE is crucial.

REFERENCES

1. Jameson JL, Fauci AS, Kasper DL, Hauser SL, Longo DL, Loscalzo J. Deep Venous Thrombosis and Pulmonary thromboembolism. In: Harrison's Principles of Internal Medicine, 20th edition. New York: McGraw-Hill Medical: New York; 2019. pp. 1911
2. Carson JL, Kelley MA, Duff A, Weg JG, Fulkerson WJ, Palevsky HI, et al. The clinical course of pulmonary embolism. N Eng J Med 1992; 326(19):1240-5.

3. Oullette, Daniel R. "Pulmonary embolism.eMedicine." Medscape.emedicine.medscape.com/article/300901-overview (2015).
4. Konstantinides SV, Meyer G, Becattini C, Bueno H, Geersing GJ, Harjola VP, et al. 2019 ESC Guidelines for the diagnosis and management of acute pulmonary embolism developed in collaboration with the European Respiratory Society (ERS). Eur Heart J. 2020;41(4):543-603.
5. Kakkar N, Vasishta RK. Pulmonary embolism in medical patients: an autopsy based study. Clin Appl Thromb Hemost. 2008;2:159-67.
6. Kamerkar DR, John MJ, Desai SC, Dsilva LC, Joglekar SJ. Arrive: A retrospective registry of Indian patients with venous thromboembolism. Indian J Crit Care Med. 2016;20(3):150-8.
7. Chaudhary N, Khan UH, Shah TH, Shaheen F, Mantoo S, Qadri SM, et al. Prevalence and predictors of pulmonary embolism in patients with acute exacerbation of chronic obstructive pulmonary disease. Lung India. 2021;38(6):533-9.
8. Wendelboe AM, Raskob GE. Global burden of thrombosis: epidemiologic aspects. Circ Res. 2016;118(9):1340-7.
9. Raskob GE, Angchaisuksiri P, Blanco AN, Buller H, Gallus A, Hunt BJ, et al. Thrombosis: a major contributor to global disease burden. Arterioscler Thromb Vasc Biol. 2014; 34(11):2363-71.
10. Horlander KT, Mannino DM, Leeper KV. Pulmonary embolism mortality in the United States, 1979-1998: an analysis using multiple-cause mortality data. Arch Intern Med. 2003;163(14):1711-7.
11. Morrone D, Morrone V. Acute pulmonary embolism: focus on the clinical Picture. Korean Circ J. 2018; 48(5): 365-81.
12. Stein PD, Henry JW. Clinical characteristics of patients with acute pulmonary embolism stratified according to their presenting syndromes. Chest. 1997;112:974-9.
13. Thames MD, Alpert JS, Dalen JE. Syncope in patients with pulmonary embolism. JAMA. 1977;238:2509-11.
14. Islam M, Filopei J, Frank M, Ramesh N, Verzosa S, Ehrlich M, et al. Pulmonary infarction secondary to pulmonary embolism: an evolving paradigm. Respirology. 2018:29577524.
15. Rodger M, Makropoulos D, Turek M, Quevillon J, Raymond F, Rasuli P, al. Diagnostic value of the electrocardiogram in suspected pulmonary embolism. Am J Cardiol. 2000;86(7):807-9, A10.
16. Worsley DF, Alavi A, Aronchick JM, Chen JT, Greenspan RH, Ravin CE. Chest radiographic findings in patients with acute pulmonary embolism: observations from the PIOPED Study. Radiology. 1993;189(1):133-6.
17. Kurnicka K, Lichodziejewska B, Goliszek S, Dzikowska-Diduch O, Zdończyk O, Kozłowska M, et al. Echocardiographic pattern of acute pulmonary embolism: analysis of 511 consecutive patients. J Am Soc Echocardiogr. 2016;29:907-13.
18. Kurzyna M, Torbicki A, Pruszczyk P, Burakowska B, Fijałkowska A, Kober J, et al. Disturbed right ventricular ejection pattern as a new Doppler echocardiographic sign of acute pulmonary embolism. Am J Cardiol. 2002;90:507-11.
19. Righini M, Goehring C, Bounameaux H, Perrier A. Effects of age on the performance of common diagnostic tests for pulmonary embolism. Am J Med. 2000;109:357-61.
20. Howick J, Cals JW, Jones C, Price CP, Plüddemann A, Heneghan C, et al. Current and future use of point-of-care tests in primary care: an international survey in Australia, Belgium, The Netherlands, the UK and the USA. BMJ Open. 2014;4:e005611
21. Kingma AEC, van Stel HF, Oudega R, Moons KGM, Geersing GJ. Multi-faceted implementation strategy to increase use of a clinical guideline for the diagnosis of deep venous thrombosis in primary care. Fam Pract. 2017;34:446-51.
22. Henzler T, Roeger S, Meyer M, Schoepf UJ, Nance JW Jr, Haghi D, et al. Pulmonary embolism: CT signs and cardiac biomarkers for predicting right ventricular dysfunction. Eur Respir J. 2012;39(4):919-26.
23. Horlander KT, Leeper KV. Troponin levels as a guide to treatment of pulmonary embolism. Curr Opin Pulm Med. 2003;9(5):374-7.
24. Qanadli SD, Hajjam ME, Mesurolle B, Barré O, Bruckert F, Joseph T, et al. Pulmonary embolism detection: prospective evaluation of dual-section helical CT versus selective pulmonary arteriography in 157 patients. Radiology. 2000;217:447-55.
25. Ghaye B, Szapiro D, Mastora I, Delannoy V, Duhamel A, Remy J, et al. Peripheral pulmonary arteries: how far in the lung does multi-detector row spiral CT allow analysis? Radiology. 2001;219(3):629-36.
26. Stein PD, Hull RD. Multidetector computed tomography for acute pulmonary embolism. N Engl J Med. 2006;354(22):2317-27.
27. Becattini C, Agnelli G, Vedovati MC, Pruszczyk P, Casazza F, Grifoni S, et al. Multidetector computed tomography for acute pulmonary embolism: diagnosis and risk stratification in a single test. Eur Heart J. 2011;32(13):1657-63.
28. Righini M, Le Gal G, Aujesky D, Roy PM, Sanchez O, Verschuren F, et al. Diagnosis of pulmonary embolism by multidetector CT alone or combined with venous ultrasonography of the leg: a randomised non-inferiority trial. Lancet. 2008;371:1343-52.
29. Reid JH, Coche EE, Inoue T, Kim EE, Dondi M, Watanabe N, et al. International Atomic Energy Agency Consultants' Group. Is the lung scan alive and well? Facts and controversies in defining the role of lung scintigraphy for the diagnosis of pulmonary embolism in the era of MDCT. Eur J Nucl Med Mol Imaging. 2009;36(3):505-21.
30. Glaser JE, Chamarthy M, Haramati LB, Esses D, Freeman LM. Successful and safe implementation of a trinary interpretation and reporting strategy for V/Q lung scintigraphy. J Nucl Med. 2011;52(10):1508-12.
31. Anderson DR, Kahn SR, Rodger MA, Kovacs MJ, Morris T, Hirsch A, et al. Computed tomographic pulmonary angiography vs ventilation-perfusion lung scanning in patients with suspected pulmonary embolism: a randomized controlled trial. JAMA. 2007;298(23):2743-53.
32. Perrier A, Bounameaux H. Ultrasonography of leg veins in patients suspected of having pulmonary embolism. Ann Intern Med. 1998;128:243.
33. Kearon C, Ginsberg JS, Hirsh J. The role of venous ultrasonography in the diagnosis of suspected deep venous thrombosis and pulmonary embolism. Ann Intern Med. 1998;129:1044-9.
34. Messika J, Goutorbe P, Hajage D, Ricard JD. Severe pulmonary embolism managed with high-flow nasal cannula oxygen therapy. Eur J Emerg Med. 2017;24:230-2.
35. Lacroix G, Pons F, D'Aranda E, Legodec J, Romanat PE, Goutorbe P. High-flow oxygen, a therapeutic bridge while awaiting thrombolysis in pulmonary embolism? Am J Emerg Med 2013;31:463.e1-2.

36. Cossette B, Pelletier ME, Carrier N, Turgeon M, Leclair C, Charron P, et al. Evaluation of bleeding risk in patients exposed to therapeutic unfractionated or low-molecular-weight heparin: a cohort study in the context of a quality improvement initiative. Ann Pharmacother. 2010;44:994-1002.
37. Büller HR, Davidson BL, Decousus H, Gallus A, Gent M, Piovella F, et al. Fondaparinux or enoxaparin for the initial treatment of symptomatic deep venous thrombosis: a randomized trial. Ann Intern Med. 2004;140:867-73.
38. Büller HR, Davidson BL, Decousus H, Gallus A, Gent M, Piovella F, et al. Subcutaneous fondaparinux versus intravenous unfractionated heparin in the initial treatment of pulmonary embolism. N Engl J Med. 2003;349:1695-702.
39. Robertson L, Jones LE. Fixed dose subcutaneous low molecular weight heparins versus adjusted dose unfractionated heparin for the initial treatment of venous thromboembolism. Cochrane Database Syst Rev. 2017;2:CD001100.
40. Agnelli G, Buller HR, Cohen A, Curto M, Gallus AS, Johnson M, et al. Oral apixaban for the treatment of acute venous thromboembolism. N Engl J Med. 2013;369:799-808.
41. EINSTEIN-PE Investigators; Büller HR, Prins MH, Lensin AW, Decousus H, Jacobson BF, Minar E, et al Oral rivaroxaban for the treatment of symptomatic pulmonary embolism. N Engl J Med. 2012;366:1287-97.
42. Schulman S, Kakkar AK, Goldhaber SZ, Schellong S, Eriksson H, Mismetti P, et al. Treatment of acute venous thromboembolism with dabigatran or warfarin and pooled analysis. Circulation. 2014;129:764-72.
43. Hokusai-VTE Investigators; Büller HR, Décousus H, Grosso MA, Mercuri M, Middeldorp S, Prins MH, et al. Edoxaban versus warfarin for the treatment of symptomatic venous thromboembolism. N Engl J Med. 2013;369:1406-15
44. Schulman S et al. Dabigatran versus warfarin in the treatment of acute venous thromboembolism. N Engl J Med. 2009;361:2342-52.
45. Schulman S, Kearon C, Kakkar AK, Mismetti P, Schellong S, Eriksson H, et al. Acenocoumarol and heparin compared with acenocoumarol alone in the initial treatment of proximal-vein thrombosis. N Engl J Med. 1992;327:1485-9.
46. Hull RD, Raskob GE, Rosenbloom D, Panju AA, Brill-Edwards P, Ginsberg JS, et al. Heparin for 5 days as compared with 10 days in the initial treatment of proximal venous thrombosis. N Engl J Med. 1990;322:1260-4.
47. Marti C, John G, Konstantinides S, Combescure C, Sanchez O, Lankeit M, et al. Systemic thrombolytic therapy for acute pulmonary embolism: a systematic review and meta-analysis. Eur Heart J 2015;36:605-14.
48. Ghignone M, Girling L, Prewitt RM. Volume expansion versus norepinephrine in treatment of a low cardiac output complicating an acute increase in right ventricular afterload in dogs. Anesthesiology. 1984; 60:132-5.

CHAPTER 11
Acute Exacerbation of Asthma

Sanjukta Dey

INTRODUCTION

Acute severe asthma is defined as asthma unresponsive to standard treatment, i.e., when the patient stops responding to multiple courses of beta-agonist therapy such as inhaled albuterol or salbutamol.[1]

It is one of the most common medical emergencies in clinical practice that requires immediate diagnosis and treatment.

Treatment should be instituted as early as possible and that includes oral, inhaled, and sometimes parenteral as need may be because the effects may take up to 6 and sometimes 12 hours.

CAUSE

- Upper respiratory infections
- Nonadherence to medication and improper use of inhalers
- Exposure nonsteroidal anti-inflammatory drug (NSAID) in aspirin-allergic patients
- Exposure to allergens like dog or cat dander (pet allergy)
- Inhalation of smoke, paint, fumes, mosquito repellants, pesticides, and occupational exposure
- Exercise, and also insufficient use of inhaled or oral corticosteroids.

HISTORY[1-8]

The patient history should be focused on concurring the diagnosis and the cause of the exacerbation by taking a quick and detailed history that will include:

- Detailed medication history
- Number of times the patients has visited accident and emergency (A&E) and hospitalizations
- Intensive treatment unit (ITU) admissions
- The frequent use of reliever drugs like salbutamol
- Night-time symptoms
- Exercise intolerance
- Smoking both active and passive
- Occupational exposure
- Pets and exposure to other allergens
- Significant family history
- Current medications
- Other coexistent conditions like allergic bronchopulmonary aspergillosis (ABPA)
- Significant medical conditions and comorbidities.

APPROACH TO A PATIENT WITH ACUTE SEVERE ASTHMA

It is important to do a quick and thorough examination and to pick up the warning signs. These include any evidence of critical obstruction such as use of accessory muscles, pulsus paradoxus inability to lie down, tachycardia, and diminished air entry and breath sounds. As subjective assessments of airway obstruction may vary with experience, it is important to have a more objective measure of airway obstruction. This can be done by using a peak flow meter, which measures the forced expiratory volume in 1 second (FEV1) and pulse oximetry. Saturations or pulse oximetry values >90% are less commonly associated with problems although this does not give an idea of CO_2 retention. Additionally peak expiratory flow rate (PEFR) values that are <25% of personal best or that are <25% of the peak flow using Wright's peak flow nomogram.

If we go by the Global Initiative for Asthma (GINA) guidelines then a patient with acute exacerbation of asthma can be divided into three broad headings.[1-7,9]

Mild or moderate exacerbation is defined as the patient being able to talk in phrases, prefers sitting not, lying not agitated, and has an increased respiratory rate. Accessory muscles of respiration are not used at this stage and in adults the pulse rate is between 100 and 120 bpm. O_2 saturation on air is 90–95% peak expiratory flow (PEF) >50% predicted or best.

Severe exacerbation on the other hand will be characterized by a patient able to talk in words (not phrases), agitated respiratory rate >30 breaths/minute and accessory muscles will be in use. Pulse rate will be raised and O_2

saturation in air will be <90%. PEF ≤50% predicted of best or less.

In Life-threatening asthma, the patient will be confused and drowsy and usually has what is known as a silent chest. Saturations will be <90% and the patient will be no situation to perform a peak flow.

■ BRITTLE ASTHMA[10]

This is a rare form of severe asthma where there is wide variability in peak flow that makes it difficult to predict acute decompensation and the attacks are usually severe and life-threatening.

In type 1 brittle asthma, it affects females usually between age 15 and 55 years. There is wide peak flow variability and usually there is food allergy and strong history of atopy. These patients have usually frequent hospital admissions.

In type 2 brittle asthma, there are acute attacks that need intensive care unit (ICU) admissions and even mechanical ventilation and these patients are at a risk of sudden death.

EARLY DIAGNOSIS AND APPROACH TO PATIENT[1,10,11]

It is to be noted that patients with acute severe asthma usually have severe respiratory distress that has developed over few hours and sometimes days. Frequently, these patients may have a previous history of mechanical ventilation, repeated visits to the A&E department and they usually have used of systemic corticosteroids, and have a history of severe allergies or anaphylaxis.

However it is important to remember that in young adults the first presentation of asthma could be an acute exacerbation.

If the physician fails to obtain a thorough history, it may hinder recognition of those patients who are prone to decompensations and acute exacerbations.

IMMEDIATE APPROACH TO PATIENT PRESENTING WITH ACUTE EXACERBATION OF ASTHMA[1,10,12]

Firstly, determine whether the patient has a severe asthma exacerbation with what is known as "silent chest" when there is no audible wheeze. This is due to severe airway obstruction and they are extremely tired and they are unable to generate enough airflow to wheeze. This is an ominous sign and is a precursor to impending respiratory failure.

■ PHYSICAL EXAMINATION[1,7,12]

Vitals
- Conscious or altered mental state
- Ability to speak, in sentences or unable to speak at all
- Presence of tachypnea
- Tachycardia
- Saturations
- Significant wheezing
- Blood pressure (BP) normally, between inspiration and expiration the difference in systolic blood will not exceed 15 mm Hg. However in patients with severe asthma, the difference in systolic blood pressure (SBP) between expiration and inspiration is higher with a difference of >25 mm Hg usually indicating severe airway obstruction.
- Initially, wheezing is heard only during expiration, but wheezing later occurs during expiration and inspiration.
- Patients ability to perform the peak flow (PEFR) and if there is a best documented peak flow for the patient, then the decrease in peak flow can establish severity of the attack.

Chest
- Hyperexpanded
- Use of accessory muscles of respiration leading to classic features of the tracheal tug and subcostal intercostal recession due to overuse of sternocleidomastoid, scalene, and intercostal
- Wheeze or the absence of wheeze, which may indicate severe airflow obstruction and if untreated the prolonged airflow obstruction may lead to bradycardia and also cardiorespiratory arrest.

Higher Mental Function

The patients mental state can give an idea of the severity of the situation; a patient may be irritable, agitated, and this can progress to lethargy and unresponsiveness and in severe cases of hypoxia may even lead to seizures and coma.

In cases where the airway obstruction is prolonged and increase in respiratory effort may eventually lead to fatigue, and terminally result in bradycardia, and cardiorespiratory arrest.

So patient with severe untreated asthma who is unresponsive and has bradycardia and decreased air entry leading to decreased wheeze is a candidate for immediate ITU admission.

■ STAGING

Acute severe asthma may be divided into stages based on arterial blood gas (ABG) progressions.

Patients in stage 1 or 2 can be hospitalized, guided by other issues including comorbidities, history of progression to severe acute asthma rapidly, and if they are brittle asthmatics.

The use of PEF values or FEV1 after treatment (>50% but <70% of predicted values) can also guide the need for admission.

Patients with ABG determinations characteristic of stages 3 and 4 require admission to an ICU. The PEF value or FEV1 is <50% of the predicted value after treatment.

Stage 1 (Mild)
- Hyperventilation
- Normal partial pressure of oxygen (PO_2)

In case these patients have been hospitalized, they may be given ipratropium treatment via a nebulizer in the emergency setting in addition to beta-agonists, but these are preferably stopped after 24–48 hours to prevent drying up of secretions **(Flowcharts 1 and 2)**.

Stage 2 (Moderate)
- Hypoxemia
- Hyperventilation

Usually these patients can be discharged from the hospital after adequate bronchodilator treatment, but they require systemic corticosteroids. **Table 1** shows commonly used corticosteroids in asthma.

Stage 3 (Severe)
- Hypoxemia
- Normal partial pressure of carbon dioxide (PCO_2) due to respiratory muscle fatigue which is a very serious sign

This is generally an indication for electively intubating the patient and for mechanical ventilation, keeping in mind that in asthma mechanical ventilation will also entail maintaining some degree of permissive hypercapnia.

Treatment will include intravenous corticosteroids, continued, sometimes hourly use of an inhaled beta-2-adrenergic bronchodilator, and where available intravenous (IV) salbutamol. These patients may benefit from magnesium sulfate as well.

Stage 4 (Severe and life-threatening)
- Hypoxemia
- Hypercapnia
- Hypoventilation with fatigue
- Possible silent chest

These patients have <20% of predicted PEFR though technically they will be unable to perform a PEFR or FEV1 and they will urgently require intubation and mechanical ventilation **(Flowchart 3)**.

Patients in stage 4 need admission to an ICU facility. Inhaled beta-2-agonists and anticholinergics need to be given via mechanical ventilator tubing along with parenteral corticosteroids, IV salbutamol, or magnesium sulfate **(Flowcharts 1 and 2)**.

■ DIFFERENTIAL DIAGNOSES[13,14]
- Allergic bronchopulmonary aspergillosis
- Aspiration syndromes
- Bronchiectasis
- Bronchiolitis
- Bronchiolitis obliterans
- Chronic bronchitis
- Chronic obstructive pulmonary disease (COPD)
- Eosinophilic granulomatosis with polyangiitis (Churg-Strauss syndrome)
- Croup
- Cystic fibrosis
- Emphysema
- Foreign bodies of the airway
- Gastroesophageal reflux disease
- Heart failure
- Idiopathic pulmonary arterial hypertension
- Inhalation injury
- Pulmonary artery sling
- Vocal cord dysfunction.

■ TREATMENT: OVERVIEW[1,10,13,15,16]
After confirming the diagnosis and assessing the severity of an asthma attack, direct treatment toward controlling bronchoconstriction and inflammation.
- Inhaled beta-agonists,
- Parenteral and corticosteroids
- Magnesium sulfate
- Theophylline group of medication.

Stepwise Asthma Management[1,9,10] (Flowcharts 1 to 3)
- *Fluid management*:
    - Hydration, with IV normal saline and added potassium as needed
    - Send Na^+, K^+, and phosphate if facilities are available
    - Hypokalemia is common and may result from either corticosteroid use or beta-agonist use as alkalosis drives potassium into cells and correcting hypokalemia may help to wean an intubated patient with asthma from ventilation.
- Hypophosphatemia may result from poor oral intake; it has to be corrected adequately to ensure recovery and prevent failure of extubation
    - *Antibiotics:*[1,12,14] The administration of empiric antibiotics routinely is not recommended unless there is reason to suspect associated or secondary infection such as pneumonia and chronic sinusitis
- *Oxygen monitoring and therapy:*[1,12,13]
    - Monitor saturations
    - Regular ABGs as needed and an arterial line is needed
    - Oxygen saturation may increase following the use of bronchodilators secondary to an increase in V/Q mismatch.
    - O_2 therapy is essential in all cases of acute severe asthma.

Flowchart 1: Rapid primary assessment of acute asthma in adults.

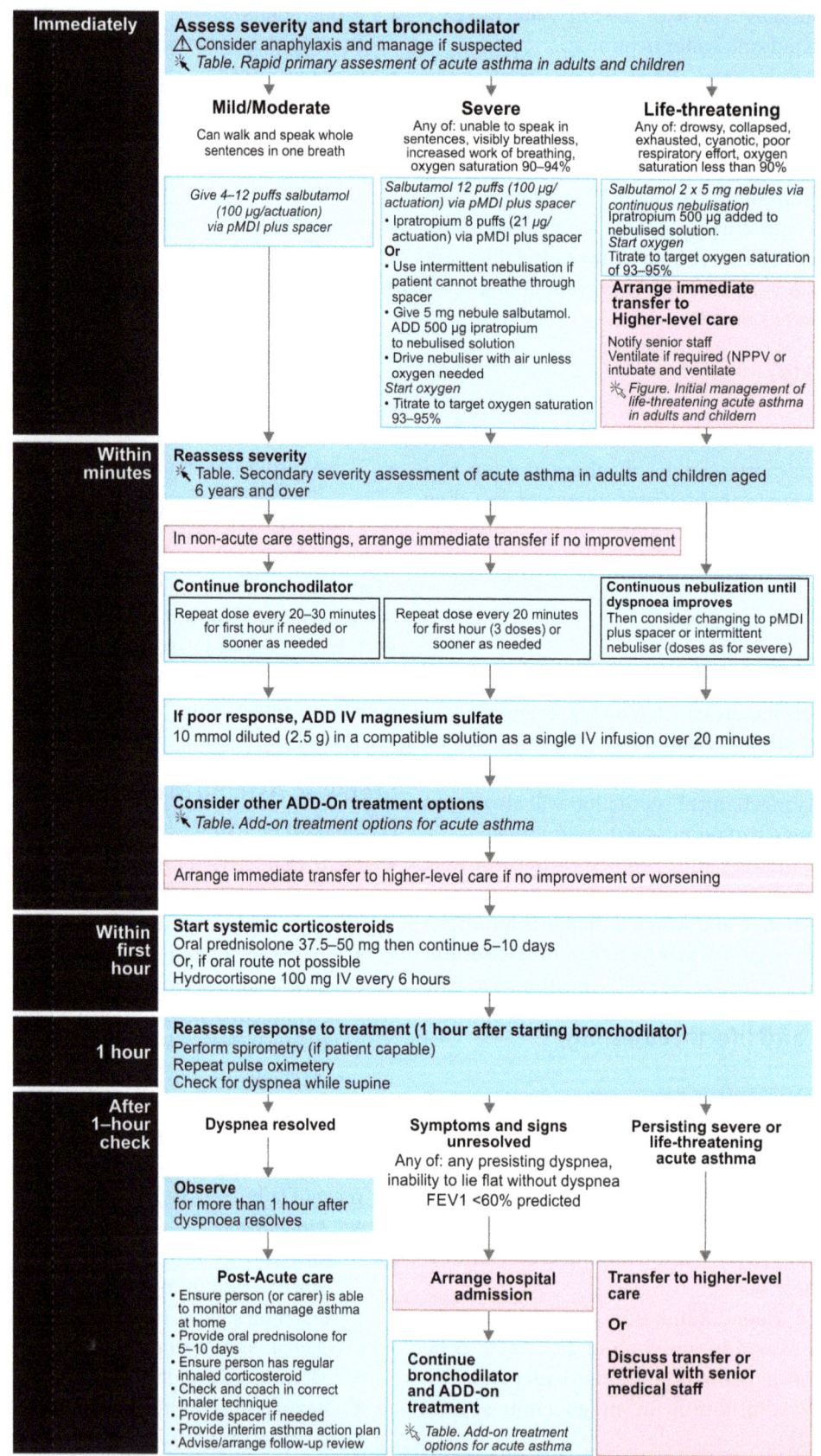

(FEV1: forced expiratory volume in 1 second; IV: intravenous; pMDI: pressurized metered dose inhaler)
Source: Australian Asthma Handbook Quick Reference Guide. asthmahandbook.org.au

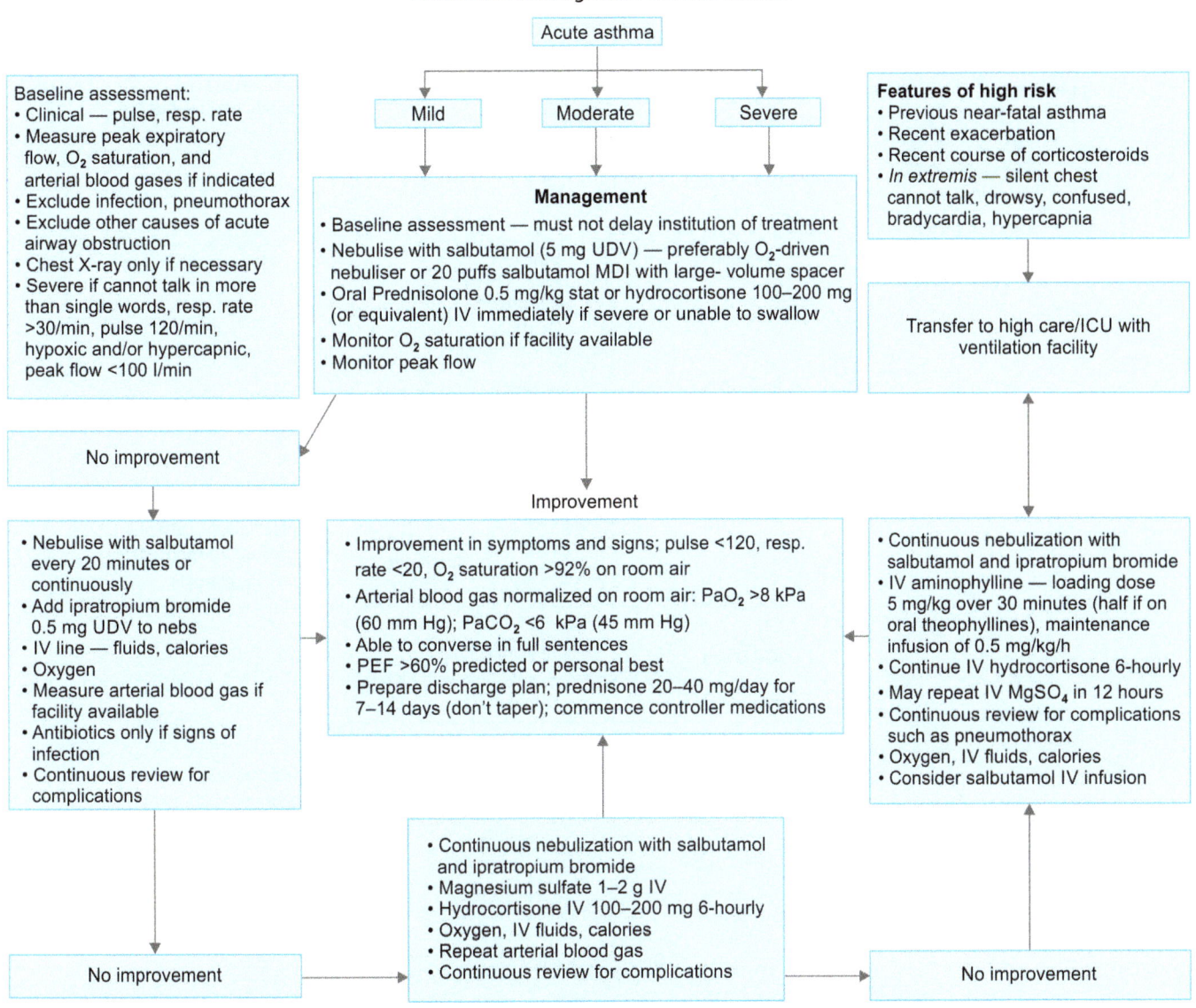

Flowchart 2: Management of acute asthma.

(ICU: intensive care unit; IV: intravenous; PaCO$_2$: partial pressure of carbon dioxide in arterial blood; PEF: peak expiratory flow; UDV: unit dose vial)
Source: Adopted from Management of Acute Severe Asthma in Adults in A & E: Form BTS Guidelines Thorax 2007

TABLE 1: Comparison of commonly used corticosteroids used in asthma.

Prescription	Potency relative to hydrocortisone	Relative sodium retention	Biological half-life (h)
Hydrocortisone	1	1	8–12
Prednisone/prednisolone	4	0.8	12–36
Methylprednisolone	5	0.5	12–36
Dexamethasone	25	0	36–72

Source: Alangari AA. Corticosteroids in the treatment of acute asthma. Ann Thorac Med. 2014;9(4):187-92.

- This can be administered via a nasal cannula or mask, although patients with dyspnea often do not like masks.
- Aim to maintain the patient's oxygen saturation above 92% (>95% in pregnant patients or those with cardiac disease).
- For significantly low saturations nonrebreathing masks (NRBMs) may be used and they deliver as much as 98% oxygen.
- Bilevel positive airway pressure (BiPAP) as a modality for acute exacerbation is useful in situations where patient is still able to generate enough tidal volume.

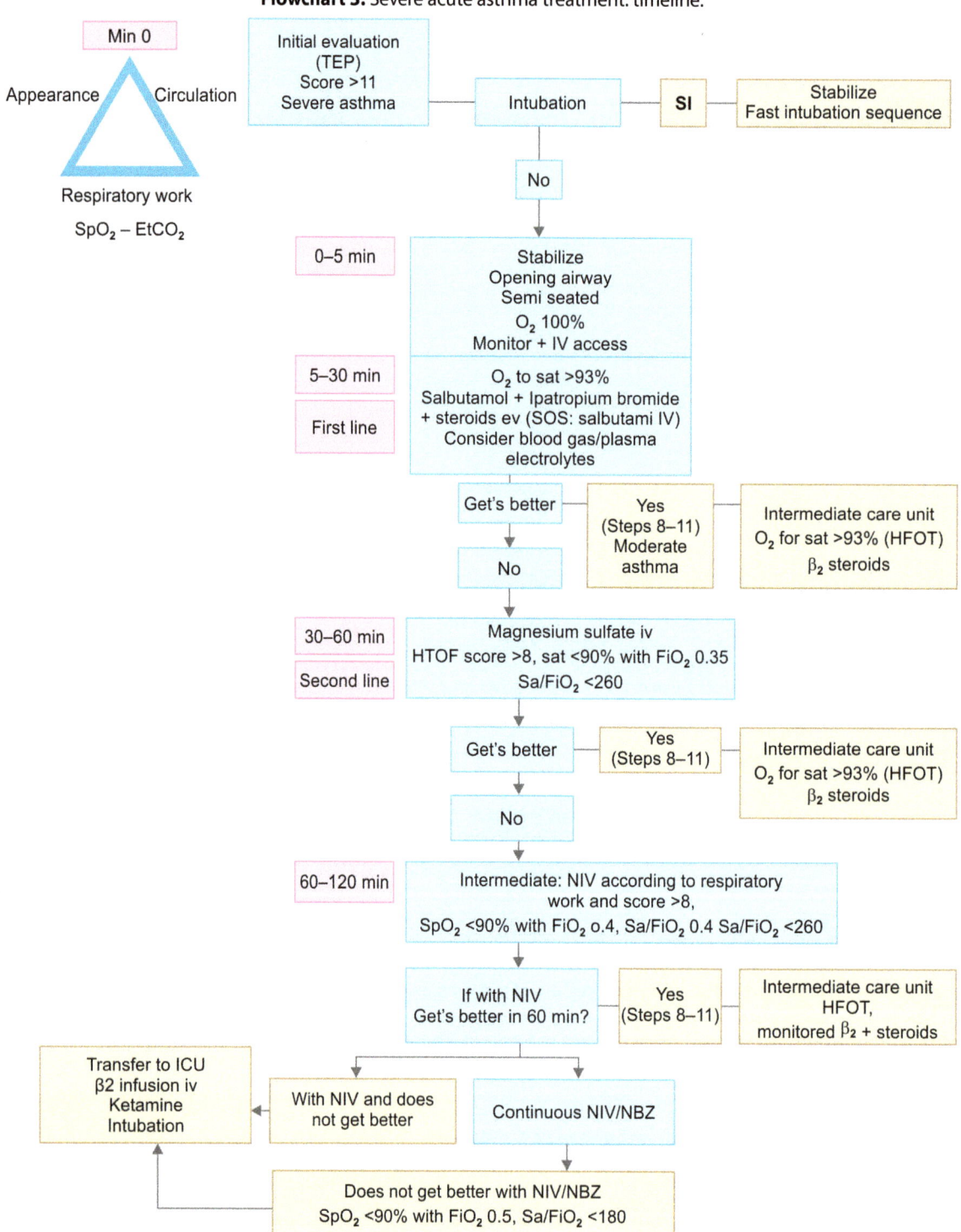

Flowchart 3: Severe acute asthma treatment: timeline.

(EtCO$_2$: end-tidal CO$_2$; FiO$_2$: fraction of inspired oxygen; HFOT: high flow oxygen therapy; ICU: intensive care unit; NBZ: nebulization; NIV: noninvasive ventilation; SpO$_2$: oxygen saturation)
Adopted from: British Guideline on the Management of Asthma sign 158: Revised July 2019

- If patients not improving with the above modalities ultimately intubation may be needed.
- *Steroids:*[1,10,14,17-19]
  - Systemic corticosteroids are the mainstay of treatment of acute exacerbation of asthma in emergency settings.
- All asthma guidelines such as GINA and Expert Panel Report 3 (EPR3) recommend this as they reduce hospitalizations

Dose of systemic steroids in asthma:
  - There is no added benefit from systemic corticosteroids when given at doses above

60–80 mg/day or 2 mg/kg/day in terms of lung function, reduction in rate of admission, or length of hospital stay.
- Studies have compared 1–6 mg/kg/day methylprednisolone in adults hospitalized with severe acute asthma dose over the low dose and found no difference between the different doses.
- Studies surprisingly also showed no difference in the efficacy or onset of action between oral and IV administration and this is especially important in treating asthma on an outpatient department (OPD) basis.
- When adults with severe acute asthma were treated with either IV hydrocortisone or prednisolone it was found that there was no difference in their peak flow measurements 24 hours after admission. In children also, oral prednisolone was found equivalent to IV methylprednisolone and IV hydrocortisone in regards to patients' length of hospital stay.
- Overall oral treatment was more cost-effective and this is particularly true for a country like India.
- The GINA guidelines prefer oral administration because it is less invasive except in patients with absorption problems or those who are not able to take orally due to the severity of their respiratory distress or because they are vomiting.

- *Magnesium sulfate:*[1,20,21]
  - Patients with an acute asthma exacerbation who have not responded to first-line therapy which includes bronchodilators and corticosteroids can also be treated effectively with intravenous magnesium sulfate which has shown benefits in both adults and children.
  - In studies done in children, magnesium sulfate reduced hospital admissions by 68%, based on a meta-analysis of three small randomized controlled trials (RCTs). In adults, magnesium sulfate reduced admissions by 25%.
  - A 2016 Cochrane review of three RCTs in children with acute severe asthma between 18 months and 18 years founds that treatment with intravenous magnesium sulfate reduced the odds of hospital admissions by 68%. Initially magnesium sulfate was given if inhaled short-acting bronchodilators and corticosteroids were ineffective in these children. Dosing was not standardized, but most studies used weight-based dosing according to guidelines from the British National Formulary for Children, which advises 40 mg/kg of body weight, up to a maximal dose of 2 g per day to be given as intravenous infusion over 20 minutes.
  - In case of adults, a 2014 Cochrane review of 14 RCTs founds a 25% reduction in hospital admissions in adults who were treated with intravenous magnesium sulfate for asthma exacerbation.
  - The most common adverse effects of intravenous magnesium sulfate were dose-related skin flushing hypotension and vasodilation when infusion rate was quicker
- *Chest tube placement:*[1,10,14,15] In patients of asthma complicated by pneumothorax chest tube may be needed.
- *Leukotriene modifiers:*[1] Leukotriene modifiers like montelukast are useful for treating chronic asthma but not acute asthma.
- *ICU admission criteria:*[1,3,7] Indications for ICU admission include the following:
  - Confusion and drowsiness including agitation
  - Markedly decreased air entry and disappearance of wheeze
  - Increasing PCO_2
  - Presence of other high-risk factors
  - Poor improvement despite adequate treatment
- Anesthesia support is needed if inhaled anesthetic agents are considered for refractory cases.
- Extracorporeal membrane oxygenation (ECMO) and extracorporeal membrane oxygenation can be considered after all modalities have failed and this requires special attention and should take place at an established ECMO center.

Take Home Messages

- In Acute Asthma Management Time is the essence.
- Peak flow monitoring at home may predict a severe exacerbation.
- Though bronchodilators and steroids remain the mainstay of asthma therapy IV magnesium sulfate may decrease ITU admissions and ITU stay.

REFERENCES

1. Global Initiative for Asthma. (2012). Global Strategy for Asthma Management and Prevention. [online] Available from https://ginasthma.org/wp-content/uploads/2019/01/2012-GINA.pdf. [Last accessed January, 2023].
2. Subbarao P, Mandhane PJ, Sears MR. Asthma: Epidemiology, etiology and risk factors. CMAJ. 2009;181:E181-90.
3. Grainge CL, Lau LC, Ward JA, Dulay V, Lahiff G, Wilson S, et al. Effect of bronchoconstriction on airway remodeling in asthma. N Engl J Med. 2011;364:2006-15.
4. Bergeron C, Al-Ramli W, Hamid Q. Remodeling in asthma. Proc Am Thorac Soc. 2009;6:301-5.
5. Holgate ST. Pathogenesis of asthma. Clin Exp Allergy. 2008;38:872-97.
6. Jackson DJ, Sykes A, Mallia P, Johnston SL. Asthma exacerbations: Origin, effect, and prevention. J Allergy Clin Immunol. 2011;128:1165-74.
7. Khetsuriani N, Kazerouni NN, Erdman DD, Lu X, Redd SC, Anderson LJ, et al. Prevalence of viral respiratory tract

7. infections in children with asthma. J Allergy Clin Immunol. 2007;119:314-21.
8. Gern JE, Busse WW. Relationship of viral infections to wheezing illnesses and asthma. Nat Rev Immunol. 2002;2:132-8.
9. Green RM, Custovic A, Sanderson G, Hunter J, Johnston SL, Woodcock A. Synergism between allergens and viruses and risk of hospital admission with asthma: Case-control study. BMJ. 2002;324:763.
10. National Asthma Education and Prevention Program. Expert Panel Report 3 (EPR-3): Guidelines for the Diagnosis and Management of Asthma—Summary Report 2007. J Allergy Clin Immunol. 120:S94-138.
11. Fuhlbrigge A, Peden D, Apter AJ, Boushey HA, Camargo CA Jr, Gern J, et al. Asthma outcomes: Exacerbations. J Allergy Clin Immunol. 2012;129:S34-48.
12. Moore WC, Bleecker ER, Curran-Everett D, Erzurum SC, Ameredes BT, Bacharier L, et al. Characterization of the severe asthma phenotype by the National Heart, Lung, and Blood Institute's Severe Asthma Research Program. J Allergy Clin Immunol. 2007;119:405-13.
13. Pollack CV Jr, Pollack ES, Baren JM, Smith SR, Woodruff PG, Clark S, et al. A prospective multicenter study of patient factors associated with hospital admission from the emergency department among children with acute asthma. Arch Pediatr Adolesc Med. 2002;156:934-40.
14. Rabe KF, Vermeire PA, Soriano JB, Maier WC. Clinical management of asthma in 1999: The asthma insights and reality in Europe (AIRE) study. Eur Respir J. 2000;16:802-7.
15. Alangari AA, Malhis N, Mubasher M, Al-Ghamedi N, Al-Tannir M, Riaz M, et al. Budesonide nebulization added to systemic prednisolone in the treatment of acute asthma in children: Double-Blind, randomized, controlled trial. Chest. 2014;145:772-8.
16. Adams JY, Sutter ME, Albertson TE. The patient with asthma in the emergency department. Clin Rev Allergy Immunol. 2012;43:14-29.
17. Camargo CA Jr, Spooner CH, Rowe BH. Continuous versus intermittent beta-agonists in the treatment of acute asthma. Cochrane Database Syst Rev. 2003;2003:CD001115.
18. Rowe BH, Edmonds ML, Spooner CH, Diner B, Camargo CA Jr. Corticosteroid therapy for acute asthma. Respir Med. 2004;98:275-84.
19. Rodrigo GJ, Castro-Rodriguez JA. Anticholinergics in the treatment of children and adults with acute asthma: a systematic review with meta-analysis. Thorax. 2005;60:740-6.
20. Alangari AA. Corticosteroids in the treatment of acute asthma. Ann Thorac Med. 2014;9(4):187-92.
21. Kokotajilo S, Degnan L, Meyers R, Siu A, Robinson C. Use of intravenous magnesium sulfate for the treatment of acute asthma exacerbation in pediatric patient. J Pediatr Pharmacol Ther. 2014;19(2)91-7.

SECTION 3
Neurological Emergencies

Section Editor: Goutam Gangopadhyay

12. **Approach to an Unconscious Patient**
    Chintha Venkata Sriram, Goutam Gangopadhyay

13. **Status Epilepticus**
    Haseeb Hassan

14. **Stroke**
    Shankha Shubhra Chaudhuri

15. **Acute Meningitis**
    Jasodhara Chaudhuri

16. **Acute Encephalitis**
    Arka Prava Chakraborty, Souvik Dubey

17. **Acute Migraine**
    Adreesh Mukherjee

CHAPTER 12: Approach to an Unconscious Patient

Chintha Venkata Sriram, Goutam Gangopadhyay

INTRODUCTION

First and foremost thing in the approach of an unconscious person is to determine if he is unresponsive or unconscious. The approach to an unresponsive person with feeble pulse or absent pulse and absent or abnormal respiration (gasping) has already been well-defined by the basic life support (BLS) protocols of the American Heart Association (AHA). In this chapter, we will discuss a practical approach to assess an unconscious person at a hospital setup.

TERMINOLOGY

Consciousness

Consciousness is a state of being fully aware of oneself and their interaction with surroundings. It is primarily composed of two parts: (1) content, and (2) arousal (level of consciousness). **Table 1** content is the culmination of all cerebral cortex activities, both cognitive and affective responses. Ascending arousal system, which consists of numerous ascending pathways arising in the mesopontine tegmentum, regulates arousal **(Table 2)**. Every level it traverses on its path to the basal forebrain, thalamus, (Relay centergates information diffusely to brain networks) and cerebral cortex it is enhanced by additional inputs.[1]

We hereby classify various disorders of consciousness **(Table 3)**. Clinically, the level of consciousness at bedside is determined by the response of a patient to the examiner. Some patients even with a preserved level of consciousness may be unresponsive during examination which may be caused by a sensory or motor impairment or a psychiatric disorder. Locked-in syndrome is a very good example of this. It is characterised by quadriplegia and anarthria with preservation of consciousness, loss of horizontal eye movement, preserved vertical eye movement and affected attention, execution in some cases.

When it comes to describing consciousness, we often hear usage of multiple terms such as coma, stupor, etc.

DEFINITIONS OF SOME IMPORTANT TERMINOLOGY

Clouding

A minimally diminished level of awareness or wakefulness is known as clouding of consciousness. It includes hyperexcitability and irritability alternating with drowsiness.

Obtundation

Obtundation literally means mental blunting or torpidity.[1] A mild to moderate decline in attentiveness and decreased interest in the environment are observed. Additionally,

TABLE 1: Features of content and level of consciousness.

	Content	Level of Consciousness
Features	• All cognitive functions, emotions • Intuitions of the brain	• Global alertness • Behavioral responsivity
Disorders	Dementia	• Clouding • Obtundation • Stupor • Coma

TABLE 2: Anatomy of consciousness.

Ascending reticular activating system (ARAS)	• Mid brain • Upper pons	• Arousal • Vigilance • Wakefulness
Diencephalon	• Thalamus • Hypothalamus	
Cerebral cortex		Awareness (Self, environment)

TABLE 3: Terms used to describe disorders of consciousness.

Acute	Subacute/chronic
Clouding	Abulic
Obtundation	Akinetic mutism
Stupor	
Coma	• Minimal consciousness • Vegetative
Delirium	Brain death
Locked-in syndrome	

these individuals respond more slowly to stimulation, have increased number of sleep hours, and may feel sleepy in between sleep sessions.

Stupor

Stupor is a state of deep sleep or equivalent behavioral unresponsiveness from which the person can only be awakened by vigorous and constant stimulation.[1] Even with maximal arousal, the level of cognitive function does not improve or may be impaired.

Coma

Coma[1] is a state of unresponsiveness in which even with strong stimulation, the patient remains unresponsive and lies with eyes closed **(Flowchart 1)**. Patient can grimace in response to painful stimuli and limbs may demonstrate stereotyped withdrawal responses, but the patient does not make localizing responses or discrete defensive movements. As coma deepens, patient's responsiveness even to painful stimuli may diminish or disappear.

■ ASSESSMENT

We provide a systematic and a comprehensive approach in the assessment of an unconscious person presenting to an emergency room. The important steps of assessment are shown in **Flowchart 2**.

Screening history and examination should be completed within first 5–10 minutes of patient arrival at the hospital without any delay. Treatment of cause can be done once it is found (Example- Hypoglycemia treated immediately) at any point/step of assessment.

Step 1: Screening History

A very brief history of the antecedent events or the presenting complaint is the best approach to begin with **(Table 4)**. This usually gives us a clue to proceed further.

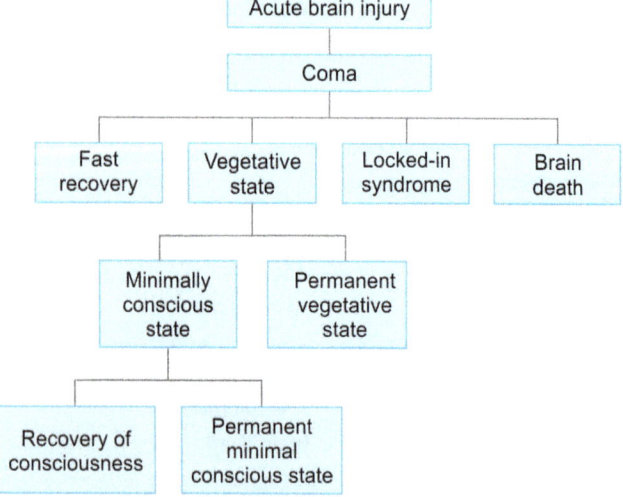

Flowchart 1: Consciousness states after coma.

Step 2: Screening Examination

A systematic screening helps effectively to arrive at an early diagnosis and for further management. All the abnormalities mentioned in **Table 5** can be caused by neurological causes as well but all other causes have to be ruled out before labeling the cause of unconsciousness as neurological.

General assessment includes a quick complete scan of the body (mainly inspection, palpation only when required to not waste any time at this point) to look or pick up for any signs that could indicate the clue to the diagnosis. For Head injury, Black eye, Bruises over the back, Frothing from mouth, Attitude of the limbs (Fracture), Torn clothes, bite marks over the leg can indicate an unknown bite.

Unknown bites are very common in India. Suraweera et al. estimated that India had 1.2 million snakebite deaths

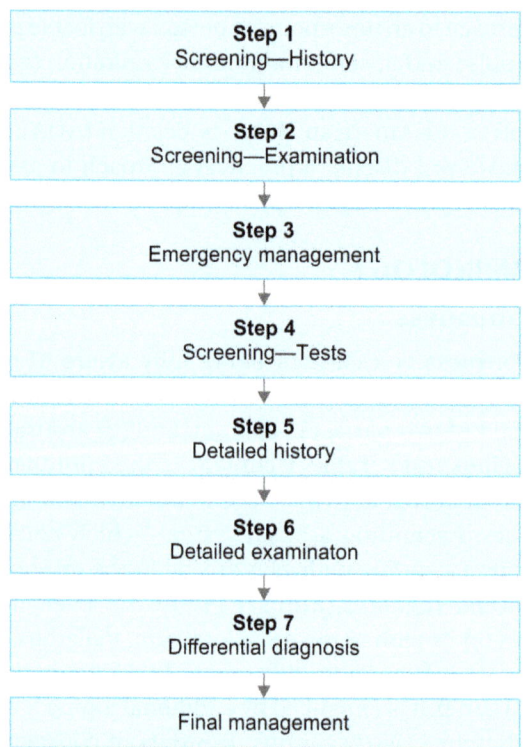

Flowchart 2: Steps of assessment.

TABLE 4: Important history.	
1.	Trauma
2.	Drug history
3.	Toxin/poison consumption or exposure
4.	Bite
5.	*Cardiac history:* Hypertension, arrhythmia pacemaker
6.	Lung disease history—Chronic obstructive pulmonary disease, Pulmonary embolism, neuro muscular disorder, pneumonia
7.	Stroke, Seizure
8.	Infections
9.	Metabolic history—Diabetes mellitus, thyroid disorder

CHAPTER 12: Approach to an Unconscious Patient

TABLE 5: Screening examination.

Parameter	Important causes	
General Assessment	General attitude	Decerebrate, decorticate, opisthotonus, color of skin
	Face	Ptosis, facial palsy, injuries
	Thorax	Any gross abnormalities, trauma
	Abdomen	
	Back	
	Limbs	Injection marks, bite, skin lesions
Smell	Unknown compounds	Explained below
Pulse	Bradycardia	Cardiac, drugs, toxins
	Tachycardia	Fever, drugs
Blood pressure	Hypotension	Cardiac, infectious, drug
	Hypertension	Primary/Secondary
Respiratory rate and Pattern	Tachypnea	Hypoxia, hypercapnia, etc.
	Bradypnea	Metabolic, toxins
Temperature	Hyperthermia	Infectious, inflammatory
	Hypothermia	Metabolic, environmental
SPO₂	Hypoxia	Respiratory, cardiac
Pupils	Constricted	Organophosphate (OP) compounds, drugs
	Dilated	Drugs
Score	Glasgow Coma Scale (GCS)	

TABLE 6: Different odours and their causes.

Odor	Some important conditions[3]
Garlic	Organophosphorus, arsenic, thallium
Bitter almond	Cyanide
Rotten apple/Acetone like	Diabetic ketoacidosis
Urine	Uremia
Amine	Hepatic encephalopathy
Malodor	Fetor hepaticus

TABLE 7: Abnormal patterns of respiration.

	Type of breathing	CNS causes[7]
1.	Cheyne-Stokes respiration	Widespread forebrain damage
2.	Central neurogenic hyperventilation	Lesions of low midbrain ventral to aqueduct of Sylvius and of upper pons ventral to the fourth ventricle
3.	Apneustic breathing	Dorsolateral tegmental lesion of middle and caudal pons
4.	Cluster breathing	*Lower pons:* Tegmental lesion
5.	Ataxic breathing	Lesion of the reticular formation of the dorsomedial part of the medulla

TABLE 8: GCS

Behaviour	Response	Score
Eye opening response	Spontaneously	4
	To speech	3
	To pain	2
	No response	1
Best verbal response	Oriented to time, place and person	5
	Confused	4
	Inappropriate words	3
	Incomprehensible sounds	2
	No response	1
Best motor response	Obeys commands	6
	Moves to localized pain	5
	Flexion withdrawal from pain	4
	Abnormal flexion (Decorticate)	3
	Abnormal extension (Decerebrate)	2
	No response	1

TABLE 9: Glasgow Coma scale (GCS) (Severity).

GCS score	Severity of brain injury
≥13	Mild
9–12	Moderate
≤8	Severe

TABLE 10A: Scales/scores other than Glasgow Coma Scale (GCS).

ACDU	**A**lert, **C**onfused, **D**rowsy, **U**nresponsive
AVPU	**A**lert, **R**esponse To **V**oice, Response To **P**ain, **U**nresponsive
FOUR SCORE COMA	• Eye response • Motor response • Brainstem reflexes • Respiration

(average 58,000/year) from 2000 to 2019,[2] so identifying a patient with a bite is very vital. Every female patient should be screened in the presence of a female attendant. Medico legal case has to be filed when in doubt (Especially doubtful history, No relative/ attendant available, rape).

Smell is not considered as a usual diagnostic tool but can be very helpful if the findings can be correlated **(Table 5 and 6)**.

Respiratory pattern and its abnormalities have been explained in **Table 7**. Teasdale and Jennett's devised the Glasgow Coma scale (*GCS*) **(Table 8 and 9)**, to categorize patients with head trauma.[6]

The GCS is scored between 3 and 15, 3 being the worst and 15 the best. It is composed of three parameters.[1]

Scale gives more neurologic detail than the GCS. However, no scale has been guidelined as a standard for a patient of unconsciousness. We advocate the use of GCS as standard for all unconscious patients irrespective of head injury.

Some important scores/scales are discussed in **Table 10A**.

ACDU and *AVPU* scales are simpler, easier and are as accurate as GCS.[5] The ACDU scale seems to be more effective at spotting early level of consciousness decline.[1]

Pupils

Examination[6] will be discussed in detail in the CNS examination section.

Step 3: Emergency Management

This can be followed similar to the AHA guidelines of BLS and advanced cardiac life support (ACLS). Airway, breathing, and circulation to be stabilized at the earliest **(Flowchart 3)**. Don't give feeding orally to an unconscious patient. Care should be taken to prevent tongue fall. Foley's catheterization and Ryles tube insertion can be done if required at this moment. Most of the cases who feign of unconsciousness will resist/become conscious on Ryle's tube or Foley's insertion.

Step 4: Screening Tests

Capillary blood glucose (CBG) should be the first and foremost test to be done in a patient presenting in an unconscious state to rule out hypoglycemia which is an easily treatable reversible cause. Prevalence of severe hypoglycemia among type 1 diabetics was reported to be around 35%.[8] Severe hypoglycemia was reported by 41.8% of all respondents, at an average rate of 2.5 events per person-year according to the InHypo-DM Study, Canada.[9]

Electrocardiogram (ECG) is the next investigation which can be done to rule out myocardial infarction, AV block, other as well. Arterial blood gas (ABG) is a resource which can be utilized when available in higher settings which can give valuable information regarding the blood gas analysis (hypoxia, poisoning) electrolytes, acid base, and lactate levels. Some additional tests such as blood ketones and bedside 2D echocardiography (ECHO) can be performed if required **(Table 10B)**.

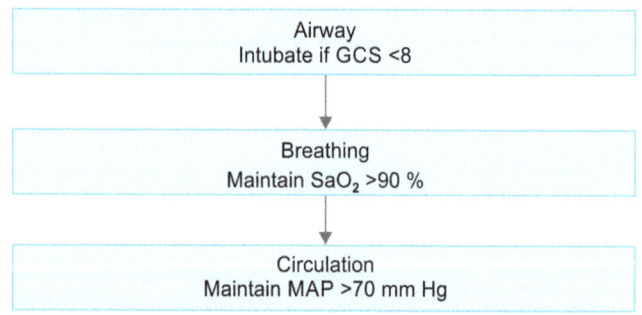

Flowchart 3: Airway management.

TABLE 10B: Screening tests.

	Test	If required
1.	Capillary blood glucose (CBG)	Blood ketone
2.	Electrocardiogram	ECHO
3.	Arterial blood gas (ABG)	FAST (Focused assessment with sonography in trauma)
4.	–	POCUS (Point of care ultrasonography)

Step 5: Detailed History

A detailed history has to be taken from the family/bystanders/attendants who brought the patient once the patient is stabilized. Some important history and their probable etiology have been explained in **(Table 11 to 13)**.

- *Occupation history:* Farmers—OP compound exposure, snake and unknown bites; forest rangers—unknown bites, insects.
- *Comorbidities history:* Diabetes mellitus, hypertension, thyroid disorder, COPD, arrhythmia, renal failure.
- *Drug and exposure history:* Medication history, drug abuse history, any toxin exposure, poisoning has to be

TABLE 11: Neurological and non-neurological symptoms.

Non-neurological	
Antecedent symptoms	Probable etiology
Chest pain	Myocardial infarction aortic dissection
Shortness of breath	Hypoxia induced
Nausea, vomiting	Poisoning
Syncope	Cardiac
Neurological	
Antecedent symptoms	Probable etiology
Thunderclap headache	SAH
Vertigo, vomiting	Posterior circulation stroke
Neck stiffness	Meningoencephalitis
Altered sensorium	
Convulsive movements	Seizure
Incontinence of bowel and bladder	
Hemiparesis	Cerebrovascular accident
Syncope	Neurological

TABLE 12: Neurological and non-neurological causes.

Antecedent symptoms	Probable etiology
Neurological	
Thunderclap Headache	SAH
Vertigo, Vomiting	Posterior circulation stroke
Neck stiffness	Meningoencephalitis
Altered Sensorium	
Convulsive movements	Seizure
Incontinence of bowel and bladder	
Hemiparesis	Cerebro vascular accident
Syncope	Neurological
Non-neurological	
Chest pain	Myocardial infarction
Aortic Dissection	
Shortness of Breath	Hypoxia induced
Nausea, Vomiting	Poisoning
Syncope	Cardiac

asked. In suspicious cases where the cause cannot be ascertained medication history in the family (suspect medication overdose), the environment where the patient stayed last or was found unconscious (suspect unknown bite/foul play/environmental exposure).
- *Family history:* Common exposure to toxin, inheritable diseases
- *Immunocompromised history:* Cancer, organ transplant, immunosuppressant medications
- *History of status of pregnancy* is very important as well—pituitary apoplexy, sinus thrombosis.
- *Psychiatric history:* Depression is a very important and often neglected history. Careful evaluation needs to be done in patients with psychiatric history and illness as their symptoms may be labeled as functional or psychiatric related and organic causes may be missed.
- *Other history:* Trauma, postoperative, fracture (fat embolism).

Step 6: Detailed Examination

General Examination

This can give a clue to the diagnosis most of the times. A detailed examination of cardiovascular, respiratory, per abdomen examination including the back should be done before proceeding to CNS examination. Some findings which can help us to get an idea of etiology are mentioned in **Table 14**.

CNS Examination

1. Glasgow Coma Scale
2. Spontaneous eye movements
3. Pupil examination
4. Optic fundus examination
5. Corneal responses
6. Oculocephalic responses (After ruling out cervical cord injury)
7. Oculovestibular responses (Caloric)
8. Skeletal muscle tone
9. Deep tendon reflexes + Plantar reflex
10. Meningeal signs

1. *Glasgow Coma Scale (GCS):* It has already been discussed earlier. It gives an idea regarding motor responses in the form of decerebrate and decorticate posturing as well which gives an idea of prognosis instantly
2. *Spontaneous eye movements:* There can be roving conjugate, roving dysconjugate, abnormal movements and absent spontaneous eye movements. We mention some common spontaneous eye movements occurring in unconscious patients **(Table 15)**.[10]

TABLE 13: Onset of symptoms or unconsciousness

	Probable etiology
Hyperacute	Vascular
Acute	Traumatic
	Infectious
Subacute	Drugs

TABLE 14: General examination findings.

Clues	
Cachexia	Chronic—Cancer, inflammatory disorders
Frank sign	Myocardial infarction
Gynecomastia, Ascites, spider nevi	Hepatic encephalopathy
Hyperpigmentation, hypotension	Addison's disease
Open wound/contusion	Trauma
Bite mark	Unknown bite

TABLE 15: Spontaneous eye examination.

1. Ocular bobbing
2. Reverse ocular bobbing
3. Ocular dipping or inverse ocular bobbing
4. Reverse ocular dipping or converse bobbing
5. Ping-pong gaze
6. Periodic alternating gaze deviation
7. Vertical myoclonus
8. Monocular movements

3. *Pupil examination*

Size	
Symmetry	
Pupillary light reflex	• Direct
	• Consensual
Ciliospinal reflex	

In patients with eye lid swelling/trauma POCUS PUPIL can be performed to look for the size and reflexes as well **(Table 15)**.

In patients with eye lid swelling/trauma POCUS (Point of care ultrasonography) PUPIL can be performed to look for the size and reflexes as well. Anisocoria can be caused by sympathetic paralysis, which causes the pupil to contract, or by parasympathetic paralysis, which causes the pupil to dilate. Stuporous or comatose patients usually have smaller than normal pupilsPupils in comatose patients have been explained in **Table 16**.

Causes of unilateral dilated and nonreactive pupil mentioned in **Table 17**. Pupillary light reflex is one of the most basic and a simple test which helps to both localize and diagnose. It is the single most significant physical sign in distinguishing between metabolic and structural coma.[1]

4. *Optic fundus examination:* It is an essential part of neurological examination and can give clues to the cause of unconsciousness.

TABLE 16: Pupils in comatose patients.[6]

Pupil size	Pupillary Reaction	Cause
Small	Reactive	Metabolic encephalopathy, drugs • Diencephalon lesions
Large	Fixed, hippus	Pretectal
Mid position	Fixed	Mid brain
Dilated	Fixed	Uncal herniation—3rd cranial nerve
Pinpoint	Sluggish	Pons

TABLE 17: Unilateral dilated and nonreactive pupil.

Etiology	Pathology
• Posterior • Communicating artery aneurysm	Oculomotor nerve compromise
Temporal lobe herniation	
Head injury	Ciliary ganglion dysfunction
Atropine drops	

TABLE 18: Oculocephalic responses.

Normal/Full response	• Brisk and tonic • Conjugate eye movements opposite to the direction of turning
Minimal response	Conjugate movements <30 degrees or inability to adduct the eyes bilaterally
Absence of response	Poorest level of function

5. *Corneal response:* Corneal response should be tested to see if present or absent. Old method of testing with a cotton wisp is not preferred now. Newer method is to use 2–3 drops of sterile saline dropped on the cornea from a height of 4–6 inches to prevent any corneal trauma.[11]
6. *Oculocephalic responses:* This test is only performed after ruling out a cervical cord injury. This test is also many times referred to as DOLL'S EYE PHENOMENON/RESPONSE. Normal responses in both horizontal and vertical directions indicate an intact brainstem pathway from the vestibular nuclei through the lower pontine tegmentum and thence the upper pontine and midbrain paramedian tegmentum (**Table 18**).[1]
7. *Oculovestibular responses (caloric):* Oculocephalic stimulation may cause sluggish or no eye movements in deeply comatose patients. In such patients, intense vestibular stimulation can be obtained by testing caloric vestibulo-ocular responses.
8. and 9. *Motor examination and reflexes:* Tone examination along deep tendon reflexes and plantar response are assessed here. These help to localize the lesion anatomically.
10. *Meningeal Signs:* A thorough examination should be done to look for meningeal irritation signs. Meningoencephalitis being a very important cause of altered level of consciousness.

Positive meningeal signs in patients of unconsciousness	
Infectious	• Meningoencephalitis • Cerebral malaria
Vascular	Subarachnoid hemorrhage
Other	Encephalitis

Methods to Elicit a Response in an Unconscious Patient

First method to elicit a response in an unconscious patient is using voice or shaking the patient vigorously. In case of unresponsiveness, the examiner then produces pain to arouse the patient. This is done laterally first on both the sides followed by midline. This provides information regarding lateralization as well.

Lateral	Midline
Nail beds	Sternum
Supraorbital ridge	
Temporomandibular joint	

Step 7: Differential Diagnosis[7]

Symmetrical

Structural	Nonstructural
Bilateral ICA occlusion	Drugs
Bilateral ACA occlusion	Toxins

Asymmetrical

Metabolic	• Hypoglycemia • Hypoxia • Hypo/hyperthermia • Hypo/hypernatremia • Hypo/hypercalcemia	
	Encephalopathy	• Uremic • Wernicke's • Hepatic • Dialysis
	Porphyria	
Vascular	• Subarachnoid hemorrhage • Subdural hemorrhage	
Infectious	• Bacterial • Viral	
Psychiatric	Catatonia	
Others	Postictal	
	Diffuse ischemia	• Myocardial infarction • Arrhythmia • Congestive heart failure
	• Hypotension • Hypertensive encephalopathy • Hypothyroidism	

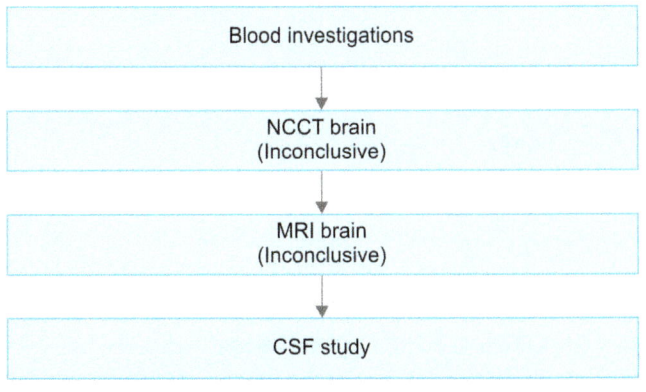

Flowchart 4: Unconsciousness evaluation.

(NCCT: noncontrast computed tomography)

Step 8: Management

Unconsciousness Evaluation: Unconscious Patient Evaluation has been Explained in **Flowchart 4**.

■ LABORATORY INVESTIGATIONS

Required for evaluation of an Unconscious patient **(Table 19)**.

Neuroimaging

Non-Contrast Computerized Tomography (NCCT) brain is the first imaging of choice in all patients of unconsciousness. It detects intracranial hemorrhage at the earliest. MRI with DWI-FLAIR mismatch is used for diagnosis of ischemic stroke especially morning awake strokes. CT angiography, MR angiography, and DSA are done when needed especially when suspecting aneurysms.

NCCT brain	• Intracerebral hemorrhage • Space occupying lesions
CT/MR angiography	• Aneurysms • Thrombosis
MRI brain	Stroke, epilepsy
MR brain contrast	Enhancing lesions
MR Spectroscopy	Prognosis
Single-photon emission computerized tomography (SPECT)	Prognostic value
Neurosonography	Intracranial Doppler sonography

Cerebrospinal Fluid (CSF)

A very essential test in a patient of unconsciousness when neuroimaging and other tests have failed to identify the etiology. CSF examination should include the following based on suspicion **(Table 20)**.

■ TREATMENT

Identifying the cause and treating it is the goal. Reversible causes should be identified and treated at the earliest before permanent brain damage occurs.

TABLE 19: Blood investigations for evaluation of an unconscious patient.

1.	Blood urea nitrogen (BUN), creatinine	Uremic encephalopathy
2.	Electrolytes including Ca^{2+}, Mg^{2+}	Metabolic
3.	Venous blood glucose	Hypoglycemia/Hyperglycemia
4.	Complete blood count	
5.	Coagulation profile	
6.	Liver function test (LFT), arterial ammonia	Hepatic encephalopathy
7.	CPKMB, Troponin	Cardiac
8.	Serum acetylcholinesterase	Organophosphorus poisoning
9.	Thyroid function tests	Myxedema coma
10.	Creatine phosphokinase (CPK)	
11.	Cultures	
12.	Adrenal function tests	Addisonian crisis
13.	CRP, procalcitonin	Bacterial sepsis
14.	Drug and toxicology screen	Drug overdose/Toxin
15.	Urine examination routine and culture	

TABLE-20: CSF examination

1.	Cell count and cytology (RBC)
2.	Protein, sugar
3.	Lactate
4.	ADA (Adenosine deaminase), CBNAAT (cartridge based nucleic acid amplification test) for tuberculosis
5.	Staining—Gram, Zn, fungal, parasitic
6.	Culture
7.	Cytology for malignant cells
8.	PCR (polymerase chain reaction)

Take Home Messages

We emphasize on a very important topic of "unconsciousness". Every patient of unconsciousness needs to be evaluated in detail before labeling the cause as neurological. We describe the definitions, anatomy and some terminology related to consciousness before proceeding to the approach. Emergency room approach to an unconscious patient is most critical as it changes the further course of management. As an age old practice we are taught to take history of the patient first. Here we describe an approach in a detailed sequence, emphasizing the role of history and examination and at which stage they would be needed. This approach covers unconsciousness as a whole and not just neurological and simplifies to arrive at a diagnosis. We also provide a proforma which can be used by the doctors working in the emergencies to aid them in managing the patients.

PROFORMA FOR UNCONSCIOUS PATIENT

I. Screening History

Presenting Complaints

1.	
2.	
3.	
4.	
5.	
6.	

1.	Trauma
2.	Cardiac history
3.	Medication and drug history
4.	Comorbidities
5.	Unknown compound
6.	Unknown bite

II. Screening Examination

1	General assessment	General attitude
		Face
		Thorax
		Abdomen
		Back
		Limbs
2	Smell	
3	Pulse	
4	Blood pressure	
5	Respiratory rate and pattern	
6	Temperature	
7	SPO$_2$	
8	Pupils	
9	GCS	

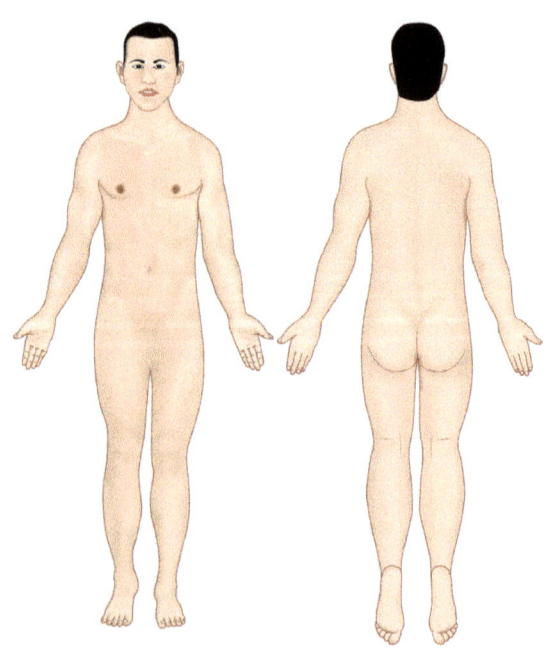

III. Emergency Management

1	Airway
2	Breathing
3	Circulation

IV. Screening Tests

1.	CBG	Blood ketone
2.	ECG	2D ECHO
3.	ABG	FAST
4.		POCUS

V. Detailed History

VI. Detailed Examination of All Systems

General examination	Built
	Nourishment
	Pallor
	Icterus
	Clubbing
	Cyanosis
	Lymphadenopathy
	Oedema
	Other
CVS	
RS	
PA	

VII. Differential Diagnosis/Impression

CNS Examination	
GCS	
Spontaneous	
Eye movements	
Pupil reaction	
Optic fundus examination	
Corneal response	
Oculocephalic response	(After C-spine injury ruled out)
Oculovestibular response	
Tone	
DTR	
Plantars	
Meningeal signs	

REFERENCES

1. Plum F, Posner JB. The Diagnosis of Stupor and Coma, 4th edition. New York: Oxford University Press; 1995.
2. Suraweera W, Warrell D, Whitaker R, Menon G, Rodrigues R, Fu SH, et al. Trends in snakebite deaths in India from 2000 to 2019 in a nationally representative mortality study. Elife. 2020;9:e54076.
3. Shirasu M, Touhara K. The scent of disease: volatile organic compounds of the human body related to disease and disorder. J Biochem. 2011;150(3):257-66.
4. Teasdale G, Jennett B. Assessment and prognosis of coma after head injury. Acta Neurochir (Wien). 1976;3(1-4): 45-55.
5. McNarry AF, Goldhill DR. Simple bedside assessment of level of consciousness: comparison of two simple assessment scales with the Glasgow Coma scale. Anaesthesia. 2004;59: 34-7.
6. Saper C. Brainstem modulation of sensation, movement, and consciousness. In: Kandel ER, Schwartz JH, Jessel TM (Eds). Principles of Neural Science, 4th edition. New York: McGraw-Hill; 2000. pp. 871-909.
7. Jankovic J, Mazziotta JC, Pomeroy SL, Newman NJ. BRADLEY and DARROFF'S—Neurology in Clinical Practice, 8th edition. New York: Elsevier; 2021.
8. Pinés Corrales PJ, Arias Lozano C, Jiménez Martínez C, López Jiménez LM, Sirvent Segovia AE, García Blasco L, et al. Prevalence of severe hypoglycemia in a cohort of patients with type 1 diabetes. Endocrinol Diabetes Nutr (Engl Ed). 2021;68(1):47-52.
9. Ratzki-Leewing A, Harris SB, Mequanint S, Reichert SM, Brown JB, Black JE, et al. Real-world crude incidence of hypoglycemia in adults with diabetes: results of the InHypo-DM Study. Canada BMJ Open Diabetes Research Care. 2018;6:e000503.
10. Leigh RJ, Zee DS. The Neurology of Eye Movements, 4th edition. New York: Oxford University Press; 2006.
11. Wijdicks EF, Bamlet WR, Maramattom BV, Manno EM, McClelland RL. et al. Validation of a new coma scale: the FOUR score. Ann Neurol. 2005;58(4):585-93.

CHAPTER 13: Status Epilepticus

Haseeb Hassan

INTRODUCTION

Status epilepticus (SE) is one of the common neurological emergencies both in pediatric and adult population. This emergent condition warrants urgent medical management to prevent devastating consequences in form of irreversible neurological damage or death. SE has varied and diverse etiology ranging from acute cerebral insult (encephalitis, stroke, trauma, etc.), remote cerebral injury (gliosis, developmental malformation, etc.) or systemic causes. An incidence of 6.2–18.3 per 100,000 population has been reported in the US.[1] There is lack of population-based data from India and most of the developing countries. Over last few decades, better understanding of SE, improved medical emergency services, improvement in critical care, and increased therapeutic choices have helped to improve care of SE and outcome. However, treatment gap is huge, especially beyond major cities due to lack of trained personnel and infrastructure.

DEFINITION

In the first International League Against Epilepsy (ILAE) classification of seizures, which was developed in 1964 and approved in 1970, SE was defined in the addendum of the publication as a *"seizure that persists for a sufficient length of time or is repeated frequently enough to produce a fixed and enduring condition".*[2] The definition was well conceptualized but was not quantified to have practical usefulness. The duration of >30 minutes was subsequently used as definition based on animal model demonstrating irreversible damage beyond this timeline. Lowenstein et al. in 1999 proposed definition as *"≥5 minutes of (1) continuous seizure or (2) two or more discrete seizures between which there is incomplete recovery of consciousness."* This definition was based on observation that almost all convulsive seizures stop in <2 minutes and continuation beyond that time frame implies failure of "normal" factors that aborts seizure. These definitions were focused mainly on generalized convulsive status epilepticus (GCSE).

The ILAE in 2015, proposed definition that encompasses both dimension and for all SE type **(Table 1)**.

TABLE 1: Operational dimensions with t1 indicating the time that emergency treatment of status epilepticus (SE) should be started and t2 indicating the time at which long-term consequences may be expected.

Type of SE	Operational dimension 1 time (t1), when a seizure is likely to be prolonged leading to continuous seizure activity	Operational dimension 2 time (t2), when a seizure may cause long-term consequences (including neuronal injury, neuronal death, and alteration of neuronal networks and functional deficits)
Tonic–clonic SE	5 minutes	30 minutes
Focal SE with impaired consciousness	10 minutes	>60 minutes
Absence status epilepticus	10–15 minutes*	Unknown

*Evidence for the time frame is currently limited and future data may lead to modifications.
(*Source:* Adapted from Trinka E, Cock H, Hesdorffer D, Rossetti AO, Scheffer IE, Shinnar S, et al. A definition and classification of status epilepticus—Report of the ILAE task force on classification of status epilepticus. Epilepsia. 2015;56:1515-23.)

"Status epilepticus is a condition resulting either from the failure of the mechanisms responsible for seizure termination or from the initiation of mechanisms which lead to abnormally prolonged seizures (after time point t1). It is a condition that can have long-term consequences (after time point t2), including neuronal death, neuronal injury, and alteration of neuronal networks, depending on the type and duration of seizures".[3]

CLASSIFICATION OF STATUS EPILEPTICUS

The ILAE has proposed classification of SE in four axes:
1. Semiology **(Box 1)**
2. Etiology **(Box 2)**
3. Electroencephalography (EEG) correlates
4. Age

> **BOX 1:** Classification of status epilepticus (SE) (based on semiology).

With prominent motor symptoms
- Convulsive SE (CSE, synonym: tonic–clonic SE)
  - Generalized convulsive
  - Focal onset evolving into bilateral convulsive SE
  - Unknown whether focal or generalized
- Myoclonic SE (prominent epileptic myoclonic jerks)
  - With coma
  - Without coma
- Focal motor
  - Repeated focal motor seizures (Jacksonian)
  - Epilepsia partialis continua (EPC)
  - Adversive status
  - Oculoclonic status
  - Ictal paresis (i.e., focal inhibitory SE)
- Tonic status
- Hyperkinetic SE

Without prominent motor symptoms [i.e., nonconvulsive SE (NCSE)]
- NCSE with coma (including so-called "subtle" SE)
- NCSE without coma
  - Generalized
    - Typical absence status
    - Atypical absence status
    - Myoclonic absence status
  - Focal
    - Without impairment of consciousness (aura continua, with autonomic, sensory, visual, olfactory, gustatory, emotional/psychic/experiential, or auditory symptoms)
    - Aphasic status
    - With impaired consciousness
  - Unknown whether focal or generalized
    - Autonomic SE

(*Source:* Adapted from Trinka E, Cock H, Hesdorffer D, Rossetti AO, Scheffer IE, Shinnar S, et al. A definition and classification of status epilepticus—Report of the ILAE task force on classification of status epilepticus. Epilepsia. 2015;56:1515-23.)

> **BOX 2:** Etiology of status epilepticus (SE).

- Known (i.e., symptomatic)
- Acute (e.g., stroke, intoxication, malaria, encephalitis, etc.)
- Remote (e.g., posttraumatic, postencephalitic, poststroke, etc.)
- Progressive [e.g., brain tumor, Lafora disease and other progressive myoclonic epilepsies (PMEs), dementias] SE in defined electroclinical syndromes
- Unknown (i.e., cryptogenic)

Semiology of SE determines the pace of irreversible neuronal damage (t2). Etiology of SE is also important determinant of outcome **(Box 2)**.

EVALUATION AND GENERAL MANAGEMENT OF STATUS EPILEPTICUS

A systematized and protocol based management is essential in improving outcome of SE. The prompt recognition and immediate treatment is starting point of SE management. The clinical presentation of SE can be broadly divided into convulsive and nonconvulsive status epilepticus (NCSE) based on motor manifestations (See **Box 1** for detailed classification).

Recognition of convulsive status epilepticus (CSE) is not very difficult. Diagnosis of SE is mainly clinical but one should be aware of pseudo-SE and other mimickers such as status dystonicus, other movement disorder (asterixis and tic), and decerebration. None of the clinical features are pathognomonic but combination of signs and symptoms help in diagnosis. Brief and target history and examination should be carried out **(Flowcharts 1 and 2)**. Along with clinical evaluation, SE management and general supportive management to be initiated simultaneously **(Flowchart 1)**. The objective of SE management is prompt termination of ongoing status along with stabilization of vital parameters, identification of etiology and precipitating factors, and management directed to it. Detailed investigation is essential but it should not delay treatment. Ensuring patent airway and adequate perfusion is utmost important. Wide bore intravenous (IV) access to be secured. Arterial blood gas analysis usually shows metabolic acidosis that improves after cessation of convulsive movement unless very prolonged or associated with underlying metabolic or renal abnormality. Intubation and ventilation may be required to secure airway **(Flowchart 1)**. In case of intubation, short-acting muscle relaxant to be used.[4] Along with antiepileptic medications (discussed in subsequent sections), 100 mg IV thiamine to be administered. Glycemic status should be checked and 50 mL of 50% of dextrose to given except in hyperglycemia. Neuroimaging is mandatory in all cases of de novo SE.[5] Patient with previous history of epilepsy, decision of neuroimaging should to individualize. In a known case of epilepsy with obvious precipitating factors and recovery to baseline after control of SE may be exempted from neuroimaging. MRI of brain is investigation of choice. However, CT scan to be done if patient is not stable, MRI is not available, or contraindicated. EEG has limited role for initial management but is mandatory after initial control of convulsive seizure.

Nonconvulsive status epilepticus is a state of continuous or repetitive seizures without convulsions. Time-based definition for CSE and NCSE remains same in most recommendations. The ILAE Task Force on Classification of SE has suggested a longer time-based definition but evidence for time cut-off is lacking.[3] It is both practical and logical to consider duration of >30 minutes as operational definition for NCSE.

Clinical presentations of NCSE are subtle and non-specific. NCSE can develop from transformation of CSE. Approximately one-third of GCSE can persist as NCSE. In high index of suspicion and timely EEG is not connected, NCSE diagnosis can be missed or delayed. It is often misdiagnosed as postictal encephalopathy or drug-induced drowsiness resulting in nontreatment or substantial delay in treatment leading to poorer outcome. Altered mental

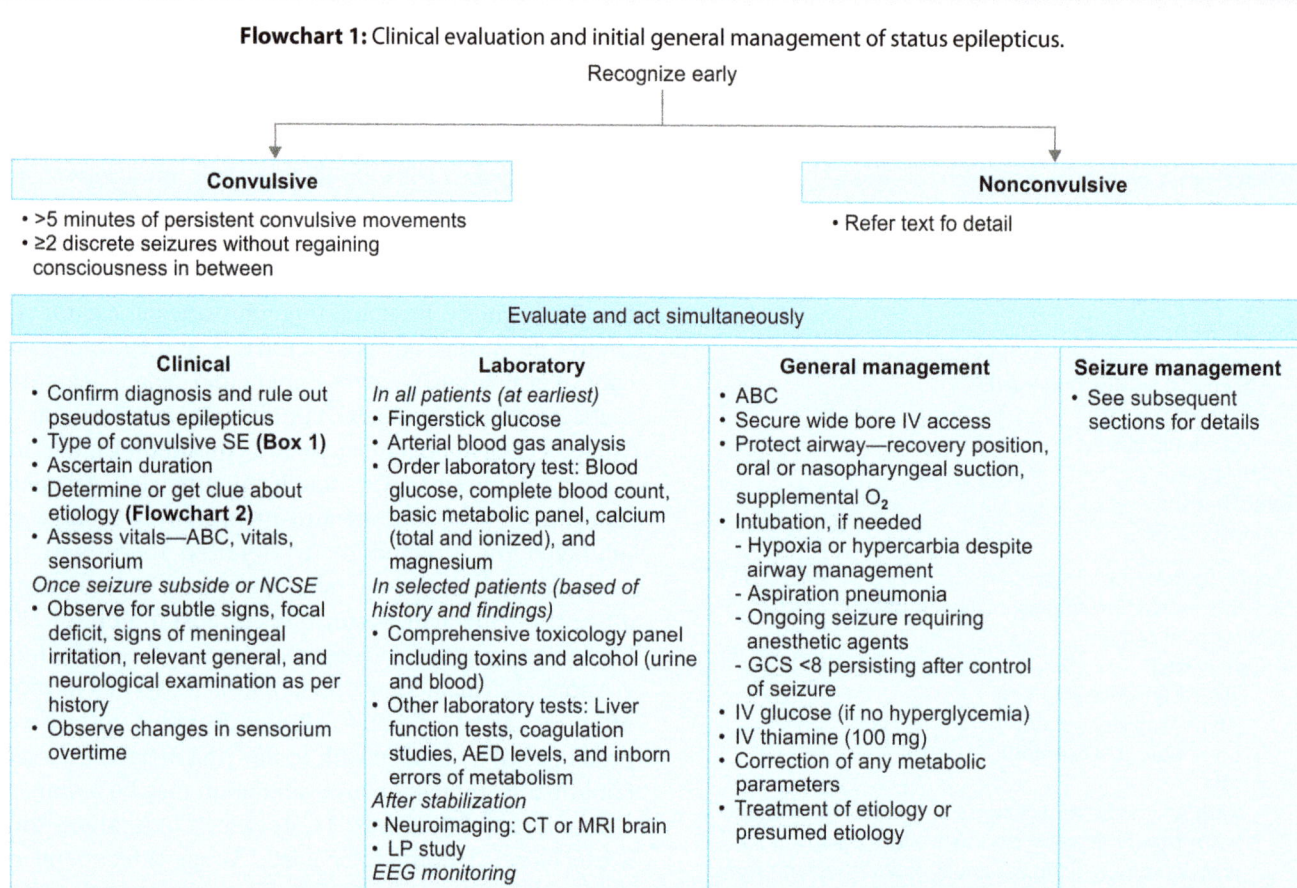

Flowchart 1: Clinical evaluation and initial general management of status epilepticus.

(ABC: airway, breathing, and circulation; AED: antiepileptic drug; EEG: electroencephalography; GCS: Glasgow Coma Scale; IV: intravenous; NCSE: nonconvulsive status epilepticus; SE: status epilepticus)

state is most common presentation that includes confusion, coma, lethargy, and memory disturbance. Other manifestations include delirium, psychosis, hallucination, extrapyramidal symptoms, and myoclonus. In emergence or persistence of these symptoms in critically ill patient without another plausible explanation should prompt for emergent EEG. Unlike CSE, NCSE diagnosis is based on EEG monitoring. However, the threshold of intubation and ventilation should be low as recovery is usually delayed.

Antiepileptic Drug Therapy in Status Epilepticus

Timely administration of antiepileptic medication is the key for successful termination of ongoing seizures. Delayed treatment not only causes brain damage but also leads to resistance to treatment due to gamma-aminobutyric acid (GABA) receptor downregulation. This makes short-acting benzodiazepines (BZDs) less effective.

First-line Antiepileptic Medication—Short-acting Benzodiazepines

Timely administration of short-acting BZDs (lorazepam, midazolam, or diazepam) can prevent cascade of events that can lead to devastating consequences **(Table 2)**. In developed world, it is used as part of prehospital management of SE. Intranasal midazolam or rectal diazepam can be useful in patients of epilepsy and caregiver can be educated in case of seizure persisting for >5 minutes before reporting to hospital. In hospital setting, either of agents can be used, but IV lorazepam is considered to be slightly better.[6] A repeat dose can be used after 5 minutes if seizure persisting. Incidence of respiratory depression is negligible and not giving short-acting BZDs are more harmful.

Second-line Antiepileptic Medication—Nonsedative Agents (10–30 Minutes) (Table 3)

Phenytoin/fosphenytoin was the gold standard antiepileptic drug (AED) for decades. Gradually, we have more antiepileptic medications that has been found equally effective and offer some advantage in form of cardiac safety and ease of administration. Levetiracetam has become very popular emergency AED for SE due to its safety profile and ease of administration. Shorter infusion time helps to use one more IV agent before anesthetic agents are considered without significant delay. Brivaracetam is theoretically very promising AED for SE due to quick onset of action, high lipophilicity leading to quicker blood-brain penetration, and higher affinity for SV2A receptor. If patient fails to respond to second-line AED, it is termed as refractory[7] status epilepticus (RSE).

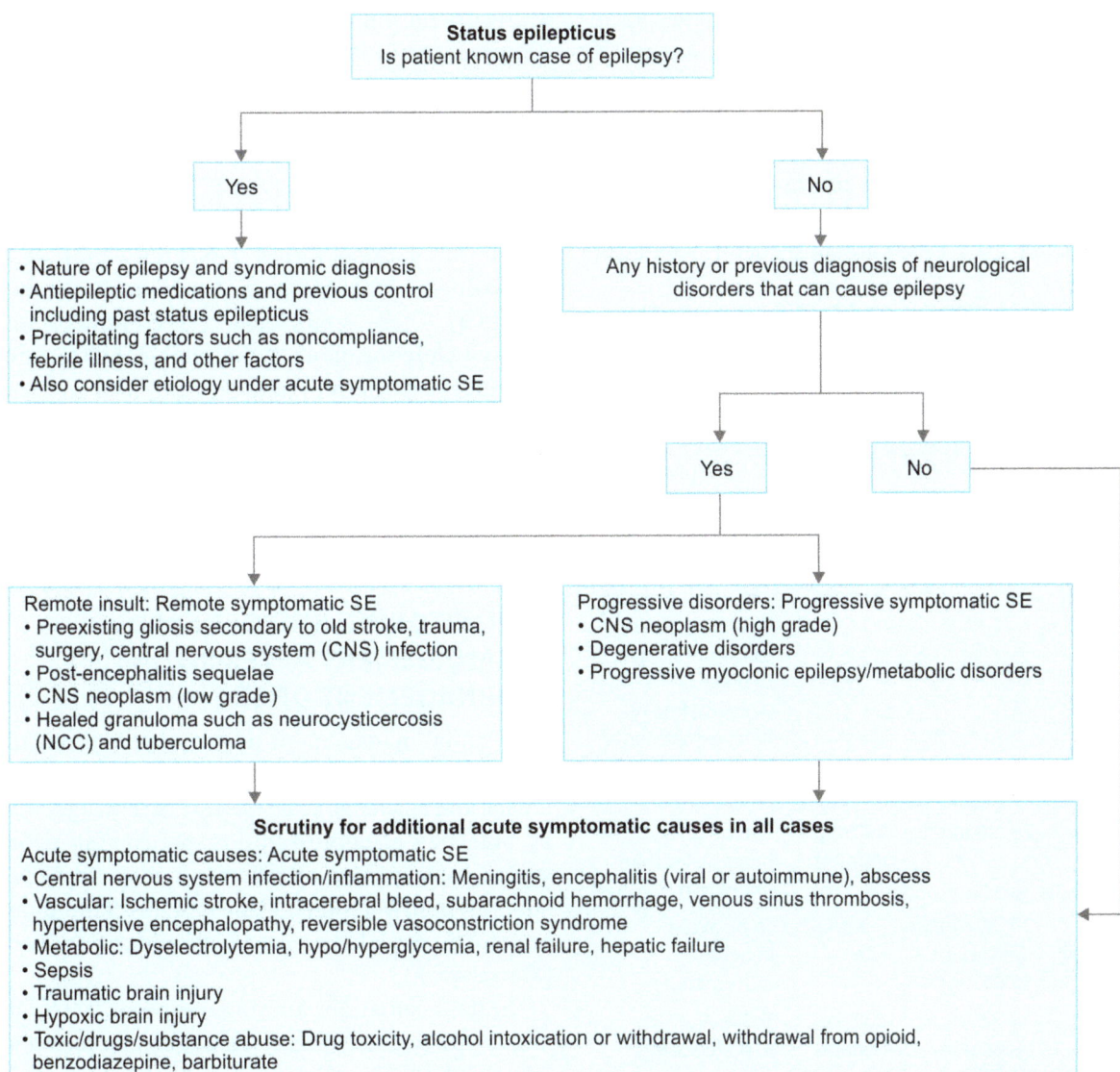

Flowchart 2: Etiology and quick approach for etiological evaluation and classification.

TABLE 2: First-line AEDs (5–10 minutes).		
BZD	**Dose**	**Route**
Lorazepam	0.1 mg/kg (maximum 4 mg)	Slow IV over 2 minutes
Midazolam	0.2 mg/kg (maximum 10 mg)	Slow IV over 3–5 minutes IM Intranasal
Diazepam	0.15–0.25 mg/kg (maximum 10 mg) 0.3–0.5 mg/kg	Slow IV over 5–10 minutes rectal

(AEDs: antiepileptic drug; BZD: benzodiazepine; IM: intramuscular; IV: intravenous)

■ REFRACTORY STATUS EPILEPTICUS

There is no single accepted definition for RSE. The most agreed upon definition is, when adequate doses of two IVs (first line and second line) antiseizure medications fail to terminate seizures, the status is said to be refractory.[8] It is common practice to use one more second-line medication before anesthetic agent is administered. Patient those respond to third medication (nonsedative) are categorized as RSE by some authors and some prefer not to label such patient as RSE.

Refractory status epilepticus needs to be managed in intensive care unit, intubated, and closing monitored. Anesthetic agents used are midazolam, thiopentone, propofol, and ketamine **(Table 4)**. Target of treatment is complete abolition of clinical as well as electrographic seizures. Hence, continuous EEG (cEEG) monitoring is desirable at this point of time. Burst suppression pattern on EEG was conventional EEG targets. However, in recent studies, control of electrographic as well as clinical seizure has similar outcome with lesser anesthetic drug toxicity; however, its use is limited mainly due to lack of this facility and trained personnel to interpret in real time.

Continuous IV anesthetic medication is real challenge. Apart from monitoring and controlling seizures and seizure-related metabolic disturbances, these agents are poorly tolerated. Hypotension, liver and/or renal dysfunction, and metabolic[9] derangements are common and need equal attention as seizures. In case of nonresponse to one agent, alternate agent is used and initial one is tapered. Parallelly, appropriate antiseizure medications are added to minimize risk of recurrence when these agents are subsequently tapered off.

SUPER-REFRACTORY STATUS EPILEPTICUS

Super-refractory SE is new term introduced in 2009 and defined as SE that continues for 24 hours or more after the initiation of anesthesia, including those cases in which the SE recurs on the reduction or withdrawal of anesthesia. These patients have highest mortality and morbidity rates and usually require intensive care unit (ICU) stays for weeks[10] to months. Data for these patients are limited to case reports and case series. Ketamine infusion has relatively better literature with fairly good success rate. Other anesthetic agents used for RSE can be recycled. Inhalational anesthetics, isoflurane and desflurane, lignocaine, IV magnesium, and pyridoxine are few options **(Table 5)**. There is empirical use of immunomodulation (IV methylprednisolone, IV immunoglobulins, and plasma exchange) especially in new-onset SE with no or presumed immunological etiology. Ketogenic diet has also been tried with variable results mainly in pediatric patients. Emergency epilepsy surgery can be considered selectively on case-to-case basis, especially with focal or hemispheric SE.

MONITORING AND GENERAL MANAGEMENT AFTER INITIAL MANAGEMENT OF SE

After initial management that is mainly protocol driven, continuous assessment and further management is equally crucial and challenging. SE has diverse etiology complicated by presence of comorbidities, preexisting neurological status, consequence of seizures, and antiepileptic drugs administered. Decision making remains continuous process and further evaluation and should be individualized **(Flowchart 3)**.

Initial evaluation, administration of BZDs (first line) and IV AEDs (second line) should be completed within 30 minutes. If SE is continued, patient should be managed as per protocol of RSE. If seizures abates and patient recovered to baseline, investigations as per clinical data need to be completed, identifiable factors to be corrected and patient should be observed for any seizure or change in mental status. In case of cessation of clinical seizures but failure to regain consciousness, patient should be evaluated further.

TABLE 3: Second-line intravenous (IV) antiepileptic medication.

IV antiepileptic drugs	Dose	Route	Comments
Phenytoin	15–20 mg/kg	50 mg/minutes	Caution in patient with cardiovascular instability, needs cardiac monitoring, to be given in dextrose free IV fluid, extravasation can cause purple hand syndrome
Fosphenytoin	25–30 mg/kg	150 mg/minutes	Can be given three times faster than phenytoin
Sodium valproate	20–40 mg/kg (Maximum 3,000 mg)	6 mg/kg/min	To be avoid in hepatic dysfunction
Levetiracetam	20–40 mg/kg (Maximum 4,500 mg)	500 mg/minutes	To be avoided in patients with psychosis
Lacosamide	200–400 mg	50 mg/minutes	No major adverse effect; may prolonged PR interval
Brivaracetam	50–400 mg	Over 2–5 minutes	Paucity of data

TABLE 4: Anesthetic agents for refractory status epilepticus (SE).

Thiopental	100–250 mg intravenous (IV) bolus (then 50 mg increments until seizures controlled) then 3–5 mg/kg/h	• Very potent with long clinical experience • Zero order kinetics • Significant cardiovascular toxicity and hepatic toxicity • Prolonged accumulation
Midazolam	0.1–0.3 mg kg/bolus then 0.05–0.4 mg/kg/h infusion	• Relatively safer but less potent • Hypotension, liver toxicity • Tachyphylaxis develops after 48 hours
Propofol	2 mg kg^{-1} IV bolus, then 5–10 mg kg^{-1} h^{-1}	• Rapid onset and rapid recovery even after prolonged use • Propofol infusion syndrome
Ketamine	0.4 mg kg^{-1} h^{-1} then titrate up to response (up to 7.5 mg/kg/h)	• Limited experience • No cardiac depressant property but can cause hypertension

TABLE 5: List of treatment options for super-refractory status epilepticus (SRSE).

Pharmacological	Nonpharmacological
Pentobarbital/thiopental	Hypothermia
Midazolam	Ketogenic diet
Propofol	Transcranial magnetic stimulation
Ketamine	Vagal nerve stimulation
Inhalational anesthetics	Resective neurosurgery
Magnesium	Deep brain stimulation
Pyridoxine	Electroconvulsive therapy
Steroids/immunotherapy	Cerebrospinal fluid (CSF) drainage

Clinical examination to be repeated and signs of subtle SE should be specifically looked for. Sings of meningeal irritation, any focal deficit, and systemic examination for etiological cue need to be done. Emergent EEG should be connected. Based of stability of the patient, imaging should be ordered and urgently pursued. In acute setting, only CT brain is feasible in most cases. Once EEG is connected, presence of NCSE need to ruled out. If NCSE or subtle CSE is present, type of NCSE to be noted and management in line of RSE need to be considered.[11] In absence of NCSE, EEG should be analyzed for etiological and prognostic clue. Presence of periodic lateralized epileptiform discharges (PLEDs) (encephalitis and stroke), asymmetrical focal or asymmetric slowing (structural cause), generalized slowing (systemic cause, postictal, and drug induced), beta comma (BZD overdose), TRIPHASIC waves (metabolic/hepatic/renal/autoimmune) can give lead to etiology. cEEG surveillance need to be continued for at least 24 hours if altered mental state is persisting for appearance of NCSE or discrete electrographic seizure. Based on CT scan of brain, laboratory evaluation, if etiology for altered mental state in controlled SE cannot be explained, once should proceed

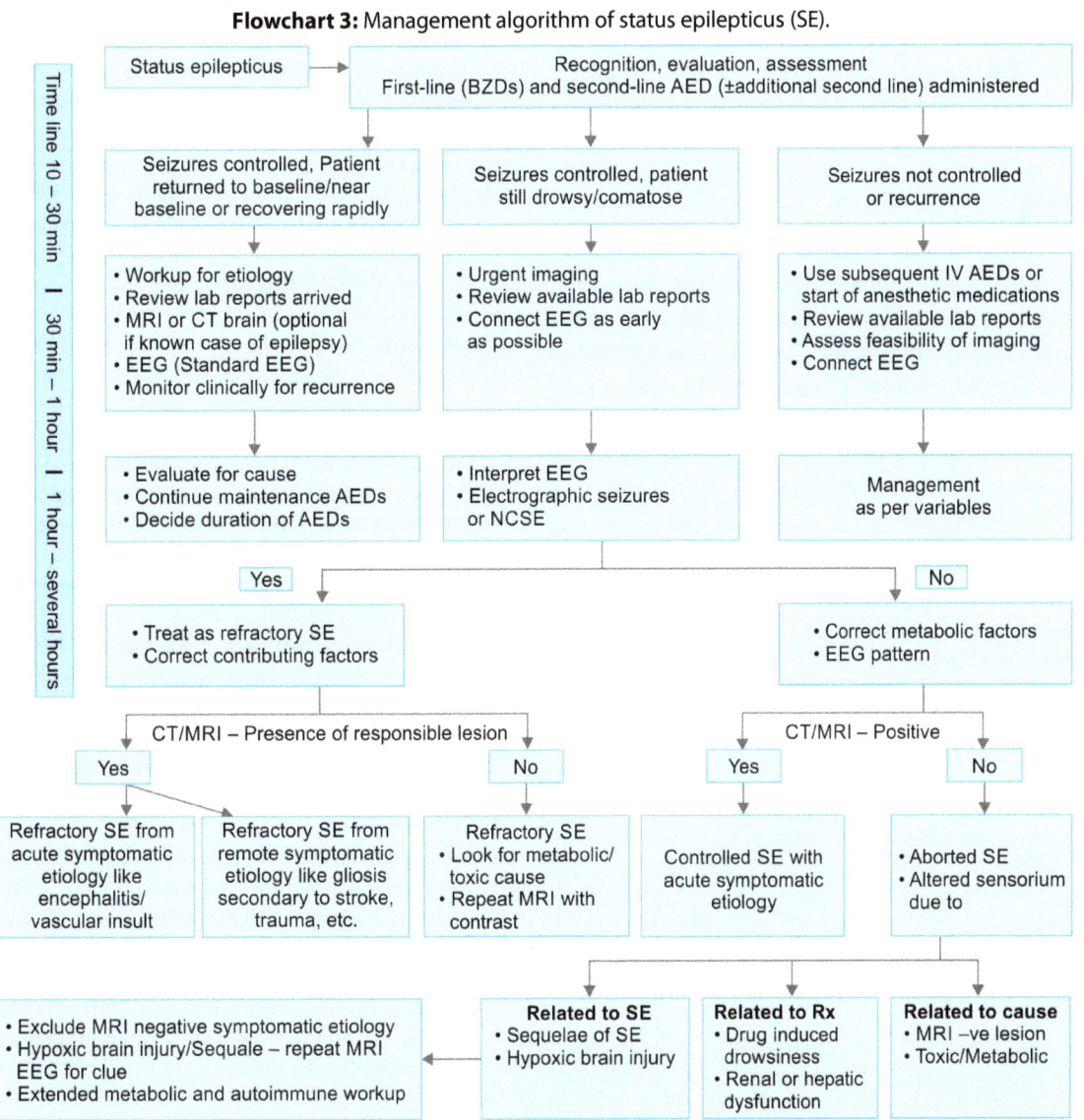

Flowchart 3: Management algorithm of status epilepticus (SE).

(AED: antiepileptic drug; BZD: benzodiazepine; EEG: electroencephalography; IV: intravenous; NCSE: nonconvulsive status epilepticus)

for cerebrospinal fluid (CSF) study and MRI of the brain. Preexisting neurological status (advanced dementia, other degenerative disorder, and multi-infarct state) and duration of SE may hint toward sequelae of SE as cause of obtunded state. Renal and hepatic dysfunction may delay clearance of medication as reason for slow recovery. MRI brain sometime can hint toward hypoxic sequelae secondary to prolonged SE. Extended laboratory workup (toxicology screen, autoimmune workup, lactate level, ammonia, and paraneoplastic workup) should be considered is altered sensorium persists.

Meanwhile, supportive care, nutritional support, and other critical care management need to be continued. The general and critical care management are equally important and appearance of systemic complication can further worsen the outcome, especially in refractory and super-refractory SE. Daily monitoring of electrolytes, basic hematological parameters and frequent monitoring of renal function and hepatic function need to be undertaken. Majority of antiepileptic medications are protein bound and hence serum protein and albumin level monitoring are very important. Ventilator-associated pneumonia, paralytic ileus, and sepsis are also common and need prompt recognition and management.

OUTCOME

Mortality from SE in various studies is up to 20%. The important determinants of the outcome in SE are the underlying[12] etiology, seizure type, age, and consciousness level. Poor infrastructure, delayed treatment, and prolonged seizures are also important determinant of outcome. There are many prognostic scoring systems but "Status Epilepticus Severity Score" (STESS) is the most important clinical score to predict in-hospital mortality of patients with SE. STESS of 0–2 is associated with good prognosis and 3–6 with bad prognosis. Mortality risk increase with increase in STESS score.[13]

Consciousness	
• Alert or somnolent/confused	0
• Stuporous or comatose	1
Worst seizure type	
• Simple-partial, complex-partial, absence, myoclonic	0
• Generalized-convulsive	1
• Nonconvulsive status epilepticus in coma	2
Age	
<65 years	0
≥65 years	2
History of previous seizures	
Yes	0
No or unknown	1
	Total 0–6

Take Home Messages

- SE is a heterogeneous group of disorders with varied etiology.
- Early recognition and prompt treatment is essential to minimize morbidity and mortality.
- Protocol driven initial management is must to minimize treatment delay.
- Detection of NCSE is challenging but crucial for outcome.
- Early EEG is essential in patients who do not recover quickly to baseline.
- Neuroimaging of brain should be done in all cases of de novo SE at earliest.
- Management of refractory and super-refractory SE is challenging.
- General intensive care management is equally important.

REFERENCES

1. DeLorenzo RJ, Pellock JM, Towne AR, Boggs JG. Epidemiology of status epilepticus. J Clin Neurophysiol. 1995;12:316–25.
2. Gastaut H. A propos d' une classification symptomatologique des etats de mal epileptiques. In: Gastaut H, Roger J, Lob H, editors. Les etats de mal epileptiques. Paris: Masson; 1967. pp. 1–8.
3. Trinka E, Cock H, Hesdorffer D, Rossetti AO, Scheffer IE, Shinnar S, Shorvon S, Lowenstein DH. A definition and classification of status epilepticus—Report of the ILAE Task Force on Classification of Status Epilepticus. Epilepsia. 2015;56:1515-23.
4. Brophy G, Bell R, Claassen J, Alldredge B, Bleck TP, Glauser T, et al. Guidelines for the evaluation and management of status epilepticus. Neurocrit Care. 2012;17:3-23.
5. Walker M. Status epilepticus: an evidence based guide. BMJ. 2005;331:673-7.
6. Alldredge BK, Gelb AM, Isaacs SM, Corry MD, Allen F, Ulrich S, et al. A comparison of lorazepam, diazepam, and placebo for the treatment of out-of-hospital status epilepticus. N Engl J Med. 2001;345:631–7.
7. Santamarina E, Carbonell BP, Sala J, Álvaro Gutiérrez-Viedma, Miró J, Asensio M et al. Use of intravenous brivaracetam in status epilepticus: a multicenter registry. Epilepsia. 2019;60(8):1593-1601.
8. Jagoda A, Riggio S. Refractory status epilepticus in adults. Ann Emerg Med 1993; 22: 1337– 48.
9. Sutter R, Marsch S, Fuhr P, Kaplan PW, Rüegg S. Anesthetic drugs in status epilepticus: risk or rescue? A 6-year cohort study. Neurology. 2014; 82:656-64.
10. Shorvon S. Super-refractory status epilepticus: an approach to therapy in this difficult clinical situation. Epilepsia. 2011;52 (Suppl 8):53-56.
11. Sutter R, Rüegg S, Kaplan PW. Epidemiology, diagnosis, and management of nonconvulsive status epilepticus — opening Pandora's box. Neurol Clin Pract. 2012; 2: 275–86.
12. Towne AR, Pellock JM, Ko D, DeLorenzo RJ. Determinants of mortality in status epilepticus. Epilepsia. 1994; 35:27-34.
13. Rossetti AO, Logroscino G, Milligan TA, Michaelides C, Ruffieux C, Bromfield EB. Status Epilepticus Severity Score (STESS): a tool to orient early treatment strategy. J Neurol. 2008;255(10):1561-1566.

Stroke

Shankha Shubhra Chaudhuri

INTRODUCTION

Despite major breakthroughs in the understanding of its pathophysiological mechanisms and management, stroke remains a major public health issue because of its high incidence rate, high case fatality rate, and devastating residual physical and neuropsychological disabilities leading to direct and indirect costs.

The term stroke signifies an acute, focal, central nervous system neurodeficit caused by a vascular lesion, either from vascular occlusion leading to an ischemic stroke, or from vessel or aneurysm rupture causing spontaneous intracerebral hemorrhage (ICH) or subarachnoid hemorrhage, respectively. Symptoms of stroke are of sudden onset and last >24 hours if the patient survives; they reflect the loss of function arising from the part of the brain affected viz., unilateral motor or sensory loss, ataxia, aphasia, agnosia, and visual disorders as well as global disorders of consciousness.

Unfortunately, many people fail to recognize the signs and symptoms of a stroke or they will attribute them to a less serious cause and thus fail to seek timely advice.

In this chapter, we will focus on acute ischemic stroke and parenchymal hemorrhage, discussing the general assessment, the specific treatment where available, and the prevention and treatment of some common complications.

ACUTE ISCHEMIC STROKE

The concept of ischemic penumbra, first described four decades ago, revolutionized the management of stroke, transforming a "preventable disease" to a "treatable disease".[1,2]

The penumbra includes hypoperfused brain areas that recover spontaneously (benign oligemia) and areas that progress to irreversible changes without effective treatment (penumbra)—this is the target area for intervention. Rate of progression to infarction depends on the arterial collateral supply, the functional and cellular state and crucially, the duration of the ischemic insult; hence the utmost importance of urgency of treatment and the aphorism "time is brain" (Fig. 1).[2,3]

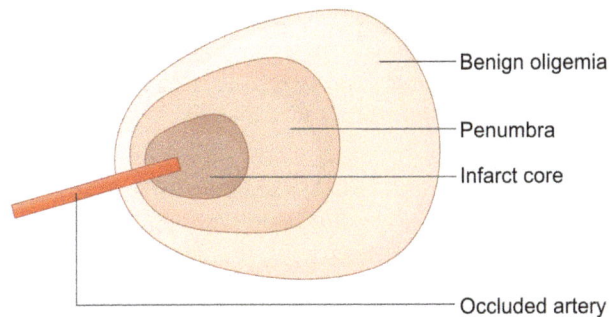

Fig. 1: In the immediate aftermath of an arterial occlusion.

In fact, it is estimated that in a typical large vessel ischemic stroke, 1.9 million neurons, 14 billion synapses, and 12 km of myelinated fibers are lost each minute.[4]

MANAGEMENT OF ACUTE ISCHEMIC STROKE[5,6]

In order to provide the fastest and most appropriate treatment, hospitals should have a designated stroke team in place, comprising emergency physicians/neurologists, nurses, laboratory, and radiology staff.

Where in-hospital consultants are unavailable, telemedicine is an acceptable alternative, both for diagnosis and initiation of thrombolytic therapy.

Patients require immediate evaluation when presenting to the emergency with suspected stroke or transient ischemic attack (TIA). The diagnosis of stroke should be confirmed, stroke mimics ruled out, and eligibility for reperfusion therapy should be determined.

A stroke severity scale is necessary as part of the initial neurological examination; the National Institute of Health Stroke Scale (NIHSS) is the preferred stroke assessment tool.

Neuroimaging[5,6]

Once airway and circulatory stability is assured, emergency brain imaging is mandatory in all suspected stroke/TIA patients prior to definitive therapy; this should be done as quickly as possible in patients who may be candidates for reperfusion therapy.

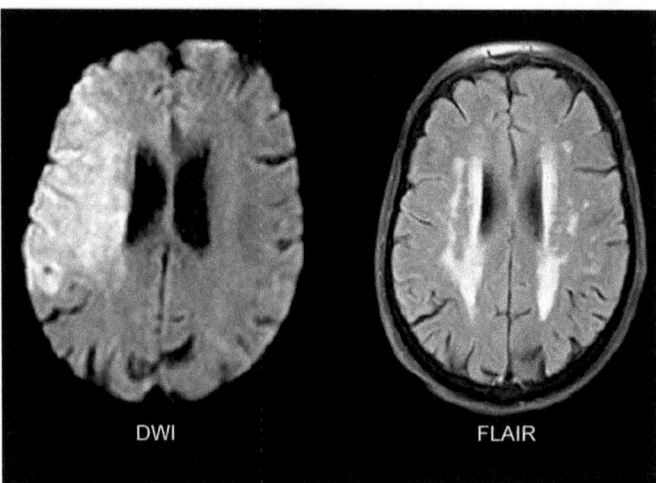

Fig. 2: The diffusion-weighted imaging (DWI) image (L) shows extensive acute right middle cerebral artery (MCA) territory ischemia while the fluid-attenuated inversion recovery (FLAIR) image (R) only shows chronic periventricular ischemic changes.

A noncontrast CT (NCCT) scan or MRI of the brain should be done as the first line, either one should be done as quickly as possible. A NCCT brain is sufficient for initiation (or not) of intravenous (IV) alteplase. In patients with acute ischemic stroke who wake up with a stroke or have unclear time of onset >4.5 hours from last known well, MRI to identify diffusion positive but fluid-attenuated inversion recovery (FLAIR) negative lesions can be useful for selecting candidates for IV alteplase within 4.5 hours of symptom recognition **(Fig. 2)**.

In highly selected cases, CT angiography with CT perfusion or MR angiography with diffusion-weighted MRI with or without MRI perfusion studies may be useful for selecting candidates for mechanical thrombectomy between 6 and 24 hours after symptom onset.

Other Investigations[5,6]

- Only the assessment of blood glucose is mandatory before initiation of IV alteplase.
- Baseline electrocardiogram (ECG) and troponin assessment is recommended but should not delay initiation of IV alteplase.
- Baseline investigations such as complete blood count, electrolytes, creatinine, and coagulation parameters should be performed but must not delay neuroimaging or initiation of therapy.

General Supportive Care[5,6]

- Airway support and ventilator assistance are recommended for patients with decreased consciousness or with bulbar dysfunction.
- Supplemental oxygen is indicated to maintain oxygen saturation (SpO_2) >94%, it is not recommended for nonhypoxic patients.

Blood Pressure Management in Acute Ischemic Stroke[5,6]

- Hypotension and hypovolemia should be corrected to maintain systemic perfusion.
- Early treatment of hypotension to lower blood pressure (BP) by 15% in the first 24 hours is indicated in patients with comorbid conditions (e.g., acute coronary event/acute heart failure/aortic dissection/postthrombolysis ICH) and in patients with BP >220/120 mm Hg.
- In patients with BP <220/120 mm Hg who are not undergoing reperfusion therapy, treatment of hypertension in the first 48–72 hours is not recommended.
- For patients who are candidates for thrombolytic therapy since elevated BP [systolic blood pressure (SBP) ≥185 mm Hg/diastolic blood pressure (DBP) ≥110 mm Hg] is a contraindication, BP must be reduced to avoid hemorrhagic complications.

Managing High Blood Pressure Before, During, and After IV Alteplase[5]

- Prior to administration, if BP >185/110 mm Hg, administer
- Labetalol 10–20 mg IV over 1–2 minutes may repeat once, or
- Nicardipine 5 mg/h titrate up by 2.5 mg/h every 5–15 minutes up to 15 g/h to maintain desired BP, or
- Clevidipine 1–2 mg/h titrate by doubling the dose every 2–5 minutes up to 21 mg/h to maintain desired BP
- Hydralazine or enalaprilat may be used instead.

If BP is not maintained ≤185/110 mm Hg, alteplase should not be given.

- During and after IV alteplase or acute reperfusion therapy, monitor BP every 15 minutes for the first 2 hours after initiation of alteplase, then every 30 minutes for 6 hours and then hourly for 16 hours.
- If BP remains high (SBP >180–230 mm Hg or DBP >105–120 mm Hg) after reperfusion therapy, nicardipine or clevidipine in the above mentioned doses may be used or use labetalol 10 mg IV followed by 2–8 mg/min IV infusion.
- IV nitroprusside may be used if BP cannot still be controlled.

Temperature[5]

Sources of hyperthermia (temperature ≥38°C) should be identified and appropriate medications including antipyretics and antibiotics if indicated should be applied.

Blood Glucose[5]

Both hypoglycemia (blood glucose <60 mg/dL) and hyperglycemia need to be avoided. A blood glucose level between 140 and 180 mg/dL is recommended.

Intravenous Alteplase

It is now well-established from several international randomized trials that treatment with IV alteplase within 4.5 hours of symptom onset improves stroke outcome, reducing death and/or disability substantially.[7]

The benefit of treatment with IV alteplase is time dependent; hence, treatment should begin as soon as possible after determining a patient's eligibility. The risks and benefits of treatment should be discussed with the patient/patient relatives and informed consent taken before initiation of IV alteplase.

Intravenous alteplase should be administered using a dose of 0.9 mg/kg (maximum dose 90 mg) over 60 minutes, giving the initial 10% of the dose as a 1 minute bolus to all patients >18 years of age who present with symptom onset of 4.5 hours from last known normal or from baseline status.[8]

For patients with ischemic stroke of 4.5-9 hours duration (known onset time) and with CT or MRI core/perfusion mismatch, and who are not candidates for mechanical thrombectomy, IV alteplase is recommended. However, this requires access to advanced CT/MRI perfusion studies and expert, case-by-case appraisal.[8]

Exclusion Criteria for Intravenous Alteplase[5,6]

- Inability to achieve or maintain BP <185/110 mm Hg
- Mild nondebilitating stroke [National Institutes of Health Stroke Scale (NIHSS) score 0-5] even in otherwise eligible patients presenting in the prescribed time window
- CT criteria:
  - Acute ICH/subarachnoid hemorrhage
  - Evidence of extensive ischemic damage
- Ischemic stroke within 3 months
- History of intracranial hemorrhage
- Recent severe head trauma within 3 months
- Intracranial/intraspinal surgery within 3 months
- Gastrointestinal (GI) malignancy or GI bleed within 21 days
- *Coagulopathy:* In patients without a history of thrombocytopenia or recent use of heparin or direct oral anticoagulants, IV alteplase may be started but should be stopped if platelet count is <100,000/mm^3 or international normalized ratio (INR) >1.7.
- *Low-molecular-weight heparin (LMWH):* IV alteplase is contraindicated in patients who have received a full treatment dose of LMWH in the previous 24 hours.
- Thrombin inhibitors or factor Xa inhibitors. Alteplase should be administered only if appropriate coagulation tests/direct factor Xa activity assays are normal or if the patient has not taken a dose in the previous 48 hours and renal function is normal.
- Major surgery in the past 14 days, e.g., abdomen, chest, skull, well-vascularized tissue, or major artery.
- Arterial puncture in a noncompressible site in the past 7 days.
- ST elevation myocardial infarction in the past 7 days
- Infective endocarditis
- Intracranial intra-axial neoplasms
- Infective endocarditis
- Aortic arch dissection.

Care during and after Administration of Intravenous Alteplase[5]

- The patient should be in an intensive care unit (ICU) or stroke unit
- Discontinue the infusion and obtain an emergency CT scan of the brain if there is severe headache, nausea or vomiting, or neurological deterioration.
- Measure BP and perform a neurological examination every 15 minutes for 2 hours, then every 30 minutes for 6 hours, then hourly for 24 hours.
- A CT or MRI brain should be done 24 hours after infusion and before starting antiplatelets or anticoagulants.
- Delay placement of nasogastric tubes intra-arterial times and catheterization if possible.

Managing Intracranial Hemorrhage Occurring in the First 24 Hours Post IV Alteplase[5]

- Stop IV alteplase.
- Get emergency NCCT head
- Obtain complete blood count (CBC), prothrombin time (PT)/INR/activated partial thromboplastin time (aPTT)/fibrinogen levels
- Arrange blood group and crossmatch
- Arrange hematology and neurosurgery referrals
- Either cryoprecipitate 10 units infused over 10-20 minutes or
- Tranexamic acid 1,000 mg IV over 10 minutes or
- ε-aminocaproic acid 4-6 g IV over 1 hour can be used

Other Intravenous Thrombolytics[5,6,8]

A single dose of IV tenecteplase (0.25 mg/kg, maximum dose of 25 mg) instead of IV alteplase may be reasonable for those patients eligible for mechanical thrombectomy. For a patient with minor neurologic impairments and one major intramural occlusion, a single IV bolus of tenecteplase 0.4 mg/kg may be considered as an alternative to IV alteplase.

Acute Endovascular Thrombectomy Treatment[5,6]

Endovascular thrombectomy treatment (EVT) may be offered to patients who arrive within 6 hours (and in highly selected cases, up to 24 hours) of symptom onset.

Endovascular thrombectomy treatment is indicated in patients based on imaging selection with NCCT head and CT angiography (including extramural and intramural arteries) or MRI and MR angiography.

Recent guidelines recommend mechanical thrombectomy with a stent retriever for a patient who meets all of the following criteria:
- Prestroke Modified Rankin Scale (MRS) score of 0 to 1
- Causative occlusion of the internal carotid artery (ICA) or middle cerebral artery (MCA) segment I (MI)
- Age 18 or older
- NIHSS score of 6 or higher
- Alberta Stroke Program Early CT Score (ASPECTS) of 6 or higher
- Treatment can be initiated within 6 hours of symptom onset.

Antiplatelet Therapy

Antiplatelet therapy is not indicated in the first 24 hours after thrombolytic therapy.[5]

For all other patients with acute ischemic stroke, antiplatelet therapy should be started ideally within 12 hours of symptoms onset, or as early as possible after neuroimaging. Based on recent studies, dual antiplatelet therapy is recommended for the initial 21 days for patients with minor stroke to prevent early recurrence. A loading aspirin dose of 160 mg and a loading clopidogrel dose of 300–600 mg are recommended continuing with a daily acetylsalicylic acid (ASA) dose of 80 mg and 75 mg of clopidogrel daily for the initial 21 days with either continuing indefinitely thereafter.[6]

■ MANAGEMENT OF COMPLICATIONS

Brain Swelling[5]
- Osmotic therapy is reasonable for patients with clinical deterioration from brain swelling.
- Use brief moderate hyperventilation (PCO_2 target 30–34 mm Hg) in patients with acute severe neurological deterioration while awaiting more definitive therapy.
- Corticosteroids are not recommended.
- Patients <60 years of age who deteriorate neurologically in the first 48 hours from brain swelling due to unilateral MCA infarctions despite medical therapy are candidates for decompressive craniectomy.

In patients with cerebellar infarctions either ventriculostomy or decompressive craniectomy or both may be required to relieve obstructive hydrocephalus and/or brainstem compression.

Seizures[5]

Seizures after stroke should be treated as they would be in any other acute neurological condition and antiepileptics chosen according to patient and seizure characteristics.

Prophylactic use of antiepileptic drugs is not recommended.

Deep Vein Thrombosis Prophylaxis[5]
- In immobile stroke patients without contraindications [e.g., gangrene, dermatitis, severe edema or peripheral vascular disease or signs of existing deep vein thrombosis (DVT)], intermittent pneumatic compression along with routine case (aspirin and hydration) is recommended.
- The benefit of subcutaneous heparin is uncertain.
- Elastic compression stockings are of no benefit and should not be used in ischemic stroke.

■ ACUTE INTRACEREBRAL HEMORRHAGE

Spontaneous ICH refers to nontraumatic bleeding in the brain parenchyma. The high 1 month case fatality rate of ~40% and poor long-term outcome makes it a major contributor to global mortality and morbidities.[9]

Approximately 85% of cases secondary to cerebral small vessel disease, predominantly hypertensive arteriopathy, and cerebral amyloid angiopathy, while the remainder is due to a macrovascular [e.g., arteriovenous (AV) malfunction, carcinoma, aneurysm, and venous thrombosis] or neoplastic cause.[9]

Acute Evaluation[10,11]

A rapid and focused history of the time of onset, presence of vascular risk factors, trauma, and concomitant antiplatelet or anticoagulant intake should be taken. In case of trauma, an attempt should be made to determine whether the bleed is the result of trauma or otherwise.

A standardized severity score should be used. The NIHSS score, commonly used in ischemic stroke, may also be in ICH. However, in view of the alteration of sensorium that is common in these patients, the Glasgow Coma Scale is equally useful. The ICH score was developed as a tool to improve standardization and is useful for prognostication **(Table 1)**.[12]

The diagnosis is easily and reliably made by a CT scan which should be done as rapidly as possible. In addition to diagnosis, the CT scan is an invaluable tool for prognostication. Calculation of the hemorrhage volume may be done from the CT parameters **(Fig. 3)**.[13]

Further Neuroimaging[10,11]

A CT angiography or MR angiography is needed in patients in whom macrovascular causes of ICH are suspected, viz.,:
- Younger age (<50 years)
- No history of hypertension
- Lobar location
- No CT signs of small vessel disease
- Primary intraventricular hemorrhage

The presence of certain radiological features suggests vascular abnormality, viz., presence of subarachnoid hemorrhage, enlarged vessels or calcifications at the ICH margins, disproportionate edema, unusual hematoma shape or location, and the presence of a mass.

TABLE 1: Calculating the intracerebral hemorrhage (ICH) score.	
Component	ICH score points
Glasgow Coma Scale (GCS) score	
3–4	2
5–12	1
13–15	0
ICH volume [mL]	
>30	1
<30	0
Intraventricular hemorrhage (IVH)	
Yes	1
No	0
Infratentorial origin	
Yes	1
No	0
Age (years)	
>80	1
<80	0
ICH score	0–6

Note: GCS score is the score at presentation, ICH volume and presence of IVH are noted from the initial CT.

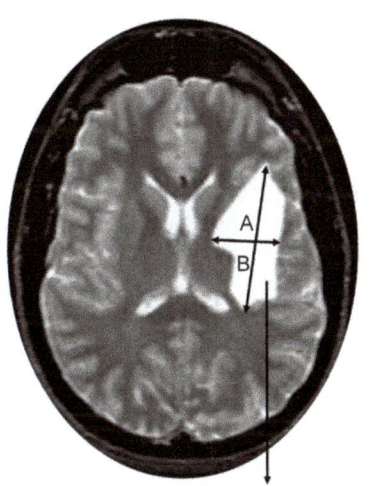

- Select the CT image with the largest area of ICH
- A is the largest ICH diameter (in centimeters)
- B is the largest diameter perpendicular to A (in centimeters)
- Multiply the slice thickness by the number of slices in which the hemorrhage is visible to obtain C (in centimeters)
- Multiply A x B x C and divide by 2 to obtain volume in cm³ or mL.

Fig. 3: Calculating the intracerebral hemorrhage (ICH) volume from the CT scan (ABC/2 formula).

Digital subtraction angiography may be required in patients with a high degree of suspicion but negative CT/MR angiography.

Other Investigations[10,11]

Routine blood tests must include coagulation parameters, especially so that treatment of coagulopathies may not be delayed.

Acute Management[10,11]

Intracerebral hemorrhage is a neurological emergency. The principle of "time is brain" also firmly applies to ICH. Hematoma expansion occurs early in about a third of patients and independently predicts a poor outcome.[14] The rapid delivery of care consisting of intensive BP management, anticoagulant reversal, intracranial pressure (ICP) control, and neurosurgery if required are the mainstays of ICH management and can substantially improve 30 days case fatality rates.

Management of High Blood Pressure[10,11]

High BP in acute ICH is associated with hematoma expansion and poor clinical outcome. There have been concerns for many years that aggressive treatment of high BP may reduce cerebral perfusion; however, recent studies assure that it is safe to reduce BP rapidly in ICH. There is still uncertainty whether this translates to functional or mortality benefit, however, especially in patients with large and severe hematomas, so caution is warranted. Based on existing guidelines, the recommendations for patients with mild-to-moderate hematomas are:

- Reduce BP in people with acute ICH who have a SBP of 150-220 mm Hg with symptom onset within the last 6 hours.
- Aim for a SBP of 130–140 mm Hg, sustained thereafter for at least 1 week.
- In most cases, aim to achieve the target BP within 1 hour of starting treatment.
- For patients with SBP >220 mm Hg, aggressive treatment with IV medication may be considered.

Rapid BP lowering should be avoided if elevated ICP is suspected, the GCS <6 or neurological evaluation is pending.

There is no particular BP lowering agent recommended but hydralazine and nitroprusside should be avoided for fear of raising ICP. IV medication may be used initially followed by oral or nasogastric medication.[15]

Hemostasis and Coagulation[10,11]

Coagulation abnormalities need to be identified and treated, if necessary with reversal agents for direct acting anticoagulants.

- Patients with a severe coagulation factor deficiency or severe thrombocytopenia should receive appropriate factor replacement therapy or platelets, respectively.
- Protamine sulfate may be considered to reverse heparin in patients with acute ICH.
- For patients taking warfarin, vitamin K 10 mg IV infusion followed by four-factor prothrombin complex concentrate (PCC) with INR-based dosing, repeating INR every 3-6 hours to achieve INR <1.3 is recommended. PCC is superior to fresh frozen plasma (FFP) in normalizing INR and has fewer complications than FFP.

Management of ICH Patients on Direct Oral Anticoagulants[16]

- Oral activated charcoal (50 g) if intake <4 hours

- Manage BP aggressively maintaining SBP <140 mm Hg but >100–120 mm Hg
- For patients on dabigatran immediate reversal with idarucizumab [2 × 2.5 g]
- For factor Xa inhibitor associated ICH, andexanet alfa should be used for reversal. Prothrombin platelet concentrate may also be used in these patients.
- Although recombinant Factor VIIa showed initial promise in limiting hematoma expansion it also increases thromboembolic events and is not recommended

Raised Intracranial Pressure[10,11]

Intracranial pressure monitoring is indicated in patients with GCS <8, those with clinical evidence of transtentorial herniation or those with significant intraventricular hemorrhage or hydrocephalus.

Though there is no clear evidence of benefit in ICH patients, general measures such as elevation of the head end of the bed by 30°,[17] mild sedation, and analgesia and osmotic therapy (mannitol/hypertonic saline) may all be used.[18]

Corticosteroids are not recommended for treatment of raised ICP in ICH patients.

Deep Vein Thrombosis Prophylaxis[10]

- Patients with ICH should have intermittent pneumatic compression for DVT prophylaxis and prevention of venous thromboembolism from the day of admission
- After documentation of cessation of bleeding, low dose subcutaneous LMWH or unfractionated heparin (UHF) may be considered in immobile patients after 1–4 days from onset.
- Compression stockings are not beneficial and are not recommended.

Seizures[10,11]

Clinical seizures should be treated with antiseizure drugs; antiepileptic drugs are also indicated in patients with a change in mental status who have electrographic seizures on electroencephalogram (EEG). Continuous EEG monitoring is probably indicated in patients with depressed mental status out of proportion to the ICH. Prophylactic antiepileptics are not recommended.

Role of Neurosurgery[10,11]

The rationale of clot removal surgery is to reduce direct and secondary brain damage. The location of ICH has a large role in decision making.

Neurosurgical intervention is generally recommended for infratentorial bleeds despite a lack of randomized evidence. Clinical guidelines recommend posterior fossa decompressive evacuation for cerebellar ICH >3 cm in diameter or for smaller hematomas associated with brainstem compression or hydrocephalus. Management of hydrocephalus by external ventricular drainage alone is not recommended and may be harmful.

For supratentorial hemorrhage however, the results of several large trials have failed to show benefit in the primary outcome,[19] so best medical management is usually pursued. However, it may be considered as a lifesaving measure for patients with ICH.

Decompressive craniectomy with or without hematoma evacuation might reduce mortality for patients with supraterritorial ICH who are in a coma, have large hematomas with significant midline shift, or have elevated intracerebral pressure resistant to medical therapy.

CONCLUSION

The last few decades have seen a significant advance in the therapy of stroke, especially ischemic. Nevertheless, there is a lack of dissemination of this knowledge, both among the general public, as well as, unfortunately, among professionals. Thus, the benefits of the recent advances reach only a minuscule proportion of patients.

Take Home Messages

- There must be widespread multimedia public health campaigns highlighting the symptoms of stroke and the need for urgency in seeking medical advice. More generally, there must also be extensive public education for the amelioration of risk factors, viz., practicing a healthy lifestyle including diet and exercise, cessation of smoking, and control of modifiable risk factors such as hypertension, diabetes, and dyslipidemia.
- Hospitals must have systems in place so that patients presenting with stroke symptoms are rapidly assessed and appropriate therapy may be started.
- Only a noncontrast CT brain and blood glucose estimation is necessary to decide on initiation of IV alteplase; with proper education and sensitization, this is achievable in many health institutions.
- More advanced procedures like mechanical thrombectomy, however, require more sophisticated institutional care, both for diagnosis as well as therapy.
- Using alternative thrombolytic agent or alternate, smaller doses of alteplase as well as refining strategies for targeting salvageable tissue are under investigation.
- For ICH, medical advance has not kept pace with that in acute ischemic stroke. However, early pressure reduction, reversal of anticoagulation, and timely surgical intervention may reduce mortality and morbidity. Strategies for prevention of early hematoma expansion and minimally invasive surgical procedures hold promise for the future.

REFERENCES

1. Astrup J, Siesjö BK, Symon L. Thresholds in cerebral ischemia—the ischemic penumbra. Stroke. 1981;12(6):723-5.
2. Ramos-Cabrer P, Campos F, Sobrino T, Castillo J. Targeting the ischemic penumbra. Stroke. 2011;42(1 Suppl):S7-11.
3. Bandera E, Botteri M, Minelli C, Sutton A, Abrams KR, Latronico N. Cerebral blood flow threshold of ischemic

penumbra and infarct core in acute ischemic stroke: a systematic review. Stroke. 2006;37(5):1334-9.
4. Saver JL. Time is brain—quantified. Stroke. 2006;37(1):263-6.
5. Powers WJ, Rabinstein AA, Ackerson T, Adeoye OM, Bambakidis NC, Becker K, et al. Guidelines for the Early Management of Patients With Acute Ischemic Stroke: 2019 Update to the 2018 Guidelines for the Early Management of Acute Ischemic Stroke: A Guideline for Healthcare Professionals From the American Heart Association/American Stroke Association. Stroke. 2019;50(12):e344-418.
6. Boulanger JM, Lindsay MP, Gubitz G, Smith EE, Stotts G, Foley N, et al. Canadian Stroke Best Practice Recommendations for Acute Stroke Management: Prehospital, Emergency Department, and Acute Inpatient Stroke Care, 6th Edition, Update 2018. Int J Stroke. 2018;13(9):949-84.
7. Wardlaw JM, Murray V, Berge E, del Zoppo GJ. Thrombolysis for acute ischaemic stroke. Cochrane Database Syst Rev. 2014;2014(7):CD000213.
8. Berge E, Whiteley W, Audebert H, De Marchis GM, Fonseca AC, Padiglioni C, et al. European Stroke Organisation (ESO) guidelines on intravenous thrombolysis for acute ischaemic stroke. Eur Stroke J. 2021;6(1):I-LXII.
9. Feigin VL, Lawes CM, Bennett DA, Barker-Collo SL, Parag V. Worldwide stroke incidence and early case fatality reported in 56 population-based studies: a systematic review. Lancet Neurol. 2009;8(4):355-69.
10. Hemphill JC 3rd, Greenberg SM, Anderson CS, Becker K, Bendok BR, Cushman M, et al. Guidelines for the Management of Spontaneous Intracerebral Hemorrhage: A Guideline for Healthcare Professionals From the American Heart Association/American Stroke Association. Stroke. 2015;46(7):2032-60.
11. McGurgan IJ, Ziai WC, Werring DJ, Al-Shahi Salman R, Parry-Jones AR, et al. Acute intracerebral haemorrhage: diagnosis and management. Pract Neurol. 2020;21(2):128-36.
12. Hemphill JC 3rd, Bonovich DC, Besmertis L, Manley GT, Johnston SC. The ICH score: a simple, reliable grading scale for intracerebral hemorrhage. Stroke. 2001;32(4):891-7.
13. Kothari RU, Brott T, Broderick JP, Barsan WG, Sauerbeck LR, Zuccarello M, et al. The ABCs of measuring intracerebral hemorrhage volumes. Stroke. 1996;27(8):1304-5.
14. Davis SM, Broderick J, Hennerici M, Brun NC, Diringer MN, Mayer SA, et al. Hematoma growth is a determinant of mortality and poor outcome after intracerebral hemorrhage. Neurology. 2006;66(8):1175-81.
15. Qureshi AI, Palesch YY, Martin R, Toyoda K, Yamamoto H, Wang Y, et al. Interpretation and Implementation of Intensive Blood Pressure Reduction in Acute Cerebral Hemorrhage Trial (INTERACT II). J Vasc Interv Neurol. 2014;7(2):34-40.
16. Kuramatsu JB, Sembill JA, Huttner HB. Reversal of oral anticoagulation in patients with acute intracerebral hemorrhage. Crit Care. 2019;23(1):206.
17. Anderson CS, Arima H, Lavados P, Billot L, Hackett ML, Olavarría VV, et al. Cluster-Randomized, Crossover Trial of Head Positioning in Acute Stroke. N Engl J Med. 2017;376(25):2437-47.
18. Balami JS, Buchan AM. Complications of intracerebral haemorrhage. Lancet Neurol. 2012;11(1):101-18.
19. Sondag L, Schreuder FHBM, Boogaarts HD, Rovers MM, Vandertop WP, Dammers R, et al. Neurosurgical Intervention for Supratentorial Intracerebral Hemorrhage. Ann Neurol. 2020;88(2):239-50.

CHAPTER 15

Acute Meningitis

Jasodhara Chaudhuri

■ INTRODUCTION

Meningitis defined as the inflammation of meninges (which consists of dura mater, arachnoid mater, and pia mater) may be caused by infectious as well as non-infectious inflammatory process.

According to the 2016 Global Burden of Disease (GBD) Study, the incidence of meningitis has increased globally from 2.50 million (2.19–2.91) in 1990 to 2.82 million (2.46–3.31) in 2016.[1,2] More than 1.2 million people are affected by bacterial meningitis each year across the globe.[3] Studies depict that in India the prevalence of meningococcal meningitis is around 1.5%.

■ ETIOLOGY

The most common causes of meningitis in immunocompetent subjects are viruses and bacteria. Viruses are responsible for nearly half of the cases. Enterovirus is the commonest with herpes simplex and varicella zoster the next frequent. *Streptococcus pneumoniae* and *Neisseria meningitidis* (*N. meningitidis*) are the commonest bacteria, together accounting for approximately one-quarter of cases. Other causes such as *Haemophilus influenzae* (*H. influenzae*), *Listeria monocytogenes* (*L. monocytogenes*), *Mycobacterium tuberculosis* (*M. tuberculosis*) and fungi (typically cryptococci) are less frequently detected.[4]

■ EARLY DIAGNOSIS AND DIFFERENTIALS

Age-wise Clinical Features

In less than a year olds: Acute bacterial meningitis in infants and neonates may present with nonspecific symptoms such as lethargy, anorexia, jitteriness, jaundice, hypotonia, apnea, diarrhea, and general weakness. Temperature fluctuations can be seen in many neonates. Seizures may occur in 34% of the neonates.[5] A bulging fontanelle may be present and hydrocephalus may be present and neck stiffness is unusual.[6] Neonates especially preterm neonates have immature immune system and hence they are more prone to meningitis.

Children: The manifestations may include fever, headache, lethargy, irritability, seizures, and alterations in mental status. Patients might be having focal neurological deficits and rash from meningococcal and streptococcal rash. Complications of meningitis in children include convulsions (17%), empyema (3%), brain abscess (5%), ischemic stroke (14–25%), hydrocephalus (3–5%), and venous sinus thrombosis (1%).[6]

Adults: Adults usually present with typical clinical characteristics of acute bacterial such as headache, stiff neck, fever, and altered mental status. In elderly population of 65 years and above, there may be an uncommon presentation such as fever, headache and neck stiffness may not be present and often there may be nonspecific confusion. A 2013 study found that in older adults, they had fewer meningococcal infections with more *L. monocytogenes* and had more pulmonary and renal complications.

Healthcare-associated meningitis: Often patients exposed to prolonged hospital stay, neurosurgical procedures, develop healthcare-associated meningitis. These patients develop some features that are difficult to diagnose. Cases may mature as a serious issue of head trauma, craniotomy, cerebrospinal fluid (CSF) leakage; develop from spread from a faraway infection site, such as pneumonia or sinusitis, otitis media, or arise in patients with compromised immune structure, due to cancer and its treatment/transplantation.

Acute Bacterial Meningitis in Children: Risk Factors

- Asplenia
- Poverty leading to ill hygiene and malnutrition
- Primary immunodeficiency
- Sickle cell anemia
- CSF leak
- Recurrent respiratory tract infection
- Lack of immunizations
- Cochlear implant.

Acute Bacterial Meningitis in Elderly and Adult Age Group: Risk Factors

- Pulmonary disease
- Malignancy
- Diabetes mellitus
- Immune deficiency [human immunodeficiency virus (HIV) infection], primary immune deficiency
- Chronic renal disease, chronic liver disease
- Autoimmune disease.

Differential Diagnoses

- Subdural hematoma
- Cerebrovascular accident
- Cerebral abscess (might accompany with meningitis)
- Subarachnoid hemorrhage
- Metastatic brain disease.

PATHOPHYSIOLOGY

Meningitis may spread by two mechanisms.

Inoculation by two routes:
- *Hematogenous seeding:* The bacteria enter the bloodstream after mucosal invasion after colonizing with the nasopharynx. The bacteria go to the subarachnoid space, then cross the blood-brain barrier, and cause an inflammatory reaction directly as well as an immune-mediated reaction.
- *Direct contiguous spread:*
  - Organisms may come in contact with the CSF during operative procedures or through adjacent anatomic composition (otitis media and sinusitis) and external objects (penetrating trauma, therapeutic devices).
  - Viruses can enter the central nervous system (CNS) through retrograde signaling by hematogenous seeding or through neuronal pathways.

APPROACH TO THE DIAGNOSIS

History and Clinical Examination

Meningitis may have a varied presentation depending on the age and immune status of the host. Symptoms include fever, neck stiffness, vomiting, and photophobia. More non-specific symptoms include headache, dizziness, confusion, delirium, irritability, and nausea and vomiting.

Signs of Increased Intracranial Pressure

The following risk factors should lower the threshold of clinical suspicion:
- Incomplete vaccinations
- Close contact (college hostel rooms and military dormitories)
- Children <5 years and adults >65 years
- Immunosuppression
- Alcohol addiction.

It is recommended to ascertain a history of sexual interactions, contact with animals, neurosurgical procedures, latest journey details, and other exposures. Most viral cases develop in the summer and rainy seasons.

The physical investigation is based on recognizing meningeal signs (Brudzinski and Kernig signs) and focal neurological deficits and specifically in case of meningococcal meningitis, pathognomonic skin lesions (petechiae and purpura). In 10-20% patients cranial nerve abnormalities are seen.

As mentioned earlier, there is a paucity of signs and symptoms in newborns and toddlers, who can come up without having any fever or hypothermia or with lower oral intake, crankiness, tense or bulging fontanelle, or lethargy. A full perinatal history and immunization records should be obtained mandatorily.

Vaccines can prevent meningitis causes such as:
- Pneumococcus
- *Haemophilus influenzae* (*H. influenzae*) type B
- Meningococcus, measles
- Varicella-virus.

Diagnosis of Bacterial Meningitis

Suspicion of meningitis is based on clinical features and diagnosis, and the etiology is established by performing a CSF study, where a lumbar puncture (LP) needle is placed in the lumbar spine. The lumbar subarachnoid space is chosen because the adult spinal cord parenchyma usually ends about T12 or L1. The spinal cord parenchyma in infants slopes down to L2. There are various risk factors while positioning/inserting the needle into the subarachnoid space. A risk of causing a localized subarachnoid hemorrhage (SAH) or epidural hematoma is increased when the patient is prone to bleeding or is on anticoagulants, especially if a radicular vein is hit by the LP needle inside the subarachnoid space. Therefore, individuals having elevated raised international normalized ratio (INR) has a threat of SAH. Similarly, in case of patient having a platelet level <50,000/mm^3 and having thrombocytopenia, there may be a higher risk of a subarachnoid bleed. Guidelines of the American Association of Blood Banks and the British Committee for Standards follow a limit for risk at about 50,000/mm^3, 21,000 mm^3 and 20,000/mm^3, respectively.[7,8]

A risk of brain herniation is there in patients who have raised intracranial tension. Meningeal inflammation arises from acute meningitis and consequent raises the CSF pressure. Opening CSF pressures >200 mm CSF are usual, although opening pressure might be >300 mm CSF. Usually, before subsiding, the CSF pressure increases in the initial 24-36 hours.

The suggested *physiopathology* of herniation in brain is that, after removing the LP needle, removing CSF along with ensuing lumbar CSF leakage via dural opening reduces the CSF pressure in the lumbar space in contrast to the supratentorial space. Such condition can accelerate herniation syndrome, the actual risk of herniation and some series report that increased risk is as high as up to 5%.[9] Risk factors from terminal cases indicate:

- Markedly reduced mental condition to coma or semicoma[9]
- Recent seizures
- Pupils dilated
- Papilledema
- Decorticate or decerebrate posturing
- Respiratory abnormalities
- Focal neurologic signs.

In case of herniation, most commonly it appears in <5 hours of LP. Managing the herniation syndrome on emergency is tricky, but application of hyperosmolar agents and ventricular drainage are perceived to be most beneficial.[10] Computed tomography (CT) brain is commonly used before an LP detecting a midline shift, which indicates that the risk of herniation could be increased if the LP is performed.

Technique of Lumbar Puncture

Cerebrospinal fluid kits which are commercial, generally comes with a 21-gauge LP sharp needle for doing an LP. There is less incidence of headaches after LP with smaller-gauge LP needles, but this issue is less pertinent in a patient having meningitis-associated headache and the smaller-gauge needles may be difficult to maneuver. Extremely difficult LPs may be needed to be performed under fluoroscopy. Fluoroscopy is required while performing extremely difficult LPs. Obtaining sufficient CSF is recommended for all tests.

Analysis of Standard Cerebrospinal Fluid Test

A CSF analysis must be done rapidly for diagnostic information to avoid deterioration of white blood cells in the CSF post 30 minutes and because increased counts of white blood cell can lower the level of CSF glucose by metabolizing it.

Identification of Etiological Bacteria

The standard method to identify etiological bacteria is to streak the sheep's blood and chocolate agar plates, followed by incubating the plates in 3–5% carbon dioxide or to inoculate the CSF into enriched broth media. Bacterial growth in an incubator typically takes 24–72 hours. Such bacteria are Gram stained and subcultured in a special antibiotic media in order to determine the sensitivities of the antibiotic. Bacteria such as *L. monocytogenes*, usually grow within a window of 5 days.

Alternate diagnostics are there such as latex agglutination and coagglutination. These tests work better in case the bacteria are actively proliferating and shedding polysaccharide. These tests are comparatively having a lesser sensitivity for bacterial detection in the blood or urine however they are rapid and simple to perform. The pace and precision of diagnosing may be improved with newer technology. Laser desorption ionization time-of-flight mass spectrometry which is matrix-assisted, is currently availed to recognize the specific bacteria in blood cultures swiftly. Recent advances in polymerase chain reaction (PCR) assays and deoxyribonucleic acid (DNA) sequencing are making error-free and quick diagnoses of a vast number of contagious diseases.

Major Bacteria Causing Acute Bacterial Meningitis

Streptococcus pneumoniae (S. pneumoniae): It is one of the commonest causative organisms in the west. The prevalence of *S. pneumoniae* meningitis is highest in the juveniles and the elderly. Ceftriaxone or cefotaxime and vancomycin along with early adjunctive corticosteroids normally constitute the antibiotic management. In the developing countries, the fatality of the cases of pneumococcal meningitis is much higher ranging from 30–40%. Also up to 30% of survivors have permanent neurologic sequeale.[11]

Neisseria meningitidis: N. meningitidis present in the nasopharynx is spread through immediate contact with oral or nasal discharge or via inhalation. Congenital deficiencies related to immunoglobulins such as agammaglobulinemia or complement deficiencies increase the risk of meningitis in individuals.[12]

Haemophilus influenzae: H. influenzae, an encapsulated Gram-negative bacterium, disburses through the respiratory channel to anyone who subsequently has a bacteremia that invades the meninges. The type B serotype shows >90% of the meningitis cases. Before the extensive vaccination, *H. influenzae* meningitis amounted to about 48% of the cases under bacterial meningitis. The clinical features of *H. influenzae* meningitis are similar to the other forms of acute bacterial meningitis. Although ampicillin or amoxicillin is used normally for treatment, occasionally chloramphenicol is also availed.[6]

Staphylococcus aureus (S. aureus): S. aureus is a Gram-positive bacterium that reports 5% of meningitis and has a high mortality rate of 30%. Meningitis due to *S. aureus* occurs via two major pathogenic mechanisms—as a postoperative complication and via hematogenous spread. In postoperative *S. aureus* meningitis, bacteria are introduced following neurosurgical procedures and also head trauma. From foci of infections outside the CNS such as dermatological infections, peritonitis, pneumonia, endocarditis or urinary tract infections, spread of hematogenous, *S. aureus* meningitis to the CNS is seen. An underlying disease is often found in individuals having hematogenous acquisition, example, cardiovascular disease, diabetes mellitus, malignancy, HIV, or primary immune deficiencies; malignancy, use intravenous (IV) drugs; or are immunosuppressed from chemotherapy.[6]

Listeria monocytogenes: L. monocytogenes is a facultatively anaerobic, nonspore-forming motile, gram-positive bacillus that causes about 9% of acute bacterial meningitis cases worldwide.[13] Patients with *L. monocytogenes* meningitis might be having a late presentation with lesser typical signs of meningitis, more uncertainty, and disorientation and thus may cause delay in diagnosis.

Tubercular Meningitis

Tuberculous meningitis (TBM) occurs as a manifestation of extrapulmonary tuberculosis caused by the seeding of the meninges with the bacilli of *M. tuberculosis* (MTB). The clinical presentation includes low grade fever for days, headache, vomiting, altered sensorium, focal cognitive decline, neurological deficits, and seizures. Diagnosis is done by CSF study and neuroimaging. CSF usually reveals elevated protein, low glucose, and modestly elevated white blood cell (WBC) count with a lymphocytic predominance. Imaging can assess vascular lesions, cerebral edema, and meningeal enhancement. CT brain is used to rule out the emergent complication of TBM-related hydrocephalus that could culminate in the need for immediate neurosurgical intervention. Therapy is by steroids and antitubercular drugs for a longer duration of approximately 12–18 months.

Anaerobic Bacterial Meningitis

Usually uncommon, it mostly occurs in infants whose mothers have amniotic fluid infection, intrapartum issues, and in children and adults with sinusitis, pulmonary infections, otitis media. The most common bacteria are as follows[14]:
- Bacteroides species
- Fusobacterium species
- Clostridium species
- Peptostreptococcus
- Actinomyces
- Veillonella
- Propionibacterium species.

CHALLENGES IN SELECTION OF ANTIBIOTIC THERAPY

It depends on the clinical team to choose the appropriate antibiotic because different microorganisms are sensitive to various antibiotics and also there are factors like toxicity. Patient-related factors to consider are:
- Nature and duration of symptoms
- Vaccination status
- Age

- Prior health status
- Allergies to certain antibiotics (allergic to sulfa drugs, special health conditions forbidding certain antibiotics such as glucose-6-phosphate dehydrogenase (G6PD) deficiency, myasthenia)
- Recent journey status.

The clinician should also verify if any other member of the patient's family or community is having meningitis or illnesses which might lead to meningitis.

Adjunctive Therapy for Acute Bacterial Meningitis

Dexamethasone therapy should be administered early (minutes before or immediately after antibiotics are given) in the course and should be in high dose in order to minimize the mortality and morbidity of acute bacterial meningitis. Also, the antibiotics given should be able to permeate the blood-brain barrier and diminish the bacteria. When the presumed infectious etiology is incorrect and the antibiotics are not working, giving corticosteroids may lead to a worse outcome.[15]

Outcome of Acute Bacterial Meningitis

The outcome of bacterial meningitis varies across countries with lower mortality and morbidity in developed countries to higher mortality and morbidity in developing countries and also depends upon the causative organism and the immune status of the host. Hearing loss, cognitive impairment, and epilepsy are the most usual sequelae reported.[16]

Case fatality rate is the highest in *S. pneumoniae*-associated acute bacterial meningitis, having a range of 20–37% in the developed countries and 50% in the developing countries.[16] High incidence of neurologic sequelae is associated with pneumococcus infection. Focal neurologic deficits normally arise due to cerebrovascular events but at times it is caused by cerebral abscesses, intracranial bleeds, subdural empyemas or severe meningeal inflammation. Focal deficits in children may include ataxia, paresis, and aphasia in around 10% of survivors. In adults, about 12% experience a cerebrovascular accident at admission neuroregression especially cognitive decline is common, especially in children. Seizures may occur prior to admission and continue in the course of hospitalization and after discharge. Since several seizure disorders resolve after meningitis over the time, anticonvulsants are advisable in some cases but are often can be discontinued 2 years after illness. Hearing loss, which is normally sensorineural, has an incidence of 14% for mild hearing loss [>25 decibel (dB)] and 5% for severe hearing loss (>75 dB). The hearing loss develops typically in the first few days of the meningitis and is usually caused by bacteria and inflammatory toxins crossing the cochlear aqueduct from the meninges to reach the cochlea.[16] Hearing loss improves spontaneously in 24%

but is permanent in some. The loss is especially common in pneumococcal meningitis, but adjunctive dexamethasone therapy can reduce its incidence and severity. Thus, a hearing assessment must be conducted in all childhood survivors of acute bacterial meningitis.[15]

CONCLUSION

Acute bacterial meningitis occurs globally across all age groups, leading to a severe life-threatening illness if not instantly managed appropriately. It is normally obtained in a community setting but may also be obtained following head trauma or invasive procedures. In individuals suspected of meningitis, the diagnosis is usually made clinically with CSF examination. The CSF classically shows a neutrophilic pleocytosis, low glucose level, and increased CSF protein. The diagnosis is confirmed by culture of the CSF, which is still the gold standard. Based on the clinical records and CSF Gram stain, fast decisions are opted to administer one or more antibiotics that cross the blood-brain barrier. When suitable, early adjunctive administration of dexamethasone may benefit the improvement of the outcome thereby reducing the sequelae in survivors. Patients are preferred to be kept in the intensive care unit of a hospital, where they are carefully monitored for 14 days of antibiotics. Even though most of the patients experience a positive outcome, few may die (depending on the offending bacteria). Few patients might experience hearing loss, cognitive impairment, or seizures.

Take Home Messages

- Clinician should detect bacterial meningitis early as late detection has been associated with adverse outcome.
- We should have an institutional algorithm for meningitis and appropriate choice of antibiotic with or without steroids depending on the case.
- Also there should be an institutional protocol for antibiotics that should be based on the local data and world literature so that uniformity is maintained.
- Early diagnosis and adequate treatment of meningitis usually means survival without neurological sequelae.

REFERENCES

1. Zunt, JR, Kassebaum, NJ, Blake, N. Global, regional, and national burden of meningitis, 1990-2016: a systematic analysis for the Global Burden of Disease Study 2016. Lancet Neurol. 2018;17:1061-82.
2. World Health Organization. (2019). Defeating meningitis by 2030: baseline situation analysis. [online] Available from https://www.who.int/immunization/sage/meetings/2019/april/2_DEFEATING_MENINGITIS_BY_2030_baseline_situation_analysis.pdf (Last accessed February, 2023).
3. Centers for Disease Control and Prevention. (2010). Chapter 2: Epidemiology of meningitis caused by Neisseria meningitidis, Streptococcus pneumoniae, and Haemophilus influenzae. [online] Available from https://www.cdc.gov/meningitis/lab-manual/chpt02-epi.pdf (Last accessed February, 2023).
4. Turtle L, Jung A, Beeching NJ, Cocker D, Davies GR, Nicolson A, et al. An integrated model of care for neurological infections: the first six years of referrals to a specialist service at a university teaching hospital in Northwest England. BMC Infect Dis. 2015;15:387.
5. Ku LC, Boggess KA, Cohen-Wolkowiez M. Bacterial meningitis in infants. Clin Perinatol 2015; 42(1):29–45, vii–viii. doi:10.1016/j.clp.2014.10.004.
6. Van de Beek D, Cabellos C, Dzupova O, Esposito S, Klein M, Kloek AT, et al. ESCMID guideline: diagnosis and treatment of acute bacterial meningitis. Clin Microbiol Infect. 2016;22(suppl 3):S37-62.
7. Kaufman RM, Djulbegovic B, Gernsheimer T, Kleinman S, Tinmouth AT, Capocelli KE, et al. Platelet transfusion: a clinical practice guideline from the AABB. Ann Intern Med. 2015;162(3): 205-13.
8. British Committee for Standards in Haematology, Blood Transfusion Task Force. Guidelines for the use of platelet transfusions. Br J Haematol. 2003;122(1):10-23.
9. Joffe AR. Lumbar puncture and brain herniation in acute bacterial meningitis: a review. J Intensive Care Med. 2007;22(4):194-207.
10. Lindvall P, Ahlm C, Ericsson M, Gothefors L, Naredi S, Koskinen LO. Reducing intracranial pressure may increase survival among patients with bacterial meningitis. Clin Infect Dis. 2004;38(3):384-90.
11. Koedel U, Scheld WM, Pfister HW. Pathogenesis and pathophysiology of pneumococcal meningitis. Lancet Infect Dis. 2002;2(12):721-35.
12. Tzeng YL, Stephens DS. Epidemiology and pathogenesis of Neisseria meningitidis. Microbes Infect. 2000;2(6):687-700.
13. Pagliano P, Ascione T, Boccia G, De Caro F, Esposito S. Listeria monocytogenes meningitis in the elderly: epidemiological, clinical and therapeutic findings. Infez Med. 2016;24(2):105-111.
14. Pittman ME, Thomas BS, Wallace MA, Weber CJ, Burnham CA. Routine testing for anaerobic bacteria in cerebrospinal fluid cultures improves recovery of clinically significant pathogens. J Clin Microbiol. 2014;52(6):1824-9.
15. Brouwer MC, McIntyre P, Prasad K, van de Beek D. Corticosteroids for acute bacterial meningitis. Cochrane Database Syst Rev. 2015;(9):CD004405.
16. Lucas MJ, Brouwer MC, van de Beek D. Neurological sequelae of bacterial meningitis. J Infect. 2016;73(1):18-27.

CHAPTER 16

Acute Encephalitis

Arka Prava Chakraborty, Souvik Dubey

INTRODUCTION

Encephalitis is inflammation of the brain parenchyma. Fever with encephalopathy with or without seizures and focal neurological deficits are very commonly encountered in an emergency setup of any hospital. Presence of altered mental status and focal signs are requisite for differentiating encephalitis from meningitis. Seizures can be present in meningitis and thus not diagnostic of encephalitis. Though there are hundreds of causes, a proper triage and identification of the broad spectrum of such illness is needed to plan further course of action. Broadly speaking, to simplify, such presentation most commonly occurs due to three groups **(Table 1)** of illnesses for which management protocols are entirely different, apart from routine supportive care. One group which is mainly important in the endemic areas is due to infective causes and needs urgent intervention with antimicrobials. Usually the cause of encephalitis is a virus. Less commonly they can also be of bacterial, rickettsial, or protozoal origin and may have the coexistent involvement of the meninges as well. Second group consists of the immune-mediated encephalitides for which a lot of new advancements in research have been done over the last decade. Many of them respond quite well to immunotherapy. The third group per say is not due to encephalitis and mainly due to systemic infection or metabolic derangements or toxin exposure. It is relevant to mention them in this chapter as they form a close differential and many patients often get treated in the line of infective encephalitis harboring such systemic insult.

The World Health Organization (WHO) defines[1] an acute encephalitis syndrome as *"a person of any age, at any time of the year with an acute onset of fever and a change in mental status (including symptoms such as confusion, disorientation, coma, or inability to talk) and/or new onset of seizures (excluding simple febrile seizure)"*. This was given in 2008 mainly as a case definition for surveillance purposes, mainly keeping in mind the infective encephalitides. What we encounter in the emergency of a tertiary center may be somewhat different. For example, many patients of herpes simplex encephalitis or N-methyl-D-aspartate (NMDA) encephalitis may present without any history of fever.[2] These cases may be missed. Thus it is necessary to have a comprehensive idea regarding these conditions. In this chapter, we have tried to elucidate the cues from clinical history, examination, and relevant investigations in identifying these diseases and framing a treatment protocol.

TABLE 1: Common causes of fever with encephalopathy.

Infective	Autoimmune	Mimickers of encephalitis
Viral • Herpes simplex virus 1 and 2 • Dengue • Cytomegalovirus, Epstein–Barr virus, human herpes viruses • Varicella-zoster virus • Japanese encephalitis • West Nile and Saint Louis virus • Nipah and Hendra virus • Human immunodeficiency virus (HIV) • Adenovirus, measles, mumps, enteroviruses *Nonviral Causes* • Tubercular • Pneumococcal, *Haemophilus influenzae*, malaria, tick-borne encephalitis, scrub typhus, *Acanthamoeba*, *Naegleria fowleri*	• NMDA • AMPA • LGi2 • CaSPR2 • GABAA and B • DPPX • GlyR • IgLon5	• Pneumonia, urosepsis, gastrointestinal sepsis • Electrolyte disturbances • Hypo- or hyperglycemia • Subdural empyema • Intracranial hemorrhage • Subarachnoid hemorrhage • Neuroleptic malignant syndrome • Malignant hyperthermia • Serotonin syndrome • Cocaine, amphetamines, salicylates • Thyrotoxic encephalopathy • Hashimoto's encephalopathy

PREVALENCE

The average incidence across multiple studies has been reported as 3.5–7.4 per 100,000 patient years, worldwide.[3] Though it affects all the age groups, it is usually higher in children. The incidence of autoimmune encephalitis (AE) on the other hand is 1.2 per 100,000 patient years. Higher incidence rates[4] have been reported over time due to the advent of improved serological techniques for the diagnosis of autoimmune antibodies. Moreover, an AE disease process can follow an infection by a viral antigen. It has been reported in 27% patients following herpes simplex viral encephalitis with detectable antibodies against the NMDA receptor.[5]

In India, about 10,000–13,000 cases are reported to the National Vector Borne Diseases Control Programme (NVBDCP) each year.[6] Case fatality remains as high as up to 30% with disabling neurological sequelae reported in up to 30–50% of the survivors. Though a lot of new diagnostic modalities have been incorporated in the management of acute encephalitis, a lot of etiologies still remain undiagnosed in the country.

APPROACH TO THE PROBLEM
Clinical History and Examination
General Clues from History

Seasonal variation can occur in the presentation of certain viral encephalitis. Herpes simplex virus encephalitis (HSVE) has no seasonal predilection, while the enteroviral and arboviral encephalitis have a tendency to occur in the summer or fall. Mumps and measles-related encephalitis usually occurs in the winter, while Japanese encephalitis (JE) clusters around June-August. Working or staying near paddy fields with water logging can harbor mosquito bites and arboviral infections such as JE and West Nile viral encephalitis. Exposure to bats or pigs or eating contaminated mangoes bitten by bats can give rise to Nipah encephalitis. Other zoonotic exposures with horses and birds leads to Hendra and avian influenza encephalitis, respectively. Presence of painful parotitis (mumps), flaccid paralysis (polio), eschar (scrub typhus), hydro/aerophobia (rabies), or grouped vesicles in dermatomal pattern (herpes zoster) are other important markers. Oropharyngeal candidiasis, thin hair, skin pigmentation, and generalized wasting points toward an underlying immunocompromised state like human immunodeficiency virus–acquired immunodeficiency syndrome (HIV-AIDS).

Systemic features of weight loss, hemoptysis, heavy smoking, new onset lump, etc., prompt us toward the identification of a paraneoplastic encephalitis syndrome. Recurrent hyponatremia (LGI2), prominent weight loss and chronic diarrhea (anti-DPPX antibody encephalitis), muscle cramps (CASPR2), and sleep disturbances (IgLoN5 disease) are other pointers which are important helpers in clinical diagnosis. Similarly, on initial screening at the emergency room one must not exclude the ingestion of any toxic substance leading to such encephalitis-like syndrome. The 2019 Bihar outbreak of encephalitis ("Muzaffarpur encephalitis") in children was thought to be due to the ingestion of large amounts of the fruit "lychee" (Lychee encephalitis) causing hypoglycemia.[7]

Cognitive and Psychiatric Features

Personality changes, lethargy, confusion, stupor, and coma are a spectrum of mental status that may be encountered in all encephalitis syndromes. Behavioral changes reported in HSVE include hypomania, Klüuver–Bucy syndrome and varying degrees of amnesia; all pointing toward the affliction of the limbic system.[8] Aphasia can also be a presentation of HSVE, though it is a rare presentation.[9] Most often patients present with global encephalopathy and delirium which makes the identification of any cognitive domain indiscernible.

Memory deficits (anterograde, affective, and working memory) and confusion are the dominant presentation in patients of AE followed by executive dysfunction. Though reviews of anti-NMDA receptor encephalitis have shown the presence of aphasia, impaired attention, apraxia, and retrograde and anterograde memory deficits.[10] Selective autobiographical memory impairment has been described well in LGI2 encephalitis.[11] Episodic, verbal, visual, and working memory impairment are seen in NMDAR encephalitis, anterograde, and episodic memory impairment in CASPR2 and anterograde memory loss in AMPAR encephalitis have been reported. Language dysfunction is a prominent and clinically appealing presentation in patients of AE, so much so that it has made a place in the diagnostic criteria of NMDA receptor AE as a separate domain.[12] Studies involving adolescent population have described language dysfunction as the most frequent finding and reported decreased verbal output in these patients. This may lead to progressive mutism in these patients. These cognitive deficits in early stage can be mistaken as a psychiatric syndrome and often lead to repeated psychiatric consultations before landing up in the hospital emergency.

Most important psychiatric manifestations reported till date in encephalitis was of mood dysfunction, aggression, agitation, delusions, and auditory/visual hallucination.[13] Mood dysfunction ranges from frank mania, hypomania, and anxiety to depression. Catatonia is a well-recognized feature of NMDAR encephalitis. Others not so commonly reported symptoms are of a schizoaffective syndrome, homicidality, and suicidality. Confabulations and Capgras delusions have also been reported in literature.[14]

Extrapyramidal Features and Movement Disorders

Secondary parkinsonism has been described as the presentation and sequelae of *Flavivirus*[15] associated encephalitis mainly JE, West Nile and Saint Louis viruses, as the brunt of lesions are on the basal ganglia and thalamus. This is a secondary parkinsonian syndrome mainly comprising of hypokinesia and rigidity. Descriptions of parkinsonism[16] from viral factors date back to the late 1910s when Von Economo described 14 patients presenting with acute onset psychiatric features and parkinsonism. This was described as "encephalitis lethargica" due to H1N1 virus (Spanish flu). Other viruses causing parkinsonism are coxsackieviruses, herpes virus, and HIV. Dancing eyes and opsoclonus-myoclonus syndrome have been described in West Nile virus encephalitis syndrome.[17]

Autoimmune encephalitis commonly can present with movement disorders.[18] Most commonly found in NMDAR AE which may present with choreoathetosis, rigidity, or tremor. Paraneoplastic encephalitis also can present in an isolated fashion as a movement disorder. They can be of central or peripheral origin **(Table 2)**. Other immune-mediated movement disorders can be seen in systemic lupus erythematosus (SLE), Sydenham's chorea, antiphospholipid syndrome, etc., which are out of the scope of this chapter.

Seizures

Acute symptomatic or unprovoked seizures are common in viral encephalitis. Focal seizures with impaired awareness are the most common types of seizures seen in encephalitis. They may or may not generalize. They are most commonly seen with HSVE, where seizures are found in about 50% of the cases. JE can also present with seizures in 7–46% of the cases. Others like Nipah are known to cause seizures in late onset and relapsing forms.[19]

Faciobrachial dystonic seizures[20] are brief, involuntary, repetitive, nonrhythmic, AND high-frequency jerky movements of one upper limb and face, which are highly specific for LGI2-related encephalitis. They are usually resistant to antiepileptics and commonly are mistaken as myoclonus. They can precede the development of encephalopathy in these patients.

New onset refractory status epilepticus (NORSE) and febrile illness related epilepsy syndrome (FIRES)[21] are new concepts evolving in understanding of new onset seizures. NORSE is usually termed when a patient goes into a refractory status epilepticus (RSE) without any prior history or identifiable structural, metabolic/toxic cause. Routine investigations done within 72 hours are unyielding in identifying an etiology in NORSE. It usually has higher mortality and higher chance of developing epilepsy. Viral causes (excluding HSV-1) and AE are implicated in causation. When no cause can be identified, immunotherapy can still be tried in management. FIRES are a subcategory of NORSE, where RSE develops with a history of a preceding febrile illness 2 weeks to 24 hours preceding ictus. Etiological contributor is same in this case.

Other Neuraxis Involvement

Cerebellar involvement is common in brainstem encephalitis, scrub encephalitis, NMDAR AE, and many paraneoplastic encephalitis due to antibodies such as Yo, Hu, Ri, Ma2, GAD-65, CV2, and SOX-1. spinal cord involvement may be seen in glycine receptor encephalitis, Hu, and CV2-related encephalomyelitis. Peripheral neuropathy can be caused by anti-Hu-mediated paraneoplastic syndrome. Progressive encephalomyelitis with rigidity and myoclonus has been described in relation to DPPX antibodies. Ganglionopathy and sensory neuropathies are also reported but they may occur without the presence of encephalitis.

■ INVESTIGATIONS

Laboratory Assessment

Routine blood investigations may reveal leukocytosis, prerenal azotemia, and hyperCKemia (due to rhabdomyolysis). Immunocompromised patients may show a decreased leukocyte count. Coexistent arterial blood gas abnormalities may be present due to ensuing systemic inflammatory state and hypoventilation. Decision for intubation and mechanical ventilation is to be guided by arterial blood gas and bedside evaluation of patient's airway and sensorium. Other tests needed to rule out mimickers can be tests for blood glucose, electrolytes, malarial parasite, blood culture, liver function tests, thyroid function, anti-thyroid peroxidase (TPO) antibodies, blood, and urinalysis for toxins.

Cerebrospinal fluid (CSF) examination[22] forms an important test to detect intracranial infection. All of them show a mononuclear pleocytosis with increased protein. West Nile virus may show a polymorphonuclear pleocytosis, whereas enteroviruses, influenza, and John Cunningham

TABLE 2: Antibody-mediated encephalitis and movement disorders.

Central	
CRMP5	Chorea
NMDA	Orofacial dyskinesias, chorea, dystonia, stereotypies
Ma2	Parkinsonism
GAD	Stiff person syndrome
DPPX	Hyperekplexia, PERM
Yo, VKCC	Tremor, ataxia
Ri	Opsoclonus-myoclonus
IgLon5	Progressive supranuclear palsy phenotype, gait problems
VGKC	Faciobrachial dystonic seizures
Peripheral	
CaSPR2	Neuromyotonia, peripheral nerve hyperexcitability
Hu	Pseudoathetosis (neuropathic)

(JC) viruses may have a normal CSF. Mumps may have a very high pleocytosis with decreased sugar. Decreased sugar is also found in HSV and varicella-zoster virus (VZV). AE usually have a lymphocytic pleocytosis and an increased protein.[23]

Cerebrospinal Fluid-based Neuroviral Diagnostic Tests

Multiple panel-based polymerase chain reaction (PCR) tests are available[24] for the diagnosis of multiple encephalitis causative viruses. They have sensitivity ranging from 85 to 100%, but have less specificity. Confirmation by agent-specific PCR tests may be more reliable than panel based testing, however incurring a lot of cost. CSF HSV PCR is an important test for diagnosis of HSVE. They have a sensitivity of 98% and a specificity of 94%. Usually they can come negative if done within first 72 hours of symptom or after 7–10 days of antiviral treatment. Serology employing enzyme-linked immunosorbent assay (ELISA) for CSF immunoglobulin M (IgM) West Nile virus, JE, and IgG VZV are some examples where serology is preferred over PCR. IgM JE can be found positive starting from 3 to 8 days of illness and persisting up to 90 days after convalescence. Thus, if clinical suspicion is high, a convalescent sample must be retested to avoid false negatives in an early sample.[25]

Cerebrospinal Fluid-based Autoimmune Encephalitis Panels

Assays available for the diagnosis of autoantibodies can be tissue-based, cell-based, or immunoprecipitation.[23] First a tissue-based assay which employs mouse-brain cells coated with the patient's sera tagged with a marker which is detected by indirect immunofluorescence (IIF). Second is a cell-based assay, where a vector cell is transfected with a plasmid containing the deoxyribonucleic acid (DNA) for target antigen of concern, which is bathed with the patient sera and detected by IIF. Immunoassays are used for cell-surface antibodies and immunoblotting is used for onconeural antibodies. Sensitivity of kits in assessing some forms of encephalitis are high (e.g., 100% sensitivity and specificity for NMDAR encephalitis), whereas for others it is not so high. Many a times no antibody can be found. The combined sensitivity for all autoantibodies is 60–80%. There is heterogeneity in presentation and serology. Mismatch between clinically suspected antibody and serologically confirmed antibody has been reported to be 30%.[26] Testing of serum has no role in diagnosis of AE. IgG subclass of antibodies have a higher diagnostic value than IgM or IgA.

Magnetic Resonance Imaging

Magnetic resonance imaging (MRI) is an important tool for diagnosis of encephalitis[27] but in any way should not delay the CSF testing, diagnosis, and empirical treatment. Many diagnostic patterns and clues can be obtained by seeing the MRI alone. Such common patterns are summarized in **Table 3**.

TABLE 3: Common radiologic features of encephalitis.

Viral encephalitis	
Herpes simplex virus (HSV)	Asymmetric temporal, insular and inferofrontal. Basal ganglia spared
Varicella-zoster virus	Grey-white junction lesions, multiple infarcts (hemorrhagic) secondary to large and medium vessel vasculopathy
Cytomegalovirus	Periventricular discrete/patchy hyperintensities ± ventriculitis
Human herpesvirus 6	Mesial temporal involvement
Japanese encephalitis	Bilateral thalamic hyperintensities (microbleeds)
Nipah virus	Small, discrete lesions deep white matter, temporal lobes, pons, peduncles
NMDAR encephalitis	Medial temporal, cerebellum, basal ganglia, and brainstem
CV2/CRMP5 encephalitis	Bilateral basal ganglia (caudate, putamen), bilateral mesial temporal
GABA A and B	Bilateral cortical and subcortical, frontal and temporal
D2r encephalitis	Bilateral basal ganglia

Electroencephalogram

Focal discharges and diffuse slowing of background activity are common findings in electroencephalogram (EEG) in any type of encephalitis. Focal attenuation may be present over affected area. Important findings on EEG, especially HSVE are periodic lateralized epileptiform discharges (PLEDs) and bilateral independent PLEDs (BiPLEDs). They are defined[28] as patterns of repetitive slow or sharp waves, unilateral or bilateral coming at intervals of 0.5–3 seconds. They can be found in any destructive lesion of the cortex and mainly described in stroke, hemorrhages, tumors, and inflammatory diseases. AE can have focal slowing coming out from temporal regions. Delta brush is a common finding in the EEG of premature neonates. A pattern of extreme delta brush (EDB) has been defined in NMDAR encephalitis.[28] When present EDB is associated with higher rates of hospitalization, higher duration of disease and increased mortality and morbidity. Electroencephalographic epileptiform activity in an unconscious patient without any convulsion can suggest "nonconvulsive status epilepticus" and dictates treatment with intravenous (IV) antiepileptic. This necessitates the use of continuous EEG (cEEG) monitoring in any neurocritical setup.

Other differentials like Hashimoto's encephalopathy can also be picked up by EEG showing frontal rhythmic slowing, triphasic waves or positive sharp waves. Hepatic encephalopathy can also give rise to triphasic waves with background delta waves.

Positron Emission Tomography

This investigation has no such use in the acute phase of the disease, but plays an important role in detection of an occult malignancy triggering paraneoplastic encephalitis. Also, after the acute phase, positron emission tomography (PET) can be utilized in detecting pattern of brain metabolism. It also helps in understanding affection of brain in MRI-negative cases.

Treatment

Supportive treatment begins by initial evaluation of airway compromise, hypoventilation, and hemodynamic compromise and their correction.

Viral encephalitis is usually treated with antivirals and other supportive therapy. HSVE, when suspected should be treated with IV acyclovir as early as possible. Ganciclovir is an alternative and is also used for cytomegalovirus. For other viral encephalitides, the outlook for antiviral treatment is grim. No particular antiviral has been recommended for use. Though there are reports of use of intrathecal ribavirin and interferon α2b, results are not conclusive. But still, due to lack of antiviral treatment for other viruses and a high mortality of untreated HSVE, empirical treatment with IV acyclovir is warranted.

Autoimmune encephalitis is usually treated by IV methyl-prednisolone (IVMP) (1 g) for 5 days. If there is no adequate response, it should be followed up by IV immunoglobulin (IVIG) or plasmapheresis (PLEx) depending on patient's eligibility and comorbidity. In severe cases, patients should be started with IVMP + IVIG/PLEx for better results. If there is no adequate response even after 2–3 weeks, a second-line therapy with rituximab for cell surface antibody-mediated encephalitis and cyclophosphamide for onconeural antibody-mediated encephalitis needs to be tried.[29] Long-term immunomodulation for relapse prevention should also initiated when applicable. Seizures should be treated as per general protocol.

■ OUTCOME MEASURES

After discharge from hospital, patients should be regularly followed up for cognitive, psychiatric, motor, and general well-being. Quantitative assessments can be done with widely available cognitive, psychiatric, and general well-being scales. Rehabilitative measures to be undertaken in a multidisciplinary approach. Treatment of psychiatric symptoms, prevention of self-harm, support for care giver, antispasticity treatment, and seizure control to be clinically titrated.

■ CONCLUSION

To conclude, dealing with fever and encephalopathy is not only limited to encephalitis but has a myriad of other causes. Proper history and clinical examination along with clues obtained from them are indispensable in identifying and managing such patients. Proper stratification of the exact nature of etiology helps to initiate appropriate empirical therapy, however delay of investigational aids should never lead to therapeutic delay, which may be life saving. We have come a long way in the understanding of seronegative encephalitides and newer research is expected to deliver better detection techniques which will surely reduce their proportion. Also we emphasize posthospitalization rehabilitation measures including cognitive and psychiatric rehabilitation, which will ensure a good quality of life in the survivors.

Take Home Messages

- Evolving from the previous grim outlook of encephalitides which were mainly thought to be of infective origin, we have ushered into an era of treatable encephalitis mainly of autoimmune origin. Hefty insight into potential clinical and radiological markers substantiated by appropriately directed biological markers help to identify the putative pathology.
- Intensive in-hospital care combined with expert neurological decision making in treatment are pillars in the management of these patients.
- Comprehensive motor and cognitive rehabilitation, management of psychiatric comorbidity as well as monitoring and protecting against disease relapse should be the essential trends in posthospital care.
- Research is further needed for new molecular markers or more sensitive methods for older markers to solve the enigma of the various seronegative encephalitides.

■ REFERENCES

1. National Vector Borne Disease Control Programme. (2006). Guidelines for Surveillance of Acute Encephalitis Syndrome (With Special Reference To Japanese Encephalitis). [online] Available from http://www.nvbdcp.gov.in/Doc/AES%20guidelines.pdf. [Last accessed January, 2023].
2. Vachalová I, Kyavar L, Heckmann JG. Pitfalls associated with the diagnosis of herpes simplex encephalitis. J Neurosci Rural Pract. 2013;4(2):176-9.
3. Granerod J, Crowcroft NS. The epidemiology of acute encephalitis. Neuropsychol Rehabil. 2007;17(4-5):406-28.
4. Dubey D, Pittock SJ, Kelly CR, McKeon A, Lopez-Chiriboga AS, Lennon VA, et al. Autoimmune encephalitis epidemiology and a comparison to infectious encephalitis. Ann Neurol. 2018;83(1):166-77.
5. Armangue T, Spatola M, Vlagea A, Mattozzi S, Cárceles-Cordon M, Martinez-Heras E, et al. Frequency, symptoms, risk factors, and outcomes of autoimmune encephalitis after herpes simplex encephalitis: a prospective observational study and retrospective analysis. Lancet Neurol. 2018;17(9):760-72.
6. Vasanthapuram R, Shahul Hameed SK, Desai A, Mani RS, Reddy V, Velayudhan A, et al. An algorithmic approach to

identifying the aetiology of acute encephalitis syndrome in India: results of a 4-year enhanced surveillance study Lancet Glob Health. 2022;10(5):e685-93.
7. Slater J. (2019). Could the humble litchi fruit be behind a mysterious sickness that has killed nearly 100 children in India?. [online]. Available from https://nationalpost.com/news/world/could-the-humble-litchi-fruit-be-behind-a-mysterious-sickness-that-has-killed-nearly-100-children-in-india. [Last accessed January, 2023].
8. Kumar A, Mendez MD. Herpes Simplex Encephalitis. Treasure Island (FL): StatPearls Publishing; 2022.
9. Win T, Maham N, Kumar S. Herpes encephalitis: a stroke mimicker. J Community Hosp Intern Med Perspect. 2019;9(4):333-5.
10. Staley EM, Jamy R, Phan AQ, Figge DA, Pham HP. N-methyl-d-aspartate receptor antibody encephalitis: a concise review of the disorder, diagnosis, and management. ACS Chem Neurosci. 2019;10:132-42.
11. Gibson LL, McKeever A, Coutinho E, Finke C, Pollak TA. Cognitive impact of neuronal antibodies: encephalitis and beyond. Transl Psychiatry. 2020;10:304.
12. Graus F, Titulaer MJ, Balu R, Benseler S, Bien CG, Cellucci T, et al. A clinical approach to diagnosis of autoimmune encephalitis. Lancet Neurol. 2016;15(4):391-404.
13. Hansen N, Timäus C. Autoimmune encephalitis with psychiatric features in adults: historical evolution and prospective challenge. J Neural Transm (Vienna). 2021;128(1):1-14.
14. Chakraborty AP, Pandit A, Ray BK, Mukherjee A, Dubey S. Capgras syndrome and confabulation unfurling anti NMDAR encephalitis with classical papillary thyroid carcinoma: First reported case. J Neuroimmunol. 2021;357:577611.
15. Jang H, Boltz DA, Webster RG, Smeyne RJ. Viral parkinsonism. Biochim Biophys Acta. 2009;1792(7):714-21.
16. Taubenberger JK. The origin and virulence of the 1918 'Spanish' influenza virus. Proc Am Philos Soc. 2006;150:86-112.
17. Papageorgiou E, Xanthou F, Dardiotis E, Tsironi EE. Dancing eyes syndrome from West Nile virus encephalitis. Postgrad Med J. 2020;96:442.
18. Panzer J, Dalmau J. Movement disorders in paraneoplastic and autoimmune disease. Curr Opin Neurol. 2011;24(4):346-53.
19. Misra UK, Tan CT, Kalita J. Viral encephalitis and epilepsy. Epilepsia. 2008;49:13-8.
20. Simabukuro MM, Nóbrega PR, Pitombeira M, Cavalcante WCP, Grativvol RS, Pinto RF, et al. The importance of recognizing faciobrachial dystonic seizures in rapidly progressive dementias. Dement Neuropsychol. 2016;10(4):351-7.
21. Sculier C, Gaspard N. New onset refractory status epilepticus (NORSE). Seizure. 2019;68:72-8.
22. Ekmekci H, Ege F, Ozturk S. (2013). Cerebrospinal fluid abnormalities in viral encephalitis. [online] Available from https://www.intechopen.com/chapters/41749. [Last accessed January, 2023].
23. Lee SK, Lee ST. The Laboratory diagnosis of autoimmune encephalitis. J Epilepsy Res. 2016;6(2):45-50.
24. Ramachandran PS, Wilson MR. Diagnostic Testing of neurologic infections. Neurol Clin. 2018;36(4):687-703.
25. Centers for Disease Control and Prevention. (2019). Japanese Encephalitis Virus. [Online] Available from https://www.cdc.gov/japaneseencephalitis/healthcareproviders/healthcareproviders-diagnostic.html#:~:text=Laboratory%20diagnosis%20of%20JE%20is,longer%20persistence%20has%20been%20documented. [Last accessed January, 2023].
26. Wandinger KP, Leypoldt F, Junker R. Autoantibody-mediated encephalitis. Dtsch Arztebl Int. 2018;115(40):666-73.
27. Gaillard F, Weerakkody Y. (2022). Encephalitis due to herpesvirus family. [online]. Available from https://doi.org/10.53347/rID-10717. [Last accessed January, 2023].
28. Hernández-Fernández F, Fernández-Díaz E, Pardal-Fernández JM, Segura T, García-García J. Periodic lateralized epileptiform discharges as manifestation of pneumococcal meningoencephalitis. Int Arch Med. 2011;4(1):23.
29. Abboud H, Probasco JC, Irani S. Ances B, Benavides DR, Bradshaw M, et al. Autoimmune encephalitis: proposed best practice recommendations for diagnosis and acute management. J Neurol Neurosurg Psychiatry. 2021;92:757-68.

CHAPTER 17: Acute Migraine

Adreesh Mukherjee

INTRODUCTION

Headache is a common neurological symptom, and it is classified as primary or secondary.[1] Even in the emergency department (ED), primary headache disorders are usually more common than secondary disorders.[2] Despite tension-type headache (TTH) being the most common primary headache disorder, migraine forms the majority of primary headache cases presenting to the ED.[3] Migraine has a 1-year prevalence of around 15% in the general population, and according to the Global Burden of Disease Study, contributes to significant disability among the neurological disorders.[4]

DIAGNOSTIC CRITERIA

The third edition of the International Classification of Headache Disorders (ICHD-3) of the International Headache Society has specified a set of diagnostic criteria for migraine **(Table 1)**.[1] Migraine is characterized by attacks of pulsating, usually unilateral headache associated with nausea, vomiting, photophobia, and phonophobia and are exacerbated by physical activity.[5] About one-third have migraine with aura, and a significant number of patients experience a premonitory phase.[5] Aura usually precedes the headache, although, it may start when the headache phase is ongoing. The most common aura is visual, often in the form of a fortification spectrum. It is a zigzag figure near the point of fixation that may gradually spread right or left with a scintillating edge, followed by variable degrees of scotoma.[1] Other types of auras include sensory, speech and/or language, motor (hemiplegic migraine), brainstem, and retinal. Chronic migraine is defined as headache occurring on ≥15 days/month for >3 months, which, on at least 8 days/month, has the features of migraine headache.[1] Interestingly, patients with chronic migraine visit the ED more frequently than patients with episodic migraine.[6]

COMPLICATIONS

Rarely, patients may present to the ED with complications of migraine. Among these, status migrainosus denotes a

TABLE 1: ICHD-3 diagnostic criteria for migraine.[1]

Migraine without aura	• At least five attacks fulfilling criteria B–D • Headache attacks lasting 4–72 hours (when untreated or unsuccessfully treated) • Headache has at least two of the following four characteristics: 　– Unilateral location 　– Pulsating quality 　– Moderate or severe pain intensity 　– Aggravation by or causing avoidance of routine physical activity (e.g. walking or climbing stairs) • During headache at least one of the following: 　– Nausea and/or vomiting 　– Photophobia and phonophobia • Not better accounted for by another ICHD-3 diagnosis
Migraine with aura	• At least two attacks fulfilling criteria B and C • One or more of the following fully reversible aura symptoms: 　– Visual 　– Sensory 　– Speech and/or language 　– Motor 　– Brainstem 　– Retinal • At least three of the following six characteristics: 　– At least one aura symptom spreads gradually over ≥5 minutes 　– Two or more aura symptoms occur in succession 　– Each individual aura symptom lasts 5–60 minutes 　– At least one aura symptom is unilateral 　– At least one aura symptom is positive 　– The aura is accompanied, or followed within 60 minutes, by headache • Not better accounted for by another ICHD-3 diagnosis

(ICHD-3: Third edition of the International Classification of Headache Disorders of the International Headache Society)

debilitating migraine attack lasting for >72 hours.[1] Persistent aura without infarction is the presence of aura symptoms for ≥1 week without evidence of infarction on neuroimaging.[1] Migrainous infarction is the occurrence of ≥1 migraine aura symptoms (persisting for >60 minutes) in association with an ischemic brain lesion in the appropriate territory demonstrated by neuroimaging, with onset during the course of a typical migraine with aura attack.[1] Migraine aura-triggered seizure is a seizure occurring during or within one hour after an attack of migraine with aura.[1]

DIFFERENTIATING FROM OTHER HEADACHE DISORDERS

History

The diagnosis of migraine appears relatively straightforward when a patient presents with distinct episodes of typical migraine headaches. However, one has to be careful to distinguish from other primary headache disorders such as TTH and cluster headache, and not to miss an underlying secondary cause of headache. This can usually be achieved by a detailed history and focused clinical examination followed by relevant investigations. The distinguishing features of the primary headache disorders are mostly clinical. Hence, it is imperative to take a good headache history. Some of the important aspects to be enquired about include the presence of any previous episodes of headache, age at onset of headache, onset, duration and frequency of headache episodes, pain characteristics (location, quality, severity, aggravating, and relieving factors), associated symptoms (photophobia, phonophobia, nausea, vomiting, lacrimation, rhinorrhea, and conjunctival injection), any aura symptoms.[2,4] It is also important to note any history of altered sensorium, seizure, focal neurodeficit, blurring of vision/double vision/visual obscuration, neck pain, fever, and other systemic symptoms. Any history of acute or preventive medication use should also be recorded. From this information, migraine can be differentiated clinically from TTH and cluster headache (**Table 2**). This is essential as the treatment approach is different for each headache disorder.

Clinical Examination

Initial clinical examination in a case of acute headache in the ED includes a rapid assessment of mental status, meningeal signs, papilledema, fever, any signs of trauma, and localizing or lateralizing abnormalities.[6] Measurement of blood pressure is mandatory in a patient of acute headache. In patients over 50 years of age, temporal artery pulsation or tenderness should be checked (giant cell arteritis). Fever indicates central nervous system (CNS) or systemic infection. Presence of other systemic symptoms such as weight loss, polyarthralgia, etc., may point to an underlying etiology. Meningeal signs include nuchal rigidity, Kernig's sign, and Brudzinski's sign. Another important aspect is the examination of cranial nerves, especially ophthalmologic evaluation. For initial screening, examination of the pupils, visual acuity and fields and fundoscopy (especially papilledema) are essential.[6] Ptosis, diplopia, and restriction

TABLE 2: Comparison of clinical features of migraine, tension-type headache and cluster headache.[4,7-9]

Clinical features	Migraine (with or without aura)	Tension-type headache	Cluster headache
Patient characteristics	• Females > males • Onset usually in adolescence/young adulthood	• Slightly more common in women • Prevalence is highest in the fourth decade	• Males > females • Onset usually at 20–40 years age
Pain location	Usually unilateral (can be bilateral)	Usually bilateral/circumferential	Unilateral (orbital, supraorbital, and temporal)
Pain quality	Pulsating (throbbing or banging)	Pressing or tightening	Usually severe, incapacitating
Pain intensity	Moderate to severe	Mild to moderate	Severe or very severe
Duration of headache	4–72 hours (adults)	30 minutes to 7 days (may be unremitting)	15–180 minutes
Associated symptoms	• Photophobia, phonophobia, nausea, vomiting • Aura	Often none	Ipsilateral to the headache—autonomic symptoms, such as conjunctival injection, lacrimation, nasal congestion, Horner syndrome
Frequency of headache	Recurrent with variable frequency (Chronic migraine—≥15 days/month for >3 months)	Infrequent to daily (Chronic tension-type headache—≥15 days/month for >3 months)	1 every other day to 8 per day Attacks occur at specific times of the day or night, "cluster" together occurring daily or almost daily for 2–3-month bouts
Effect on activities	Aggravated by routine activities, prefers dark and quiet room	Not aggravated by routine activities	Restlessness or agitation

of eye movements are also important. Presence of conjunctival injection, lacrimation or signs of angle-closure glaucoma should be noted. Any new neurologic finding in a patient with acute headache suggests a thorough evaluation for a secondary cause.[6] Examination should focus on any focal neurodeficit, speech, or gait impairment.

Secondary Headache Disorders

Identifying an underlying cause is crucial in a patient of acute headache. Clinical clues indicating the possibility of a secondary cause of headache are useful in the ED to plan investigations and treatment. The acronym $SNOOP_4$ (sometimes expanded to $SNNOOP_{10}$) is helpful to remember "red flags" for secondary headache **(Table 3)**.[3,10,11] While some features of headache such as a "thunderclap" headache raises suspicion of a secondary cause, sometimes a secondary headache can mimic the characteristics of a primary headache disorder such as migraine. When a new headache occurs for the first time in close temporal relation to another disorder that is known to cause headache, the new headache is considered as a secondary headache, even if the headache characteristics appear similar to migraine or other primary headache disorder. On the other hand, in a patient with preexisting migraine, if the headache becomes significantly worse in close temporal relation to a causative disorder, an additional secondary headache diagnosis should be given.

INVESTIGATIONS

Investigations for a patient of acute headache are directed by the history and clinical examination, especially if there is possibility of a secondary headache disorder. Specific etiologies considered after the initial evaluation will guide subsequent investigations such as blood tests, cerebrospinal fluid (CSF) analysis, and neuroimaging. For example, the presence of fever and nuchal rigidity indicates the possibility of meningitis, which requires analysis of CSF along with neuroimaging. Although routine blood tests are usually uninformative, a raised erythrocyte sedimentation rate (ESR) and C-reactive protein (CRP) might indicate giant cell arteritis or other inflammatory causes of headache. In the case of acute migraine, additional investigations are usually normal.

Neuroimaging is commonly performed in the ED in acute headache. The imaging modality may include computed tomography (CT) scan of the head or magnetic resonance imaging (MRI). According to the clinical setting, the CT/MRI may be contrast-enhanced, or angiography/ venography may be obtained. These modalities are useful in diagnosing a secondary headache. In acute migraine,

TABLE 3: "Red flags" for secondary headache using the SNOOP4 mnemonic.[3,10]

	Warning symptom/sign	Respective features	Possible causes
S	Systemic	• *Symptoms:* Fever, night sweats, chills, weight loss, jaw claudication • *Diseases:* Malignancy, immunosuppression, chronic infection (HIV, tuberculosis)	Metastases, infection (CNS, systemic), CVST, giant cell arteritis
N	Neurologic symptoms/signs	Confusion, focal neurologic symptoms/signs, meningism, diplopia, transient visual obscurations, pulsatile tinnitus	Structural lesion (neoplastic or non-neoplastic), stroke, hydrocephalus, inflammatory, infectious, idiopathic intracranial hypertension
O	Onset	Headache that reaches peak intensity in <1 minute (thunderclap)	RCVS, subarachnoid hemorrhage, CVST, arterial dissection, pituitary apoplexy
O	Older (age at onset >50 years)	New onset headache after age 50 years	Neoplastic, infectious CNS disease, giant cell arteritis
P	Pattern change/progressive or recent onset of headache	• New onset or change to persistent/daily headache • Change in headache pattern, intensity or duration	Neoplastic, infection, Inflammatory or vascular disorder, medication-overuse headache
P	Postural/positional aggravation	Worse on standing or lying or with change in position	Intracranial hypotension from CSF leak (worse when standing), mass lesion, CVST, sinus pathology
P	Precipitated by Valsalva maneuver	Cough, sneeze, bending, straining	Chiari malformation, structural lesions that obstruct CSF flow, intracranial/posterior fossa mass, CSF leak, intracranial hypotension
P	Papilledema	Visual obscurations, diplopia or field defects	Intracranial hypertension
(P)	Pregnancy/postpartum	New onset during pregnancy	CVST, preeclampsia, RCVS, stroke, pituitary lesion

(CNS: central nervous system; CSF: cerebrospinal fluid; CVST: cerebral venous sinus thrombosis; HIV: human immunodeficiency virus; RCVS: reversible cerebral vasoconstriction syndrome)

MRI is usually normal, although, it may show white matter foci of T2-weighted hyperintensity. Rarely, an infarct may be revealed in a patient of migraine (especially with aura) with complications. Importantly, MRI can reveal clinically insignificant abnormalities (such as white matter lesions and arachnoid cysts), which, though not responsible for the acute headache, can raise concern and lead to additional unnecessary investigations.[4]

ACUTE TREATMENT

Goals of Acute Treatment

Generally, medications used to reduce the pain of migraine should be administered early in the headache phase of an attack.[12] The goals of acute treatment include a rapid and consistent freedom from pain and associated symptoms without recurrence or need for repeat dosing, restored ability to function and optimal self-care, with minimal or no adverse events.[5] However, along with the acute treatment for migraine, education of the patient is essential to reduce the risk of medication-overuse headache (MOH). It is usually seen when the migraine attacks are recurrent and the patient uses acute medications too frequently. MOH is defined as headache occurring on ≥15 days/month in a patient with a preexisting primary headache and developing as a consequence of regular overuse of acute headache medication (on ≥10 or ≥15 days/month, depending on the medication) for >3 months.[1]

Therapeutic Approach

Stratified Approach

Several therapeutic options are available for the acute treatment of migraine **(Table 4)**. In a stratified approach, selection of initial acute treatment is based on features of a specific attack (pain intensity, migraine-associated disability, presence of associated symptoms including nausea, and vomiting). Use of nonspecific treatment such as nonsteroidal anti-inflammatory drugs (NSAIDs) or acetaminophen (paracetamol) should be considered for mild-to-moderate attacks. For moderate or severe attacks and mild-to-moderate attacks that respond poorly to nonspecific therapy, migraine-specific agents (triptans, gepants, and ditan) are useful **(Flowchart 1)**.[5] The small molecule CGRP receptor antagonists (gepants) and selective serotonin (5-HT1F) receptor agonist (ditan) are newer

TABLE 4: Acute treatment medications in migraine.[4,7]

Class	Drug	Dosage	Adverse effects	Contraindication/caution
Analgesic	Paracetamol	10,00 mg oral	Nausea, vomiting, and insomnia	Hepatic disease and renal failure
NSAIDs	• Ibuprofen • Diclofenac • Naproxen	• 400 mg oral • 50 mg or 100 mg oral • 500 mg oral	Nausea, vomiting, constipation, diarrhea, reduced appetite, dizziness, rash, and drowsiness	Gastrointestinal bleeding/peptic ulcer disease, heart failure, poorly controlled hypertension, and coronary artery disease
Triptans	• Sumatriptan • Zolmitriptan • Almotriptan • Rizatriptan • Naratriptan • Frovatriptan • Eletriptan	• 50 or 100 mg oral • 6 mg subcutaneous • 10 or 20 mg intranasal • 2.5 or 5 mg oral • 5 mg intranasal • 12.5 mg oral • 10 mg oral tablet • (5 mg if treated with propranolol) • 10 mg mouth-dispersible wafers • 2.5 mg oral • 2.5 mg oral • 20, 40, or 80 mg oral	• Nausea, dizziness, somnolence, paresthesia, dry mouth, flushing, and heaviness sensation • Theoretical risk of serotonin syndrome when used with other serotonin drugs	Cardiovascular or cerebrovascular disease, uncontrolled hypertension, hemiplegic migraine, and migraine with brainstem aura
Gepants	• Ubrogepant • Rimegepant	• 50, 100 mg oral • 75 mg oral	Nausea and somnolence	Contraindicated with strong CYP3A4 inhibitors Avoid coadministration with inhibitors of P-glycoprotein or BCRP Caution for hypersensitivity to rimegepant
Ditans	Lasmiditan	50, 100, or 200 mg oral	• Dizziness, fatigue, paresthesia, and sedation • Avoid driving for 8 hours after use	Concomitant use with drugs that are P-glycoprotein substrates

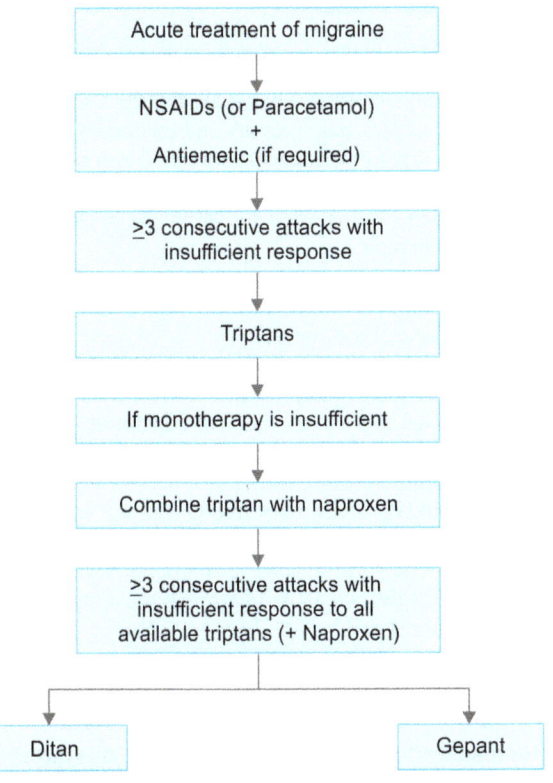

Flowchart 1: Acute treatment of migraine.

(NSAIDs: nonsteroidal anti-inflammatory drugs)

medications that are usually advised in patients who had adverse effects, or inadequate response, or contraindications to triptans.

Stepped Care Approach

The acute treatments can be classified as first-line, second-line, third-line, and adjunct. The first-line medications are NSAIDs (acetylsalicylic acid, ibuprofen, and diclofenac potassium). Paracetamol may also be used, although it has less efficacy. If these are ineffective, triptans are used as second-line agents. Triptans are selective serotonin 5-HT1B/D agonist. Triptans are most effective when taken early in an attack, when the headache is still mild. Upon relapse, patients can repeat the triptan treatment or combine it with fast-acting NSAID (naproxen sodium). If one triptan is ineffective, others might still be useful.[4] In case of headache rapidly reaching peak intensity or inability to take oral triptans because of vomiting, subcutaneous injection of sumatriptan may be helpful. If there is inadequate response to triptans (at least three consecutive attacks) or their use is contraindicated, ditan (lasmiditan) or gepants (ubrogepant and rimegepant) may be used as third-line medications. However, these are newer molecules and not widely available. For patients who experience nausea/vomiting during migraine attacks, prokinetic antiemetics such as domperidone and metoclopramide are useful oral adjuncts.[4]

An emerging option for acute treatment of migraine is noninvasive neuromodulation. Four devices are approved for use—external trigeminal nerve stimulation, single-pulse transcranial magnetic stimulation, noninvasive vagus nerve stimulation, and remote electrical neuromodulation. These may be useful in patients who have adverse effects or contraindications to current therapy, prefer nondrug therapy or are overusing acute medications. However, the cost is high and these are not widely available in India.

Status Migrainosus

Although, status migrainosus is defined by an attack lasting for >72 hours, its treatment often begins earlier. When attacks are severe at onset with high risk for progression to status migrainosus, the use of intranasal or subcutaneous triptans are preferred because these have faster onset of effect. Another method for attacks that are severe from onset is acute combination therapy consisting of NSAID, triptan, and antidopaminergic agent. As a next step, one can consider options such as ketorolac (NSAID), gepants and ditans, or steroids (oral dexamethasone, prednisolone, or methylprednisolone) along with maintenance of adequate hydration. If the headache is still persisting, parenteral medications may be useful such as antidopaminergic agents (metoclopramide), NSAIDs (ketorolac), paracetamol, and intravenous corticosteroids (dexamethasone or methylprednisolone).

Specific Situations

Children and Adolescents

Migraine is common among children, although the criteria are slightly different and the duration of migraine attacks can be 2–72 hours. In children, the attacks are often shorter and the headache is more often bilateral and may not be pulsating. In children with attacks of short duration, bed-rest alone might suffice. When needed, ibuprofen is recommended as first-line medication. For adolescents aged 12–17 years, multiple NSAIDs and triptans are approved.

Migraine in Women

Paracetamol should be used as the first-line medication for acute treatment of migraine in pregnancy. Migraine medication therapy in the postpartum period also requires caution because of potential risks to the infant. Paracetamol is the preferred acute medication, although ibuprofen and sumatriptan are also considered safe.[4] In women with menstrual migraine, about 8% experience migraine attacks that are exclusively related to their menstruation, referred to as pure menstrual migraine. If acute medication therapy is inadequate, perimenstrual preventive treatment may be used which includes a long-acting NSAID (naproxen) or triptan (frovatriptan or naratriptan) for 5 days, beginning 2 days before the expected first day of menstruation.

Medical Comorbidities

Some medical conditions preclude use of certain acute therapies or require additional monitoring such as the use of NSAIDs in kidney dysfunction or gastrointestinal bleeding/ulcers, paracetamol in liver dysfunction, triptans in cerebrovascular/cardiovascular disease, and antiemetic in cardiac dysrhythmia.

RESPONSE TO TREATMENT

Resolution or improvement of headache at 2 hours with medication is considered good control. Some patients can experience relapses, which are defined as a return of symptoms within 48 hours after apparently successful treatment.[4] They can repeat the triptan treatment or combine the triptan with fast-acting NSAID (naproxen). However, repeating the treatment does not prevent further relapses and ultimately increases the risk of MOH.

Initiation of Preventive Treatment

In patients who have at least 2 migraine days/month and adverse effects despite therapy, preventive treatment should be considered. The aim of preventive treatment is to reduce the frequency, duration, or severity of migraine attacks. It also improves responsiveness to and avoid escalation in use of acute treatment. This is helpful in MOH. Several medications are available for preventive treatment including beta blockers (atenolol, bisoprolol, metoprolol, or propranolol), topiramate, candesartan, flunarizine, amitriptyline, sodium valproate, and the newly introduced CGRP monoclonal antibodies.

CONCLUSION

Migraine is a common primary headache disorder. The attacks can be severe enough to bring the patient to the ED. In such cases, migraine should be differentiated from other causes of headache, both primary and secondary. In a known patient of migraine, a recent aggravation of headache should be investigated properly to ensure an underlying cause is not missed. Several medications are available for the acute treatment of migraine, and a stratified or stepped care approach may be followed for their optimal use. The selection of an appropriate medication is guided by the headache characteristics as well as the demographic profile and comorbidities of the patient. While the goal of acute treatment is rapid and consistent freedom from pain and associated symptoms, it is also important to prevent MOH by providing proper guidance to the patient and implementing adequate preventive treatment when required.

Take Home Messages

- The diagnosis of migraine is clinical—a good headache history is of utmost importance.
- An acute attack of migraine has to be differentiated from other headache disorders, both primary and secondary, especially in the case of a first-ever headache or a worst-ever headache.
- Neuroimaging (and other investigations) is useful in a case of acute headache, but is not a substitute for good history and clinical examination.
- Acute medication should be offered to everyone who experience migraine attacks, and it should be used early in the headache phase of the attack.
- A stratified or stepped care approach should be followed for the optimal use of acute medications.
- Selection of an appropriate medication should be guided by the headache characteristics as well as the demographic profile and comorbidities of the patient.
- Patients should be advised that frequent, repeated use of acute medication can lead to MOH.
- In patients who have at least 2 migraine days/month and adverse effects despite acute treatment, preventive treatment should be considered.

REFERENCES

1. Headache Classification Committee of the International Headache Society (IHS). The International Classification of Headache Disorders, 3rd edition. Cephalalgia. 2018;38:1-211.
2. Chinthapalli K, Logan AM, Raj R, Nirmalananthan N. Assessment of acute headache in adults—what the general physician needs to know. Clin Med (Lond). 2018;18:422-7.
3. Dodick DW. Diagnosing Secondary and Primary Headache Disorders. Continuum (Minneap Minn). 2021;27:572-85.
4. Eigenbrodt AK, Ashina H, Khan S, Diener HC, Mitsikostas DD, Sinclair AJ, et al. Diagnosis and management of migraine in ten steps. Nat Rev Neurol. 2021;17:501-14.
5. Ailani J, Burch RC, Robbins MS; Board of Directors of the American Headache Society. The American Headache Society Consensus Statement: Update on integrating new migraine treatments into clinical practice. Headache. 2021;61:1021-39.
6. Orr SL, Friedman BW, Dodick DW. Emergency Headache Diagnosis and Management, 1st edition. United Kingdom: Cambridge University Press; 2017.
7. McNeil M. Headaches in Adults in Primary Care: Evaluation, Diagnosis, and Treatment. Med Clin North Am. 2021;105: 39-53.
8. Weaver-Agostoni J. Cluster headache. Am Fam Physician. 2013;88:122-8.
9. National Institute for Health and Care Excellence. Headaches in over 12s: diagnosis and management. NICE Guideline, No. 150. London: National Institute for Health and Care Excellence (NICE); 2012.
10. Dodick DW. Pearls: headache. Semin Neurol. 2010;30:74-81.
11. Do TP, Remmers A, Schytz HW, Schankin C, Nelson SE, Obermann M, et al. Red and orange flags for secondary headaches in clinical practice: SNNOOP10 list. Neurology. 2019;92:134-44.
12. Ashina M. Migraine. N Engl J Med. 2020;383:1866-76.

SECTION 4

Gastrointestinal Emergencies

Section Editor: Jayanta Mukherjee

18. **Acute Abdomen: Approach**
    Jayanta Mukherjee

19. **Acute Gastrointestinal Hemorrhage: Approach**
    Jayanta Mukherjee

20. **Acute Pancreatitis: Approach**
    Jayanta Mukherjee

21. **Acute Hepatic Failure**
    Vikas Prakash

CHAPTER 18

Acute Abdomen: Approach

Jayanta Mukherjee

■ INTRODUCTION

The abdomen is a Pandora's box. An "acute abdomen" in the emergency is a challenge to the junior doctor on duty and is like a jigsaw puzzle in which you try to solve the puzzle fast and correctly except here we are dealing with a human life. The approach to the problem should be with an open mind and without any bias toward a specific diagnosis and the "ego" should not be hurt if the diagnosis changes after re-evaluation.

Pain is the most common presentation of an acute abdomen, though rarely the situation may present painlessly especially in the extreme of ages and occasionally in pregnancy.[1] Majority of the cause of pain abdomen need a surgical intervention but quite a few can be managed by nonsurgical measures. Approximately 40% of these patients have nonspecific findings. In a small number of patients, the etiology of acute abdomen is life-threatening and the evaluation must be efficient and accurate so that there is no delay in treating seriously ill patients and resources are not overused in less critical patients.

Abdominal pain can be:[2]
- *Visceral pain:* Vague in onset and localization and perceived as a dull sensation in the abdominal midline. The visceral pain is usually the result of stretch and distension of the organs.
- *Parietal pain:* It is more intense, and well localized and is due to noxious stimulation of the peritoneum, skin or muscles.
- *Referred pain:* It is perceived at a point distant from the primary source of pain and may be situated away from the abdomen.[1]

■ EVALUATION

An evaluation of a patient with an acute abdomen requires a careful and expeditious history taking and a physical examination and followed by investigations—imaging and blood tests.

As in all cases of a medical emergency a rapid assessment of the patients overall physiological state looking for clues that the patient is in shock or at the edge of hemodynamic instability. An early identification of patients who are unstable or in shock is essential to expedite treatment and improve the likelihood of a satisfactory outcome.[2]

History

A proper history taking remains the most important component of the initial evaluation of a patient with acute abdominal pain.

Chronology

The initiation of pain and its progress helps to identify the possible cause of pain. Rapid onset of pain is often a measure of the severity of the underlying disorder. Pain that is sudden in onset is usually the result of an intra-abdominal catastrophe such as a perforated viscus, mesenteric infection or a ruptured aneurysm. Affected patients usually recall the exact moment of pain. Progression of pain is also an important factor. In some disorders pain is self-limited. Whereas in others pain is progressive. A wavy pattern of pain usually points toward obstruction of a hollow viscus. The duration of pain is also important. A pain persisting for an extended period usually suggests a less life-threatening cause of pain than those who present within hours to days of their symptoms.[3]

Location

The location of pain provides a clue to interpreting the cause. A noxious stimulus may lead to a combination of visceral, somatoparietal or referred pain thereby leading to confusion in interpretation. A proper knowledge of the neuroanatomical pathways is required to evaluate the location. A pain starting in the abdomen and radiating to the back usually points toward pancreatic or a duodenal pain.[3]

Intensity and Character

Acute abdominal pain usually follows one of the three patterns.[1,4]

1. Pain, that is severe in intensity and physically incapacitates the sufferers and is usually due to severe

life-threatening disease such as perforated viscus, ruptured aneurysm or severe pancreatitis.
2. The second type of pain is called a colic and is a crescendo-decrescendo type of pain pointing toward a hollow viscus.
3. The third pattern is a gradually increasing discomfort poorly localized initially but becomes more localized as the pain intensifies. Symptoms in the elderly and children can be subtle in spite of the presence of a life-threatening pathology making this group particularly challenging.[5]

Aggravating and Relieving Features

The relationship of pain with positional change, meals, bowel movement and stress may yield diagnostic clues. Patients with parietal pain prefer to lie motionless whereas those with colic may writhe in an attempt to be comfortable. Intake of food precipitating pain suggests the possibility of gastric ulcer, pancreatitis, biliary colic or a mesenteric ischemia. Pain relieved by intake of food points toward the duodenal ulcers. Relief of pain with passage of flatus and stool usually suggests a colonic or small intestinal pathology.[5]

Associated Symptoms

An extensive list of constitutional symptoms such as fever, chills, weight loss, joint pains, anorexia, nausea, vomiting, flatulence, constipation or diarrhea jaundice, dysuria, changes in menstruation and pregnancy should be sought for. These associated symptoms in addition to the primary complaint may help to reach a possible diagnosis.

Past History

A careful review of the patients additional medical or surgical problems often gives clue to the cause of acute pain abdomen. Recurrences of pain suggests a previously existing problem like subacute obstructions, renal calculi or pelvic inflammatory disease. Intestinal obstruction in the absence of previous history or surgery in the abdomen points toward a surgical pathology like hernia or neoplasm. Few medical illnesses such as vasculitis scleroderma or sickle-cell disease can present with acute abdomen. A list of medications being consumed by the patient needs to be evaluated too to identify a possible culprit.[6]

Physical Examination

The physical examination of a patient of acute abdomen begins as soon as the patient is first seen by the physician. The patient's appearance, method of lying, position of limbs gives the first clue. A patient unwilling to move suggests parietal pain while an uncomfortable continuously changing position suggests a visceral pain. A shallow breathing or deep sighing respiration breathing pattern may suggest a parietal pain or metabolic acidosis, respectively. A rapid assessment for signs of sepsis or shock is essential.[6]

Abdominal Examination

A careful inspection of the exposed abdomen should be done, to assess for abnormal protrusions visible peristalsis or swellings. An auscultatory examination for bowel sounds should precede any maneuvers that disturbs abdominal contents. The examiner should listen for at least 2 minutes before concluding that the abdomen is silent. In intestinal obstructions a high tinkling sound is audible. The auscultation is a good method to assess for tenderness too. If tenderness is detected an assessment for rebound tenderness should be carried out to look for peritonitis. A palpation is perform next do identify involuntary guarding or muscle rigidity. Patients with a rigid abdomen rarely reveal any additional findings.[3,7]

Genital, Rectal and Pelvic Examination

The physical examination of an acute abdominal pain is incomplete if the genital, rectal and pelvic examination is not done properly. A gynecological pathology needs to be excluded in all women with acute abdominal pain.[3,7]

Laboratory Data

The history and physical examination is supported by the laboratory data to find the etiology of acute abdominal pain. All patients of acute abdominal pain should have a:
- Complete blood count with a differential count
- Urine analysis
- Serum electrolytes
- Renal function tests
- Glucose
- Fluid and acid base status
- Urine for a pregnancy testing should be performed in all women of reproductive age presenting with pain abdomen
- Liver biochemistry
- Serum amylase and lipase is required in all patients of upper abdominal pain[1]

■ IMAGING

The basic imaging in the emergency department is an X-ray of the abdomen in supine and erect position supported by an ultrasonography (USG) examination.

X-ray

An X-ray of the abdomen is the basic imaging to be done in an acute abdominal pain. Intestinal obstruction, hollow viscus perforation, renal calculi and occasionally gallstone disease can be identified by this basic test which is often forgotten in lieu of advanced tests.[8]

Ultrasonography

A USG done properly has the capability of identifying a large majority of the causes of acute abdominal pain.

The advantage of a USG is that it can be performed in the emergency suite or even at the bedside of the patient. Gallstone disease and its complications, pancreatitis, fluids in the abdomen, ureteric calculus, appendicitis and torsion of testis and ovary and ruptured ectopic pregnancy are the major pathological problems identified by a USG.[8]

Computed Tomography

The development of high-speed helical computed tomography (CT) has revolutionized the evaluation of acute abdominal pain. The request for a CT scan in the emergency by the attending physician depends upon the inability of identifying the cause of acute abdomen in spite of the basic imaging such as X-ray and USG. The arguments against routine CT scan in evaluation of acute abdominal pain are the selection of CT protocols such as noncontrast computed tomography (NCCT) or CT with oral, IV or rectal contrasts, which requires a radiologists attention. Exposure to radiation and its inability to identify gallstone disease and cholangitis in majority are also a hindrance to its excessive use.

An algorithm to remember in the emergency room is mentioned here (Flowchart 1).[1]

An acute abdomen can be a nightmare to deal with, unless a swift and an accurate diagnosis is made and therefore providing proper care.

In our hospital, the common causes of acute pain are—acute pancreatitis, acute cholecystitis, acute appendicitis, renal colic, and intestinal obstruction. The less common causes seen in our hospital are ectopic pregnancy, diverticulitis, intestinal ischemia, acute myocardial infarction (AMI), pneumonia (referred pain), diabetic ketoacidosis (DKA) to name a few. Functional pain presenting as an acute abdomen may require an astute physician to identify the problem to avoid unnecessary utilization of resources

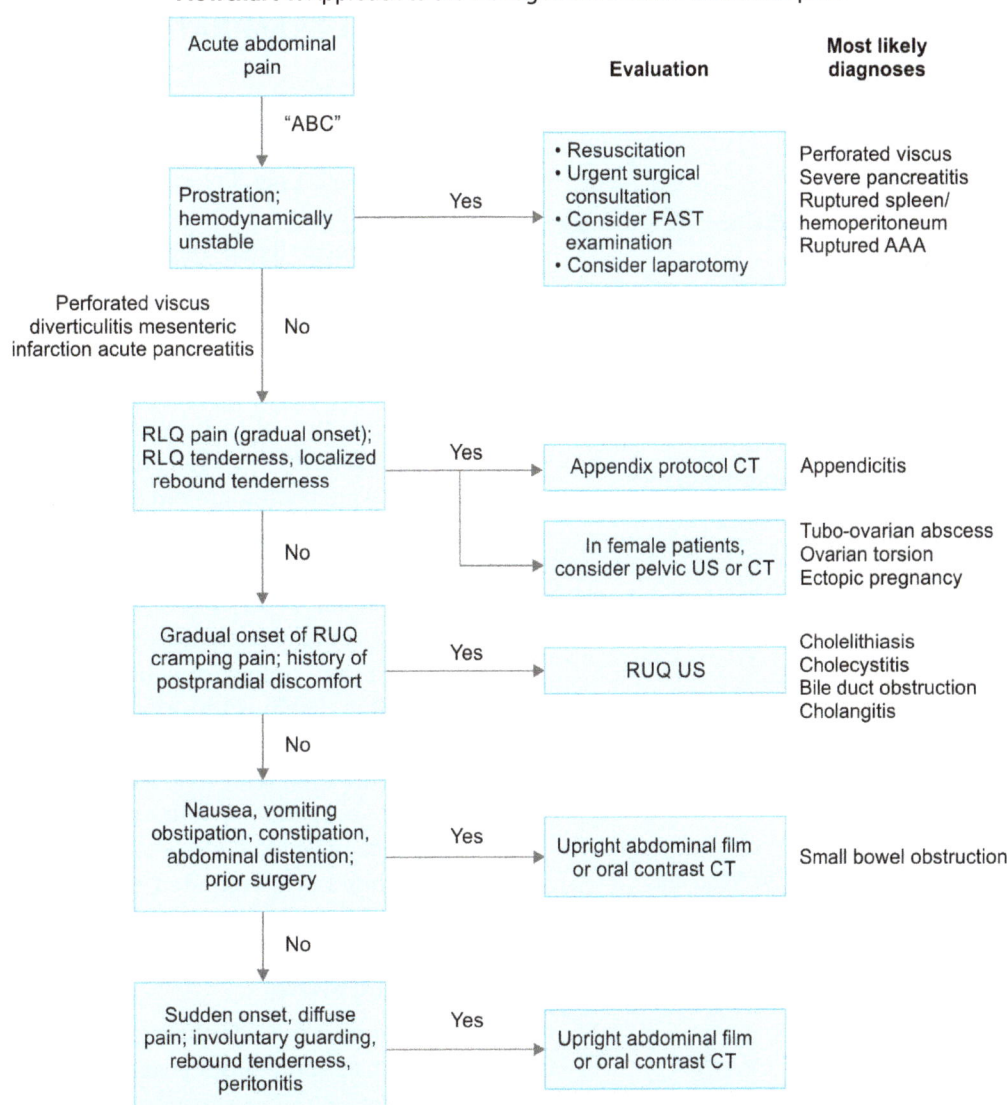

Flowchart 1: Approach to the management of acute abdominal pain.

(AAA: abdominal aortic aneurysm; ABC: airway, breathing, circulation; FAST: focused abdominal sonogram for trauma; RLQ: right lower quadrant; RUQ: right upper quadrant)

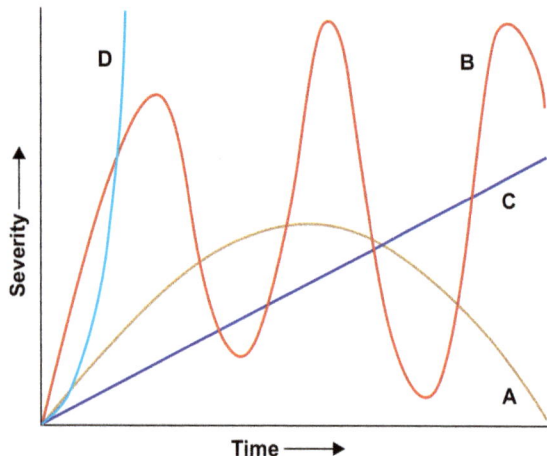

Fig. 1: Patterns of pain. A—pain subsides spontaneously with time-gastroenteritis; B—colic-intestinal, renal, biliary pain; C—progressive pain–appendicitis, diverticulitis; D—catastrophic onset—ruptured aortic aneurysm.

In certain cases, the physician needs to attend to an acute abdomen patient in his chamber where there is the scarcity of basic investigations. A rapid assessment of the patient will determine need of urgent admission to a hospital or whether an OPD evaluation may be possible.

FEATURES OF "PAIN"

These help to identify the causes of pain, which are discussed here.

Position

- *Upper abdomen:* Pancreatitis, cholecystitis, peptic ulcer disease (PUD)
- *Mid abdomen:* Renal colic (flanks), intestinal colic
- *Lower abdomen:* Renal colic, ectopic pregnancy
- *Right side of abdomen:* Appendicitis
- *Left side of abdomen:* Diverticulitis

Duration of Pain (Fig. 1)

- Upper abdomen
  - *Less than an hour or two:* Biliary colic and PUD (recurrent episode)
  - *>2 hours but <6–8 hours:* Acute cholecystitis
  - *In days:* Pancreatitis
- Mid abdomen
  - *In minutes to hours:* Intestinal or renal colic
- Lower abdomen
  - *Hours to days—continuous:* Appendicitis, diverticulitis, ectopic pregnancy

Type of Pain/Relation

- Upper abdomen
  - *Continuous pain with related to food:* Cholecystitis, pancreatitis, and PUD
- Mid abdomen
  - *Colic related to food:* Intestinal pathology
  - *Colic not related to food:* Renal colic
- Lower abdomen
  - *Continuous pain:* Appendicitis, diverticulitis, and ectopic pregnancy

RELIEVING FACTORS

- Vomiting reduces pain
- *Small volume vomiting:* Cholecystitis
- *Large volume vomiting:* Intestinal colic and PUD with gastric outlet obstruction
- *Crouched posture and self-compression:* Colic—intestinal, renal
- *Crouched and avoiding touch (tenderness):* Pancreatitis, and cholecystitis
- Flatus and stool
- Intestinal colic, and diverticulitis

CLINICAL EXAMINATION

- Abdomen
- *Rigid:* Peritonitis
- Soft tender (upper) cholecystitis
- PUD (lower) appendicitis
- Diverticulitis
- *Soft nontender:* Renal colic
- Firm tender (upper) pancreatitis
- *Lower:* Appendicitis with complications, ectopic pregnancy
- *Distended nontender:* Intestinal obstruction
- Peristalsis-hurried-early intestinal obstruction
- *Tinkling sounds:* Intestinal obstruction
- *Absent:* Pancreatitis, prolonged intestinal obstruction
- Hemodynamic evaluation
- Presence of tachycardia and hypotension would suggest dehydration, sepsis or severe pain and warrants urgent hospitalization irrespective of the clinical diagnosis.

Though the etiology of acute abdomen are varied, a proper and meticulous history and a clinical examination will help identify majority of the causes prior to admission and the remaining after few basic tests and the rest after detailed investigation. While attempting a diagnosis, the triage and management also should start at the emergency and continued and upgraded to the required level after admission.

CONCLUSION

Acute abdomen is a life-threatening emergency. A rapid assessment, triaging, hospitalization and stabilization of the patient along with investigation guided further treatment decides the outcome of the event, which in the majority of the individuals is satisfactory but in others may lead to prolonged hospitalization, ICU care, surgery, significant morbidity and even mortality.

Take Home Messages

Common causes of acute pain are:
- Acute pancreatitis, acute cholecystitis, acute appendicitis, renal colic and intestinal obstruction.
- Less common causes are ectopic pregnancy, diverticulitis, intestinal ischemia, AMI, pneumonia (referred pain), DKA to name a few.
- Functional pain presenting as an acute abdomen may require an astute physician to identify the problem to avoid unnecessary utilisation of resources.

The protocol which we ask our residents to follow are:
- A proper clinical history and examination for triage regarding admission (OPD management, hospitalization in a general bed or in the ICU).
- A basic series of tests—ECG, urine ketone, and an X-ray abdomen in erect position is done in the emergency helping us to diagnose or exclude certain causes of acute abdomen.
- It is followed by the series of common tests in all— USG abdomen, blood biochemistry and urine examination.
- If yet inconclusive then advanced tests like CT abdomen, endoscopy, MRI and others are advised.

REFERENCES

1. Feldman M, Friedman LS, Brandt LJ. Sleisenger and Fordtran's Gastrointestinal and Liver Disease: Pathophysiology, Diagnosis, Management, 11th edition. Philadelphia: Saunders; 2015.
2. Falch C, Vicente D, Häberle H, Kirschniak A, Müller S, Nissan A, et al. Treatment of acute abdominal pain in the emergency room: a systematic review of the literature. Eur J Pain. 2014;18(7):902-13.
3. Andersen DK, Billiar TR, Brunicardi FC, Dunn DL, Hunter JG, Matthews JB, et al. Schwartz's Principles of Surgery. New York: McGraw-Hill Education; 2015.
4. Trentzsch H, Werner J, Jauch KW. Acute abdominal pain in the emergency department—a clinical algorithm for adult patients. Zentralbl Chir. 2011;136(2):118-28.
5. Prystupa A, Kurys-Denis E, Krupski W, Mosiewicz J. Diagnostics of acute pain in abdominal right upper quadrant. J Pre-Clin Clin Res. 2011;5(2):56-9.
6. Martin RF, Rossi RL. The acute abdomen: an overview and algorithms. Surg Clin North Am. 1997;77(6):1227-43.
7. Squires RA, Postier RG. Acute abdomen. Sabiston Textbook of Surgery, 19th edition. Philadelphia: Elsevier Saunders; 2012.
8. Kamin RA, Nowicki TA, Courtney DS, Powers RD. Pearls and pitfalls in the emergency department evaluation of abdominal pain. Emerg Med Clin North Am. 2003;21(1):61-72.

CHAPTER 19

Acute Gastrointestinal Hemorrhage: Approach

Jayanta Mukherjee

■ INTRODUCTION

Gastrointestinal (GI) bleeding, an acute and horrifying event, especially if per oral, for the patient and their relatives brings a patient to emergency room (ER) earlier than majority of the other GI emergencies. For >50 years the mortality from upper gastrointestinal (UGI) bleeding was reported at 5–14%. Recent data suggests in-hospital mortality around 2%, likely due to advance in medical and endoscopic treatment.[1]

The cause of bleeding can be broadly distributed into an UGI or a lower GI bleeding and an evaluation at the emergency needs to be done by the ER resident to triage the patient, irrespective of the etiology for outpatient department (OPD) evaluation or institutionalization, and if admitted—general ward or intensive care unit (ICU) for monitoring and urgent treatment.

The "UGI" bleeding, historically suggested as bleeding proximal to the ligament of Treitz and "lower GI" bleeding distal to this ligament. Since 2006, the definition of lower GI bleeding has been modified to bleeding from a source distal to the ileocecal valve.

A new terminology—"mid gut" bleeding has been proposed for the bleeding arising from the small bowel.[1]

Approximately 50% of admissions for GI bleeding are for UGI bleeding, 40% for lower GI bleeding, and 10% are for obscure (small bowel) bleeding.[2]

■ DEFINITIONS

Severe Gastrointestinal Bleeding

Documented GI bleeding [hematemesis, hematochezia, melena, or positive nasogastric (NG) lavage] accompanied by shock or orthostatic hypotension, a decrease of hematocrit by at least 6%, hemoglobin by 2 g/dL, or transfusion of at least two units of packed red blood cell (PRBC).[1,3]

Overt Gastrointestinal Bleeding

It is defined as visible blood loss from GI tract.

Hematemesis

It is defined as vomiting of blood—source of bleeding form nasopharynx, esophagus, stomach, and duodenum. Bright red blood suggests recent or ongoing bleeding and dark material suggests bleeding that stopped some time ago.

Melena

It is defined as black tarry stool, resulting from degradation of blood to hematin by intestinal bacteria. It usually occurs when the bleeding is >50–100 mL in the UGI tract.

Hematochezia

It refers to bright red bleed from rectum.

Occult Gastrointestinal Bleeding

It is defined as bleeding that is not clinically visible.

Obscure Gastrointestinal Bleeding

It refers to GI bleeding that is not apparent after a routine upper gastrointestinal endoscopy (UGIE), lower gastrointestinal endoscopy (LGIE), and possibly a push enteroscopy.[1]

■ UPPER GASTROINTESTINAL BLEEDING

The causes can be broadly distributed as variceal and nonvariceal suggesting the urgency and mode of treatment and prognosticating the possible outcome and additional treatment, especially in cases of portal hypertension.[2,4]

■ INITIAL ASSESSMENT AND MANAGEMENT OF GASTROINTESTINAL BLEEDING

History

A proper medical history regarding possible:
- Liver dysfunction
- Medications causing ulceration or bleeding

- Prior GI surgery along with features suggesting the source of bleed[5]
- Esophageal source is suspected with a history of gastroesophageal reflux disease (GERD), dysphagia, odynophagia, pill ingestion, and alcohol abuse
- Painless rectal bleeding is more suggestive of diverticular or hemorrhoidal bleeding
- Presence of abdominal cramps may suggest an infectious or an inflammatory cause of lower GI bleeding[6]
- On a background of cardiovascular disease and ischemic cause of GI bleed may be favored.

Examination

Initially, physical examination should focus on:[4]
- The patient's vital signs, with attention to signs of hypovolemia such as hypotension, tachycardia, and orthostasis.
- The abdomen should be examined for surgical scars, tenderness, and masses.
- Signs of chronic liver disease include spider telangiectasias, palmar erythema gynecomastia, ascites, splenomegaly, caput medusae, and Dupuytren contracture.
- The skin, lips, and buccal mucosa should be examined for telangiectasias, which are suggestive of hereditary hemorrhagic telangiectasia (HHT), or Osler-Weber-Rendu disease.
- Changes of the skin of the fingers may indicate scleroderma (systemic sclerosis), which is associated with gastric antral vascular ectasia (GAVE) or UGI.
- Pigmented lip lesions may suggest Peutz-Jeghers syndrome.
- Purpuric skin lesions may suggest Henoch-Schönlein purpura.
- Acanthosis nigricans may suggest underlying malignancy, especially gastric cancer.
- The patient's feces should be observed to identify melena or maroon and red stool; however, the subjective description of stool color varies greatly among patients and physicians.

Resuscitation and Monitoring

General

Adequate resuscitation and stabilization is an essential and first step in managing patients with GI bleed.
- Venous access by two large caliber intravenous catheters or a central venous catheter is essential.
- Fluids should be infused to restore normal circulating volume.
- Vasopressor therapy should be considered in patients with shock after replenishing intravenous fluid.
- Supplemental oxygen via nasal cannula is often given.
- Hemodynamically stable patients may be admitted to a regular ward.
- Those with hemodynamic instability, respiratory problems or with multiple comorbidities, or have active ongoing bleeding are to be admitted in ICU.
- Prophylactic intubation in select patients may be required.
- Unlike UGI bleeding, hemodynamic instability is a rare presentation of lower GI bleed.
- Presence of hemodynamic compromise in a case of lower GI bleed might indicate an UGI source of bleeding which is found in about 15% of patients of lower GI bleeding.[6,7]

Nasogastric Tube

Nasogastric tube aspirate visually characterize gastric contents and is useful for determining the presence or absence of large amounts of red blood, coffee-ground material, or nonbloody fluid.[8] It is particularly useful in patients with melena in the absence of hematemesis. Patients who have coffee-ground emesis or fresh bloody emesis that is witnessed do not require placement of an NG tube for diagnostic purposes, but may need an NG tube to help clear the gastric blood for better endoscopic visualization and to minimize the risk of aspiration.

Although, NG lavage has been associated with an earlier time to endoscopy, this does not affect clinical outcomes such as mortality or need for surgery or transfusion.[8,9] Due to its lack of patient benefits and its adverse events including pain, current guidelines do not recommend routine NG tube placement or lavage in the early management of patients with suspected nonvariceal UGI bleed.

Nasogastric tubes are not contraindicated in suspected variceal bleeding.

Proton Pump Inhibitors

Proton pump inhibitor (PPI) plays an important role in managing nonvariceal UGI bleeding. An 80 mg intravenous (IV) bolus followed by 8 mg/h continuous infusion for 72 hours stabilizes the clot, prevents rebleeding, reduces the length of hospitalization, number of blood transfusions, and need for surgery.[2,10]

Blood Transfusion

Transfusion of packed red cells is a key element in the initial management of GI bleed. Patients with ongoing significant bleed will require blood transfusion regardless of hemoglobin levels at presentation as the hemoglobin has not yet had time to equilibrate in cases of rapid bleeding.[5]

A restrictive policy of blood transfusion for subjects with GI bleeding with the threshold of hemoglobin level <7 g/dL aiming for 9-10 g/dL, except in cases of massive active bleeding or cardiovascular comorbidities that may necessitate a more individualized strategy with higher transfusion thresholds of 9–10 g/dL.[10]

Platelet transfusion should be considered when the count is <50,000/dL.

Drugs to Reduce Portal Hypertension

Drugs such as somatostatin, octreotide, and terlipressin are often infused prior to endoscopic therapy, especially in suspected portal hypertensive patients or those with a prior episode of variceal bleeding. The bleeding may be arrested prior to endotherapy with these drugs and thereby helps in visualization of the bleeding vessels. These drugs are occasionally used in lower GI bleeding in order to reduce the portal pressure and arrest the bleeding.[1]

Antibiotics

Antibiotics are preferably given in suspected variceal bleeding with oral rifaximin to prevent hepatic encephalopathy.[4,5]

For algorithms to follow in cases of upper GI bleeding[1] see **Flowchart 1**.

For algorithm in case of lower GI bleeding see **Flowchart 2**.[1]

Postresuscitation–Endoscopy

In case of UGI bleeding, an endoscopy is a critical step in the management. Current guidelines recommend that endoscopic be performed within 24 hours of presentation. However, the role of an emergency endoscopy remains controversial. In general, endoscopy perform within 12 hours of presentation identified more high-risk lesions without any improvement in clinical outcomes but endoscopic performed within 24 hours decrease the length of hospital stay and the need for surgery.[9,11]

Patients of lower GI bleeding with high-risk features who have evidence of ongoing bleed should undergo an urgent colonoscopy within 24 hours of presentation with bowel cleansing, whereas in the absence of high-risk features without any signs of active bleeding a colonoscopy can be deferred.[6,11]

Take Home Message

- In our hospital, the most common causes of UGI bleed are usually ulcers and erosions in the stomach, duodenum or esophagus, varices, and malignancy. Whereas the common causes of lower GI bleeding are hemorrhoids, inflammatory bowel disease, malignant lesions, and left colonic diverticula in the elderly population, while bleeding from rectal polyps and anal fissure are more common in the younger generation. Usually a rapid evaluation of the history and clinical status of a patient presenting with GI bleeding for triaging and early admission and resuscitation along with targeted medical, endoscopic, or surgical intervention is the protocol to follow to have a successful outcome.

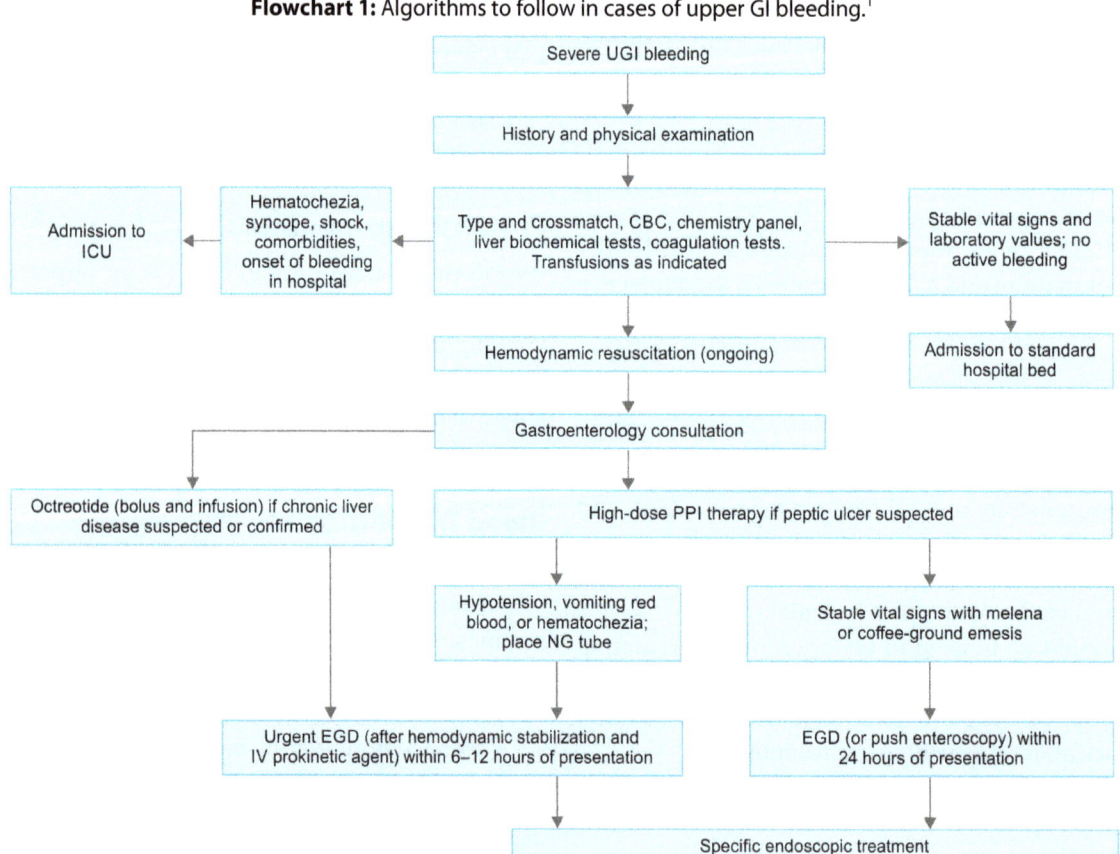

Flowchart 1: Algorithms to follow in cases of upper GI bleeding.[1]

Flowchart 2: Algorithm in case of lower GI bleeding.[1]

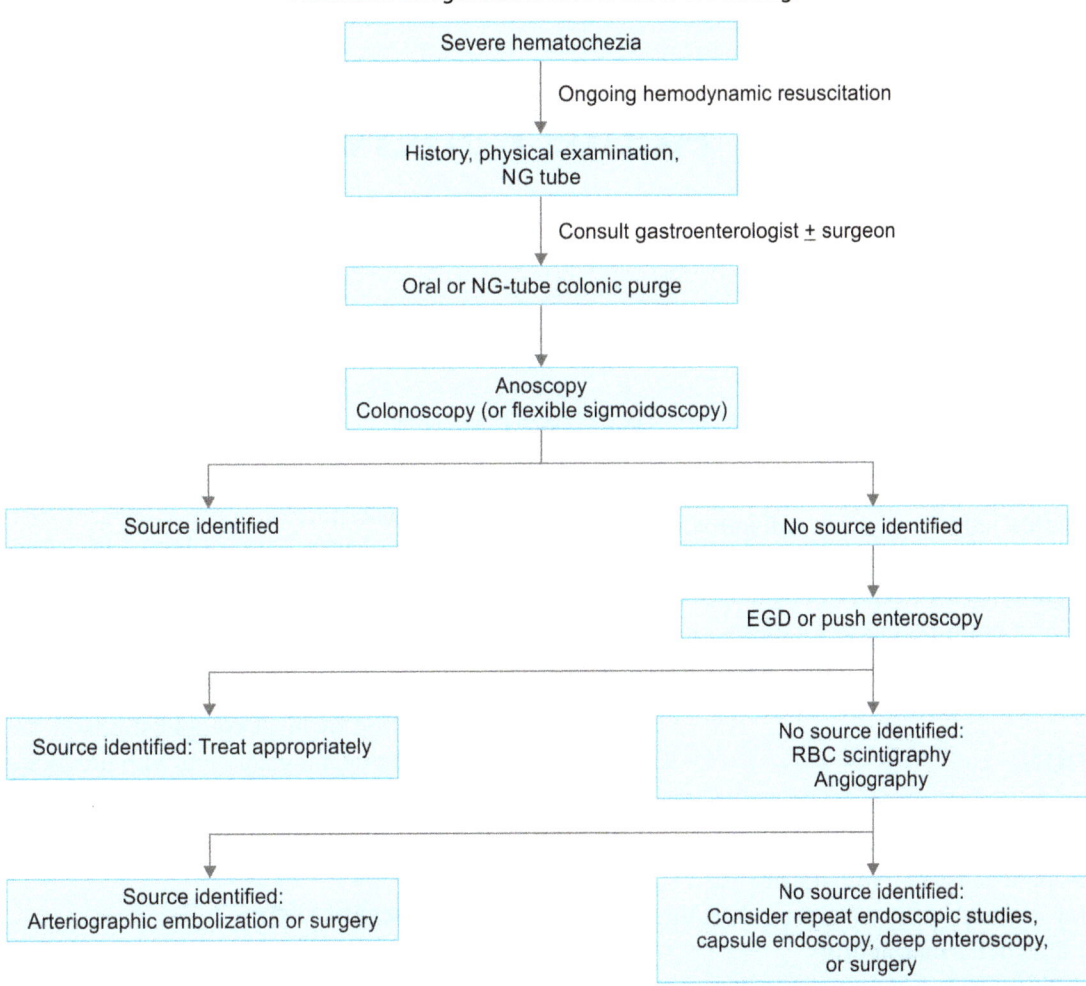

REFERENCES

1. Sleisenger and Fordtran-11th Edition.
2. Laine L, Jensen DM. Management of patients with ulcer bleeding. Am J Gastroenterol. 2012;107:345-60.
3. Stanley AJ, Ashley D, Dalton HR, Gaya DR, Thompson E, Warshow U, et al. Outpatient management of patients with low-risk upper-gastrointestinal haemorrhage: Multicentre validation and prospective evaluation. Lancet. 2009;373:42-7.
4. Longstreth GF. Epidemiology of hospitalization for acute upper gastrointestinal hemorrhage: a population-based study. Am J Gastroenterol. 1995;90:206-10.
5. Hawkey GM, Cole AT, McIntyre AS, Long RG, Hawkey CJ. Drug treatments in upper gastrointestinal bleeding: value of endoscopic findings as surrogate end points. Gut. 2001;49:372-9.
6. Jensen DM, Machicado GA. Diagnosis and treatment of severe hematochezia. The role of urgent colonoscopy after purge. Gastroenterology. 1988;95:1569-74.
7. Chait MM. Lower gastrointestinal bleeding in the elderly. World J Gastrointest Endosc. 2010;2:147-54.
8. Barkun AN, Bardou M, Kuipers EJ, Sung J, Hunt RH, Martel M, et al. International consensus recommendations on the management of patients with nonvariceal upper gastrointestinal bleeding. Ann Intern Med. 2010;152:101-13.
9. Gralnek IM, Barkun AN, Bardou M. Management of acute bleeding from a peptic ulcer. N Engl J Med. 2008;359: 928-37.
10. Carson JL, Guyatt G, Heddle NM, Grossman BJ, Cohn CS, Fung MK, et al. Clinical practice guidelines from the AABB: red blood cell transfusion thresholds and storage. JAMA. 2016;316:2025-35.
11. Longstreth GF. Epidemiology and outcome of patients hospitalized with acute lower gastrointestinal hemorrhage: a population-based study. Am J Gastroenterol. 1997;92: 419-24.

CHAPTER 20

Acute Pancreatitis: Approach

Jayanta Mukherjee

■ INTRODUCTION

Acute pancreatitis (AP) is an acute inflammation of the pancreas due to various factors, setting off a sequence of events starting from various degree of pain upper abdomen and vomiting and culminating to a rapid and successful recovery or in few cases to prolonged hospitalization and even death.

■ DEFINITION[1]

The diagnosis of AP is most often established by the presence of two of the three following criteria:
1. Abdominal pain consistent with the disease,
2. Serum amylase and/or lipase greater than three times the upper limit of normal, and/or
3. Characteristic findings from abdominal imaging.

Contrast-enhanced computed tomography (CECT) and/or magnetic resonance imaging (MRI) of the pancreas should be reserved for patients in whom the diagnosis is unclear or who fail to improve clinically within the first 48–72 hours after hospital admission or to evaluate complications.[2]

The inflammatory event has two different phases:
1. Early (within 1 week), characterized by the systemic inflammatory response syndrome (SIRS) and/or organ failure; and
2. Late (>1 week), manifested by local complications.

Disease severity is identified by the number of organ failures and its recovery over time, by medication and support.[3]

- Organ failure is defined as shock [systolic blood pressure (SBP) <90 mm Hg]
- Pulmonary insufficiency [partial pressure of arterial oxygen (PaO_2) <60 mm Hg]
- Renal failure (creatinine >2 mg/dL after rehydration)
- Gastrointestinal GI bleeding (>500 mL of blood loss/24 hours)

Local complications such as peripancreatic fluid collections, pancreatic and peripancreatic necrosis (sterile or infected), pseudocysts, and walled-off necrosis (sterile or infected) usually develop later.

Mild pancreatitis is suggested by the absence of organ failure and/or pancreatic necrosis and local complications.

Severe AP (15–20%) is now defined entirely on the presence of persistent organ failure. An intermediate grade of severity has been suggested—moderately severe AP, that is characterized by local complications in the absence of persistent organ failure. Patients with moderately severe AP may have transient organ failure, lasting <48 hours.

■ DIAGNOSIS

Clinical Presentation

Patients usually rapid in onset and is usually epigastric on left upper quadrant in position which is constant in nature with radiation to back, chest, or flanks. The intensity is usually severe but maybe of lesser intensity. The duration of pain in few hours suggests a disease other than pancreatitis, like acute cholecystitis of peptic ulcer disease (PUD) pain.

Patients typically acquire a crouched position during pain. Recurrent nonvoluminous vomiting with abdominal distension is an associated complaint. Physical findings vary with the severity of pancreatitis. Patients with a mild attack may not appear acutely ill; whereas, in severe pancreatitis, patients look severely ill with abdominal distension, tenderness, and rarely rigidity. Bowel sounds are usually attenuated or absent. Tachypnea and tachycardia with disorientation, hallucination, agitation, or coma is seen in severe pancreatitis. Hypertension is usually due to third space fluid loss and systemic toxicity. Body temperature is usually normal, but fever can be expected in the first week of illness due to the inflammatory process.

Laboratory Parameters

Serum amylase and lipase are the two common markers used to identify pancreatitis. Amylase generally rises within a few hours of symptoms and returns to normal within

3-5 days whereas serum lipase rises later and persists longer. Amylase concentrations maybe normal in alcoholic AP and hypertriglyceridemia. Serum amylase may rise in the absence of pancreatitis in patients with chronic renal failure (CRF), acute appendicitis, acute cholecystitis, intestinal obstruction, PUD, and gynecological disease. An absolute value of more than three times the upper limit of normal of these enzymes favors the diagnosis of AP. In lesser values, the clinical conditions are to be assessed and imaging of the pancreas may give a definitive clue.

Abdominal Imaging

Imaging in the form of ultrasonography and CECT provides a higher sensitivity and specificity for the diagnosis of AP. CT scan also gives an assessment of the severity of pancreatitis. MR of the abdomen is helpful in patients with contrast allergy and renal insufficiency to identify pancreatic necrosis.

Etiology

The most common causes of AP are gallstones (40-70%) and alcohol (25-35%).[2,4] Other causes such as medications, infectious agents, and metabolic causes such as hypercalcemia, hypertriglyceridemia (1-4%), and hyperparathyroidism. Pancreatitis may also be caused by iatrogenic surgical trauma and after endoscopic retrograde cholangiopancreatography (ERCP). Other rare causes would include anatomical and physiology anomalies of the pancreas like sphincter of Oddi dysfunction (SOD), pancreas divisum, and annular pancreas. Genetic defects with abnormal mutations in the physiological pathways of the pancreas lead to pancreatitis from an early age and runs in families.

Admission

Patients having clinical evidence of severe pancreatitis with organ damage should be admitted in the intensive care unit (ICU) while those with mild pancreatitis can be admitted in the regular ward, though a strict monitoring may be required for early detection of progress toward a severe pancreatitis and early transfer to the ICU may be essential for a better outcome.[5,6]

TREATMENT

In spite of multiple trials no medication has been shown to be effective in treating AP. A supportive care is required along with management of complications, if they develop.

Fluids[5,7]

Aggressive hydration (250-500 mL of isotonic crystalloid solution) within 12-24 hours of the attack remains the cornerstone of treating early pancreatitis. Hydration is expected to reduce the possibility of pancreatic necrosis and combat the early organ failure which is secondary to severe intravascular volume depletion.

The amount of fluid is assessed by laboratory parameters such as:
- Hematocrit (suggesting hemodilution)
- Blood urea nitrogen (BUN) (suggesting adequate renal perfusion)
- Maintaining a normal creatinine and urine output during the first day of hospitalization
- In the ICU setting with severe pancreatitis, a central line to assess fluid deficit is the usual intervention.

The fluid of choice is lactated Ringer's solution which was noted to be more beneficial than normal saline (NS) in order to avoid SIRS and maintain a better electrolyte balance. A cautious approach to aggressive hydration is preferable in the high-risk group like the elderly and those with a history of cardiac or renal disease to avoid volume overload and its consequences such as abdominal compartment syndrome, pulmonary edema, and congestive failure. Remember, patients not responding to aggressive hydration in the first 6-12 hours are unlikely to benefit from continued aggressive hydration.

Analgesics[2,8]

Apart from hydration the major role is played by the various analgesics. Nonopioid [nonsteroidal anti-inflammatory drugs (NSAID)] or opioid (tramadol, morphine or its analogs) medication are the mainstay of pain management. Patient controlled analgesia pumps are widely used.

Additional Treatment[2]

Ryles tube is not routinely used, but it is effective only in cases with intractable nausea and vomiting, or in cases of gastric and intestinal ileus. Patients are usually keeps nil per os (NPO) unless nausea and vomiting have subsided.

Oxygen via a nasal cannula is required in majority of patients. If nasal cannula is unable to correct hypoxemia, noninvasive pressure ventilation (NIPV) or invasive ventilation is an early intervention. Acute respiratory distress syndrome (ARDS) is a dreaded complication without any specific treatment, requiring invasive oxygen support, and renal replacement therapy.

Antibiotics[2]

Majority of the guidelines do not support early antibiotic therapy unless a severe pancreatitis with possibility of an infected necrosis is suspected. Imipenem, fluoroquinolones, and metronidazole have shown highest penetration into the pancreatic tissue.[9]

Nutrition

Fasting adversely affects the gut mucosal barrier and allows penetration of gut bacteria into the extraluminal

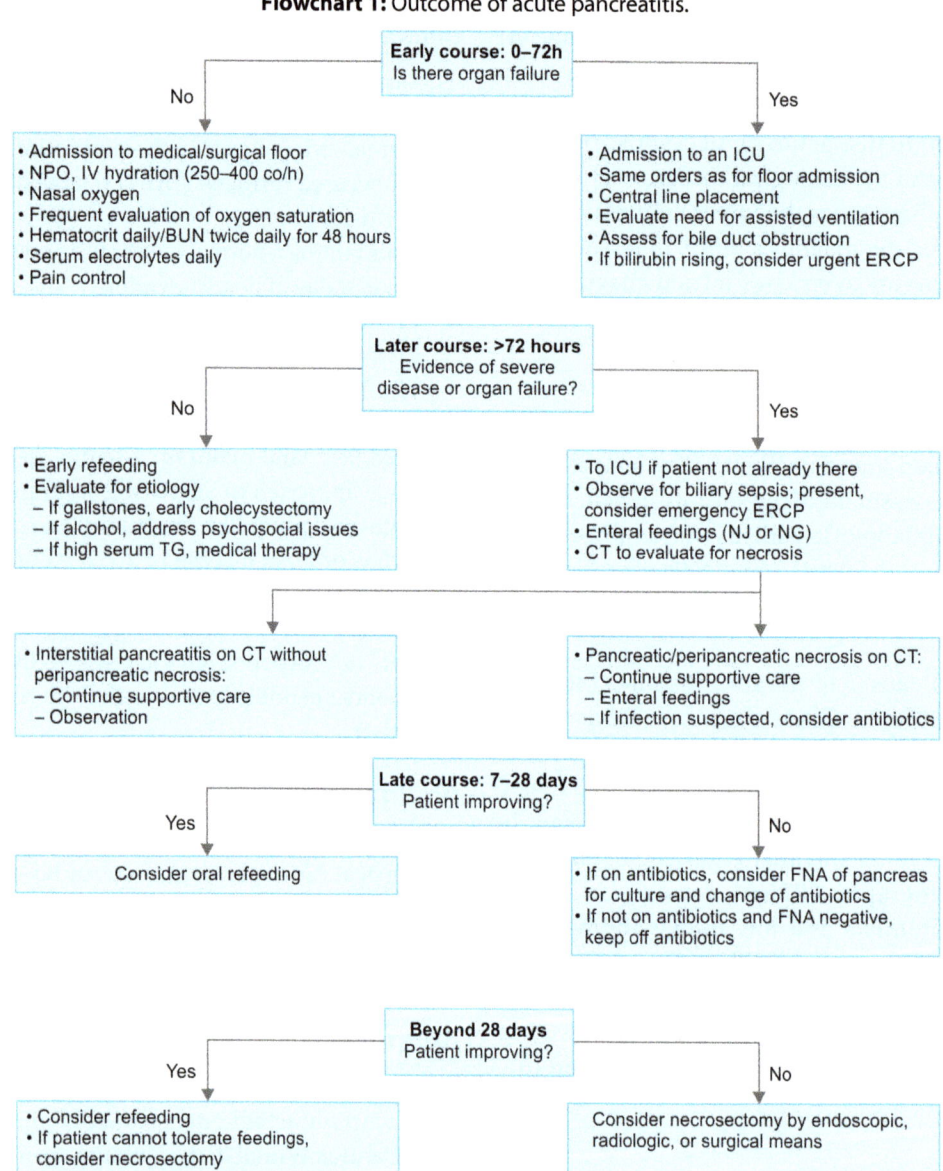

Flowchart 1: Outcome of acute pancreatitis.

(BUN: blood urea nitrogen; ERCP: endoscopic retrograde cholangiopancreatography; FNA: fine-needle aspiration; ICU: intensive care unit; IV: intravenous; NG: nasogastric; NJ: nasojejunal; NPO: nil per os; TG: thyroglobulin)

tissue.[4] In mild pancreatitis, an early feeding schedule is preferred with progression from a liquid low-calorie diet to a semisolid low fat diet. Even in cases of severe AP and early feeding schedule is preferred to total parenteral nutrition (TPN). In some cases, nasogastric or nasojejunal feeding is required if the patient is unable to feed orally. Only in rare cases TPN is indicated if the person is unable to take oral diet for a long time and if enteral feeding is not possible or not tolerated.[10]

In short, an early diagnosis of AP and a clinical assessment of the severity, therefore triaging of the patient to an ICU admission with aggressive fluid resuscitation, pain management, and early nutritional support, with additional support in the form of antibiotics will decide the outcome of pancreatitis (**Flowchart 1**).

CONCLUSION

Acute pancreatitis is an inflammatory condition of the pancreas and is a gastroenterological emergency. Majority of the patients attend the emergency room of a hospital with intolerable pain and occasionally with vomiting and clinical features of acute abdomen. An early diagnosis and a rapid intervention—mainly with fluid replacement and pain management usually leads to a satisfactory and fast recovery. Rarely, the outcome can be "stormy" with involvement of all the organ systems and lead to prolonged hospitalization and even death.

Take Home Message

- An early diagnosis of AP and a clinical assessment of the severity, therefore triaging of the patient to an ICU admission with aggressive fluid resuscitation, pain management, and early nutritional support, with additional support in the form of antibiotics will decide the outcome of pancreatitis.

REFERENCES

1. Steinberg W, Tenner S. Medical progress: acute pancreatitis. New Engl J Med. 1994;330:1198-210.
2. Banks PA, Freeman ML. Practice guidelines in acute pancreatitis. Am J Gastroenterol. 2006;101:2379-400.
3. Marshall JC, Cook DJ, Christou NV, Bernard GR, Sprung CL, Sibbald WJ. Multiple organ dysfunction score: a reliable descriptor of complex clinical outcome. Crit Care Med. 1995;23:1638-52.
4. Uhl W, Müller CA, Krähenbühl L, Schmid SW, Schölzel S, Büchler MW, et al. Acute gallstone pancreatitis: timing of cholecystectomy in mild and severe disease. Surg Endosc. 1999;11:1070-6.
5. Gardner TB, Vege SS, Pearson RK, Chari ST. Fluid resuscitation in acute pancreatitis. Clin Gastroenterol Hepatol. 2008;6:1070-6.
6. Working Party of the British Society of Gastroenterology. UK guidelines for the management of acute pancreatitis. Gut. 2005;54:1-9.
7. Warndorf MG, Kurtzman JT, Bartel MJ, Cox M, Mackenzie T, Robinson S, et al. Early fluid resuscitation reduces morbidity among patients with acute pancreatitis. Clin Gastroenterol Hepatol. 2011;9:705-9.
8. Tenner S. Initial management of acute pancreatitis: critical decisions during the first 72 hours. Am J Gastroenterol. 2004;99:2489-94.
9. Beger HG, Bittner R, Block S, Büchler M. Bacterial contamination of pancreatic necrosis: a perspective clinical study. Gastroenterology. 1986;91:433-8.
10. Hartwig W, Maksan SM, Foitzik T, Schmidt J, Herfarth C, Klar E. Reduction in mortality with delayed surgical therapy of severe pancreatitis. J Gastrointest Surg. 2002;6:481-7.

CHAPTER 21

Acute Hepatic Failure

Vikas Prakash

INTRODUCTION

Acute liver failure (ALF) is a dramatic presentation of liver when its functions decline rapidly with development of coagulation disorder and alteration in mentation. It is rapidly fatal in most of cases if not treated adequately by an expert critical care team. In most cases, a liver transplant is required.

DEFINITION

Presence of jaundice and coagulopathy followed by appearance of encephalopathy within 26 weeks marks ALF.

TYPES

Based on duration we can define three types although they are not of any help in defining the prognosis.[1]
1. Hyper acute—<7 days
2. Acute—7–21 days
3. Subacute—from 21 days till 26 weeks

COMMON CAUSES OF ACUTE LIVER FAILURE

- Viral hepatitis
- Drug
- Toxins
- Autoimmune hepatitis
- Pregnancy related

INVESTIGATIONS

- Electrolytes—sodium, potassium, calcium, magnesium, phosphate, and chloride
- Liver tests—bilirubin, aspartate transaminase/alanine transaminase (AST/ALT), gamma-glutamyl transferase (GGT), and albumin
- Kidney test—urea and creatinine
- Complete blood count
- Arterial blood gas (ABG)—lactate
- Blood and urine culture
- Endotracheal (ET) tube culture, if ventilated
- X-ray chest and ultrasound abdomen
- International normalized ratio (INR)/prothrombin time
- Viral hepatitis—hepatitis B surface antigen (HBsAg), immunoglobulin M antibody to hepatitis B core antigen (anti-HBc IgM), antihepatitis E virus (HEV), antihepatitis C virus (HCV), antihepatitis A virus (HAV) IgM, herpes simplex virus (HSV), varicella zoster virus (VZV) cytomegalovirus (CMV), and Epstein-Barr virus (EBV)
- Autoimmune hepatitis— antinuclear antibody (ANA), antismooth muscle antibody (ASMA), and IgG total
- Serum ceruloplasmin

DIFFERENTIAL DIAGNOSIS

- Ischemic hepatitis.
- Malignancy
- Budd-Chiari syndrome—acute presentation
- Hepatic manifestation of systemic disease
- Infiltrative liver diseases
- Metabolic diseases in childhood and sometimes adults
- Infections like fulminant malaria

History and examination is utmost importance in ALF. Any previous history of hepatitis B or autoimmune hepatitis can be a clue. In pregnancy, urgent delivery of baby can help. Any systemic disease should be evaluated and liver involvement as secondary can be thought of. Chronic liver disease, if present on examination, can help in clinical decision making. Presence of ascites in ALF can point toward Budd-Chiari syndrome. Substance abuse drug ingestion and suicidal attempt with paracetamol should be inquired from family members.

MONITORING AND CARE OF ACUTE LIVER FAILURE PATIENT

- Pulse rate and blood pressure
- Sensorium/neurological evaluation should be done at intervals
- ABG—lactate and oxygen/carbon dioxide levels should be monitored

Initial Treatment

- An elevation of head to 30° upright angle should be done.
- Hourly urine monitoring along with serum creatinine levels should be done.
- Venous thrombosis prophylaxis should be given.
- N-acetylcysteine injection at loading dose of 150 mg/kg over 15 minutes in 5% dextrose followed by a maintenance dose of 50 mg/kg over 4 hours then 100 mg/kg infused over 16 hours should be given to both paracetamol and nonparacetamol poisoning cases.[2]
- Avoid administration of blood products to correct coagulation since INR is an important measure of prognosis and decision making. Blood products can be transfused if there is any bleeding.
- Prevention of stress ulcers and starting prophylactic treatment is important.
- Encephalopathy and its assessment is important hence sedatives should be avoided to prevent hindrance in clinical assessment.
- In ALF kidneys are at stake due to multiple factors hence nephrotoxic medications and hepatotoxic medications should be avoided.
- Bed should be raised to 30°. Surroundings should be as quiet as possible so as to provide minimal stimulation to patient which could prevent brain edema-related complications.[3]
- Empirical antibiotic prophylaxis should be stated.
- Intubation should be considered for patients with grade III encephalopathy or more.

When to refer to a tertiary care hospital?[4]

- Bilirubin >17.6 mg/dL
- Decreasing liver size
- An INR of more than 1.8
- A pH < 7.30 or HCO_3 < 18
- Development of encephalopathy, hypoglycemia, or metabolic acidosis
- Decreasing urine output or renal failure
- Hyponatremia developing Na < 130 mmol/L

Complications Seen in Acute Liver Failure

Table 1 shows complications of acute liver failure.

TABLE 1: Etiology and complications in acute liver failure.

Etiology	Complications
Cerebral edema	Brain herniation
Coagulopathy	Bleeding, low platelets
Infections	Fungal, urinary tract infection (UTI), bacterial, sepsis
Metabolic abnormalities	Hypophosphatemia, hyponatremia, hypoglycemia, hypokalemia
Pulmonary dysfunction	Overload, pneumopathy, acute respiratory distress syndrome
Kidney	Functional failure, toxic injury
Hemodynamic	Arrhythmia

Blood Pressure and Cardiovascular Monitoring

Assess for hydration. If jugular venous pressure is low and there is oliguria and renal injury suggestive of end-organ damage volume depletion is likely. Rehydration is required since most of patients are dehydrated at presentation. Initial fluid for rehydration is normal saline. Albumin can be used but should be seen as drug rather than a rehydration fluid. Overhydration should be prevented to avoid brain edema and hyponatremia. Excessive hydration leads to increased mortality if persistent.

If hypotension develops noradrenaline is the vasopressor of choice which should be started promptly to prevent ischemic hepatitis.[5] The starting dose of noradrenaline would be 0.05 lg/kg/min. Additionally a low dose of vasopressin (1–2 units/hour), can be considered if norepinephrine requirements are more and increase to >0.2–0.3 lg/kg/min.

Some patients in intensive care unit (ICU) in whom vasopressor required increase to >0.2 lg/kg/min an arterial pressure monitoring by a central arterial catheter (either axillary or femoral) can be considered to assess better and accurately as opposed to monitoring via peripheral arterial line.

The target blood pressure appropriate is controversial with not much data to support any value. In adult patients with no preexisting hypertension, a 60 mm Hg mean arterial pressure (MAP) generally is adequate. In patients having risk factors for acute kidney injury (AKI) there is evidence of a MAP > 75 mm Hg faring better.[6]

Hydrocortisone can improve blood pressure; however, does not confer a mortality benefit. It is seen that adrenal dysfunction is present in around 50% of patients with ALF when they are tested with a standard adrenocorticotropic hormone (ACTH) stimulation test.[7,8] Target hemoglobin for transfusion is around 7 g/L.

A slightly low tidal volume with appropriate positive end-expiratory pressure (PEEP) should be used for maintaining an open lung. Chest physiotherapy should be done regularly to prevent pneumonia. Hypo- or hypercarbia should be avoided. CO_2 target ranging from 34 to 41 mm Hg.[9] Tidal volumes needs to be maintained around 6 mL/kg of body weight with a maximum being 8. Acute respiratory distress syndrome (ARDS) or acute lung injury is generally not seen in ALF.[10]

Feeding

Enteral or parenteral nutrition should be instituted since in ALF resting energy expenditure is increased. Proton pump inhibitor (PPI) prophylaxis can be withheld once enteral nutrition is started.

Electrolytes

Hyperglycemia tends to increase intracranial pressure (ICP) and should be prevented. A tight glycemic control with insulin infusion reduces mortality. A target of blood glucose between 150–180 mg/dL is optimal.[11]

Hyponatremia has to be prevented and maintaining a relative hypernatremia by infusing hypertonic saline prevents raised ICP. However, if the serum sodium levels increase above 150 mmol/L, it may cause cell damage and should better be avoided. Targets therefore would be to maintain sodium at 140-145 mmol/L. Rapid changes in sodium levels are to be avoided and the rate of correction should be correlated with rate of drop, which must not exceed 10 mmol/L per 24 hours.[12]

Around 40-80% of ALF patients who are referred to a tertiary care liver units have AKI, which is associated with increased mortality and prolonged length of hospital stay. Renal replacement therapy (RRT) generally is instituted for uremia, fluid overload, and hyperkalemia; however in ALF, RRT may be started to treat acidosis, hyperammonemia, and hyponatremia. It can also facilitate temperature and metabolic control. Therefore, timely consideration of RRT has to be done with markedly elevated ammonia.[13] Continuous RRT is preferred over intermittent dialysis.

Brain Edema

Intracranial hypertension due to brain edema is classical complication of ALF. Mannitol (150 mL, 20% given over 20 minutes) or hypertonic saline can be given for intermittent surges of ICP.[14] A short-term hyperventilation with attendant risk of cerebral hypoxia should be considered. Monitored hypothermia and indomethacin (0.5 mg/kg) can be given if intracerebral hemorrhage (ICH) is uncontrolled for hyperemic cerebral blood flow.[15]

Liver Assist Devices

Liver assist devices can be used in trials only and has no recommendations for general use. Plasma exchange if available has been shown to have a mortality benefit. It is more beneficial for patients who have not been previously treated and now moving toward transplant.[16]

Liver Transplant

Patients who fulfill Clichy or Kings College criteria should be taken up for transplant.

King's College Criteria[17]

Table 2 shows King's College Criteria for paracetamol overdose and nonparacetamol acute liver failure.

CONCLUSION

Acute liver failure can have high mortality in a society which has either shortage of cadaveric donors or is economically crippled. In a society with adequate donor organs sensitization about initial assessment, adequate management by primary care physician and a timely referral can improve outcomes. Differentiation from ALF mimickers are equally important to save the patient and start empirical antibiotics and antiedema measures. Society should be sensitized about organ donation and blood donation. A timely liver transplant markedly improves the survival.

TABLE 2: King's College Criteria for paracetamol overdose and nonparacetamol acute liver failure.

Paracetamol overdose	Nonparacetamol acute liver failure
pH of <7.3 on ABG or • PT over 100 seconds (INR 6.5) • Creatinine over >3.4 mg/dL • Grade 3–4 encephalopathy (All within a 24 hours timeframe)	PT over 100 seconds (INR 6.5) or • Any three: – Age under 10, or over 40 – Bilirubin over 17.4 mg/dL – >7 days separate onset of jaundice from onset of encephalopathy – Etiology is seronegative hepatitis, or a drug-induced hepatitis – INR ≥ 3.5

(ABG: arterial blood gas; INR: international normalized ratio; PT: prothrombin time)

Take Home Messages

- Critical care management is very important in initial stages. The decision taking into account the finances and risks and the timing of liver transplant is critical. Initial 5 days are very important. In first 3 days or so various prognostic models can be applied although none of them are optimum. Subsequently a decision for transplant can be made during the "optimum window" period. A too late decision will make the patient unfit for transplant and a futile transplant is done.
- It depends on clinical sense of an astute hepatologist to decide the optimum time and need based on various clinical parameters response to treatment and the expertise available.

REFERENCES

1. O'Grady JG, Schalm SW, Williams R. Acute liver failure: redefining the syndromes. Lancet. 1993;342(8866):273-5.
2. Bernal W, Williams R. Acute liver failure. Clin Liver Dis. 2020;16(S1):45-55.
3. Wendon J, Cordoba J, Dhawan A, Larsen FS, Manns M, Samuel D, et al. EASL Clinical Practical Guidelines on the management of acute (fulminant) liver failure. J Hepatol. 2017;66(5):1047-81.
4. Droogh JM, Smit M, Absalom AR, Ligtenberg JJ, Zijlstra JG. Transferring the critically ill patient: are we there yet? Crit Care. 2015;19(1):62.
5. Russell JA, Walley KR, Singer J, Gordon AC, Hébert PC, Cooper DJ, et al. Vasopressin versus norepinephrine infusion in patients with septic shock. N Engl J Med. 2008;358(9):877-87.
6. Leone M, Asfar P, Radermacher P, Vincent JL, Martin C. Optimizing mean arterial pressure in septic shock: a critical reappraisal of the literature. Crit Care. 2015;19(1):101.

7. Etogo-Asse FE, Vincent RP, Hughes SA, Auzinger G, Le Roux CW, Wendon J, et al. High density lipoprotein in patients with liver failure; relation to sepsis, adrenal function and outcome of illness. Liver Int. 2012;32(1):128-36.
8. Marik P, Zaloga G. Prognostic value of cortisol response in septic shock. JAMA. 2000;284(3):308-9.
9. Malhotra A. Low-tidal-volume ventilation in the acute respiratory distress syndrome. N Engl J Med. 2007;357(11): 1113-20.
10. Futier E, Constantin JM, Paugam-Burtz C, Pascal J, Eurin M, Neuschwander A, et al. A trial of intraoperative low-tidal-volume ventilation in abdominal surgery. N Engl J Med. 2013;369(5):428-37.
11. Mesotten D, Wauters J, Van den Berghe G, Wouters PJ, Milants I, Wilmer A. The effect of strict blood glucose control on biliary sludge and cholestasis in critically ill patients. J Clin Endocrinol Metab. 2009;94(7):2345-52.
12. Klinck J, McNeill L, Di Angelantonio E, Menon DK. Predictors and outcome impact of perioperative serum sodium changes in a high-risk population. Br J Anaesth. 2015;114(4):615-22.
13. Davenport A. Is there a role for continuous renal replacement therapies in patients with liver and renal failure? Kidney Int Suppl. 1999;72:S62-6.
14. Canalese J, Gimson AE, Davis C, Mellon PJ, Davis M, Williams R. Controlled trial of dexamethasone and mannitol for the cerebral oedema of fulminant hepatic failure. Gut. 1982;23(7):625-9.
15. Tofteng F, Larsen FS. The effect of indomethacin on intracranial pressure, cerebral perfusion and extracellular lactate and glutamate concentrations in patients with fulminant hepatic failure. J Cereb Blood Flow Metab. 2004;24(7): 798-804.
16. Clemmesen JO, Kondrup J, Nielsen LB, Larsen FS, Ott P. Effects of high-volume plasmapheresis on ammonia, urea, and amino acids in patients with acute liver failure. Am J Gastroenterol. 2001;96(4):1217-23.
17. O'Grady JG, Alexander GJ, Hayllar KM, Williams R. Early indicators of prognosis in fulminant hepatic failure. Gastroenterology. 1989;97(2):439-45.

SECTION 5
Nephrological Emergencies

Section Editor: Pratim Sengupta

22. **Acute Renal Failure**
    Pratim Sengupta, VK Mohun, Sumanta Biswas

23. **Drugs and Kidney**
    Pratim Sengupta, VK Mohun, Sumanta Biswas

Acute Renal Failure

Pratim Sengupta, VK Mohun, Sumanta Biswas

INTRODUCTION

Nephrology emergencies frequently lead to therapeutic challenges, as well as a variety of adverse clinical outcomes. Most common renal emergencies are acute renal failure (ARF) of diverse etiologies, rapidly progressing renal failure (RPRF), renal infarction, outflow tract obstruction, renal trauma, and last but not the least the toxicological insult to kidney. Regardless of the cause, ARF requires immediate medical attention or could lead to life-threatening consequences if not treated on time. The purpose of this chapter is to cover some of these clinical scenarios from both a diagnostic and therapeutic standpoint.

DEFINITION

Conceptually the understanding ARF has dramatically changed over last one and half decade. Acute kidney injury (AKI), which is better expressive and syndromically more inclusive terminology, is preferred now than what, previously was called ARF. AKI is a condition where there is sudden deterioration or impairment of renal filtration or excretory function with or without preexisting chronic kidney disease (CKD); within a few hours or days. The consequences of which is accumulation of water-soluble metabolic waste products, especially nitrogenous one in body which are otherwise cleared by the kidney and/or significant decrease (oliguria) or complete elimination of urine (anuria), with or without electrolyte, and other hemodynamic and metabolic imbalances. Conceptually we need to understand that AKI is a syndrome rather than a single disease. By AKI we conglomerate a group of clinical situations that share a common manifestation like increase in nitrogenous waste product in body along with or without reduction in urine output (UO).

Mounting evidence suggests that acute, relatively mild injury to the kidney or impairment of kidney function, manifest by changes in UO and blood chemistries, portend serious clinical consequences.

HISTORIC UNDERSTANDING OF ACUTE KIDNEY INJURY

Eknoyn in a review stated William Heberden described ARF for the first time in 1802 under the name ischuria renalis.[1] Acute Bright's illness, which was known as ARF at the start of the 20th century, was well-described as the result of toxic substances, pregnancy, burns, trauma, or kidney surgery as described in the famous textbook of medicine by Professor William Osler (1909). The syndrome was known as "war nephritis"[2] during World War I and was recorded in a number of papers. Before Bywaters and Beall published their landmark study on crush injury victims during the Second World War, the syndrome had been ignored.[3] However, the phrase "acute renal failure" was first used by Homer W Smith. In his book "Acute Renal Failure Associated to Severe Injuries" was a chapter where he first used the term "acute renal failure" in the year 1951. However, a clear-cut clinico-pathological description or definition of ARF was never coined until recently, when the issues were addressed by scientific forums like Kidney Disease: Improving Global Outcomes (KDIGO) or Acute Kidney Injury Network (AKIN). Very recently report of one survey revealed that there are at least 35 different definitions of ARF are there in current literature.[4] This is why there is so much confusion and lack of clarity regarding proper diagnosis and reporting of incidence of ARF and its clinical significance.

RIFLE Criteria

For systematic diagnosis and classification of so called ARF, first structured and planned evidenced-based initiative was taken by the Acute Dialysis Quality Initiative (ADQI) group. ADQI developed a system based on UO, creatinine, and estimated glomerular filtration rate (eGFR) for precise diagnosis and classification of a broad spectrum of acute impairment of kidney function through a broad consensus of experts.[5] The summary of that diagnostic criteria and classification in different broad classes are depicted in the **Figure 1**.

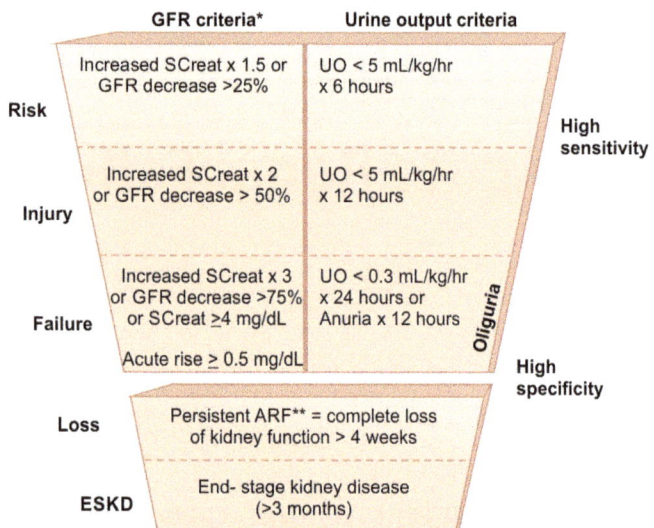

Fig. 1: The RIFLE criteria for AKI. (AKI: acute kidney injury; ARF: acute renal failure; ESKD: end-stage kidney disease; GFR: glomerular filtration rate; SCreat: serum creatinine concentration; UO: urine output)
*Glomerular filtration rate
**Acute renal failure

TABLE 1: Kidney Disease: Improving Global Outcomes (KDIGO) classification of different stages of acute kidney injury (AKI).		
Stage	SCr	UO
1.	Increase in SCr ≥0.3 mg/dL (≥26.5 µmol/L) or increase in SCr ≥150–200 % (1.5 to 1.9×)	<0.5 mL/kg/h (>6 h)
2.	Increase in SCr >200–300 % (>2 to 2.9×)	<0.5 mL/kg/h (>12 h)
3.	Increase in SCr > 300% (≥3×) or increase in SCr to ≥4 mg/dL (≥353.6 µmol/L) or initiation of renal replacement therapy	<0.3 mL/kg/h (24 h) or anuria (12 h)

SCr: serum creatinine; UO: urine output

The acronym RIFLE depicts the increasing clinical severity and ultimate outcome among the spectrum of renal impairment. Risk, injury, and failure are the three classes which present increasing severity of acute kidney insult; and the last two classes, loss and end-stage renal disease (ESRD), depict the end outcome of the acute nonrecovering renal insult.

ACUTE KIDNEY INJURY/IMPAIRMENT

Conceptually RIFLE criteria first implemented the idea of capturing the broad spectrum of changes of renal function by combining practically measurable indices of renal function with stipulated time frame and first time the RIFLE criteria moved the understanding of renal dysfunction beyond preexisting concept of ARF. Following universal acceptance of RIFLE criteria, and its popular clinical use for diagnosis and classification of spectrum of acute renal insufficiency, new terminology "AKI/impairment" has been advocated for referring the entire spectrum of the ARF, starting from minor changes in markers of renal dysfunction to the end result of acute severe kidney failure, i.e., requirement for renal replacement support. Hence by implementing the concept of AKI, as defined by RIFLE criteria, a new paradigm shift in understanding of ARF has been started. Point to be kept in mind that AKI is neither totally synonymous with acute tubular necrosis (ATN) nor it is otherwise as believed to be as renal failure. Instead, it means both and also by definition it includes other, less severe conditions of renal impairment. AKI in its definition also includes patients without actual renal damage but with functional impairment relative to physiologic demand. Such inclusion in the understanding of AKI is conceptually beneficial as it shift focus on early intervention and thereby prevention of setting up clinically significant renal damage.

PREVALENCE AND EPIDEMIOLOGICAL CONSIDERATION OF ACUTE KIDNEY INJURY

Acute kidney damage (AKI) is a common diagnosis, with a prevalence of 5–7.5% among all hospital admission, up to 30% intensive care admission and up to 50–60% in terms of prevalence among critically sick patients.[1-6] It is estimated that globally each year 13–16 million people suffer from AKI and AKI is associated with longer hospital stays, higher healthcare expenses, and higher in-hospital mortality. AKI is strongly associated with increased all cause cardiovascular mortality and major cardiovascular event, especially those admitted to intensive care unit (ICU) where hospital mortality exceeds 50%. AKI increases the risk of development or progression and worsening of preexisting CKD, and also increase long-term mortality. Evidence wise number of AKI has grown by more than three to fourfold in last two decades. The annual incidence is roughly 500 per 100,000 population culminating it as a serious public health issue.

DIAGNOSIS OF ACUTE KIDNEY INJURY

The KDIGO workgroup developed the current classification of AKI in the year 2012, which has defined AKI as an absolute rise in serum creatinine (SCr) from its baseline value to at least 0.3 mg/dL within 48 hours, an increase in SCr to more than 1.5 times the baseline, or a decrease in UO to <0.5 mL/kg/h for 6 hours.[7,8] The staging of AKI as per KDIGO based on change of creatinine and UO criteria is depicted in **Table 1**.

Limitations of Diagnosis

The current definition of AKI depends on serum creatinine and UO, but these two parameters are imperfect markers. Creatinine is nonsensitive marker for assessment of renal function as it is affected by various factors such as age of the subject, ethnicity, gender of the patient, dietary habits and

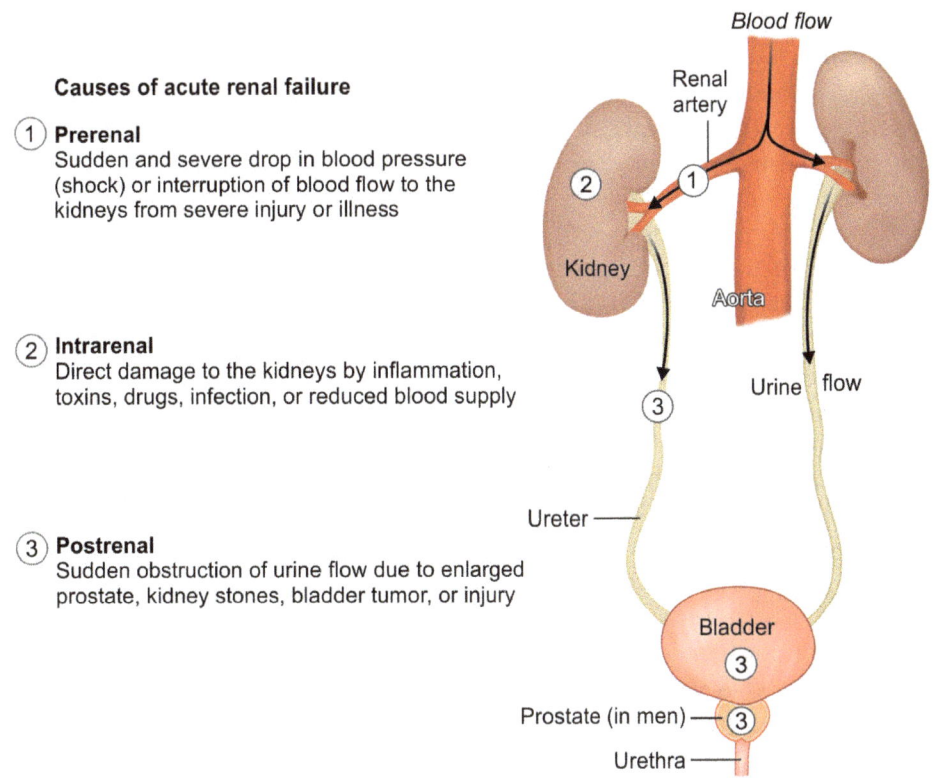

Fig. 2: Causes of acute kidney injury (AKI).

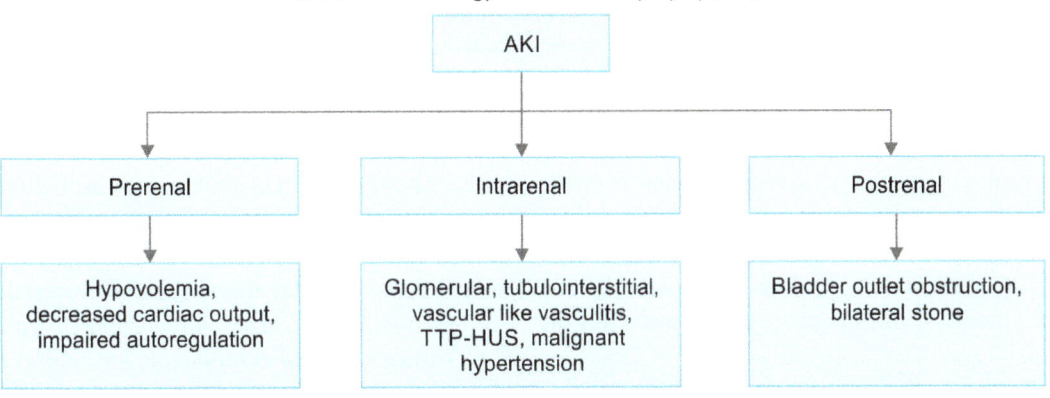

(TTP-HUS: thrombotic thrombocytopenic purpura-hemolytic uremic syndrome)

pattern, existing muscle mass, presence or absence of sepsis, and ongoing fluid therapy.[9] Therefore, creatinine cannot be considered as an accurate marker to predict overall kidney function or glomerular filtration rate (GFR). On the other hand it takes 2–3 days for the serum creatinine to rise from baseline after any acute insult in kidney.

Though UO is an early marker for AKI, it also relies on patient's urine volume and hemodynamic status and the use of diuretics, and so it is difficult to assess without a urinary catheter and its usefulness relies on an hourly assessment that is time intensive and operationally challenging. Often urinary catheter malfunctioning in a busy critical unit poses a challenge for accuracy in detection of kidney function.[10]

ETIOLOGICAL CLASSIFICATION

The age-old conceptual causal classification of AKI in prerenal, intrarenal, and postrenal cause is still worth discussing **(Fig. 2)**.

Nevertheless, it is worth mentioning that in rare clinical setting all the three or combination of more than one etiology may persist as a cause of AKI **(Flowchart 1)**.

Prerenal Acute Renal Failure

Impaired renal perfusion with a resultant fall in glomerular capillary filtration pressure is a common cause of AKI. In this setting, tubular function is typically normal, renal reabsorption of sodium and water is increased and consequently the urine exhibits low sodium concentration (<20 mmol/L) and high osmolality (>500 mOsm/kg), presuming a diuretic has not been administered. A marked reduction in renal perfusion may overwhelm autoregulation and precipitate an acute fall in GFR. Sometimes agents such as nonsteroidal anti-inflammatory drugs (NSAIDs) and angiotensin-converting enzyme (ACE) or angiotensin receptor blockers (ARBs) can cause AKI due to impaired afferent arteriolar dilation causing disruption in renal autoregulation. Prerenal AKI is often secondary to extracellular fluid volume depletion as a result of gastrointestinal (GI) losses (diarrhea, vomiting, and prolonged nasogastric drainage), renal losses (osmotic diuresis in hyperglycemia), dermal losses (burns and extensive sweating), or sequestration of fluid, sometimes known as third-spacing (e.g., acute pancreatitis and muscle trauma) or when there is systemic arterial vasodilation with redistribution of cardiac output to extrarenal vascular beds (e.g., sepsis and liver cirrhosis). Prerenal AKI can be corrected if the extrarenal factors causing the renal hypoperfusion are rapidly reversed.

Intrarenal Acute Renal Failure

The most common intrarenal causes of AKI are the glomerular diseases of diverse etiology, especially glomerulonephritis, toxic insult to kidney due to different environmental agents, drug-induced nephrotoxicity, acute tubulointerstitial diseases, vasculitis, and renal microthrombotic disorders like hemolytic uremic syndrome-thrombotic thrombocytopenic purpura (HUS-TTP). The primary glomerular diseases or systemic diseases with glomerular insults are most common among this group. Drug and contrast-induced nephrotoxicity leading to AKI needs special consideration due to their preventability and adverse consequences if not diagnosed or intervened on time.

Postrenal Acute Renal Failure

Obstruction of the extrarenal collection system at any level (renal pelvis, ureters, bladder, or urethra) can increase intratubular pressure, which opposes glomerular filtration pressure and decrease GFR. Obstructive nephropathy is more common in older men with prostatic disease, in patients with a single kidney, and in those with intra-abdominal or pelvic cancer. All types of renal obstruction are also associated with inflammation and fibrosis and can result in permanent injury. If treatment or intervention is early, prognosis of postrenal ARF is often good.

■ APPROACH TO THE PROBLEM

Once a patient is diagnosed with AKI or suspected for having AKI or at risk of AKI, a detailed clinical assessment is needed that must comprises of a vivid medical history, including history of exposure to all current or recent medications and exposures to any nephrotoxins, as well as a thorough physical examination. The clinical and laboratory evaluation should be targeted and executed in phased manner keeping in mind the clinical context.

It is worth remembering that patients with AKI may present with symptoms and signs resulting directly from diminished kidney function. These typically include edema, hypertension, and/or decreased UO or, in severe AKI, anuria. However, many patients have no clinical symptoms, and an increase in creatinine is detected by laboratory tests that are routinely obtained among hospitalized patients.

After the detailed history and clinical examination, the understanding regarding the fluid status and the evaluation for presence of acute or chronic heart failure, sepsis, and urological causes like outflow tract obstruction must be assessed.

The preliminary investigations must comprise serum creatinine, blood urea nitrogen (BUN), Na, K, and other electrolytes, complete hemogram, C-reactive protein (CRP), procalcitonin, liver function tests (LFTs), blood glucose level, urine routine and microscopic examination, and an ultrasound of kidney ureter and bladder. Based on results of preliminary examination the tire-2 investigations to specify the exact etiology must be planned. Measuring time-based UO is must. A simple chest X-ray sometimes can reveal of potential causes of AKI, such as pneumonia, clues to pulmonary renal syndrome, and it is also useful to understand pulmonary congestion or central volume overload. A 2D echocardiogram to evaluate the inferior vena cava (IVC) diameter also provides a clear picture of patient's volume status. If there is fever, rash, joint pains, pulmonary abnormalities, significant proteinuria, or microhematuria, then tire-2 investigations like markers for collagen vascular disease must be considered. In this context, testing myeloperoxidase (MPO) and proteinase 3 (PR3) antineutrophil cytoplasmic antibodies (ANCA), anti-glomerular basement membrane (anti-GBM) antibodies, antinuclear antibodies (ANAs), antidouble-stranded DNA (anti-dsDNA) antibodies, and complement factors are necessary and reveals specific groups of collagen vascular diseases. Specific environmental and tropical diseases, which are common in South-East Asia such as snake bite, bee bite, malaria, and *Leptospira* are usually evident from the history and clinical examination and demand a special approach in terms of investigation and management. The overall intention of the preliminary workup should be to identify the etiology to establish whether prerenal, intrarenal, or postrenal factors are playing a role or not, and also to identify the holistic clinical status so that proper intervention can be planned. Nevertheless it is wise to remember that cardiorenal syndrome, hepatorenal syndrome in earlier stages, and alteration of renal autoregulation by ACEi or ARBs and NSAIDs often lead to diagnostic challenge if proper medical history and clinical examination are not carried out.

In nutshell, the evaluation approach of AKI in hospitalized patients is depicted in **Flowchart 2**.

■ LABORATORY ASSESSMENT

As mentioned earlier, except the preliminary laboratory assessment, the advanced assessment must be in continuum and congruent with the clinical context. The preliminary

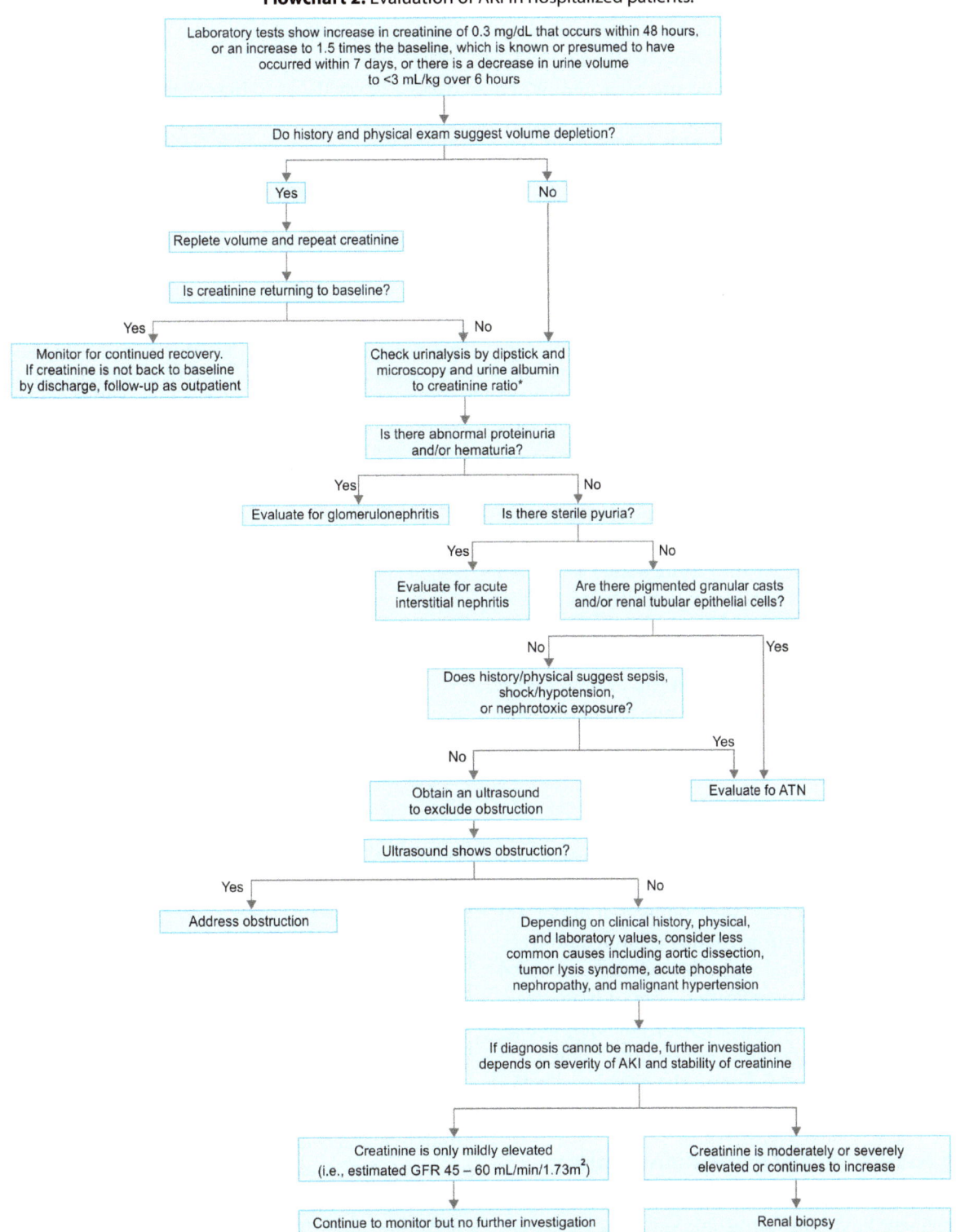

Flowchart 2: Evaluation of AKI in hospitalized patients.

(ATN: acute tubular necrosis; AKI: acute kidney injury; GFR: glomerular filtration rate: SPEP: serum protein electrophoresis; UPEP: urine protein electrophoresis)
*For patients who are at higher risk for multiple myeloma, we also cheek SPEP, UPEP with immunofixation, and a serum free light chain assay. Higher-risk patients include all patients >40 years who have no other obvious cause for increased creatinine.

laboratory assessment should be primarily with blood, urine, and imaging, however renal failure indices, urinary osmolality assessment, and kidney biopsy and biomarkers has their respective place in appropriate clinical context.

Blood Workup

Blood workup must consider complete hemogram, uric acid, urea creatinine, electrolytes, arterial blood gas analysis, LFT, and sepsis markers such as CRP and procalcitonin. When indicated, blood culture and complement level along with collagen vascular markers such as ANA, ANCA, and anti-GBM antibody are also considered. Anemia is common in AKI. Peripheral eosinophilia is often associated with acute interstitial nephritis, atheroembolic renal disease, polyarteritis nodosa, and Churg–Strauss syndrome. Severe anemia without any evident bleeding may reflect red blood cell (RBC) breakdown due to hemolysis, marrow disorders like multiple myeloma, or TTP/HUS complex. Schistocytes in peripheral smear and thrombocytopenia are also indicative of TTP/HUS and mandates further assessment of lactate dehydrogenase (LDH), which is high in TTP/HUS and also haptoglobin and ADAMTS-13 level to confirm the diagnosis. Patients with history of trauma and muscle injury, rhabdomyolysis needs to be ruled out by measuring further uric acid, creatinine kinase, and urinary or blood myoglobin. In AKI, normally the anion gap may be increased as a result of retention of anions such as phosphate, hippurate, sulfate, and urate. The concurrent rise in anion gap along with osmolar gap and urinary oxalate crystalluria is suggestive of ethylene glycol poisoning, low anion gap in this context suggestive of multiple myeloma where due to unmeasured serum cationic proteins serum anion gap becomes low.

Urinalysis

Measurement of UO and laboratory assessment of urine is one of the most important windows through which the etiological interpretation of AKI can be done easily and must be considered in all AKI cases. Most simple but important tests to be considered are urine routine examination (RE), microscopic examination for cast, active sediment, crenated RBC, and urinary protein quantification. Urinary biomarkers are opening new horizon of understanding pathophysiology of AKI and will be dealt in subsequent section. **Table 2** will help us to understand and interpret the urinalysis in the setting of AKI.

Imaging Assessment of Acute Kidney Injury

Ultrasonography of whole abdomen and urogenital system is must, echocardiography, ultrasonic volume assessment by IVC diameter and collapsibility with respiration, ascitic and pleural space assessment for third space fluid accumulation, and serial chest X-ray. USG is efficient in diagnosis of bladder outlet obstruction, prostatomegaly, by

TABLE 2: Interpretation of urinalysis in acute kidney injury (AKI).

Urinary patterns associated with different kidney diseases

Urinary pattern	Kidney disease suggested by pattern
Hematuria with dysmorphic red blood cells, red blood cell casts, varying degrees of albuminuria	Proliferative glomerulonephirtis (e.g., IgA nephropathy, ANCA-associated vasculitis, lupus nephritis)
Heavy albuminuria with minimal or absent hematuria	Nonproliferative glomerulopathy (e.g., diabetes, amyloidosis, membranous nephropathy, focal segmental glomerulosclerosis, minimal change)
Multiple granular and epithelial cell casts with free epithelial cells	Acute tubular necrosis in a patient with underlying acute kidney injury
Isolated pyuria	Infection (bacterial, mycobacterial) or tubulointerstitial disease
Abnormal kidney function with normal dipstick and sediment containing few cells, no casts, and no or minimal proteinuria	• Prerenal acute kidney injury due to either volume contraction or an effective decrease in circulating volume (e.g., heart failure, liver disease) • Hypercalcemia • Light chain cast nephropathy in multiple myeloma • Tumor lysis syndrome • Vascular disease that produces glomerular ischemia but not infarction (e.g., hypertensive emergency, scleroderma, thrombotic microangiopathies) or that affects extraglomerular vessels (e.g., cholesterol atheroemboli, polyarteritis nodosa) • Urinary tract obstruction

(ANCA: antineutrophil cytoplasmic antibody; IgA: immunoglobulin A)

finding hydroureteronephrosis, and thickened bladder wall. Retroperitoneal fibrosis encasement with tumor may need further imaging by either CT scan or MRI. Normal sized kidneys are usually expected in AKI; however, preexisting CKDs are often detected based on shrunken kidney. Enlarged kidneys are indicative of acute tubule interstitial disease, diabetic kidneys, and renal infiltrative disorders like amyloidosis.

Renal Failure Indices

Multiple markers and indices have been applied in clinical practice to differentiate prerenal azotemia from intrinsic AKI when the tubules are not functioning properly. BUN/creatinine ratio, fractional excretion of Na (FeNa), and fractional excretion of urea (FeUr) are the popular renal failure indices.

The low tubular flow rate and rise in recycling of urea at the medullary compartment of tubule is usually seen in prerenal azotemia, which usually causes the disproportionate elevation of BUN compared to creatinine. In this context, it is wise to keep in mind upper GI bleed, use of steroid, increased tissue catabolism, and hyperelementation also may cause similar pattern of disproportionate BUN rise in comparison to creatinine rise.

The FeNa is the fraction of the filtered Na load that is reabsorbed by tubule. FeNa <1% suggestive of avid tubular Na reabsorption and sign of prerenal azotemia. However, FeNa is influenced by external factors such as diuretic use, salt intake, effective intravascular volume, and preexisting CKD. FeNA may be >1% despite volume depletion due to treatment with diuretic, hence diuretic history is mandatory before interpreting FeNa. On the other side, low FeNa can be observed in glomerulonephritis and hence should not be taken as prima facie evidence of prerenal azotemia. In ischemic AKI, FeNa may be >1% because of tubular injury, and side by side nephrotoxin-associated AKI, sepsis which are primarily intrarenal may have low FeNa. Henceforth low FeNA therefore suggestive but not synonymous with intravascular volume depletion and interpreted with caution.

Understanding the sensitivity issues of FeNa in diagnosis prerenal versus intrarenal AKI, nowadays FeUr is considered better marker in this regard and not directly influenced by diuretic use.

Urine Osmolality

The production of concentrated urine by kidney is totally dependent on good tubular function in different parts of nephron. Patients not taking diuretic urinary osmolality >500 mOsm/kg are indicative of good tubular function and suggestive of prerenal azotemia. Loss of concentrating ability is common in most intrinsic forms of AKI, that affects tubule and interstitium, resulting urine osmolality <350 mOsm/kg. Though urinary osmolality has decent sensitivity it lacks specificity due to lots of external influencing factors like age or preexisting CKD.

Kidney Biopsy

In laboratory evaluation of AKI, when cause of AKI is not apparent from clinical context, physical examination, laboratory studies, and radiological evaluation, kidney biopsy must be considered. The histopathological and immunofluorescence study of biopsy sample can provide diagnostic and prognostic information about AKI. Addition of electron microscopy further helps in diagnosing rare glomerular and immunotactoid glomerulopathies. However in acute critical setting, biopsy has some inherent operational issues and bleeding risk.

NOVEL BIOMARKERS IN ACUTE KIDNEY INJURY

Since inception of understanding of kidney disease urea and creatinine are considered as age-old traditional functional biomarkers of overall GFR. Urea and creatinine however do not reflect specific tissue injury therefore suboptimal for diagnosing acute parenchymal injury to kidney. BUN and creatinine rises after a significant time after an acute kidney insult. A large number of biomarkers have been investigated earlier and show promise for accurate diagnosis and prognostication of AKI. Understanding AKI being a continuum and syndrome **(Fig. 3)**, roles of biomarkers are prudent to identify at early stage.

Recently few potential urinary and serum biomarkers of AKI have been pointed out. Cystatin-C, neutrophil gelatinase-associated lipocalin (NGAL), N-acetylglucosaminidase (NAG), kidney injury molecule-1 (KIM-1), interleukin-6

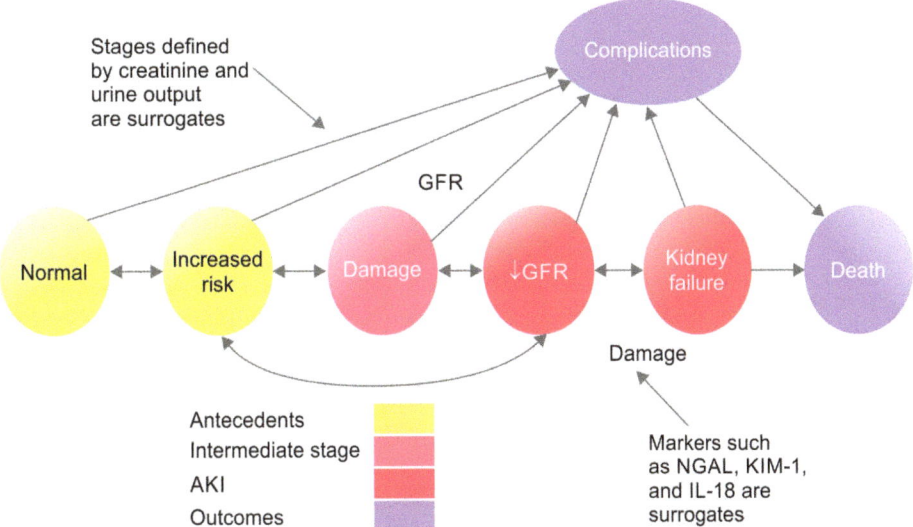

Fig. 3: Spectrum of AKI and relation to GFR and biomarkers. (AKI: acute kidney injury; GFR: glomerular filtration rate; IL-18: interleukin-18; KIM-1: kidney injury molecule-1; NGAL: neutrophil gelatinase-associated lipocalin)

(IL-6), interleukin-8 (IL-8), interleukin-18 (IL-18), liver-type fatty acid-binding protein (L-FABP), and calprotectin (TIMP-2) are some of them. Among the above-mentioned markers, maximum data and clinical correlation has been evidenced with NGAL and IGFBP7 with TIMP-2. However, their exorbitant cost and lack of widespread availability limits their widespread use in clinical settings.[11,12]

As these biomarkers reflect different stages of spectrum of AKI, using panels of these biomarkers in clinical settings will give a better early diagnostic picture for management of AKI **(Fig. 4)**.

The greatest benefits of the biomarkers are diagnostic timing and prognostication. In relation to time scale, the urea and creatinine rises late in the course of AKI, hence early diagnosis of AKI or patients who are at risk cannot be identified based on urea creatinine elevation. However, it is observed in clinical and experimental models that the novel biomarker rises much earlier than the urea creatinine rises **(Fig. 5)**, helping clinicians to identify the risk or earlier diagnosis of AKI.

■ MANAGEMENT OF ACUTE KIDNEY INJURY

The first goal for the treatment of AKI is to attain hemodynamic stability, identification of the cause of AKI, and early identification of the complications of AKI. Medication list must be thoroughly reviewed and if there is any drug that has proven nephrotoxicity must be stopped immediately.

If there is evidence of sepsis with high procalcitonin, then prompt initiation of broad-spectrum renal friendly

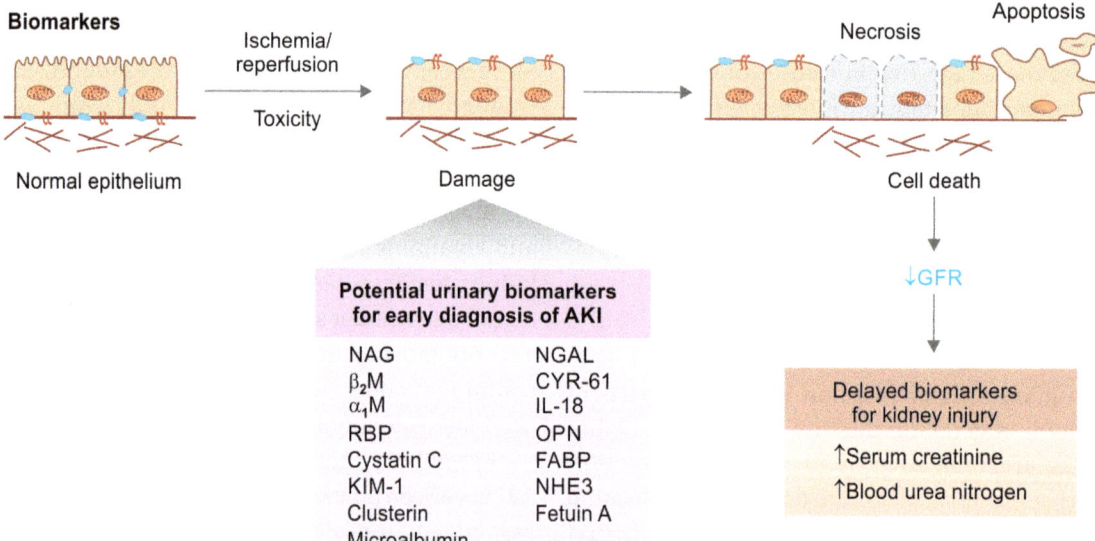

Fig. 4: Biomarkers for acute kidney injury (AKI).

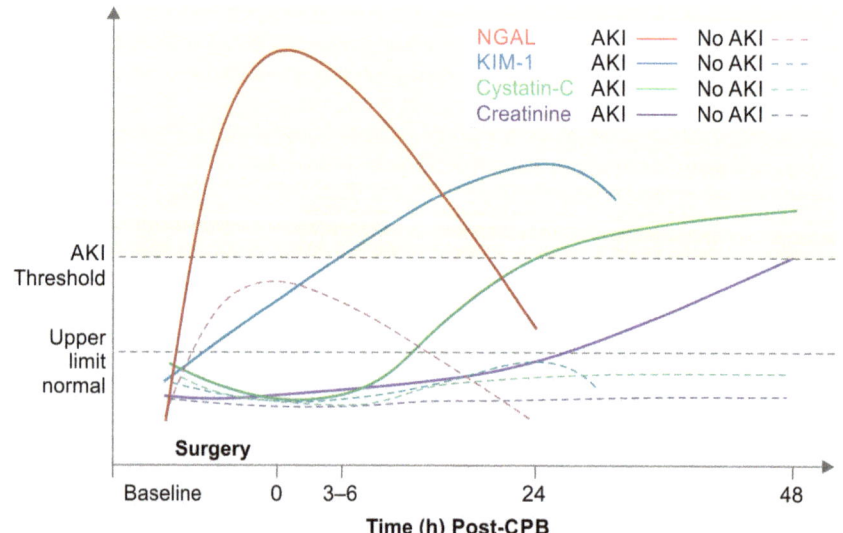

Fig. 5: Time line of different biomarker rise in acute kidney injury (AKI).

antibiotic coverage is needed until the culture-guided specific antibiotic is considered.

It is always imperative to quickly identify and treat other life-threatening associated complications in patient with AKI, such as high potassium, metabolic acidosis, low hemoglobin (Hb), and fluid overload.

Fluid Therapy

Stabilization of the hemodynamic of the patient and correction of any fluid deficit will have a great preventive impact on kidney function. Fluid resuscitation should be done while monitoring UO, blood pressure, or central venous pressure (CVP) dynamic changes as endpoints to avoid excessive fluid administration.

It is advised to use isotonic crystalloids rather than colloids (albumin or starches) as the initial therapy for expansion of intravascular volume in patients at risk for AKI or with AKI if hemorrhagic shock is not present.

Colloid solutions such as albumin can be used in patients with hypoalbuminemia along with fluid volume deficit, hypotension, and AKI.

Patients with liver cirrhosis who also have AKI in the form of hepatorenal syndrome should receive albumin infusions in addition to vasopressors.

Vasopressors

It is not clear till date, efficacy wise which vasopressor is best for prevention of AKI in a patient at risk or for treatment of patients with AKI and especially in the setting of septic shock. Among all the available vasopressors, maximum evidence is available with norepinephrine, dopamine, and vasopressin either in isolation or in combination. In septic shock with AKI, norepinephrine is the vasopressor of choice with target mean arterial pressure of 65–70 mm Hg. In patients with vasomotor shock, vasopressors in conjugation with fluids are the best choice of therapy.

Dopamine, when used in low dose, usually increase renal salt and water excretion in prerenal states but clinical trials has failed to show any benefits in patients with intrinsic AKI. As we all know dopamine is arrhythmogenic and known to cause bowel ischemia, use of dopamine for prevention of AKI in prerenal azotemic states are no more recommended.

Fenoldopam and Natriuretic Peptide

In absence of definitive conclusive evidence, these two agents are not recommended to use for prevention of AKI.

Diuretics

As a common practice diuretics are frequently prescribed in critical and noncritical care setting for patients who are at risk of developing AKI, with the notion to prevent AKI. However, controlled studies proved that diuretics have no role in prevention of AKI on the contrary for patients at risk diuretics increase the risk of AKI. Hence, KDIGO in its latest guideline clearly recommends not to use diuretic for prevention of AKI. The role of diuretics in the management of established AKI is limited to management of volume overload and prevention of pulmonary edema. Since volume overload is one of the major manifestations of AKI, diuretics are main armamentarium in noninvasive fluid management in AKI. Use of diuretics in this context permits safe administration of parenteral or enteral nutrition and intravenous medications without further volume overload. In patients with hypervolemia and decompensated heart failure, loop diuretics should be the treatment of choice. In resistance cases, combination of loop diuretic and thiazide or distally acting diuretic may be used.

Mannitol in Prevention of Acute Kidney Injury

The age-old practice of using mannitol for prevention of AKI is no longer advocated nowadays due to lack of adequately powered and properly designed randomized controlled study data in this regard. Whatever data are available in this context are retrospective and underpowered. The practice of prophylactic use of mannitol, especially in surgical cases, is mainly opinion based with anecdotal doubtful beneficial observations, henceforth no more recommended.

Electrolyte Imbalance

Electrolyte imbalances such as hyponatremia, hypernatremia, hypokalemia or hyperkalemia, hyperphosphatemia, and hypermagnesemia are extremely common in AKI. Addressing these electrolyte imbalances along with concomitant acid base disorder is extremely important for treating a patient with AKI. When serum K levels is 6.5 mEq per L (6.5 mmol per L) or greater, it is considered as severe hyperkalemia; which indeed is a life-threatening condition. Hyperkalemia leads to electrocardiogram (ECG) changes and can lead to cardiac arrest. ECG changes typical of hyperkalemia are tall, peaked T waves, bradycardia, sine-wave pattern, prolonged QR interval, and presence of any of them needs immediate intervention. In severe hyperkalemia, glucose insulin drip is live saving. Intravenous 25–50% dextrose mixed with 5–10 units of regular insulin shift potassium from circulation to the intracellular space. In this situation along with glucose insulin drip, intravenous calcium gluconate (10 mL of 10% solution infused intravenously over 5 minutes) is concomitantly used to stabilize the membrane and reduce the risk of arrhythmias. In hyperkalemia without ECG changes, infusion of calcium gluconate as mentioned is not usually required. In these situations, modest and slow potassium reduction by oral sodium polystyrene sulfonate (Kayexalate) and use of loop diuretics for renal potassium loss are standard clinical practice. For long-term potassium control dietary modification, lower potassium intake must be advocated. Hyperphosphatemia is another common abnormality observed in AKI, usually treated with phosphate chelating agents or phosphate binders like sevelamer carbonate or calcium acetate.

Acidosis

Acidosis is common in AKI; however, unless pH reaches to <7.2 or HCO_3 <15 mmol/L, active intervention may be avoided. Acidosis is treated with oral or intravenous sodium bicarbonate supplementation; however, constant watch on overcorrection is necessary in view of alkalosis and associated problems such as hypocalcemia, hypokalemia, and volume overload. Resistant and severe metabolic acidosis demands renal replacement therapy (RRT).

Anemia

Anemia in AKI are multifactorial, more of due to erythropoietin (EPO) resistance, acute overt or covert bleeding, hemolysis, nutrient utilization defect, and marrow suppression. EPO response often inadequate in AKI due to EPO resistance. Indication of transfusion depends on clinical context understanding dilutional factors and volume overload in interpreting low Hb and cardiac condition or ongoing bleeding. Hb level of 7 g/dL or less is reasonable indication for red cell transfusion.

Glycemic Control

In any critical care setting, stress hyperglycemia is common same applicable in AKI. Proinflammatory cytokines and counter-regulatory hormones play a pivotal role in stress hyperglycemia. Achieving glycemic control through exogenous insulin administration is extremely important in these situations to reduce morbidity and mortality. Extensive evidence are there where it has been shown a consistent, almost linear, relationship between blood glucose levels in patients hospitalized with acute coronary syndrome or sepsis and adverse clinical outcomes, even in nondiabetic patients. Having said that it is also observed low spontaneous blood sugar, i.e., hypoglycemia was also associated with increased mortality, especially in extremes of ages. In prevention of AKI, tight glycemic control is frequently used in patients at risk of AKI and in the management of those who develop AKI. It has been proposed that tight glycemic control can reduce the incidence and severity of AKI. KDIGO in its latest guideline recommends stringent blood sugar control to the tune 110–149 mg/dL (6.1–8.3 mmol/L) in critical care setting with insulin therapy whenever required.

Discontinuation of Nephrotoxic Medications

All medications that may potentially affect renal function by direct toxicity or by hemodynamic mechanisms should be discontinued, if possible. For example, metformin should not be given to patients with diabetes mellitus who develop AKI. The dosages of essential medications whose drug clearance is mostly through kidney should be adjusted. Whenever possible iodinated contrast media and gadolinium should be avoided, if imaging is at all needed, noncontrast studies should be preferred. NSAIDs are strictly prohibited. Several antibiotics such as aminoglycosides and penicillins have potential nephrotoxicity and must be avoided.

Supportive Therapies

Supportive therapies, e.g., antibiotics, maintenance of adequate nutrition, mechanical ventilation, prevention of deep venous thrombosis, and pressure sore should be pursued based on standard management practices. In patients with rapidly progressive glomerulonephritis, confirming the diagnosis by proper collagen vascular marker tests and kidney biopsy is urgently necessary. Treatment with pulse steroids, cytotoxic therapy, or a combination should be considered without delay for prevention of permanent damage. Patient with AKI should receive a basic intake of 0.8–1.0 g of protein/kg body weight/day if not catabolic and a total energy intake of 20–30 kcal/kg/day as recommended by KDIGO guideline.

Renal Replacement Therapy

Renal replacement therapies are indicated when the medical management fails to control fluid overload, electrolyte imbalance, especially hyperkalemia, metabolic acidosis, and in some special situations like AKI due to toxic ingestions. The severe complications of uremia such as uremic encephalopathy, asterixis, and uremic pericarditis are also indication of initiation of RRT. Timing of initiation dialysis is also in a debate as late initiations risks volume overload, chest congestion whereas early initiation has risk of hypotension and hemodynamic instability access-related complications, arrhythmia, infections, and membrane bioincompatibility. Thus, overall approach should be based on patient's clinical condition and clinicians' expertise on predictability of worsening or improving AKI.

Regarding most optimal modality of RRT, there are multiple options and depending on the clinical context and expertise the preferred modality is choose in managing AKI in a given situation. Hemodialysis may be intermittent or continuous. Based on the clinical context, diffusive clearance or regular hemodialysis or convective clearance (hemofiltration) is chosen. Sometimes combination of both diffusive and convective clearance (hemodiafiltration) is chosen. Patients who are in AKI and hypotensive, having significant brain edema and gross volume overload; if expertise is available, continuous renal replacement therapy (CRRT) is the best option. Continuous venovenous hemofiltration (CVVH) is the preferred mode in this situation, however in absence of CRRT machine, continuous venovenous hemodialysis (CVVHD) could be an alternative option. Where this expertise is not available, slow low efficient extended hemodialysis (SLEED) is a reasonable alternative for CRRT. Intermittent hemodialysis or hemodiafiltration are considered for hemodynamically stable patients. In newborns and children with AKI, peritoneal dialysis is the preferred option for RRT when clinically or metabolically indicated. Because of its continuous nature apart from children, some centers prefer peritoneal dialysis over intermittent hemodialysis among hemodynamically unstable adult patients also.

OUTCOME AND PROGNOSIS

Development of AKI in any admission or in community is always associated with significant increase in in-hospital and long-term mortality and morbidity. For the survivors of AKI, the hospital stays and cost of care is significantly higher than those who do not had AKI in any hospital stay.[13] Among the different etiologies of AKI, postrenal AKI has better prognosis, in comparison to prerenal or intrarenal AKI.[14] Survivors of AKI who required RRT are at higher risk of progressing to CKD and up to 10% develop end-stage renal failure, requiring maintenance hemodialysis or renal transplantation.

CONCLUSION

The most frequent causes of AKI are fluid volume deficits or renal hypoperfusion, shock, inflammatory states, or nephrotoxic medications. To prevent further development of AKI and mortality, early recognition of the pathophysiology of AKI through careful review of the patient's history, intravascular volume assessment, past medicinal history, supplemented by urine biochemical analysis, and urine microscopy, should be the basis for management strategy.

Take Home Messages

Being one of the most common and serious day-to-day affairs in all discipline of medicine we need to deal AKI with due care. Early diagnosis and prevention are most important along with multidisciplinary team approach for the management of the established AKI, to prevent mortality or arrest progression to CKD. In this regard author's recommendations are as follows:
- Periodic CME involving all ICU medical and paramedical staff regarding early diagnosis of AKI is mandatory in each licensed critical care Unit. The role of education of nurses, brothers, and resident doctors is most important for introducing the culture of high index of suspicion, and early identification of those who are at risk or already in asymptomatic AKI so that prompt intervention can reverse the course.
- Nationwide standardized data keeping and periodic audit of AKI data from all critical care units will help to understand gap in care.
- Availability of biomarkers in critical care units may help in early diagnosis and timely preventive intervention.
- Pan country AKI task force development to formulate strategy for AKI prevention and optimized care.

REFERENCES

1. Eknoyan G. Emergence of the concept of acute renal failure. Am J Nephrol. 2002;22:225-30.
2. Davies F, Weldon R. A contribution to the study of "war nephritis". Lancet. 1917;190:118-20.
3. Bywaters EGL, Beall D. Crush injuries with impairment of renal function. BMJ. 1947;1:427-32.
4. Kellum JA, Levin N, Bouman C, Lameire N. Developing a consensus classification system for acute renal failure. Curr Opin Crit Care. 2002;8:509-14.
5. Bellomo R, Ronco C, Kellum JA, Mehta RL, Palevsky P; Acute Dialysis Quality Initiative workgroup. Acute renal failure—definition, outcome measures, animal models, fluid therapy and information technology needs: the Second International Consensus Conference of the Acute Dialysis Quality Initiative (ADQI) Group. Crit Care. 2004;8:R204-12.
6. Susantitaphong P, Cruz DN, Cerda J, Abulfaraj M, Alqahtani F, Koulouridis I, et al. Acute Kidney Injury Advisory Group of the American Society of Nephrology. World Incidence of AKI: A Meta-Analysis. Clin. J. Am. Soc. Nephrol. 2013;8:1482-93 .
7. Lameire N, Van Biesen W, Vanholder R. The changing epidemiology of acute renal failure. Nat Clin Pract Nephrol. 2006;2:364-77.
8. Khwaja A. KDIGO Clinical Practice Guidelines for Acute Kidney Injury. Nephron. 2012;120:c179-84.
9. Fujii T, Uchino S, Takinami M, Bellomo R. Validation of the Kidney Disease Improving Global Outcomes Criteria for AKI and Comparison of Three Criteria in Hospitalized Patients. Clin J Am Soc Nephrol. 2014;9:848-54.
10. Luo X, Jiang L, Du B, Wen Y, Wang M, Xi X. A comparison of different diagnostic criteria of acute kidney injury in critically ill patients. Crit Care. 2014;18:R144.
11. Ostermann M, Philips BJ, Forni LG. Clinical review: Biomarkers of acute kidney injury: Where are we now? Crit Care. 2012;16:233.
12. Kashani K, Cheungpasitporn W, Ronco C. Biomarkers of acute kidney injury: The pathway from discovery to clinical adoption. Clin Chem Lab Med. 2017;55:1074-89.
13. Bagshaw SM, George C, Bellomo R. Changes in the incidence and outcome for early acute kidney injury in a cohort of Australian intensive care units. Crit Care. 2007;11:R68.
14. Rodrigues FB, Bruetto RG, Torres US, Otaviano AP, Zanetta DMT, Burdmann EA. Incidence and Mortality of Acute Kidney Injury after Myocardial Infarction: A Comparison between KDIGO and RIFLE Criteria. PLoS One. 2013;8:e69998.

CHAPTER 23

Drugs and Kidney

Pratim Sengupta, VK Mohun, Sumanta Biswas

■ INTRODUCTION

We all know that the kidney is the main excretory organ and eliminates all water soluble metabolic waste products, many drugs and its metabolites from our body. In kidney disease, the excretory capacity of kidneys gets diminished, and hence many drugs and its metabolites get accumulated in our body. To avoid toxicity of the drugs, we need dose adjustment in renal impairment. Apart from kidney liver is another organ which metabolizes drugs in our body. Those drugs which are primarily metabolized or converted to active metabolites by liver, active metabolic components also gets accumulated in renal insufficiency. Here lies the importance of adjusting optimum exposure of drug either by dose reduction or increasing the gap between two doses of drugs in renal insufficiency to avoid toxicity. We all are aware about therapeutic index of any drug. Proper knowledge regarding the therapeutic index of any individual drug helps us to decide the precise dose reduction policy. Drugs which have wide therapeutic range like cephalosporins antibiotics, dose adjustment for those drugs in renal insufficiency may not require equal precision as it required for drugs which have very narrow therapeutic range like aminoglycosides or digitalis. Patients who are undergoing extracorporeal renal replacement therapy (RRT) (hemodialysis, hemofiltration) or undergoing peritoneal dialysis due to end-stage renal disease (ESRD), drug dose adjustment is a separate challenge. Drugs which are removed by dialysis demand supplemental dose after the procedure to maintain the stable drug level in blood. For the drugs which are not removed, removal of fluid during dialysis may change the volume of distribution (Vd) of the drug.[1] For dialyzable drugs, the factors which impact on to what extent the drug will be removed during dialysis procedure is quite complex and depends on multiple conditions. For example, the molecular size of the drug and dialyzer pore size, depending on the protein-binding nature of the drug and surface affinity for adsorption of the drug to the dialysis membrane material in given acid base situation influence the dialyzability of a drug in a given situation. Keeping on account these complex interactions of multiple factors even in a same class of chemical prior prediction of removal rate in any dialysis session is often impossible. Hence serial serum drug concentrations complemented by published data in given set of therapy modalities are only means to predict dose adjustment policies in these groups of patients.

In this chapter, we will discuss the framework for drug dose adjustment in renal impairment, principles of drug dosing in patients with renal insufficiency and how different drugs lead to kidney injury, especially acute kidney injury (AKI).[2,3] Guidelines for appropriate dosing of any drugs in patients with renal dysfunction, including dialysis, are available in multiple online resources readers are requested to access those prior prescribing as this is beyond the scope of this chapter. As a general rule, it is considered if 30% or more of a drug is excreted through urine unchanged, in healthy volunteers then, in presence of renal insufficiency the accumulation of the drug will be of clinical concern. However based on therapeutic index as discussed earlier this baseline rule varies drug to drug. In general an accumulation of endogenous organic acids in plasma is must in renal failure. These organic acids compete with drugs and its metabolites for binding to plasma protein. As a result protein binding of drugs or its metabolites gets diminished. Hypoalbuminemia, another common problem in proteinuric and nonproteinuric renal insufficiency, results in diminished binding of drugs to albumin which is major plasma protein. These results in major alteration in the concentration of unbound fraction of pharmacologically active drugs in plasma and also its pharmacokinetic behavior in renal insufficiency.

In dialysis whatever be its modality, blood is passed through a semipermeable membrane. Through diffusion or convection substances are removed from blood. Now there are some specific characteristics which dictate drug removal through dialysis membrane during dialysis. For example drugs which are bound to circulatory proteins are less likely to get filtered through dialysis membrane, on the other hand drugs with small molecular size, lesser than the membrane pore diameter are more likely to get filtered out through dialysis membrane. Regarding Vd of a drug it should be kept in mind that drugs, those are widely distributed in tissues, may readily cross a permeable membranes used in dialysis, though it is obvious that the amount removed during dialysis is clinically insignificant. Understanding the pharmacokinetic characteristics of a drug is the framework on which the following discussion is based. This allows predictions that can be helpful in clinical situations in which insufficient dosing information is available.

DRUG DOSE ADJUSTMENT: PRINCIPLES

Loading Dose

When rapid achievement of therapeutic level of a drug is necessary for a clinical context, loading dose is common clinical practice. Usually, it is well known that in any given situation when loading dose is not given roughly 4–5 half-life of a drug is necessary to achieve a therapeutic plateau of a drug level. Depending on the clinical need, urgency to achieve therapeutic drug level and half-life of drug loading dose is employed.[4] The loading dose is directly proportional to the Vd of any drug. The initial blood concentration ($C_{initial}$) also has some bearings on calculating loading dose. Loading dose is calculated by the following formula:

$$\text{Loading dose} = (C_{initial}) \times (Vd)$$

For example, if the Vd for a drug such as an ampicillin antibiotic is 14.2 L/kg and the desired peak serum concentration is 3.5 µg/L, the necessary loading dose can be calculated as follows:

$$\text{Loading dose} = (3.5\ \mu g/L) \times (14.2\ L/kg) = 49.7\ mg/kg$$

In day-to-day clinical practice, a therapeutic guideline for loading dose based on pharmacokinetic studies of any drug in its published literature is usually considered instead calculating it from Vd. Because Vd varies based on fluid load status and serum protein level and other clinical condition of the patient.

Maintenance Dose

The steady state therapeutic drug concentration otherwise as known as maintenance dose is the drug concentration which is desired in blood for any treatment with a drug.[4] Maintenance dose is determined by multiplying the targeted average drug concentration ($C_{average}$), with the rate of clearance (Cl) of the drug from the body:

$$\text{Maintenance dose} = (C_{average}) \times (Cl)$$

Half-life

Once we take any drug our body starts excreting the drug from the system. The time required to fall the concentration of the drug to half (50%) is called half-life ($t\frac{1}{2}$) of a drug. Most drugs (except few like phenytoin or salicylates) follow a linear pattern in rate of elimination and rate of elimination does not depend on initial drug concentration. This otherwise means that for most drug the $t\frac{1}{2}$ is independent of the initial or later serum concentration. Hence for most of the drug, especially those who follows linear pattern of elimination rate, the time for a drugs concentration to decrease from 200 to 100 units of concentration is the same as for a decrease from 100 to 50 units. $t\frac{1}{2}$ in other way indicates the rate of clearance of a drug from body. If there is rise in $t\frac{1}{2}$ that means there is proportional decrease in clearance. The maintenance dose in this condition needs to be calculated appropriately keeping long $t\frac{1}{2}$ in mind. In renal insufficiency as the renal clearance decrease, naturally the $t\frac{1}{2}$ of a drug which otherwise gets eliminated by kidney is increased. And we need to calculate the maintenance dose accurately.

Point to be kept in mind that any change in $t\frac{1}{2}$ can lead to a change in Vd, or a change in Cl, or can change both. Ideally, a correct dosing regimen must be adjusted depending on the above mentioned factors.

Dosing Regimens

Every clinical context requires specific dosing regimen. The situations where need of loading doses are eminent, depending on the Vd changes in the loading dose may be imperative. Whenever possible the serum drug concentration must be monitored to understand the adequacy of area under the curve for better clinical efficacy of any drug. If monitoring shows serum drug concentrations have been too low, a supplementary dose can be given. On the other side, if the serum drug concentration is high the following maintenance dose may be delayed to avoid drug toxicity. The main objective is to maintain the similar mean drug concentration in a patient without renal disease. In day-to-day clinical practice as maximum number of drugs follows linear or first-order elimination kinetics, any change in clearance of the drug due to renal failure can be easily compensated by a proportional change in the dosing rate:

Usual maintenance dose/modified maintenance dose
= Usual clearance/Patient's clearance

or,

Modified maintenance dose = (Patient's clearance/ Usual clearance) × Usual maintenance dose

Therefore, for a given drug if the clearance of that drug in a patient with renal insufficiency is one-third of what is seen otherwise person with the "normal" renal function, then the maintenance dose of that drug in renal insufficiency should be one-third of what usually administered in a person with normal renal function. Appropriate dose modifications in this way will maintain a normal average steady state drug concentration of the drug.

The maximum length of a dosing interval cannot be uniform and it is imperative that no general rule can be applied here into; in routine clinical practice 24 hours seem to be a reasonable interval. In my opinion 24 hours interval likely be helpful for patient adherence and compliance. If response to a drug is not as expected even though selection of the drug for the clinical context is appropriate, the possible inappropriate dosing regimen must be considered. On the other side, when any features of toxicity is experienced shortly after administration of an individual drug, either delaying the next dose or administration of smaller dose may be incorporated in the dosing regimen.

■ DIALYSIS

End-stage renal disease patients cannot survive without dialysis. Patients who are treated with RRT either hemodialysis or peritoneal dialysis or continuous renal replacement therapy (CRRT), as blood is filtered through semipermeable membrane in RRT, have an additional path through which drugs can be eliminated from their body. If substantial elimination of any drug by these routes takes place, without giving supplemental dose after RRT session steady state drug concentration cannot be maintained. The supplemental dose is calculated as the amount of drug removed during the procedure. In case of continuous ambulatory peritoneal dialysis (CAPD) as slow dialysis mode goes on over hours, drug removal is a continuous process during the entire treatment time. In this scenario, achieving steady state needs different principles of supplemental dose. Low dose frequent supplementation or in fluid addition for intraperitoneal absorption are two common modalities of maintaining steady state concentration. Here one point to be kept in mind, for those who has some residual renal function, total clearance of a drug is the sum of the clearance by residual renal function and clearance via RRT modalities.

Couple of time we encounter a situation where exact information regarding how much drug is cleared through dialysis is not available, in those scenario pharmacokinetic parameters of the drug may give us some idea or insight regarding its dialyzability. If molecular size of the drug is larger than pore size of dialysis membrane, it is obvious that the drug will not pass through dialysis membrane. For example, molecular size of vancomycin is 3.2/2.2 nm and standard pore size of a dialysis membrane is 1–10 nm, hence, it is quite understandable that vancomycin will not be removed by dialysis. Protein boundness of any drug again is another factor which dictates its dialyzability irrespective of its molecular size. Majority of plasma proteins are large enough to not to pass through dialysis pore, now the drugs which are by nature bound to plasma protein by >90%, even its molecular size is less then dialysis membrane pore size, it is unlikely that the drug will be eliminated by dialysis. On the other hand, water soluble drugs are freely filtered through dialysis membrane provided their molecular size lesser than pore size. Lastly, drugs which have large Vd, they get themselves distributed in different compartment, and a small portion stays in vascular compartment, naturally they have minimal dialyzability. Points to be noted for drugs with large Vd, once dialysis ends, and a significant amount of drug from the tissues and other compartments of body bounce back to vascular compartment to maintain equilibrium.

The ultimate clearance of the drug depends on the modality of RRT chosen, hence, the drug dosing is also dependent on dialysis modalities and types. RRT modalities where filtration is the main methods of toxin removal, clearance of drug is much more than the RRT modalities which depend on diffusion. In convection-based therapies such as continuous venovenous hemodiafiltration (CVVHDF) and continuous veno-venous hemofiltration (CVVHF), removal of drugs depends upon the sieving coefficient (SC) of the dialyzer membrane.[5] SC is considered as one property of membrane through which its filterability is measured. SC is measured by ratio of ultrafiltrate to plasma solute concentration. Therapies such as routine hemodialysis and sustained low efficiency dialysis (SLED), diffusion is the main principle of clearance. In diffusion, the gradient of solute between the dialysate and the plasma compartments determines the rate of clearance. The mass transfer coefficient (KoA) is one parameter which determines the efficiency of a dialyzer, otherwise means the maximum theoretical clearance of any solute through a dialyzer in milliliter per minute at infinite blood and dialysis solution flow rates. It is the one yard stick by which capability of a dialyzer to remove small molecular weight (MW) substances such as urea, is estimated and KoA is dependent on the surface area of a dialyzer.

Based on KoA dialyzers are classified as low, moderate, and high efficiency dialyzers. Those with KoA <500 is considered as "low efficiency" and low efficiency dialyzers are used for small framed patients or in those patients who are elderly, having low muscle mass and presumed to be at high risk of dialysis disequilibrium syndrome. Dialyzers with a KoA between 500 and 800 are considered as moderate efficiency dialyzers and dialyzers with a KoA >800 are referred as high efficiency dialyzers.

Dialyzer flux is another dialyzer-related factor which plays a significant role on determining appropriate drug dosing in a patient who is on RRT. Flux of a dialyzer is directly proportional to water permeability of the membrane. Based on water permeability, dialyzer membranes are classified as low flux (<10 mL/min), medium flux (10–20 mL/min), and high flux (>20 mL/min). In most clinical settings, dialyzers with flux >20 mL/min are preferred. Molecules or solutes with MW >1,000 Da are negligibly cleared by low flux dialyzer where as high-flux dialyzers are capable of significant removal of solutes having MW >1,000 Da, irrespective of whether diffusion- or convection-based modalities of RRT are chosen or not.

Dosing Recommendations

In renal insufficiency, the Vd of a drug gets significantly altered. As a consequence to have optimal therapeutic concentration, the loading dose needs to be appropriately adjusted. Similarly, keeping in mind the compromised clearance due to renal failure maintenance dose also needs to be optimized to maintain expected therapeutic concentration and avoid toxicity. The common practice is either changing the each individual dose, or changing the interval between doses, or both. Choice of strategy depends on the nature of the drug, the clinical context and clinician's expertise, and experience on dosing regimen.

Drug Dosing Considerations for Patients with AKI

- The first and foremost target should be identifying who are at risk of AKI. In this regards, the guidelines for AKI identification by KDIGO AKI (Kidney Disease: Improving Global Outcomes Acute Kidney Injury) criteria, or AKIN (Acute Kidney Injury Network) criteria, or RIFLE (Risk, Injury, Failure, Loss, and End-stage renal failure) criteria should be prospectively applied to early or quick identification of AKI risk.
- For nephrotoxic medications or other drugs with narrow therapeutic index, there is always the possibility of potential toxic complications due to supratherapeutic serum concentrations due to low clearance in renal insufficiency. The possibility of such situation should be assumed proactively to avoid unnecessary drug toxicities and better patient safety.
- In AKI due fluid retention, third spacing of fluid, capillary leakage Vd often increases to a great extent. Hence, larger loading doses may be needed to achieve quick therapeutic level. On the other hand, renal clearance is diminished hence maintenance dose requirement may be less or interval between two dose may be more.
- Therapeutic drug monitoring which is mainstay for monitoring optimal drug exposure must be implemented whenever possible.
- Serum creatinine, cystatin C, urea, and urine output along with volume status as assessed by either clinically or noninvasive and invasive techniques are the real guide to understand the status of progress or deterioration of AKI. These indices should be analyzed to guide drug dosing when an AKI is setting in.
- Because of logistic issue when therapeutic drug monitoring is not possible, close monitoring of drugs pharmacodynamic property may be a useful to monitor drug dosing.
- With advent of bioinformatics electronic validated tools are available for understanding drug-drug or drug-nutrient interaction. Whenever possible use of these tools must be implemented for better drug dosing consideration.
- Whenever possible a patient-centered team approach with mission of best clinical outcome and better drug dosing must be created. Role of ICU pharmacist in this team is most crucial to solve some complex puzzles related to safer drug delivery to a patient.

Drug Dosing Considerations—Hemodialysis

- As all modalities of dialysis have enhanced elimination of some drug, it is common practice to give the dose after dialysis to ensure active drug levels until next dosing. An appropriate supplementary dose in addition is always considered to compensate the amount eliminated during dialysis.
- Patients who are undergoing extended dialysis regimens with high diffusive or convective membranes have been associated with extensive drug clearances. In these situations, supplementary dose may need to be escalated proportionately.

To conclude for critical patients especially those who are at risk of AKI, or those who already has AKI, the usage of drugs needs careful intensive monitoring. Depending on the clinical context doses of certain drugs needs to be continuously adjusted. Patients with RRT whatever be its form need further special attention by appropriate timing, dosing, and supplemental drug dose increment based on modalities of RRT.

DRUG-INDUCED AKI

Kidney being one of the most vulnerable organs for drug toxicity, drug-induced AKI is a serious problem in day-to-day clinical practice. It is estimated that around 20% of AKI among hospitalized patients are secondary to drugs. Drug-induced nephrotoxicity mainly damages either tubules of nephrons leading acute tubular necrosis (ATN) or interstitium of kidney leading to acute interstitial nephritis (AIN). ATN is believed to be resulting from direct drug toxicity on tubular cells and AIN is secondary to allergic response of renal interstitium to drugs.

Platinum-based chemotherapeutic drugs such as cisplatin, carboplatin, aminoglycosides, and amphotericin-B are classical example of direct tubulotoxic drugs which cause ATN. Whereas penicillin antibiotics, Nonsteroidal anti-inflammatory drugs NSAIDs, and proton pump inhibitors are allergic to renal interstitium and commonly leads to AIN.

Crystal deposition in intratubular space is another way of nephrotoxicity by some groups of drug otherwise known as crystalline nephropathy. Identification of crystals or crystal containing cast in urine or in kidney biopsy specimen is often found in crystal nephropathy patients. Drugs like acyclovir, indinavir are commonly known for crystalline nephropathy.

We have to keep in mind antimicrobial agents, chemotherapeutic agents, calcineurin inhibitors, contrast agents, and NSAIDs are common classes of drugs which are known to cause drug-induced AKI. There are some known risk factors for drug-induced AKI. Intravascular volume depletion, preexisting kidney disease, acidosis, hyperuricemia, high-dose diuretic requirements, and advanced age are some of the common risk factors. Before onset of drug-induced AKI, where tubules get affected, tubular dysfunction occurs in phases. First the drug is actively transported in proximal tubule. Organic anionic transporters such as OAT1 and OAT3 play an active role in this process. Subsequently, secretion of drug takes place in the tubular lumen by apical membrane transporter such as MRP2 and MRP4. Then the drugs again get incorporated inside the tubular cells where by inhibiting mitochondrial function the final cellular damage takes place, which ultimately leads to ATN and AKI.

Without renal biopsy confirmed diagnosis of drug-induced AIN cannot be done. The main pathological findings are interstitial inflammation and infiltration of inflammatory cells within tubule known as tubulitis. Lymphocytes and monocytes, smaller numbers of eosinophils, plasma cells, neutrophils, and histiocytes are the main interstitial infiltrate commonly observed in drug-induced AIN.

Drug-induced AIN often clinically asymptomatic or presents with minimal nonspecific symptoms like malaise, loss of appetite, pain at flank region, myalgia, arthralgia, etc. High index of suspicion is necessary to identify drug-induced AIN. Unexplained new onset urinary abnormality with or without renal insufficiency in a subject who is newly exposed to drugs known to cause AIN are the candidates who need further evaluation in that line. Rarely, myositis and arthritis may be presenting symptoms. Fever rash and eosinophilia so-called the classic triad of AIN together with renal insufficiency is typically observed <6–10% of all drug-induced AIN.

Renal manifestation of drug-induced AIN is an increase in blood urea nitrogen (BUN) level and rise in serum creatinine. Urine output never be compromised in drug-induced AIN (nonoliguric AKI), in some time the patients may present with polyuria due to renal concentrating defect. There is usual delay of 5–10 days in between exposure to drug and clinical manifestation of drug-induced AIN. Among the metabolic abnormality, hyperkalemic hyperchloremic metabolic acidosis, inconsistent with the degree of kidney failure, is most common presenting feature. Rarely, in some variety of drug-induced AIN, renal insufficiency may be prolonged and patient may require RRT support until recovery. The mainstay of treatment is identifying the culprit drug and its discontinuation **(Table 1)**.

Drugs Known to Cause AKI

Drugs known to cause AKI is depicted in **Table 1**.

TABLE 1: Drugs known to cause acute kidney injury (AKI).

Tubular epithelial cell damage

Acute tubular necrosis
- Aminoglycoside antibiotics
- Radiographic contrast media
- Cisplatin, carboplatin
- Amphotericin B
- Cyclosporine, tacrolimus
- Adefovir, cidofovir, tenofovir
- Pentamidine
- Foscarnet
- Zoledronate

Osmotic nephrosis
- Mannitol
- Dextran
- IV immunoglobulin

Hemodynamically mediated kidney injury
- Angiotensin-converting enzyme inhibitor
- Angiotensin II receptor blockers
- Nonsteroidal anti-inflammatory drugs (NSAIDs)
- Cyclosporine, tacrolimus
- OKT3

Obstructive nephropathy

Intratubular obstruction
- Acyclovir
- Sulfonamides
- Indinavir
- Foscarnet
- Methotrexate
- Triamterene
- Indinavir

Nephrocalcinosis
- Oral sodium phosphate solution

Nephrolithiasis
- Sulfonamides

Glomerular disease
- Gold
- Lithium
- NSAIDs, cyclooxygenase-2 inhibitors
- Pamidronate

Tubulointerstitial disease

Acute allergic interstitial nephritis
- Penicillins
- Ciprofloxacin
- NSAIDs, cyclooxygenase-2 inhibitors
- Proton pump inhibitors
- Loop diuretics

Chronic interstitial nephritis
- Cyclosporine
- Lithium
- Aristolochic acid

Papillary necrosis
- NSAIDs, combined phenacetin, aspirin, and caffeine analgesics

Renal vasculitis, thrombosis, and cholesterol emboli

Vasculitis and thrombosis
- Hydralazine
- Propylthiouracil
- Allopurinol
- Penicillamine
- Gemcitabine
- Mitomycin C
- Methamphetamines
- Cyclosporine, tacrolimus
- Adalimumab
- Bevacizumab

Cholesterol emboli
- Warfarin
- Thrombolytic agents

DOSAGE MODIFICATION IN AKI

In AKI, change in volume status the body compartments and compromised organ cross talk, delayed clearance from kidney, changes the pharmacokinetic and pharmacodynamic parameters of any given drug. Hence, appropriate dosage modification and optimizing dosage frequency, keeping in mind the change in Vd, alteration in hepatic metabolism, and renal clearance are a great challenge.

Protein Binding

We all know the overall Vd of a drug is analyzed based on Vd of free or active component and Vd of the total component. The Vd of free active component of the drug (active form) is quite different from the Vd for the total drug. The concentration of the free drug is extremely sensitive to plasma protein level[6] and presence or absence of uremic toxins. There is usually an increase in plasma concentration free fraction of drugs in the context of AKI,[7] as on one hand, there is usually low albumin depicting lesser binding of free drug with protein, and on the other hand, the uremic toxins can displace drugs from their protein binding. On top of that blood flow distribution to splanchnic circulation, skeletal muscle, and fat is altered in AKI, therefore, the apparent Vd of drugs is also changed. Keeping all these factors in mind the dosage adjustment of any given drug is considered in AKI.

Amino Acids

In AKI, raised urea concentration in serum and decreased arginine production from kidney have the impact on hepatic ornithine cycle. In addition, serum concentrations of some amino acids such as dimethylarginine, methionine, and homocysteine are significantly increased in AKI. The clinical consequences of these imbalances in amino acid synthesis are not clearly known, but it is imperative that excess amino acids can exacerbate metabolic acidosis. Acidosis plays an important role in regards to protein binding of any drug also amino acids sometimes comes with some drugs in protein bindings leading to altered free total bound drug ratio, which is important for dosage modification in AKI.

Drug Excretion in AKI

It is quite interesting to observe that in AKI not only the renal clearance of drug get hampered also the non-glomerular drug elimination is also gets significantly compromised. There are ample of evidence showing the intestinal, hepatic, and pulmonary clearance of drugs are compromised in AKI. This is supported by the fact that the drugs that are primarily hepatically eliminated also get accumulated during AKI. The possible mechanism in this regards is probably gut edema, compromised organ cross talk, influence of uremic toxins, and change in metabolic milieu during AKI. Hence, while adjusting dose it must be kept in mind that not only renally excreted drugs need attention in AKI on the contrary drugs which are eliminated by nonrenal elimination path, their clearance is also compromised in AKI.

■ CONCLUSION

Kidney plays an important role in eliminating or maintaining therapeutic levels of many drugs and their metabolites. On the other side kidney is vulnerable to self-injury due to toxic accumulation of many drugs. Hence understanding framework how a drug is handled inside our body and how its dose needs to be modified in compromised renal function is utmost important to avoid toxicity and maintaining therapeutic efficacy. Patients who are in RRT need special attention to maintain therapeutic drug levels especially for dialyzable drugs. It is often difficult to remember exact dosing in different spectrum of kidney function impairment and wise to keep online drug dosing tools handy for basic and common drugs.

Take Home Messages

- Kidney plays a crucial role in drug elimination from body, hence in renal impairment understanding principles of adjusting drug dose of individual drugs is important to avoid toxicities.
- Among patients who are on renal replacement therapy understanding pharmacokinetic principles in relation to dialysis clearance is necessary for optimum drug exposure.
- Many drugs are known to cause AKI, hence it is necessary to know potential nephrotoxic mechanism of drugs to avoid drug induced AKI.

■ REFERENCES

1. Mehta RL, Pascual MT, Soroko S, Savage BR, Himmelfarb J, Ikizler TA, et al. Spectrum of acute renal failure in the intensive care unit: the PICARD experience. Kidney Int. 2004;66(4):1613-21.
2. Hoste EA, Bagshaw SM, Bellomo R, Cely CM, Colman R, Cruz DN, et al. Epidemiology of acute kidney injury in critically ill patients: the multinational AKI-EPI study. Intensive Care Med. 2015;41(8):1411-23.
3. Liu C, Yan S, Wang Y, Wang J, Fu X, Song H, et al. Drug-Induced Hospital-Acquired Acute Kidney Injury in China: A Multicenter Cross-Sectional Survey. Kidney Dis (Basel). 2021;7(2):143-155.
4. Verbeeck RK, Branch RA, Wilkinson GR. Drug metabolites in renal failure: pharmacokinetic and clinical implications. Clin Pharmacokinet. 1981;6(5):329-45.
5. Reetze-Bonorden P, Böhler J, Keller E. Drug dosage in patients during continuous renal replacement therapy. Pharmacokinetic and therapeutic considerations. Clin Pharmacokinet. 1993;24(5):362-79.
6. Greenblatt DJ, Sellers EM, Koch-Weser J. Importance of protein binding for the interpretation of serum or plasma drug concentrations. J Clin Pharmacol. 1982;22(5-6):259-63.
7. Reidenberg MM, Drayer DE. Alteration of drug-protein binding in renal disease. Clin Pharmacokinet. 1984;9 Suppl 1:18-26.

SECTION 6

Metabolic Emergencies

Section Editor: Ghanshyam Goyal

24. **Metabolic Emergencies (Electrolyte): Hyponatremia, Hypernatremia, Hypokalemia, and Hyperkalemia**
    Pankaj Singhania, Piyas Gargari, Sujoy Ghosh

25. **Metabolic-hyperglycemic Emergencies**
    Sanjay K Shah, Vivek Shah

26. **Endocrinal (Hypoglycemia)**
    Ghanshyam Goyal, Usashi Biswas Bose, Rekha Basak Srivastava

CHAPTER 24

Metabolic Emergencies (Electrolyte): Hyponatremia, Hypernatremia, Hypokalemia, and Hyperkalemia

Pankaj Singhania, Piyas Gargari, Sujoy Ghosh

INTRODUCTION

Electrolyte imbalances are a fairly common encounter in clinical practice. They are more common and important in the emergency department and the intensive care setting. Sodium and potassium are the two most common electrolytes ordered in emergency medicine. This proves their profound effect on physiological processes and the common expression of a number of pathological entities. While it is emergent to correct these electrolyte abnormalities, an accurate etiological diagnosis is important to prevent recurrence and for sustained improvement. It is also essential to remember that uncorrected sodium and potassium levels can also prove to be fatal.[1] So, an accurate diagnosis and an algorithm-based step-wise approach is the key to the management of dyselectrolytemia. In the following pages, we have given a brief overview of the four most common electrolyte abnormalities experienced by clinicians—(1) hyponatremia, (2) hypernatremia, (3) hypokalemia, and (4) hyperkalemia.

HYPONATREMIA

Definition

Hyponatremia is defined as serum sodium concentration <135 mmol/L.

Etiology and Classification

- True hyponatremia should always be differentiated from pseudohyponatremia.
- In certain cases, such as severe hyperglycemia and serum sodium estimation may be falsely low because of dilutional effect from solvent drag.
- Therefore, the corrected serum Na$^+$ in mmol/L = measured (Na$^+$) + 2.4 × (glucose in mg/dL − 100)/100
- Also, in conditions of marked hyperlipidemia and hyperproteinemia, serum sodium can also be spuriously low.[2]
- Depending on the osmolar status and tonicity, hyponatremia can be broadly divided into—hypovolemic, euvolemic, and hypervolemic hyponatremia **(Tables 1 and 2)**.

Clinical Features

- Mild hyponatremia can be defined as serum Na$^+$ between 130 and 135 mmol/L, as measured by ion-specific electrode, moderate if 125–129 mmol/L and profound if serum Na$^+$ <125 mmol/L.[4]
- Usually, mild cognitive impairment can be seen with mild hyponatremia whereas headache, confusion, and nausea are evident when serum Na$^+$ is between 120 and 125 mmol/L and seizures at Na$^+$ <115 mmol/L.
- According to European Guidelines, symptomatology can be divided into severe and moderately-severe symptoms.
- Severe symptoms are vomiting, cardiopulmonary distress, deep somnolence, seizures, and coma (Glasgow Coma Scale <8) whereas moderately severe symptoms comprise of nausea without vomiting, confusion, and headache. Identification of these helps in therapeutic decision.
- The management also depends on the rapidity of development.
- Rapid correction in chronic hyponatremia leads to osmotic imbalance and eventually, osmotic demyelination syndrome.

TABLE 1: Etiology of hyponatremia.

Hypovolemic hyponatremia	Euvolemic hyponatremia	Hypervolemic hyponatremia
Urine Na$^+$ >40 mmol/L • Diuretics • Cerebral salt-wasting syndrome • Salt-wasting nephropathy • Mineralocorticoid deficiency *Urine Na$^+$ <20 mmol/L* • Gastrointestinal losses (vomiting/diarrhea) • Pancreatitis	• Hypothyroidism[3] • Secondary adrenal insufficiency • Syndrome of inappropriate antidiuretic hormone (SIADH) • Beer potomania • "Tea and toast" hyponatremia	• Cardiac failure • Hepatic failure • Renal failure

TABLE 2: Etiologies of SIADH.				
Malignant diseases	Pulmonary disorders	Disorders of the nervous system	Drugs	Others
• Carcinoma lung • Carcinoma oropharynx • Carcinoma of GI tract • Carcinoma of bladder, prostate, and endometrium • Lymphoma • Thymoma • Ewing's sarcoma	• Bacterial pneumonia • Viral pneumonia • Tuberculosis • Asthma • Cystic fibrosis • Respiratory failure associated with positive-pressure breathing	• Encephalitis • Meningitis • Brain abscess • AIDS • Cerebral malaria • Subdural hematoma • Stroke • Brain tumor • Hydrocephalus • Guillain–Barré Syndrome • Shy–Drager syndrome • Acute intermittent porphyria	• Selective serotonin reuptake inhibitors (SSRIs) • Tricyclic antidepressants • Carbamazepine • Oxcarbazepine • Antipsychotics • Chlorpropamide • Tolbutamide • MDMA • Nicotine • Cyclophosphamide	• Gain-of-function mutation of vasopressin V2 receptor • Idiopathic • Exercise-associated (marathon runners) General anesthesiaStress • Nausea

(AIDS: acquired immunodeficiency syndrome; GI: gastrointestinal tract; MDMA: methylenedioxymethamphetamine; SIADH: syndrome of inappropriate antidiuretic hormone secretion)

- Once hyponatremia is confirmed and causes of pseudohyponatremia are ruled out, the etiology of hyponatremia must be sought.
- Signs of hypovolemia such as dry mucous membranes and reduced skin turgor points toward hypovolemic hyponatremia.
- Urinary osmolality if <100 mOsm/kg, indicates excess water intake as the cause of hypotonic hyponatremia.[4]
- If the urine osmolality is >100 mOsm/kg, urine Na$^+$ estimation from spot sample taken simultaneously from blood would differentiate between etiologies of hypovolemic hyponatremia.
- Similarly, the presence of volume overload features such as bibasilar rales, raised jugular venous pressure (JVP), pedal edema, ascites indicates hypervolemic hyponatremia.
- In case of euvolemic hyponatremia, before stamping as syndrome of inappropriate antidiuretic hormone secretion (SIADH), cortisol, and thyroid function tests must be done to rule out hypothyroidism and hypocortisolism.

Management

Emergency Measures

There are two prongs of therapy in hyponatremic patients—(1) immediate stabilization and (2) cause-directed therapy. Therefore, it would be logical if the patient is stabilized first followed by searched for etiology. The following algorithm may be beneficial (**Flowchart 1**).

When a patient presents in the emergency with symptomatic hyponatremia with severe symptoms as described, a prompt intravenous infusion of 150 mL of 3% hypertonic saline over 20 minutes seems to be prudent followed by estimation of serum sodium after 20 minutes while starting another 150 mL of 3% hypertonic saline. In case of grossly deviant body composition, 2 mL/kg solution can be administered instead of the fixed 150 mL. This should be repeated to reach a target of rise of serum sodium of 5 mmol/L above baseline, after which 3% hypertonic saline should be stopped and 0.9% normal saline should be continued just for keeping the peripheral line open. Increase in serum sodium of 10 mmol/L during the first 24 hours and an additional 8 mmol/L for each additional day until the serum Na$^+$ concentration of 130 mmol/L should be targeted. For that reason, serum sodium should be checked every 6–12 hourly basis.

However, if the serum sodium does not rise to 5 mmol/L above baseline after the first infusions, 3% hypertonic saline infusion should be continued aiming an additional 1 mmol/L/h increase in Na$^+$ concentration, and the infusion should be stopped when symptoms improve, 10 mmol/L rise of serum Na$^+$ achieved or serum Na$^+$ becomes 130 mmol/L. Serum sodium, in this case, should be checked every 4 hours. However, it should be kept in mind that patient's mentation may not recover immediately even after electrolytes correction. In case of rapid correction, relowering of serum Na$^+$ can be attempted.

The sodium change in serum after 1 L infusion can be calculated from Adrogue-Madias formula which is as follows:

$$\text{Change in serum Na}^+ \text{ (mmol/L)} = [\text{infusate (Na+)} - \text{serum (Na+)}]/[\text{TBW} + 1],$$

where TBW is total body water and can be derived by multiplying body weight with 0.6 for adult males and 0.5 for adult females, 0.5 for elderly males and 0.45 for elderly females.

For acute hyponatremia without symptoms, nonessential fluids should be stopped, causes if found should be addressed and if serum Na$^+$ drop >10 mmol/L, a single 3% hypertonic saline of 150 mL over 20 minutes would be sufficient. Correction of serum K$^+$ level would also improve hyponatremia which should be kept in mind during correction.

Flowchart 1: Stepwise algorithm for hyponatremia management.

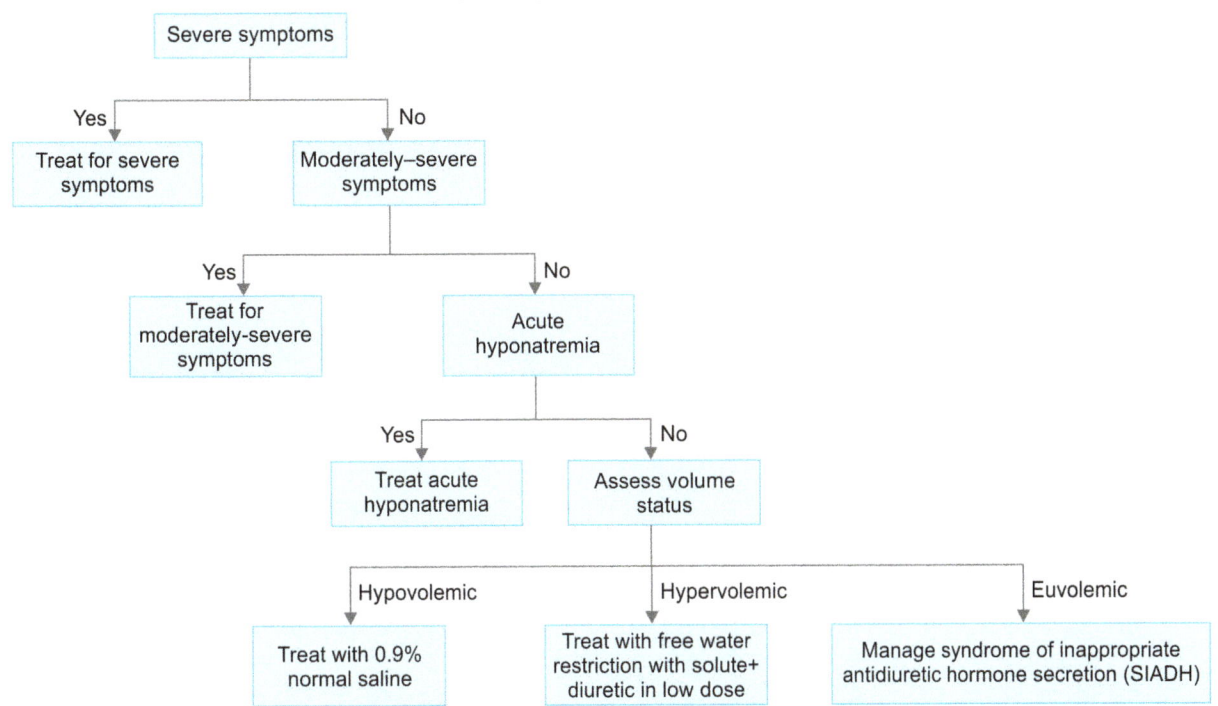

For chronic hypervolemic hyponatremia, fluid restriction is the first-line treatment. If this is not helpful, then 0.25–0.5 g/kg/day of urea or a combination of low-dose loop diuretics and oral sodium chloride is recommended.[4]

In cases of hypovolemic hyponatremia, IV infusion of 0.9% saline at 0.5–1 mL/kg/h can be given to restore extracellular volume. However, in case of hemodynamic instability need for rapid fluid resuscitation overrides risk of rapid Na^+ increase.

Chronic Management

Once stabilized, the patient should be treated for the etiology. In some cases of hypervolemic hyponatremia such as congestive cardiac failure, arginine vasopressin (AVP) antagonists play an important role in managing fluid status although not being recommended by European guidelines. Oral drug tolvaptan was approved in USA for patients with hypervolemic and euvolemic hyponatremia in those cases with serum Na^+ 125–134 mmol/L and not responding to fluid restriction alone.[5]

■ HYPERNATREMIA

Definition

Hypernatremia is defined as serum sodium concentration exceeding 145 mmol/L.

Etiology and Classification

The various etiologies are **(Flowchart 2)**
- Aging
- Impaired cognitive and higher neural function
- Vomiting
- Excessive sweating
- Hyperventilation
- Diarrhea
- Long Exercise
- Intraoperative losses of fluid
- Tubing and drains
- Drugs like demeclocycline
- Osmotic diuresis
- *Diabetes insipidus (DI):*
  - *Central:* Hereditary syndromes, pituitary surgery, tumors (craniopharyngioma, germinoma, metastases, and pinealoma), traumatic brain injury, granulomatous diseases, infection, hypophysitis, and idiopathic.
  - *Nephrogenic:* Hereditary, chronic renal disease (polycystic kidney and obstructive uropathy), hypercalcemia, hypokalemia, amyloidosis, and drugs (lithium and demeclocycline).
  - Gestational DI
  - Dipsogenic DI
- Adipsic patient (osmoreceptor malfunction)
- Conn's syndrome
- Cushing syndrome
- Inadvertent administration of hypertonic fluid administration/inappropriate formula during hospital stay
- Salt Intoxication.

Based on urine volume and urine osmolarity, a simplified algorithm for hypernatremia is proposed here.

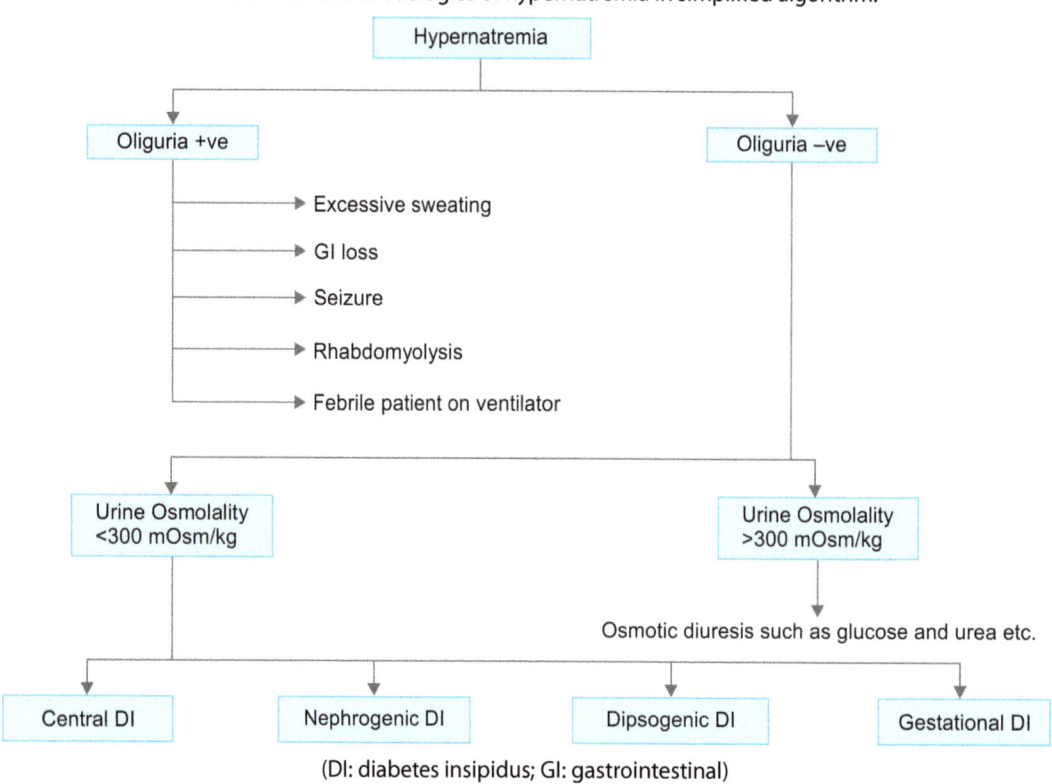

Flowchart 2: Various etiologies of hypernatremia in simplified algorithm.

(DI: diabetes insipidus; GI: gastrointestinal)

It can also be divided into mild, moderate and severe hypernatremia depending on serum sodium levels, i.e., 148–150 mEq/L, 151–154 mEq/L, and ≥155 mEq/L.[1]

Clinical Features

- Symptoms and appearance of signs largely depend on degree as well as rapidity of developmental of hypernatremia.
- Therefore, many chronic hypernatremia patients remain asymptomatic consequent to their slow rate of development.
- Age distribution is an important factor as this is particularly prevalent in younger children and older adults.
- In children, a characteristic high-pitched cry, irritability, lethargy, weakness is found followed by coma.
- The symptomatology becomes obvious when Na$^+$ level exceeds 160 mmol/L. Focal neurodeficit can also occur.
- Once hypernatremia is found, determination of hydration level seems to be useful.
- Depending on the total body Na$^+$ level compared to total body water content, it can be divided into hypovolemic, euvolemic, and hypervolemic conditions.
- The presence of polyuria may indicate renal loss and commonly diabetes insipidus. Polyuria is defined as urine volume >150 mL/kg/day at birth, >100 mL/kg/day up to age of 2 years, and >50 mL/kg/day for older adults.[2] In addition to, certain clues such as pituitary surgery, drugs points toward obvious etiologies.

Investigations

Paired serum and urine osmolality along with estimations of glycemic status seems to be the best initial screening test.

In an euglycemic individual, demonstration of urine osmolality <300 mOsm/kg in background of plasma osmolality >295 mOsm/kg is consistent with diabetes insipidus. Elevated serum Na$^+$ level >145 mmol/L may also supplant the diagnosis.[3] Determination of subtype can be found out by administration of vasopressin. Urine osmolality that improves 50% or more is associated with central DI and that does not improve, is associated with nephrogenic diabetes insipidus. When this is not a straightforward case, water deprivation test can be done in hospital setting.

Management

Emergency Measures

The basic ABCs of emergency life support must be ensured followed by etiology-directed treatment.

Treatment depends on the chronicity of the condition which is frequently unknown. In those cases, slow correction of hypernatremia with a target correction of 10 mmol/L/day is undertaken.

In all cases, management depends on two basic questions—(1) management of prevailing hypertonicity and (2) management of the underlying cause. As there is a free water deficit in most cases, the management should begin with the estimation of free water deficit which should be replaced intravenously or via feeding tube or by both in a controlled manner. Too rapid correction can lead to cerebral edema, cerebral herniation, and eventually death. Usually, it is prudent to correct at 8–12 mmol/day, i.e., 1 mmol/h in case of acute hypernatremia (that has developed within 48 hours). In case of chronic hypernatremia or in those cases where there is no documented onset, it might be prudent not to exceed 8–10 mmol/day of correction, i.e., not exceeding Na$^+$ correction beyond 0.5 mmol/h.[4]

Calculation of free water deficit in liters = TBW × (current Na$^+$ level – 140/140)

where TBW = total body water and can be calculated by multiplying 0.6 to body weight for males and 0.5 for females.

The effect of 1 L of various infusions on serum sodium can be estimated by using Adrogue–Madias formula, which is as follows:

Change of serum Na$^+$ after 1 L = (Infusate Na$^+$ – serum Na$^+$)/(TBW + 1),

where TBW is total body water.

Insensible losses (500 mL/day usually for adults, and 400 mL/m^2/day for children) and ongoing losses should be also accounted for and should be added to the total fluid required for the patient.

Chronic Management

- Once the patient has been stable and emergency measures have been taken, next the etiology should be tried to determine and etiology specific measures should be taken.
- In case of diabetes insipidus, desmopressin acetate (DDAVP), a synthetic long-acting vasopressin analog that has minimal pressor activity but twice the antidiuretic potency of AVP should be considered, especially in cases of central diabetes insipidus.
- It can be administered via intranasal spray, or more commonly, orally. In postsurgical conditions, DDAVP can be used depending on the increased output e.g., exceeding 200–250 mL for 3 hours persistently.
- For regular use, dilutional hyponatremia is a concern for which reason omission of DDAVP once weekly to allow for water diuresis.
- For nephrogenic diabetes insipidus (NDI), DDAVP is not very effective choice. Thiazide diuretics (hydrochlorothiazide 25 mg/day) or nonsteroidal anti-inflammatory drugs (NSAIDS) (ibuprofen 200 mg/24 hours) can be used in adjunct to dietary salt restriction.

■ HYPOKALEMIA

Definition

Hypokalemia is generally defined as serum potassium <3.5 mEq/L (3.5 mmol/L)

Severity of hypokalemia is enumerated in **Table 3**.

TABLE 3: Severity of hypokalemia.

Severity	Serum K level (mEq/L)
Moderate	2.5–3
Severe	<2.5

Etiology[6]

- Inadequate potassium intake
- Increased potassium excretion
- Intracellular shift of potassium.

Inadequate Intake

- Eating disorders: Anorexia, bulimia, and starvation
- Dental problems
- Potassium poor total parenteral nutrition (TPN).

Increased Potassium Excretion

- Enhanced sodium delivery to collecting ducts due to diuretic use
- Hyperaldosteronism (primary and secondary)
- Renal artery stenosis (RAS)
- Osmotic diuresis
- Genetic disorders: Congenital adrenal hyperplasia (CAH) (11-β-hydroxylase or 17-α-hydroxylase deficiency, glucocorticoid-remediable aldosteronism (GRA), Bartter syndrome, Gitelman syndrome, Liddle syndrome, hypokalemic periodic paralysis, and thyrotoxic periodic paralysis).
- Cushing syndrome
- Renal tubular acidosis (1 and 2)
- Drugs—diuretics, theophylline, verapamil, amphotericin B, gentamicin, cisplatin, and beta agonist
- GI loss—diarrhea, vomiting, and nasogastric tube (NG) suction.

Intracellular Shift

- Intravenous (IV) insulin therapy like in treated diabetic ketoacidosis (DKA)
- Alkalosis
- Beta adrenergic stimulation
- Hypokalemic periodic paralysis
- Thyrotoxic periodic paralysis
- Refeeding.

Coronavirus Disease 2019

- Increased prevalence of hypokalemia in severe coronavirus disease (COVID)
- Cause not ascertained clearly.

Clinical Features

- Mild hypokalemia may be largely asymptomatic
- Symptoms are nonspecific and related to muscular or cardiac function

- Weakness and fatigue are most common symptoms. Weakness may progress to paralysis.
- Worsening of diabetes control or polyuria (hyperglycemia or DI)
- Psychological symptoms.

History
- Poor intake
- Drug history
- Vomiting/diarrhea
- High dose insulin
- Similar episodes in past
- Family history of adrenal tumor, episodes of paralysis, hyperthyroidism or surgery of pituitary or adrenal.

Physical Examination
- Generally normal
- Tachycardia/irregular beats/tachypnea
- Hypertension (PA/RAS/licorice/CAH/GRA/Liddle)
- Relative hypotension—laxative use/diuretic use/Bartter syndrome/Gitelman syndrome
- Depressed or absent deep tendon reflexes
- Absent/muffled bowel sounds
- Severe-bradycardia, arrhythmias, and respiratory paralysis
- Tooth erosion (bulimia).

Diagnosis[7]

Most common cause is urinary or GI loss. History and physical examination may give clues to the etiology. Urine potassium is an important test to clinch a diagnostic etiology. At initial attempt also do a serum magnesium. An electrocardiography (ECG) is a must in dealing with hypokalemia, as untreated severe hypokalemia can lead to life-threatening arrhythmias **(Fig. 1)**.

Depending on suspicion the following tests may be ordered:
- Plasma renin and aldosterone
- Serum cortisol
- Renal artery Doppler for renal artery stenosis
- Enzyme assays for CAH
- Thyroid function tests

- Evaluation for Cushing syndrome including magnetic resonance imaging (MRI) pituitary
- CT scan abdomen for source of aldosterone excess.

Spot Urine Potassium
Spot urine potassium is used for diagnosis **(Table 4)**.

24 Hours Urine Potassium
- More cumbersome but more accurate
- <20 mEq over 24 hours suggests nonrenal wasting
- Always do urine creatinine to ensure accuracy of collection.

Spot Urine Sodium
Spot urine sodium <20 mEq/L in a setting of high urine Potassium may suggest secondary hyperaldosteronism.

Urine Osmolality
High urine osmolality (>700 mOsm/kg) may mislead urine potassium values and high urine potassium values may not represent renal potassium wasting.

Transtubular Potassium Gradient
- Useful because it takes into account potentially cofounding effect of urine concentration on urine potassium

$$\text{Transtubular potassium gradient (TTKG)} = \frac{\text{urine potassium} \times \text{serum osmolality}}{\text{Serum potassium} \times \text{urine osmolality}}$$

- TTKG <3 = nonrenal potassium loss
- TTKG >7 = renal potassium loss.

Other Metabolic Profile
- *Serum sodium:* Low serum suggests diuretic use or GI loss. High serum sodium suggests nephrogenic DI or hyper aldosteronism.
- *Serum bicarbonate:* Low serum bicarbonate suggests renal tubular acidosis (RTA), diarrhea, and acetazolamide use.
- High serum bicarbonate suggests hyper aldosteronism, Bartter, and Gitelman or Liddle syndrome.
- Creatine kinase may be elevated in profound muscle weakness or rhabdomyolysis

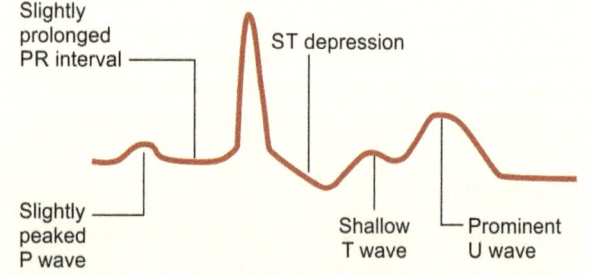

Fig. 1: Electrocardiography (ECG) findings of hypokalemia.

TABLE 4: Differentiation of various etiologies of hypokalemia with spot urine K^+.

Spot urine potassium (mEq/L)	Diagnosis
<20	Gastrointestinal (GI) loss, poor intake, and intracellular shift
>40	Renal loss

Arterial Blood Gases

- *Alkalosis suggests*—vomiting, Bartter syndrome, Gitelman syndrome, or hyperaldosteronism
- *Acidosis suggests*: RTA or presence of toxins like toluene.

Treatment

The treatment of hypokalemia is four pronged **(Table 5)**.

Decreasing Potassium Loss

- Stop diuretics, use potassium sparing diuretics
- Treat diarrhea/vomiting
- Treatment of hyperglycemia.

Replenishment of Potassium

- Every 1 mEq/L decrease in serum potassium = 200–400 mEq potassium deficit.
- *Mild hypokalemia*—oral potassium replacement therapy unless serious cardiac arrythmias needs to be addressed.
- *Severe hypokalemia*—IV potassium should be given with continuous ECG monitoring and serial potassium checking.
- Oral potassium is well absorbed but limited by GI intolerance.
- IV potassium can be given at 20 mEq/h by peripheral line and 40 mEq/h by central line.

Medications

- Oral potassium chloride is used
- IV injection—injection potassium chloride (KCl) available as 10 mEq or 20 mEq ampoules. Never give IV shot, always dilute in normal saline.

Surgery for Hypokalemia

Renal artery stenosis, adrenal adenoma, intestinal obstruction, Cushing's disease, and villous adenoma are surgically amenable causes of hypokalemia.

Complications

- Cardiovascular—atrial and ventricular arrhythmias and hypertension
- Muscular—weakness, depressed deep tendon reflexes, flaccid paralysis, and rhabdomyolysis
- Renal—nephrogenic DI, metabolic alkalosis, cystic degeneration, and interstitial scarring

- Metabolic—decreased insulin release and peripheral insulin sensitivity.

HYPERKALEMIA

Definition

Hyperkalemia is defined as serum potassium level >5.0–5.5 mEq/L in adults. The upper limit may be as high as 6.5 mEq/L in young or premature infants.

Severity (Table 6)

Etiology[8]

Hyperkalemia can result from the following:
- Excess intake of potassium
- Decreased excretion of potassium
- Shift of potassium from intracellular to extracellular space
- Combination of the above.

Excess Intake of Potassium

- Very uncommon if estimated glomerular filtration rate (eGFR) >60 mL/min
- Most common source is IV or potassium supplementation
- PRBC transfusion can also lead to hyperkalemia.

Decreased Excretion

This is the most common cause of hyperkalemia. The common etiologies are as follows:
- Renal failure
- Medications such as NSAIDs, angiotensin-converting enzyme (ACE) inhibitors, potassium sparing diuretics, cyclosporine, heparin, ketoconazole, pentamidine, metyrapone, trimethoprim—sulfamethoxazole.
- *Hypoaldosteronism*:
  - Reduced aldosterone production
  - Distal tubule resistance to aldosterone (RTA 4, sickle cell anemia, and urinary tract obstruction)
  - Addison's disease
  - Salt wasting CAH
  - Pseudohypoaldosteronism.

Shift from Intracellular to Extracellular Space

- Insulin deficiency like DKA
- Acute acidosis
- Rhabdomyolysis and tumor lysis syndrome

TABLE 5: Strategies for hypokalemia management.

Reduction of potassium loss	Replenishment of potassium store
Evaluation for potential toxicities particularly cardiac	Determination of cause and preventing recurrence

TABLE 6: Severity of hyperkalemia.

Serum potassium (mEq/L)	Severity
5.5–6.0	Mild
6.1–7.0	Moderate
≥7.0	Severe

- Malignant hyperthermia
- Hyperkalemic periodic palsy
- Drugs such as propofol, digitalis, β-blockers, epsilon-aminocaproic acid (EACA), succinylcholine, cyclosporine
- Electrical ad thermal burns
- Hyper tonicity.

Clinical Features

The symptoms of hyperkalemia are predominantly muscular and cardiac in nature. Patients often complain of weakness and fatigue. Chest pain, palpitations, nausea, vomiting, and paresthesia are other presentations.[2,9,10]

History

- Unusual eating habits consuming fruits and dried fruits.
- Very low sodium and high potassium diets as a measure for cardiac, diabetic, and hypertensive patients.
- Over the counter herbal medications, salt substitutes, or sports drinks.
- History of recent blood transfusion.
- Cardiac surgery (cardioplegic solutions).
- History of renal failure or chronic kidney disease (CKD).
- History of diabetes, sickle cell anemia, urinary tract obstruction, polycystic kidney disease (PCKD), amyloidosis (type 4 RTA).
- History of drugs causing hyperkalemia.

Physical Examination

- Vitals signs are generally normal
- Muscle weakness, fatigue, and depression are nonspecific finding
- Cardiac examination may show bradycardia, extra-systoles and pauses due to varying degrees of heart block
- Respiratory muscle weakness may present as tachypnea
- Flaccid paralysis and absent deep tendon reflexes may be present[9]
- This is an emergency and should alert the clinician to adopt urgent measures.

Diagnosis[11]

Pseudohyperkalemia due to lysis of cellular contents should always be excluded before diagnosing hyperkalemia. The common practice such as milking of extremities during phlebotomy and fist clenching can lead to pseudohyperkalemia. Thrombocytosis can also falsely elevate serum potassium levels. After excluding pseudohyperkalemia, proceed with the following:

- Kidney function test [blood urea nitrogen (BUN), serum creatinine, 24 hours urine for creatinine clearance, eGFR]
- Serum calcium (hypocalcemia can worsen cardiac arrythmias)
- ECG
- Complete blood count
- Glucose level and digoxin level
- Arterial blood gas (ABG)/venous blood gas (VBG)—for acidosis
- Serum cortisol and aldosterone levels
- Serum uric acid and phosphorus for tumor lysis syndrome.

Urine Potassium, Sodium, and Osmolality

Spot urine potassium is obtained and interpreted as soon below **(Table 7)**.

Transtubular Potassium Gradient

Calculation and interpretation are similar to hypokalemia. Refer to section on hypokalemia.

Treatment

The aggressiveness of treatment will depend on potassium levels, presence of toxicity, and cardiac rhythm status[12] **(Table 8)**.

Emergency Management

- Secure IV excess and connect cardiac monitor.
- If QRS widening seen IV bicarbonate, calcium and insulin with 25% dextrose may be administered (see below for details).
- If required dialysis may be utilized as an emergency measure.
- Measure potassium levels at frequent intervals.
- After stabilization resort to means of increasing potassium excretion such as cation exchange resins and dialysis.

Medical Management of Hyperkalemia (Table 9)

General measures: Remove sources of excess potassium intake, diet, supplements, drugs, etc.

TABLE 7: Differentiation of etiologies of hyperkalemia based on urine K^+.

Urine potassium (mEq/L)	Interpretation
<20	Impaired renal excretion
>40	Intact renal excretion

TABLE 8: Management strategies of hyperkalemia.

Targets of treatment	
Emergency management	Cardiac protection
Transcellular shift of potassium inside the cells	Increased potassium excretion and dialysis

TABLE 9: Time to action of various treatment of hyperkalemia.

Effect	Agent	Dose	Onset	Duration
Cardiac membrane stabilizers	IV calcium gluconate	10 mL of 10% injection IV over 2–3 minutes	Immediate	30–60 minutes
Shifters	• Short acting insulin • Salbutamol	• 10 U in 100 mL 25% dextrose • 10 mg in 4 mL NS nebulized over 10 minutes	• 20 minutes • 30 minutes	• 4–6 hours • 2 hours
Excretors	• Furosemide • Sodium bicarbonate • Sodium polystyrene sulfonate	• 40–80 mg IV stat • 150 mmol/L IV at variable rates • 15 g OD to QID	• 15 minutes • Hours • >2 hours	• 2–3 hours • During infusion • 4–6 hours
Definitive	Hemodialysis		Immediate	3 hours

Reducing cardiac toxicity: Intravenous calcium gluconate to counter cardiac toxicity. 10 mL of 10% calcium gluconate IV over 2–3 minutes.

Move potassium inside the cells:

- 25% IV dextrose + insulin for moving potassium inside the cells. 10 U of regular insulin in 100 mL of 25% (or 50%) dextrose is infused. May be repeated if required. Beware of hypoglycemia especially in patients with renal insufficiency. Corticosteroids and mineralocorticoids in subjects with salt wasting CAH.
- Sodium bicarbonate if acidosis is severe
- *Beta adrenergic agonists*—nebulized salbutamol (albuterol)—10mg. Particularly useful in renal failure. Parenteral preparations are not recommended.

Increase potassium excretion:

- Increase renal excretion in adequate renal function by IV normal saline along with furosemide. Maintains euvolemia.
- Renal excretion can be enhanced by using aldosterone analogue like 9-α-fluorohydrocortisone acetate. Used in cyclosporine-induced hyperkalemia in cases of solid organ transplant.
- GI excretion can be enhanced with cation exchange resins like sodium polystyrene sulfonate, administered orally or per rectal. Not useful in acute hyperkalemia. One or more daily doses of 15 g can be used. Caution to be exercised in patients with constipation or stool impaction, may cause bowel perforation.
- *Patiromer*: Patiromer sorbitex calcium is a nonabsorbable cation exchange polymer that increases fecal potassium excretion. It has a better safety profile compared to sodium polystyrene sulfonate.
- *Sodium zirconium cyclosilicate*: Another potassium binder increasing fecal potassium excretion.

Dialysis: Emergency dialysis is a final step for life-threatening and refractory hyperkalemia. This is particularly useful in patients with compromised renal function.

Once hyperkalemia has been treated, look for cause of hyperkalemia and manage accordingly.

Take Home Messages

Hyponatremia:
- Hyponatremia is fairly common among admitted patients.
- Volume status of the patient should be ascertained.
- Too rapid correction of hyponatremia should be avoided.
- Fluid balance and electrolytes should be checked strictly.

Hypernatremia:
- Hypernatremia should be checked in patients presenting with obtundation or focal neurological signs
- Too rapid correction should be avoided in cases where onset is unknown.
- Ongoing loss and insensible loss must also be added in calculating total fluid requirement.
- DDAVP can be a good choice in hypernatremia patients with polyuria in post-operative setting.

Hypokalemia:
- Pseudo-hypokalemia—sampling errors, samples taken from an arm running IV fluids[3]
- TTKG cannot be applied when the urine osmolality is less than serum osmolality
- Low urine potassium in presence of very low urine sodium (<25 mEq/L) cannot exclude renal potassium wasting
- Total body potassium deficit may not be fully representative of serum potassium concentration as conditions like hypokalemic periodic palsy may have low serum potassium caused by transcellular maldistribution not by true deficit.
- While replenishing potassium losses keep into consideration ongoing losses
- Avoid glucose containing IV fluids to prevent insulin induced intracellular shift of potassium.
- If patient is acidotic correct potassium first, as alkali may cause transcellular shift of potassium.
- IV potassium chloride for damaging peripheral veins, check for thrombophlebitis frequently. For prolonged IV infusions central line is preferred.

Hyperkalemia:
- Using a tourniquet to collect blood may cause falsely elevated serum potassium levels
- Improperly collected or hemolyzed blood samples is the most common cause of pseudohyperkalemia.
- Always take history of recent blood transfusion before diagnosing hyperkalemia
- Do not collect blood for potassium estimation upstream of an IV-line infusing potassium containing fluid.

- If urine osmolality is high (>700 mOsm/kg), the absolute value of urine potassium can be misleading.
- In DKA an initial hyperkalemia does not reflect total body potassium stores. Once treatment is initiated hypokalemia ensues requiring potassium supplementation.
- Potassium binders available currently are to be used with caution because they may cause colonic perforation particularly in constipated individuals.
- Insulin use with dextrose does not guarantee protection from hypoglycemia. Beware of hypoglycemia while using insulin + dextrose infusion.
- In case of acute and life-threatening hyperkalemia resort to fast and immediate acting measures and cardiac protection should be on top of the list.
- Dialysis is overall the most effective treatment for hyperkalemia in cases refractory to all other measures, especially in a setting of compromised renal function.

REFERENCES

1. Sturdik I, Adamcova M, Kollerova J, Koller T, Zelinkova Z, Payer J. Hyponatraemia is an independent predictor of in-hospital mortality. Eur J Intern Med. 2014;25(4):379-82.
2. Pillai BP, Unnikrishnan AG, Pavithran PV. Syndrome of inappropriate antidiuretic hormone secretion: Revisiting a classical endocrine disorder. Indian J Endocrinol Metab. 2011;15(Suppl 3): S208-15.
3. Warner MH, Holding S, Kilpatrick ES. The effect of newly diagnosed hypothyroidism on serum sodium concentrations: a retrospective study. Clin Endocrinol (Oxf). 2006;64(5): 598-9.
4. Spasovski G, Vanholder R, Allolio B, Annane D, Ball S, Bichet D, et al. Clinical practice guideline on diagnosis and treatment of hyponatraemia. Eur J Endocrinol. 2014;170(3):G1-47.
5. Reilly T, Chavez B. Tolvaptan (Samsca) for Hyponatremia: Is It Worth Its Salt? Pharm Ther. 2009;34(10):543-7.
6. UpToDate. (2020). Causes of hypokalaemia in adults (Mount DB). [online] Available from: https://www.uptodate.com/contents/causes-of-hypokalemia-in-adults. [Last Accessed January, 2023].
7. UpToDate. (2019). Clinical manifestations and treatment of hypokalaemia in adults (Mount DB). UpToDate. [online] Available from: https://www.uptodate.com/contents/clinical-manifestations-and-treatment-of-hypokalemia-in-adults. [Last Accessed January, 2023].
8. Kasper DL, Fauci AS, Hauser SL, Longo DL, Jameson JL, Loscalzo J. Harrison's Principles of Internal Medicine, 20th edition. New York: McGraw Hill Education; 2018.
9. UpToDate. (2021). Hyperkalemic periodic paralysis (Gutmann L, Conwit R). [online] Available from https://www.uptodate.com/contents/hyperkalemic-periodic-paralysis. [Last Accessed January, 2023].
10. UpToDate. (2020). Clinical manifestations of hyperkalaemia in adults (Mount D). [online] Available from: https://www.uptodate.com/contents/clinical-manifestations-of-hyperkalemia-in-adults. [Last Accessed January, 2023].
11. UpToDate. (2020). Causes and evaluation of hyperkalaemia in adults (Mount DB). [online] Available from: https://www.uptodate.com/contents/causes-and-evaluation-of-hyperkalemia-in-adults. [Last Accessed January, 2023].
12. Medscape. (2021). Hyperkalaemia (Lederer E). [online] Available from: https://emedicine.medscape.com/article/240903-overview. [Last Accessed January, 2023].

CHAPTER 25: Metabolic-hyperglycemic Emergencies

Sanjay K Shah, Vivek Shah

INTRODUCTION

Diabetic ketoacidosis (DKA) and hyperosmolar hyperglycemic state (HHS) are two distinct serious metabolic derangements which are preventable and salvageable in diabetes and at times can occur together **(Fig. 1)**; manifested by dehydration, severe hyperglycemia, absolute or relative insulin deficiency, and an increase in counter regulatory hormones.[1] A good understanding of the pathogenesis and a proper management strategy is very important to produce a successful and positive outcome.

DIABETIC KETOACIDOSIS

Definition

Diabetic ketoacidosis has three important biochemical features as the name suggests hyperglycemia, moderate-to-severe ketosis, and resulting metabolic acidosis.[2] Clinically, it can be divided according to severity as mentioned in **Table 1**.

Clinical Features

The features are of marked hyperglycemia and acidosis which includes nausea, vomiting, abdominal pain, thirst, dehydration, acidotic breathing, shortness of breath, and extreme weakness; also symptoms of the precipitating illness can be present. Early in the illness patients are mentally alert but with increasing severity they may be confused and even in coma.[3]

Precipitating Factors

There are several causes precipitating DKA; the two most common being intercurrent infections and omission of insulin. Other less common causes are psychological

TABLE 1: Diagnostic criteria in diabetic ketoacidosis (DKA) and hyperosmolar hyperglycemic state (HHS).

Diagnostic criteria	DKA mild	DKA moderate	DKA severe	HHS
Plasma glucose#	>250	>250	>250	>600
Arterial pH	7.25–7.30	7.00–7.25	<7.00	>7.30
Serum bicarbonate	15–18	10–15	<10	>18
Ketosis blood and urine		Medium to large amounts		Small
Anion gap*	>10	>12	>12	Variable
Serum osmolality^		Variable		>320

#Euglycemic DKA has been reported see text
*Anion gap calculation, see text
^Effective serum osmolality calculation, see text

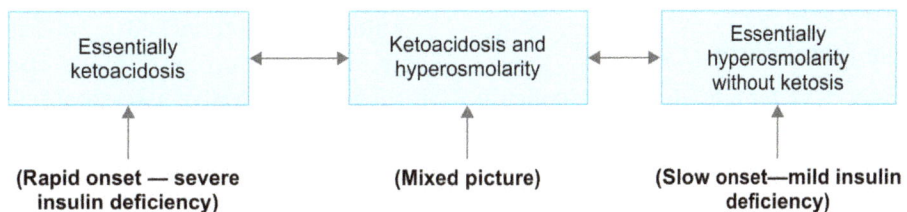

Fig. 1: The clinical spectrum of acute metabolic hyperglycemic emergencies.

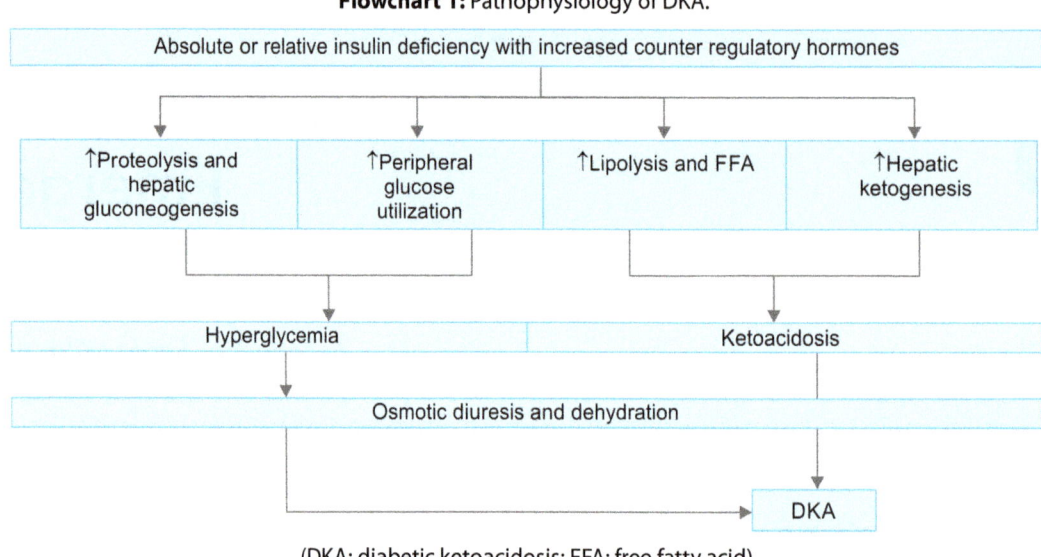

Flowchart 1: Pathophysiology of DKA.

(DKA: diabetic ketoacidosis; FFA: free fatty acid)

stress, myocardial infarction, cerebrovascular accident, alcohol abuse, trauma, and even pregnancy. Lately we have seen DKA being precipitated by coronavirus disease-2019 (COVID-19) infections and the newer drugs in oncology immune checkpoint inhibitors.[4,5]

Pathogenesis (Flowchart 1)

Marked insulin deficiency is a necessary precondition for DKA as this results in hyperglycemia due to reduced peripheral glucose uptake and increased hepatic glucose output. The counter regulatory hormones (catecholamines, cortisol, glucagon, and growth hormone) also add fuel to the fire resulting in osmotic diuresis, dehydration, and ketoacidosis. The most important biochemical abnormality ketoacidosis results from the uncontrolled lipolysis of adipose tissue resulting in the release of free fatty acids into the circulation which in turn stimulates ketogenesis and gets converted into ketone bodies by the liver as acetoacetate, 3OH butyrate and acetone. Ketone bodies form the alternate fuel source in the absence of insulin. The ketonemia in excess accumulates in circulation overwhelming the body's buffering capacity resulting in metabolic acidosis.[6] The resulting ketoacidosis produces the clinical features of DKA and respiratory compensation through hyperventilation initially but later on can lead to respiratory and circulatory depression.

Macronutrient Abnormalities

Water and Electrolyte Metabolism

The severe derangement of water and electrolyte deficit is a consequence of hyperglycemia and hyperketonemia. Hyperglycemia beyond the renal threshold for glucose (about 200 mg %) results in glucosuria, osmotic diuresis, dehydration, loss of sodium, potassium, and other electrolytes. The hyperosmolar state from hyperglycemia and the metabolic acidosis from ketonemia draw water and potassium into the circulation from the intracellular space. Potassium shifts are further exacerbated by acidosis and proteolysis from insulin deficiency. A lot of the potassium in circulation is subsequently lost through the kidneys and by vomiting.

Laboratory Evaluation and Pitfalls[6]

It is extremely important to diagnose DKA promptly and start treatment immediately. DKA is characterized by hyperglycemia (serum glucose > 250 mg/dL) ketosis and metabolic acidosis (serum bicarbonate < 18 mEq/L) with increased anion gap. On the rare occasion, blood sugars can be mildly elevated or normal as in patients using SGLT2 inhibitors and sometimes in pregnancy. Arterial blood gases will show pH levels (<7.3) with respiratory compensation in the form of low partial pressure of carbon dioxide (pCO_2). Despite total body potassium depletion described earlier, serum potassium levels initially may be elevated secondary to acidosis and volume depletion.

Total body sodium, chloride, magnesium, and phosphorous are also reduced, but may not be reflected in serum values. Elevated urea and creatinine levels are a consequence of dehydration and leukocytosis, hyperamylasemia (salivary) is commonly found without infection or pancreatitis. Serum lipase levels needs to be checked if pancreatitis is suspected.

Ketosis can be checked by measuring beta-hydroxybutyrate in serum and more conveniently urinary dipsticks for qualitative assessment of acetone bodies and acetoacetate. The resulting acidosis and the subsequent anion gap are calculated by a formula (serum sodium + serum potassium—serum chloride—serum bicarbonate). This is usually >10 in DKA.

Management and Treatment of Diabetic Ketoacidosis[3,6]

Initial management with a sense of urgency is fluid replacement and initiation of intravenous insulin. Simultaneously identifying the precipitating event and instituting treatment for the same is equally important. For the successful management of DKA frequent assessment and monitoring of fluid status, blood sugar, urine output, serum bicarbonate, serum potassium, and rarely phosphate and magnesium levels are necessary **(Box 1)**.

Once the acidosis, ketosis, dehydration, and electrolyte imbalance resolves the patient can resume oral intake and this signals the transition from intravenous insulin to subcutaneous insulin with a mix of basal and bolus insulin would be preferred as this can be used later in the outpatient setting. Even relatively brief periods of inadequate insulin administration which can commonly occur during the transition phase to subcutaneous insulin may result in relapse of DKA. This problem is addressed by injecting subcutaneous insulin half an hour to 1 hour before stopping the intravenous insulin.

Intravenous fluid replacement with normal saline is started to address the severe dehydration to the tune of 1–2 liters immediately followed by 3–4 liters of fluid for the rest of the day and subsequently daily.

Hyperglycemia resolves with the institution of IV insulin (usual starting dose of 0.1 unit/kg body weight stat and followed immediately by continuous insulin infusion at 0.1 unit/kg/hour).[7] Blood sugar is expected to be reduced by about 50–100 mg/dL/hour and hourly checking of blood sugar is usually recommended. If blood sugar reduction is unsatisfactory, then checking the insulin infusion system and increasing the dose is necessary. You can double and rarely even triple the infusion rate to get the required result. When the serum glucose values reach between 200 and 250 mg/dL intravenous glucose should be added to the intravenous fluid regime along with half strength saline infusion so that IV insulin requirements remain at a modest dose for acidosis and ketosis inhibition to continue, as the latter corrects more slowly than hyperglycemia. A cautionary note; a more rapid correction of glucose can precipitate the development of cerebral edema more so in children. The improvement in acidosis is defined by improvements in serum bicarbonate levels and an improvement in anion gap and reduction in ketone body formation as evidenced by reduction in urinary ketones.

Potassium levels initially may be high but the body stores are severely depleted as explained above. Treatment with insulin and fluids contributes to the lowering of serum potassium and can also result in hypokalemia. These factors include insulin-mediated potassium transport into cells, resolution of acidosis, and urinary losses. Potassium repletion should start immediately when normal serum potassium levels are documented. The need for 20–40 mEq of potassium in each liter of fluid is a reasonable place to start with a target to achieve normal potassium levels in the steady state.[8]

Bicarbonate replacement is usually not necessary as the above actions of fluid replacement and insulin infusion corrects the acidosis. In the presence of severe acidosis arterial pH < 6.9 and hemodynamic instability intravenous bicarbonate can be given over a couple of hours to correct the pH to just >6.9 as the use of bicarbonate can paradoxically increase cerebrospinal fluid (CSF) acidosis, rebound alkalosis, hypokalemia, and lactic acidosis. Phosphate and magnesium deficiency if severe may require supplementation.[9,10]

Intravenous insulin, intravenous fluids, correction of electrolytes and intensive care unit (ICU) care has reduced the mortality rate in DKA to <5%.[6]

Mortality is more likely to be due to the precipitating factors such as sepsis, myocardial infarction, cerebrovascular event, pancreatitis, and the like.

The list of complications of DKA and its treatment include:[11]

- Hypokalemia
- Hypoglycemia
- Cerebral edema
- DKA relapse
- ARDS
- Rhinocerebral mucormycosis

> **BOX 1:** Guide to initial management of diabetic ketoacidosis (DKA).
>
> - Arrange for two intravenous lines in the patient
> - *Fluids:* Replace 1–2 liters of normal saline over 1 hour followed by 500 mL infusion every 4 hours. Use half strength saline if serum sodium is >150 mEq/L. Use 5% dextrose infusion when blood sugar is <250 mg/dL
> - *Potassium:* No potassium in the first 1–2 liters of fluid unless initial plasma potassium levels are <3.5 mEq/L. To each liter of fluid add 20–40 mEq of KCl if potassium levels between 4 and 5.5. No KCl if there is hyperkalemia
> - *Insulin:* Start soluble insulin or rapid acting analogs of insulin intravenously at 0.1 unit/kg of body weight as a bolus dose followed by continuous infusion at the same rate hourly. We expect the capillary blood sugar to correct by 50–100 mg per hour and if this is not achieved the infusion rate can be doubled or even tripled
> - *Other measures:* Check capillary blood glucose hourly, serum potassium, bicarbonate and urinary ketone levels 8 hourly initially and the frequency can be reduced appropriately adjusted to the patient's condition
> - Once the patient is stable and blood sugars between 150 and 250 mg and acidosis is resolved insulin infusion can be reduced and transitioned to subcutaneous regime. Subcutaneous insulin should be given at least 30–60 minutes before stopping intravenous Insulin
> - If patient condition not improving, think using phosphate-magnesium therapy

- Venous thrombosis
- Gastrointestinal (GI) bleed

Transitioning to Subcutaneous Insulin[12]

Once the patient is stable hemodynamically and ketoacidosis resolves then we can think of switching the patient to subcutaneous insulin from intravenous insulin. The rule of thumb with respect to calculating the dose is to calculate the total dose of insulin administered over the last 8 hours when the patient has been stable and multiplying it by 3—that constitutes the 24 hours insulin subcutaneous dose. Half the total dose can be given as basal insulin and the other half divided into three prandial insulin shots before each meal. So if a patient needed 20 units of insulin in the last 8 hours then he will need (20 × 3) which is 60 units in 24 hours. We should give 30 units of basal insulin (glargine) and 10 units each of human regular insulin or analog before each of the three meals. Fine tuning of the dose can be done later with the data received subsequently with use. Giving subcutaneous insulin 30–60 minutes before stopping intravenous insulin has been mentioned earlier.

Sick Day Rules[13]

To prevent further recurrences of DKA an attempt at understanding the cause of the present DKA has to be appreciated and communicated to the patient and the family. Patient education and explaining the sick day rules during intercurrent illnesses is extremely important.

When unwell:
- Frequent monitoring of capillary blood sugars is recommended
- Measure urinary ketones when blood sugars are >250 mg/dL
- Drink more fluids to maintain hydration (calorie free)
- *Do not stop insulin*—continue insulin even during the illness and you may need to increase the dose in spite of not eating or drinking or eating very little
- Seek medical attention, if not well.

HYPEROSMOLAR HYPERGLYCEMIC STATE

Hyperosmolar hyperglycemic state is a very serious complication of diabetes mellitus and carries a high risk of morbidity and mortality in spite of the major advances in diabetes care. HHS typically occurs with a lesser degree of insulin deficiency than DKA. It usually occurs in patients with type 2 diabetes and tends to be in older individuals; where the onset is gradual with mild or no ketosis. DKA and HHS are two ends of the spectrum of severe hyperglycemia in a patient with diabetes and can occur together **(Table 1)**. The typical history of several days to weeks of polyuria, weight loss, poor oral intake that gradually progresses into mental confusion, lethargy, seizures, and coma.

The typical components of HHS are **(Table 1)**:
- Blood glucose >700 mg/dL
- Serum osmolality > 320 mOsm
- Arterial pH > 7.3 and bicarbonate > 15
- Urinary ketones are usually absent or weakly positive
- Prerenal azotemia

Pathophysiology (Flowchart 2)[14]

Relative insulin deficiency and inadequate fluid intake are the two most important pathophysiological factors causing HHS. Of note is that in some elderly patients' water intake is replaced by sugary solutions such as colas and similar drinks when thirsty which can raise blood sugars to dangerously high levels.[14]

Relative insulin deficiency allows for hepatic glycogenolysis and gluconeogenesis. This results in a slow and progressive rise of plasma glucose. Hyperglycemia is further aggravated by the actions of counter regulatory hormones. The osmotic diuresis that accompanies the glucosuria ultimately leads to profound dehydration. This volume loss causes reduced renal blood flow and resultant azotemia. Dehydration and hypotension further stimulates the secretion of catabolic counter regulatory hormones and becomes a vicious cycle. The absence of significant ketosis is most likely due to the relative preservation of endogenous insulin secretion in contrast to what happens in DKA; also there is inhibition of lipolysis from the hyperosmolar state.

Clinical Features and Precipitating Factors

Hyperosmolar coma can be the presenting feature of diabetes. Symptoms of intense thirst, polyuria, and gradual clouding of mentation are common. Vomiting is usually absent. The signs of dehydration, postural hypertension, focal neurologic deficits, seizures, and even coma can occur.

Hyperosmolar hyperglycemic state has many precipitating factors which can coexist in a particular patient:[15]
- Infection
- Myocardial infarction
- Acute pancreatitis
- Cerebrovascular event
- Renal failure
- Excessive alcohol consumption
- Noncompliant with insulin therapy
- Certain drugs such as furosemide, beta-blockers, steroids, phenytoin, and antipsychotic drugs

Laboratory Diagnosis and Pitfalls

The diagnosis is readily confirmed by a markedly raised blood sugar, usually >700 mg% and an elevation of urea, hematocrit, and mild leukocytosis.

Serum sodium is usually high and can be normal (falsely depressed) because of high blood sugars and hypertriglyceridemia. Serum sodium levels can be corrected

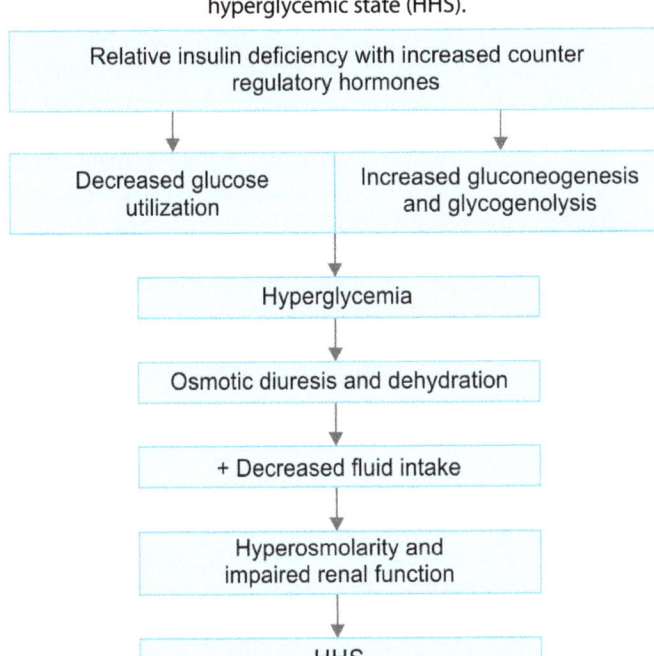

Flowchart 2: Pathophysiology of hyperosmolar hyperglycemic state (HHS).

to the nominal value by 1.6 mEq for every 100 mg/dL of increased blood sugar.[16]

Arterial pH is usually >7.3 and serum bicarbonate is >15 mEq/L.

Management of Hyperosmolar Hyperglycemic State

Hyperosmolar hyperglycemic state and DKA share the two most common clinical features of dehydration and hyperglycemia. Careful monitoring, understanding and managing fluid status, solute load, and osmotic changes with the use of insulin for the treatment of hyperglycemia remain very important. Prompt treatment of the precipitating event is equally helpful. Mortality rates are as high as 15% in HHS reflecting the patient's age and other comorbidities present and the challenge of navigating the resuscitation.

Fluids

Initially rapid intravenous infusion of normal saline of about 1 liter/hour for 2-3 hours is needed to stabilize the patient hemodynamically. Once the hemodynamic stability has been ensured, a more conscious rehydration therapy should be adopted, keeping in mind the fluid shift due to osmotic changes and the high risk of deterioration of neurologic function.[17] The free water deficit calculated is usually 8-10 liters in the individual patient and this can be corrected slowly, with the judicious mix of normal saline and half strength saline over 2-3 days. Potassium, magnesium, and phosphate repletion may be required during the resuscitation.

Insulin Therapy

While rehydration does lower blood glucose in patients with HHS; there is still a need for intravenous insulin infusion as treatment with a usual dose of 0.05-0.1 unit/kg/hour (about 3-6 units/hour) in our patients with an aim to bringing down the blood sugars steadily as in patients with DKA and switching to 5% dextrose as IV fluid when blood sugar comes down to 250 mg/dL.[18,19]

Insulin infusion should continue till the patient is clinically much better eating and drinking. IV insulin can then be changed to subcutaneous insulin which has largely been seen to be far less than those patients who have recovered from DKA. On the odd occasion you may be able to send the patient home on oral hypoglycemic agent.

Two unique complications in HHS are thromboembolic disorders and rhabdomyolysis which needs to be identified early and subsequently prevented and treated.[20]

Sick Day Rules for Hyperosmolar Hyperglycemic State (Patient Education)

- Frequent monitoring of blood glucose
- Early treatment of hyperglycemia
- Adequate hydration
- Seek medical attention
- Refrain from insulin discontinuation.

CONCLUSION

DKA and HHS are not so uncommon medical emergencies of our times. The discovery of insulin and its judicious use and the evolution of intensive care in the management of critically ill patients together with a deeper understanding of the pathophysiology of these conditions have helped us triumph from nearly 100% mortality rates to less than 10% in HHS and less than 5% in DKA.

Take Home Messages

- Both DKA and HHS are preventable and treatable.
- Results from absolute or relative deficiency of insulin.
- Dehydration is severe.
- Start resuscitation with intravenous fluids immediately.
- Start intravenous insulin immediately.
- Frequently check both sodium and potassium levels.
- Bicarbonate supplementation usually not required in DKA
- Prevent thromboembolism.
- Overlap subcutaneous insulin and intravenous insulin during transition.
- Teach sick day rules to patients, family, carers, and paramedics.

REFERENCES

1. Kitbachi AE, Umpierrez GE, Miles JM, Fischer JN. Hyperglycemic crises in adult patients with diabetes. Diabetes Care. 2009;32:1335-43.

2. Alberti KGMM. Diabetic ketoacidosis: aspects of management. In: Ledingham JG (Ed). Advanced Medicine: Tenth: Symposium. Tunbridge Wells: Pitman Medical; 1974. pp. 68-72.
3. Eledrisi MS, Alshanti MS, Shah MF, Brolosy B, Jaha N. Overview of the diagnosis and management of diabetic ketoacidosis. Am J Med Sci. 2006;331:243-51.
4. Yousef N, Noureldein M, Daoud G, Eid AA. Immune checkpoint and diabetes: Mechanism and predictors. Diabetes Metab. 2021;47(3):101193.
5. Palermo NE, Sadhu AR, Mcdonnell ME. Diabetic ketoacidosis in COVID-19: unique concerns and considerations. J Clin Endocrinol Metab. 2020;105(8):2819-29.
6. Kitbachi AE, Fischer JN, Murphy MB, Rumbak MJ. Diabetic Ketoacidosis and hyperglycemic hyperosmolar nonketotic state. In: Kalin RC, Weir GC (Eds). Joslin Diabetes Mellitus, 13th edition. Philadelphia: Lea & Febiger; 1994. pp. 738-70.
7. Burghen GA, Ettledorf JN, Fischer JN, Kitabchi AQ. Comparison of high dose and low dose insulin by continuous intravenous infusion in the treatment of diabetic ketoacidosis. Diabetes Care. 1980;3:15-20.
8. Beigelman PM. Potassium in severe diabetic ketoacidosis. Am J Med. 1973;54:419-20.
9. Narins BRG, Cohan JJ. Bicarbonate therapy for organic acidosis: the case for its continued use. Ann Int Med. 1987;106:615-8.
10. Cohen RD, Kitbachi AE, Murphy MB. When is bicarbonate appropriate in treating metabolic acidosis including diabetic ketoacidosis? In: Gitnick G, Barnes HV, Duffy TP (Eds). Diabetes in Medicine. Chicago: Year Book Medical Publishers; 1990. pp. 200-33.
11. Alberti KG, Natrass M. Severe diabetic ketoacidosis. Med Clin North Am. 1978;62:799-814.
12. Umpierrez GE, Jones S, Smiley D, Mulligan P, Keyler T, Temponi A, et al. Insulin analogs versus human insulin in the treatment of patients with diabetic ketoacidosis: A randomized Control Trial. Diabetes Care. 2009;32(7):1164-9.
13. CDC. (2022). Managing Sick Days. [online] Available from https://www.cdc.gov/diabetes/managing/flu-sick-days.html. [Last accessed January, 2023].
14. American Diabetes Association. Hyperglycemic crises in patients with diabetes mellitus. Diabetes Care. 2001;24:154-61.
15. Pinies JA, Cairo G, Gaztambide S, Vazquez JA. Course and prognosis of 132 patients with diabetes non-ketotic hyperosmolar state. Diabete Metab. 1994;20:43-8.
16. Hillier TA, Abbott RD, Barett EJ. Hyponatremia: evaluating the correction factor for hyperglycemia. Am J Med. 1999; 106:399-403.
17. Gonsalez-Campay JM, Robertson RP. Diabetic ketoacidosis and hyperglycemic hyperosmolar non-ketotic state: gaining control over extreme hyperglycemic complications. Postgrad Med. 1996;99:143-52.
18. Wright AD, Walsh CH, Fitzerald MG, Mailins JM. Low dose insulin treatment of hyperosmolar diabetic coma. Postgrad Med J. 1981;57:556-9.
19. Carroll P, Matz R. Uncontrolled diabetes mellitus in adults: experience in treating diabetic ketoacidosis and hyperosmolar coma with low dose insulin and a uniform treatment regimen. Diabetes Care. 1983;2:635-9.
20. Lord GM, Scott J, Pusey CD, Rees AJ, Walport MJ, Davies KA, et al. Diabetes and rhabdomyolysis: a rare complication of a common disease. BMJ. 1993;307:1126-28.

CHAPTER 26

Endocrinal (Hypoglycemia)

Ghanshyam Goyal, Usashi Biswas Bose, Rekha Basak Srivastava

INTRODUCTION

Hypoglycemia is the most important acute complication of antidiabetic therapies. Most common cause of hypoglycemia is found to be iatrogenic, i.e., drug induced. Severe hypoglycemia can be life-threatening if it is not treated promptly. It is obvious that hypoglycemia is an independent risk factor for cardiovascular diseases. In addition, hypoglycemia influences the quality of life of a diabetic patient to an appreciable extent.

Hypoglycemia is a barrier to achieve optimum glycemic control in diabetic patients who are on insulin or insulin secretagogues. Thus it limits the potential to have less occurrences of both microvascular and macrovascular complications through strict glycemic control.

Intensive glycemic control is always associated with a high risk of hypoglycemic episodes. Increased incidence of hypoglycemia possesses health and economic burdens both directly and indirectly. Hypoglycemic events, even if not severe, have negative impacts on self-management of diabetes, sleep quality, and the daily activities of patients with both type 1 diabetes mellitus (T1DM) and type 2 diabetes mellitus (T2DM).

10% plagia

DEFINITION[1]

Hypoglycemia is clinically defined as a syndrome of low blood glucose concentration (70 mg/dL or 3.9 mmol/L) associated with signs and symptoms of hyperactivity of autonomic nervous system and neuroglycopenia.

MODIFIED WHIPPLE'S TRIAD FOR DIAGNOSIS OF HYPOGLYCEMIA IN DIABETES[2]

- Occurrence of symptoms +/– signs appropriate with low levels of plasma glucose
- Proven Low (<3.5 mmol/L) plasma glucose concentration
- Rapid recovery of signs/symptoms with restoration of plasma glucose concentration

CAUSES[1,3]

- Insulin excess (accidental or deliberate)
- Antidiabetic drug overdose—sulfonylureas, meglitinides
- Inadequate food intake, skipping of meals
- Excessive exercise
- Alcohol ingestion
- Autonomic neuropathy
- Immediate postpartum period
- Onset of menstruation
- Insulinomas
- Multiple endocrine neoplasia syndromes (MEN)
- Postprandial hypoglycemia
- Hormone deficiency (e.g.: growth hormone)
- Other drugs:
  - *Salicylates:* Augment sulfonylurea action
  - *β-blockers:* Diminished counter regulatory response
- Renal failure
- Liver failure (58% in liver cirrhosis)[4]
- Dumping syndrome
- *Uncommon causes:* Hypopituitarism, Addison's disease, Glycogen storage disease.

GRADES[2]

Level 1 (Mild): 54 to <70 mg/dL

Level 2 (Moderate): <54 mg/dL

Level 3 (Severe): Any level when patient needs assistance (except young children who needs assistance at any level)[1]

CLINICAL CLASSIFICATION OF ACUTE HYPOGLYCEMIA[2]

- *Mild:* Symptomatic, self-treated, no major lifestyle interference
- *Moderate:* Symptomatic, self-treated, but with significant lifestyle interference
- *Severe:* Often (but not always) asymptomatic, but patient is unable to self-treat because of cognitive impairment
  - Third-party help required but not parenteral therapy

- Parenteral therapy required (intramuscular glucagon or intravenous glucose)
- Associated with coma or seizure

SYMPTOMS[5,6]

Mild (Level 1)
- Sweating, clammy skin
- Palpitations
- Tremor
- Hunger
- Nausea
- Abnormal nocturnal behavior (primary sleep disorder, nocturnal seizures)[7]
- Headache

Moderate (Level 2)
- Drowsiness
- Confusion
- Anxious
- Slurring of speech
- Blurring of vision

Severe (Level 3)
- Loss of consciousness
- Coma
- Convulsions.

NORMAL RESPONSE TO HYPOGLYCEMIA (FLOWCHART 1)

In a nondiabetic person when blood glucose level falls below the normal range, there is activation of physiological defense mechanisms in order to overcome hypoglycemia. This mechanism comprises of a successive lowering of insulin secretion, rise in glucagon secretion, and increased secretion of adrenomedullary epinephrine (when increased glucagon secretion is absent). The signs and symptoms of hypoglycemia are derived from these counter-regulatory hormonal responses. The clinical symptoms of hypoglycemia can be classified into two groups: Autonomic (nervousness, anxiety, tremulousness, sweating, palpitation, shaking, dizziness, hunger, and tingling) and neuroglycopenic (confusion, weakness, tiredness, drowsiness, difficulty with concentration, speech difficulty, odd behavior, and incoordination).

COMPROMISED DEFENSES AGAINST HYPOGLYCEMIA (FLOWCHART 2)

Patients with type 1 diabetes and well established type 2 diabetes with β-cell dysfunction or absolute insulin deficiency have compromised defense mechanisms against hypoglycemia. This results in a deficit of endogenous insulin secretion and subsequent glucagon secretion, and impaired epinephrine release. Therefore, plasma glucose levels drop but hypoglycemic symptoms are absent, which contemplates an attenuated sympathetic neural response.

Counter-regulation[9] (the spontaneous rectification of a falling plasma glucose level) always occurs even if there is inhibition of insulin and glucagon responses. This is due to an effect of secondary defense mechanisms that stimulates the autonomic nervous system and adrenal medulla. As a result there is release of epinephrine and norepinephrine, which stimulate endogenous glucose synthesis and also inhibit peripheral glucose uptake. Glucose is synthesized primarily by hepatic glycogenolysis followed by hepatic (and renal) gluconeogenesis.

There is increase in the substrates (including non-esterified fatty acids) for gluconeogenesis, which also inhibit peripheral glucose oxidation.

- The glycemic threshold for decrease in insulin secretion is approximately 4.5 mmol/L (81 mg/dL).
- Increase in glucagon and epinephrine secretion normally starts as glucose level drops just below the physiological range [threshold is approximately 3.8 mmol/L (68 mg/dL)].
- Neuroglycopenic symptoms are seen at blood glucose level of approximately 3.0 mmol/L (54 mg/dL).
- Lower glucose levels lead to overt functional brain failure including significant cognitive impairments [threshold equal to approximately 2.8 mmol/l (50 mg/dL)].

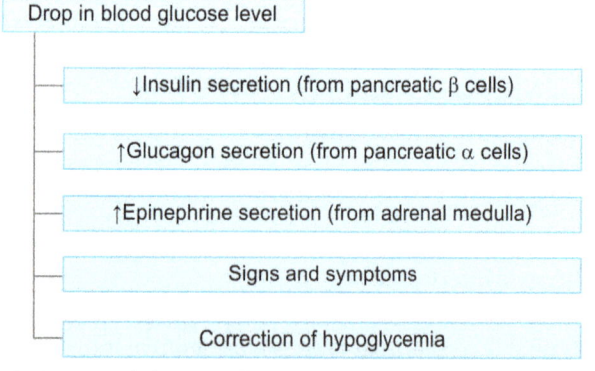

Flowchart 1: Normal response toward hypoglycemia.[8]

(T1DM: type 1 diabetes mellitus; T2DM: type 1 diabetes mellitus).

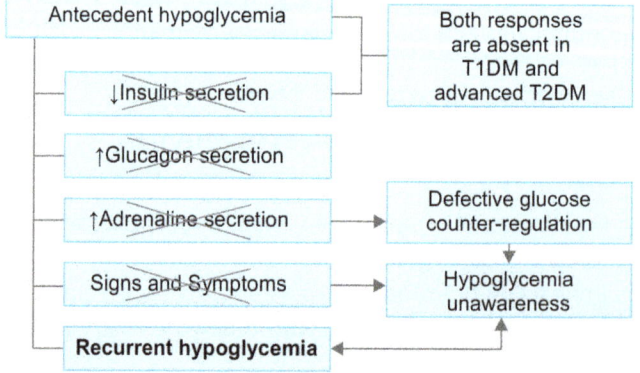

Flowchart 2: Pathophysiology of defective defense against hypoglycemia.

- Coma can occur at glucose levels in the range of 2.3–2.7 mmol/L (41–49 mg/dL)
- In a study of insulin-induced hypoglycemia in monkeys, it is observed that 5–6 hours of blood glucose concentration of <1.1 mmol/L or 20 mg/dL [average blood glucose level was 0.7 mmol/L (13 mg/dL)] leads to permanent neuronal damage in brain.[10]

■ HYPOGLYCEMIA UNAWARENESS[6,11]

Unable to produce and/or recognize hypoglycemic symptoms is known as the syndrome of hypoglycemia unawareness. The risk of severe hypoglycemia is increased by about 10-folds. Patients with long standing diabetes who are on sulfonylurea often do not get adrenergic symptoms and present in emergency with severe hypoglycemia. It is due to decreased sympathetic response with insignificant rise in circulating epinephrine and glucagon levels. The threshold which triggers the autonomic response in hypothalamus is set to a much lower level. Nocturnal hypoglycemia can lead to defective awareness of hypoglycemia the next day.

Drugs like beta blockers conceal the symptoms of hypoglycemia such as palpitation and tremor because they block the effects of norepinephrine. Hunger, irritability, and confusion may be obscured as well. However, sweating remains unmasked and it may be the only recognizable sign of hypoglycemia in people who are taking beta-blockers. Patients with type 1 diabetes, who are having very tight glycemic control, start feeling symptoms of hypoglycemia at a much lower level.

Experiments have showed that impaired awareness of hypoglycemia and counter-regulatory responses can be restored by avoiding hypoglycemia episodes cautiously in daily life. In studies it has been found that hypoglycemia when avoided for about 3 weeks can restore responses in both tightly controlled and poorly controlled Type 1 DM.

■ PSEUDOHYPOGLYCEMIA[1]

This is defined as an episode when the plasma glucose concentration remains either normal or above the normal range (i.e., no hypoglycemia), but the patient feels symptoms of hypoglycemia. It occurs in patients with long standing disease with poor glycemic control. Here the patient experiences hypoglycemic symptoms even with blood glucose >70 mg/dL.

■ POSTHYPOGLYCEMIC HYPERGLYCEMIA AND HYPOGLYCEMIA[1]

Posthypoglycemic hyperglycemia occurs due to over-correction of the hypoglycemic episode and the generation of insulin resistance as a result of hypoglycemia counter-regulation. The effect of a single episode of hypoglycemia may manifest as postprandial hyperglycemia the next day rather than as fasting hyperglycemia. There may be occurrence of ketonuria the morning after a nighttime hypoglycemic episode, which explains fasting hyperglycemia.

■ NOCTURNAL HYPOGLYCEMIA[1]

The counter-regulatory mechanisms to hypoglycemia are markedly decreased during deep sleep.

High fasting glucose following nocturnal hypoglycemia is due to loss of insulin action, possibly associated with a *dawn phenomenon*. There might be a correlation between nocturnal hypoglycemia and altered mood next morning (no evidence for cognitive impairment), failure to consolidate memory during the daytime, and reduced responses to hypoglycemia next day.

How to Prevent Nocturnal Hypoglycemia[1]?

- Use of peak less basal analogues decreases risk of nocturnal fall of blood glucose
- Taking basal insulin at bedtime delays the peak
- Bedtime glucose <110 mg/dL increases the risk of morning hypoglycemia
- Replacing multiple daily injections with CSII (continuous subcutaneous insulin infusion).

■ DAWN PHENOMENON[12]

The *dawn phenomenon* (also known as the *dawn effect*) is the term used to describe an abnormal early-morning rise in blood glucose usually between 2–8 AM in diabetic subjects. This is due to the physiological overnight release of the counter-regulatory hormones (including growth hormone, cortisol, glucagon, and epinephrine), which increase the insulin resistance, leading to elevation of blood glucose. Morning hyperglycemia is also caused by insufficient bedtime insulin in the last night, insufficient antidiabetic medication dosages or carbohydrate snack consumption at bedtime.

This is diagnosed by checking blood glucose at 3 AM, which is found to be high. Increasing the dose of night time insulin is needed to control the early morning rise of blood glucose.

■ SOMOGYI EFFECT[13]

The Somogyi effect, also known as the "Chronic Somogyi Rebound", or "Posthypoglycemic hyperglycemia", is characterized by falling of blood glucose level too low during the late night that activates counter-regulatory hormones (such as adrenaline, corticosteroids, growth hormone, and glucagon) leading to activation of gluconeogenesis and ultimately results in hyperglycemia in the early morning.

A low blood glucose measured at 3 AM is generally diagnostic of this condition. So reduction of the dose of night time insulin is needed.

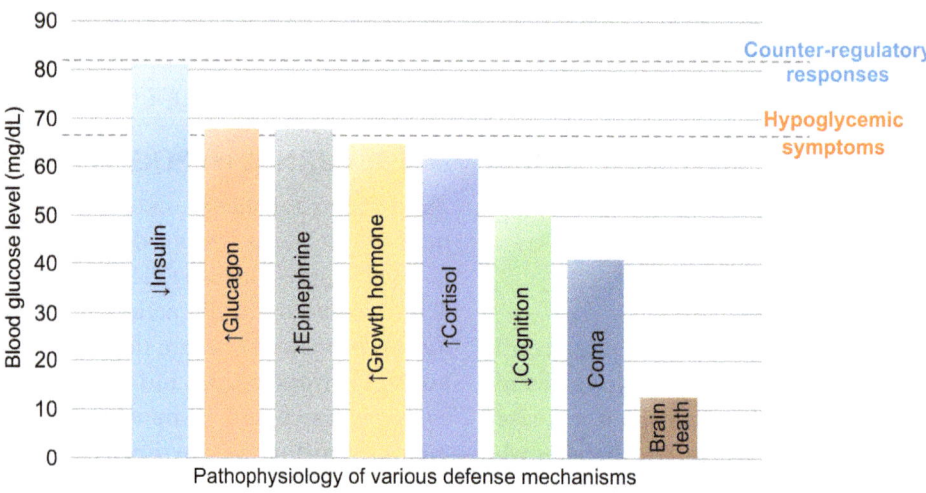

Fig. 1: Defense against hypoglycemia.

TABLE 1: Acute and chronic complications of hypoglycemia.	
Acute	**Chronic**
• Focal; neurological signs • Accidental injury • Acute vascular events • Fatal hypoglycemic coma • Unexplained diabetes-related deaths (dead in bed) • Hypoglycemic hemiplegia • Convulsions	• Permanent neurological deficit • Intellectual impairment • Behavioral changes • Precipitation of acute cerebrovascular disease • Myocardial infarction • Neurocognitive dysfunction • Retinal cell death • Loss of vision

DEFECTS IN COUNTER-REGULATION ASSOCIATED WITH DIABETES MANAGEMENT (FIG. 1)

- *Peripheral hyperinsulinemia:* Blood insulin level does not decline with dropping glucose level. This is either due to continuous absorption of exogenous insulin or glucose independent insulin secretion by sulfonylureas. This results in iatrogenic hypoglycemia.
- *Loss of glucagon response:* There is loss of the ability to increase glucagon synthesis by pancreatic alpha cells in response to hypoglycemia.
- *Loss of C-peptide:* Absence of measurable C-peptide level is associated with higher rates of severe hypoglycemia (mostly in type 1 diabetes patients).

COMPLICATIONS OF HYPOGLYCEMIA

Acute and chronic complications of hypoglycemia is depicted in **Table 1** and **Flowchart 3**.

HYPOGLYCEMIA-ASSOCIATED AUTONOMIC FAILURE[10,15]

The theory of hypoglycemia-associated autonomic failure (HAAF) is generally associated with T1DM patients, although it might occur in T2DM patients also. In these patients recent antecedent iatrogenic hypoglycemia causes both defective glucose counter-regulation and hypoglycemia unawareness. As a result there is a shift of glycemic thresholds for autonomic, symptomatic, and cognitive dysfunction responses to a lower plasma glucose concentration. This impairs the glycemic defense and is also responsible for reduced detection of hypoglycemia in the clinical setting.

Mediators of Hypoglycemia-associated Autonomic Failure (HAAF) (Flowchart 4)

- Cortisol response to antecedent hypoglycemia mediates HAAF
- Antecedent exercise, which releases cortisol reduces autonomic responses
- Plasma norepinephrine, pancreatic polypeptide (an index of parasympathetic activation), and glucagon responses to hypoglycemia are not reduced.

MANAGEMENT OF HYPOGLYCEMIA[16] (FLOWCHART 5)

Management of hypoglycemia mainly depends on the duration and severity of the hypoglycemic episode. Self-treatment with oral ingestion of rapid-acting carbohydrates is usually sufficient to treat mild-to-moderate hypoglycemia. On the contrary external help is must for the recovery from severe hypoglycemia.

Dextrose: Those patients having altered consciousness are unable to swallow glucose orally. In such a case peripheral administration of intravenous dextrose by an emergency personnel is an alternative. Usual adult dose is 60–100 mL of 25% dextrose (1 mg/kg body weight). A total of 25% dextrose solution should only be administered via a patent IV line (either peripheral or central) as it is heavily necrotic due to its hyperosmolar nature. It may lead to tissue necrosis if the IV line becomes infiltrated.

Flowchart 3: Effects of hypoglycemia[14].

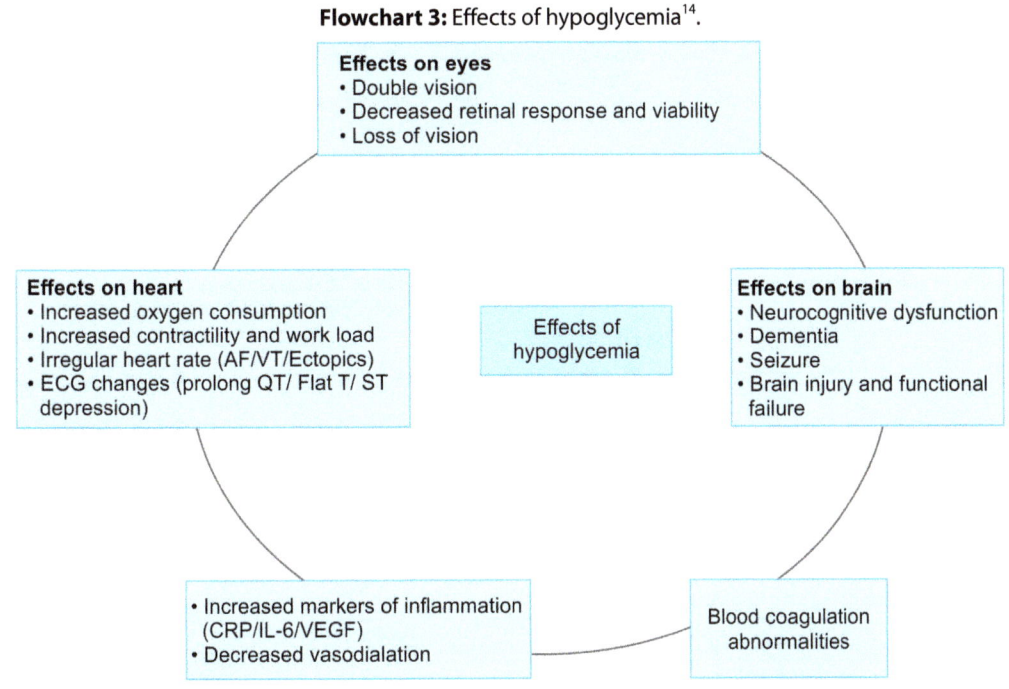

Flowchart 4: Mechanism of hypoglycemia-associated autonomic failure (HAAF).

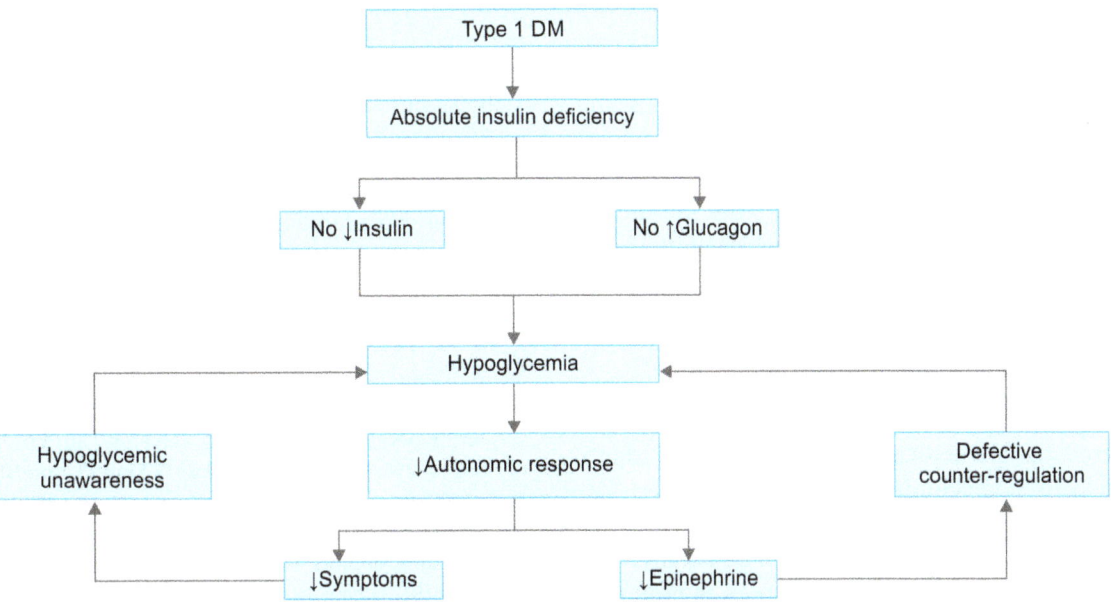

Glucagon: It is the first-line treatment for severe hypoglycemia in diabetic patients who are under insulin therapy. Glucagon can be administered by either subcutaneous or intramuscular route by trained parents or caregivers. Recombinant glucagon has a short half-life (~8–18 minutes), and maximum plasma concentration is achieved a few minutes after its administration.

- Examples of 15–20 g rapidly available carbohydrate
  - 200 mL fresh fruit juice
  - Glucose tablets
  - Glucose gel tube
  - One tablespoon of sugar, honey, or corn syrup
  - Hard candies, jellybeans, or gumdrops
- *If meal is due in next half an hour:* The patient should take reduced dose of premeal insulin.
- *If meal is not due in next half an hour:* The patient should take further 15–20 g of slowly absorbed carbohydrate.
  - Glucagon is absorbed from the rectum but does not hasten recovery from hypoglycemia in patients with type 1 diabetes.[7]
  - Glucagon should not be used to treat sulfonylurea induced hypoglycemia because it further stimulates insulin secretion dramatically.[17]

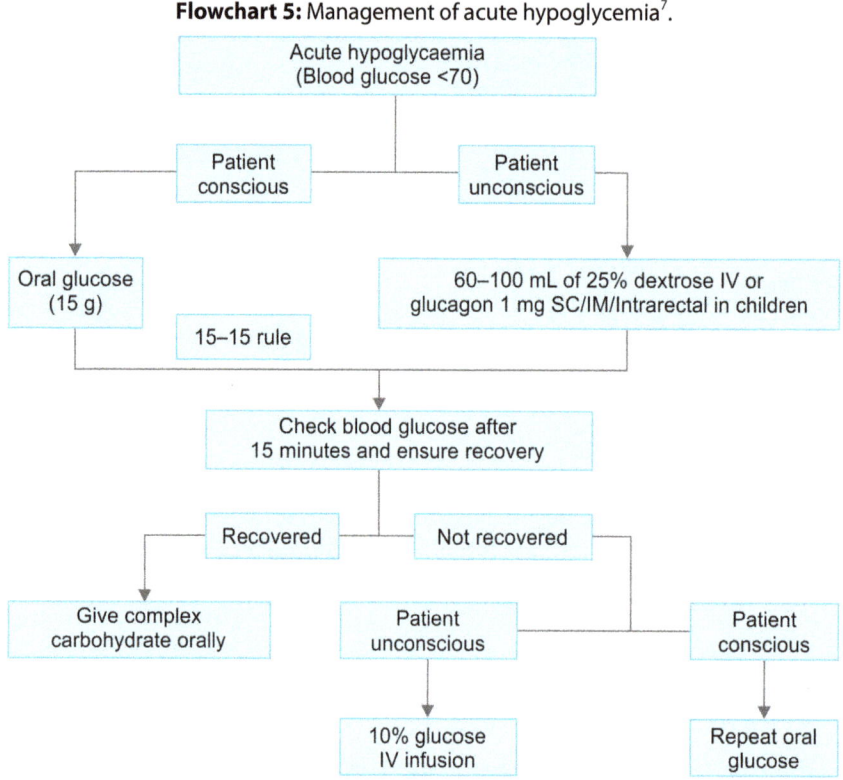

Flowchart 5: Management of acute hypoglycemia[7].

PROLONGED HYPOGLYCEMIA

In some special conditions like patient is having chronic kidney disease and patient is on sulfonylurea there is high risk of having prolonged hypoglycemia. In such situations patient is advised for admission in hospital for close monitoring because of high chances of recurrent hypoglycemic episodes. Glucose monitoring is done every hourly. Patient is treated with 5% dextrose IV infusion with 25% dextrose IV on SOS basis whenever there is hypoglycemia (<70 mg/dL).

PREVENTION[11]

- Structured patient education regarding early identification of hypoglycemic symptoms is necessary to prevent hypoglycemia.
- Self-adjustment of dose of insulin is to be taught to the patient, if hypoglycemia is occurring on a routine basis (including assessment of carbohydrate content of each food).
- Institute self-monitoring of blood glucose (SMBG) regime or real time continuous glucose monitoring (CGM) as acceptable to patient (including periodic night time blood sugar monitoring).
- Have patients wear identifications indicating diabetes.

Take Home Messages

- Hypoglycemia-associated autonomic failure is the main pathogenic mechanism behind severe hypoglycemia.
- Defective glucose counter-regulation and a lack of awareness regarding hypoglycemia are common components of HAAF in patients with diabetes.
- To prevent hypoglycemic events, the setting of glycemic goals should be individualized, particularly in elderly individuals or patients with complicated or advanced type 2 diabetes.
- Careful selection of high-risk patients for the development of severe hypoglycemia in future and successful implementation of intensive education with reinforcement are the keys to prevent hypoglycemia.

REFERENCES

1. Balijepalli C, Druyts E, Siliman G, et al. Hypoglycemia: a review of definitions used in clinical trials evaluating antihyperglycemic drugs for diabetes, Clin Epidemiol. 2017; 9: 291–296. Published online 2017 May 23. doi: 10.2147/CLEP.S129268.
2. Stephanie Anne Amiel, Iatrogenic Hypoglycemia, Joslin's Diabetes Mellitus, Fourteenth Edition p671-84.
3. Shah SN, Joshi SR. Chapter 54 Hypoglycemia. In: RSSDI Textbook of Diabetes Mellitus, 3rd edition. New Delhi: Jaypee Digital; 2014.
4. Singh D, Ali Memon HN, Shaikh TZ, Ali Shah SZ, Hypoglycemia in patients with liver cirrhosis. Professional Med J. 2015;22(4).
5. WebMD. (2022). Hypoglycemia: When Your Blood Sugar Gets Too Low. [online] Available from https://www.webmd.com/diabetes/guide/diabetes-hypoglycemia [Last accessed January, 2023].
6. American Diabetes Association. Hypoglycemia (low blood sugar). [online] Available from https://www.diabetes.org/healthy-living/medication-treatments/blood-glucose-testing-and-control/hypoglycemia [Last accessed January, 2023].
7. Parker DR, Braatvedt GD, Bargiota A, Newrick PG, Brown S, Gamble G, et al. Glucagon is absorbed from the rectum but

does not hasten recovery from hypoglycaemia in patients with type 1 diabetes. Br J Clin Pharmacol. 2008l;66(1):43-9.
8. Normal physiological and behavioral defenses against hypoglycemia in humans (https://www.kjim.org/journal/Figure.php?xn=kjim-30-6.).
9. Sprague JE, Arbeláez AM. Glucose counterregulatory responses to hypoglycemia. Pediatr Endocrinol Rev. 2011;9(1): 463-75.
10. Cryer PE. Hypoglycemia, functional brain failure, and brain death. J Clin Invest. 2007; 117(4): 868-70.
11. Mayo Clinic. (2022). Hypoglycemia. [online] Available from https://www.mayoclinic.org/diseases-conditions/hypoglycemia/symptoms-causes/syc-20373685 [Last accessed January, 2023].
12. Mayo Clinic. (2022). The dawn phenomenon: What can you do?. [online] Available from https://www.mayoclinic.org/diseases-conditions/diabetes/expert-answers/dawn-effect/faq-20057937 [Last accessed January, 2023].
13. Healthline. (2022). What Is the Somogyi Effect?. [online] Available from https://www.healthline.com/health/diabetes/what-is-the-somogyi-effect [Last accessed January, 2023].
14. Researchgate. Figure 2: Physiological impact of hypoglycemia on different systems and their counter-regulatory responses. [online] Available from https://www.researchgate.net/figure/Physiological-impact-of-hypoglycemia-on-different-systems-and-their-counter-regulatory_fig1_257251455/download [Last accessed January, 2023].
15. Philip E. Cryer, Hypoglycemia-associated autonomic failure in diabetes. Am J Physiol. 2001;281(6).
16. Nitil Kedia, Treatment of severe diabetic hypoglycemia with glucagon: an underutilized therapeutic approach. Diabetes Metab Syndr Obes. 2011;4:337-46.
17. Lheureux PE, Zahir S, Penaloza A, Gris M. Bench-to-bedside review: antidotal treatment of sulfonylurea-induced hypoglycaemia with octreotide. Crit Care. 2005;9(6): 543-9.

SECTION 7

Gynecological Emergencies

Section Editor: Aruna Tantia

27. **Gynecological Emergencies**
    Aruna Tantia, Sunipa Chatterjee, Ushasi Mukherjee

CHAPTER 27

Gynecological Emergencies

Aruna Tantia, Sunipa Chatterjee, Ushasi Mukherjee

INTRODUCTION

Emergencies can occur pertaining to any organ of our body. We are mostly aware of heart attack or brain stroke where the first hour is the crucial golden hour, whereby a life is saved if brought to hospital early during that period.

Irony is most of these occur in middle of night or at remote location where no medical person may be nearby. Mostly it is family members or friends who are left to deal though they are not trained to recognize and attend such emergencies. Delay and seeking help results in permanent disability. Let us discuss these conditions.

Health emergencies occur in women's lifetime also.

DEFINITION

Gynecological emergencies often dangers the life of affected woman including her reproduction potential.[1-3] It is relatively common and include ectopic pregnancies, adnexal torsion, tubo-ovarian abscess, hemorrhagic ovarian cysts, gynecologic hemorrhage, and vulvovaginal trauma. The aim of this text is to provide an aphoristic review of these emergencies that specialize on the evaluation and treatment choices for the patient. In several cases, other causes of an acute abdomen are in the differential diagnosis. Understanding the tenets of diagnosis helps the surgeon slender the etiology and guide applicable treatment.

Specialist emergency gynecology units present in developed countries provide fast interventions for such acute gynecological problems.

PREVALENCE

The most common morbidity cause among women of child-bearing age in India is ectopic pregnancy. Incidence is as high as 3.86 per 1,000 live birth [the Indian Council of Medical Research (ICMR) task force].

In developing countries like USA, more than 1 million visits to emergency rooms are made by women between 15 and 44 years of age gynecological emergency. Acute gynecological conditions are the topmost cause of mortality and morbidity in these developed countries.

Given the weak health infrastructure, gynecological emergencies present enormous challenge in developing countries such as India, Bangladesh, Sri Lanka, Pakistan, and Brazil. They are also the most important case of morbidity and mortality and pose as important problem to public health.

Outline of gynecological emergency conditions **(Fig. 1 and Flowchart 1)**:

Obstetric cause:
- Ectopic pregnancy
- Hyperemesis gravidarum
- Scar ectopic pregnancy
- Pregnancy with adnexal torsion
- Eclampsia
- Ruptured uterus/scar dehiscence
- Ovarian cyst hemorrhage/torsion
- Miscarriage
- Fibroids red degeneration.

Gynecological cause:
- Acute pelvic inflammatory disease

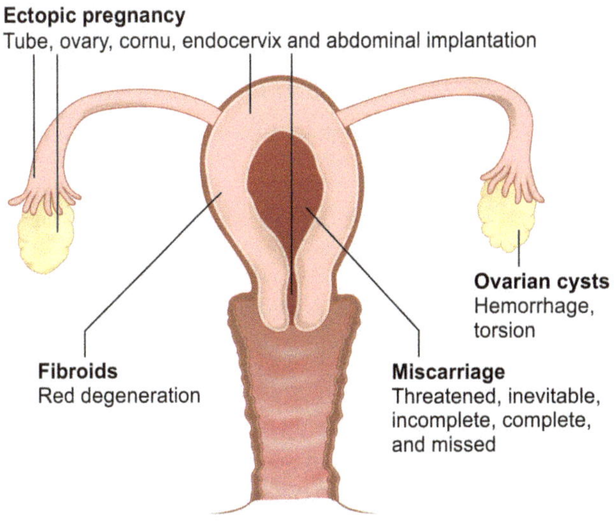

Fig. 1: Problems in pregnancy.
(*Source:* Pickrell D. Gynæcological emergencies. In: Luesley DM (Ed). Common Conditions in Gynaecology. Boston, MA: Springer; 1997.

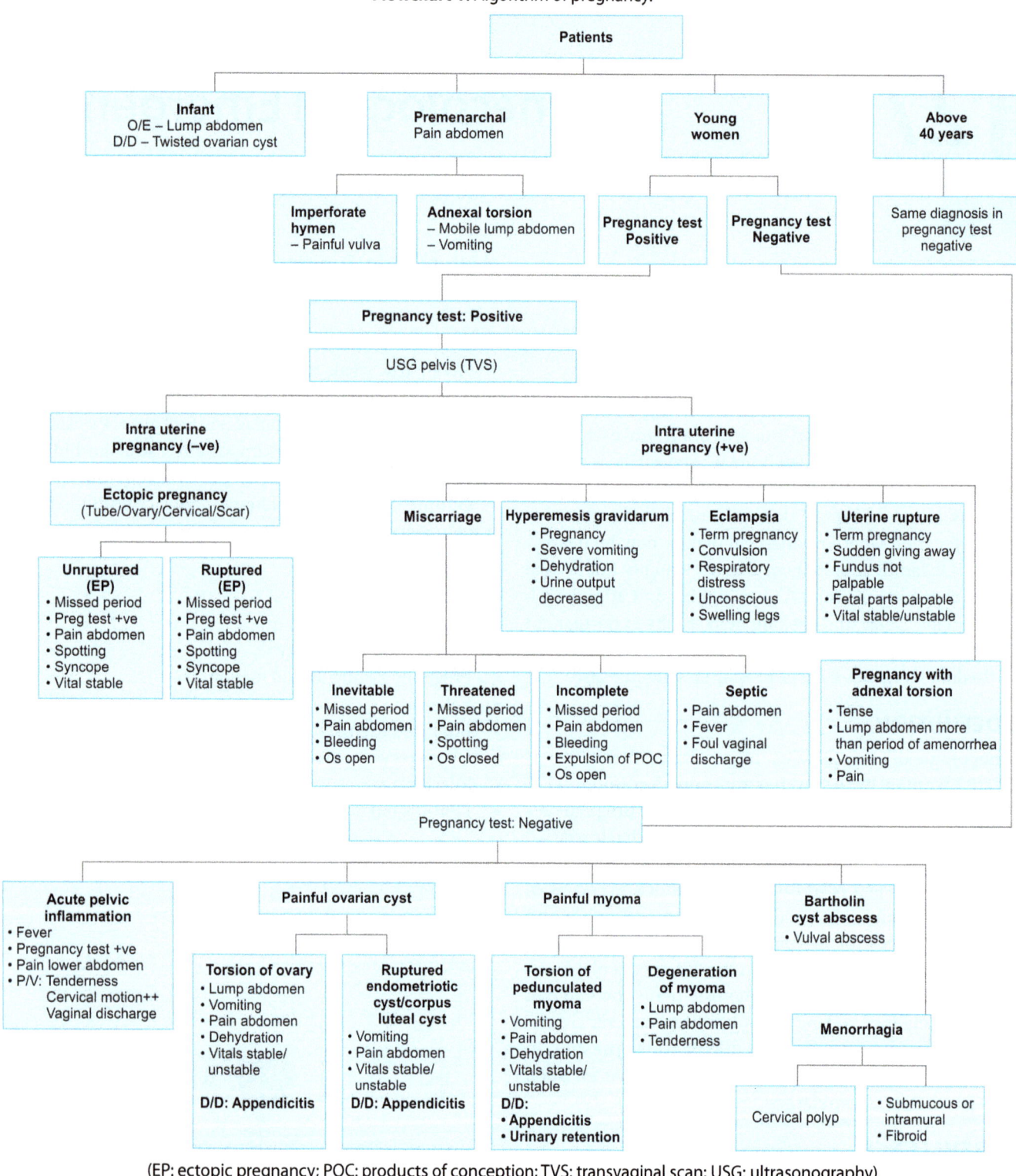

Flowchart 1: Algorithm of pregnancy.

(EP: ectopic pregnancy; POC: products of conception; TVS: transvaginal scan; USG: ultrasonography)

- Pelvic endometriosis
- Torsion or rupture of ovarian neoplasm
- Torsion or degeneration of uterine leiomyoma
- Imperforate hymen
- Vulvar/Bartholin abscesses
- Traumatic gynecological emergencies:
  - Sexual violence
  - Bicycle injuries
  - Foreign body insertion
  - Childbirth lacerations
- *Massive vaginal bleeding:*
  - Puberty menorrhagia
  - Bleeding due to fibroids
  - Bleeding due to endometrial or cervical cancer.

CHAPTER 27: Gynecological Emergencies

◼ APPROACH TO THE PROBLEM

Ectopic Pregnancy (Table 1)

Ectopic pregnancy may present with shock and moribund condition due to massive intra-abdominal bleeding. There can be sign of hemodynamic instability, lower abdominal tenderness. It is leading cause of maternal deaths in India. A life-threatening gynecological emergency like ectopic pregnancy is a dominant cause of maternal morbidity and causing a mortality rate of 3.5% in pregnancies (**Figs. 2 and 3**).[4,5]

History Taking

If there is history of missed cycle and pregnancy test is positive then ectopic pregnancy to be suspected. If pregnancy test is

TABLE 1: Outcome assessment—obstetric emergencies.			
Obstetric emergencies	**Hospital**	**Intervention**	**Outcome**
Ectopic pregnancy	• USG-pelvis, TVS • CBC, CXR, ECG • β-hCG • Blood transfusion request • Resuscitate	Laparoscopic salpingectomy Or Laparoscopic salpingostomy	• Patient stable • Hemorrhage arrested • β-hCG level decreases
Rupture uterus	• USG • CBC/blood requisition	• Urgent laparotomy • Repair/cesarean hysterectomy	Saving of life of mother and baby

• Miscarriage
  – Inevitable
  – Incomplete
  – Threatened
  – Septic
	• USG-pelvis
	• CBC
	• Antibodies
	• Fluids
		• Cervical encirclage for inevitable abortion
		• D&C for incomplete abortion
		• D&C for septic abortion
		• Conservative management for threatened abortion
			• Pregnancy continued
			• Hemorrhage stops
			• Fever subsides
			• Bleeding stops

Eclampsia	• CBC, urea, creatinine • USG–obstetric • CTG for fetal monitoring • Catheterization • Channel for fluid • Eye–fundoscopy	• Conservative • MgSO$_4$ IV/LM 14 mg • Catheterization • Mouth gag • Monitor RR/knee jerk • Uric output • LUCS if term	• Pregnancy continued if less • Live baby • Mother saved
Scar ectopic	• CBC, CXR, ECG • USG-pelvis, TVS • Blood requisition	Laparoscopic/laparotomy—excision of scar ectopic	• Scar cleared of ectopic • Scar repaired • Massive hemorrhage averted

(β-hCG: β-human chorionic gonadotropin; CBC: complete blood count; CTG: cardiotocography; CXR: chest X-ray; D&C: dilation and curettage; ECG: electrocardiogram; LUCS: lower segment cesarean section; TVS: transvaginal scan; USG: ultrasonography)

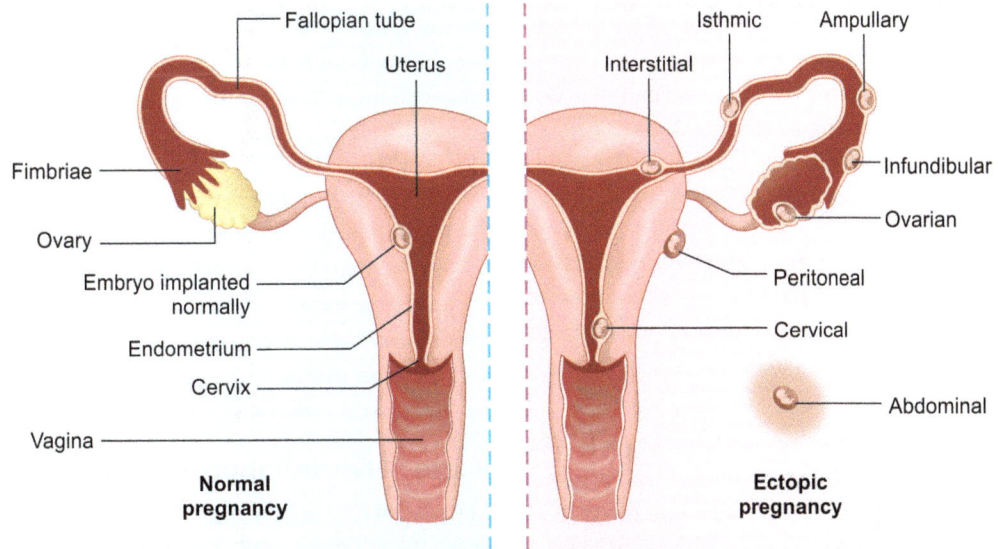

Fig. 2: Type of pregnancy.

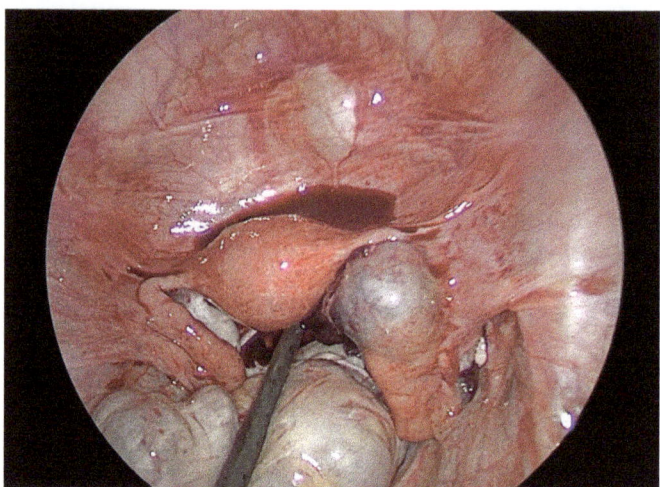

Fig. 3: Ectopic pregnancy.

positive and severe bleeding per vagina with pain then it is suspected as miscarriage. The first symptoms of an ectopic pregnancy may be terribly the same as typical pregnancy symptoms.

However, you may experience additional symptoms during an ectopic pregnancy, including:
- Vaginal bleeding
- Pain in your lower abdomen, pelvis, and lower back
- Dizziness or weakness.

If the fallopian tube ruptures, pain and bleeding could be severe enough to cause additional symptoms. These can include:
- Fainting
- Low blood pressure (hypotension)
- Shoulder pain
- Rectal pressure
- Muscle guarding.

Laboratory Assessment
- Urine for pregnancy test.
- *Ultrasonography (USG) pelvis by transvaginal scan (TVS):* Ultrasound can generally detect intrauterine pregnancies that are 5–6 weeks along. A negative pelvic ultrasound (that is, not seeing anything) does not mean that there is no ectopic pregnancy, since approximately 15–26% of women with an ectopic pregnancy will have a negative ultrasound.
- *Blood test of complete blood count (CBC):* Any mass in adnexal region, may be tubal pregnancy or free fluid in abundance may suggest hemoperitoneum or hemorrhage.

Role of Biomarker
A blood test [beta-human chorionic gonadotropin (β-hCG)]: An ectopic pregnancy should be suspected if transvaginal USG shows no intrauterine gestational sac when the β-hCG level is >1,500 mIU per mL (1,500 IU per L). If the β-hCG level plateaus or fails to double in 48 hours and the ultrasound examination fails to identify an intrauterine gestational sac, uterine curettage may determine the absence of chorionic villi.

Prehospital Care at Home
- If patient have vaginal bleeding—injection Pause can be given intramuscularly
- If patient experience some stomach pain—paracetamol
- Do pregnancy test strip for confirmation of pregnancy
- In shocked or hemodynamically compromised patient, start IV fluid and arrange blood donors, shift immediately to hospital with intensive care unit (ICU) and occupational therapy (OT) facility.

When tube bursts, patient may feel sharp lower abdominal pain. This is a medical emergency and one needs to rush to hospital. In case of any delay, one may lose patient.

Miscarriage (Fig. 4 and Table 1)
Most (75%) miscarriages occur before 16 weeks of gestation and 26% occur within first 8 weeks.[6] Unsafe abortions are from important cause leading to maternal deaths and more than three-fourths occur in developing nations.[7-9]

Laboratory Assessment
Serum beta (β)-hCG, bedside pregnancy or urine test, and ultrasound may point toward diagnosis.

Exclusion criteria of a viable intrauterine gestation:
- Crown–rump length of 7 mm or greater and no heartbeat
- Mean sac diameter of 25 mm or greater and no embryo
- Absence of embryo with heartbeat 2 weeks or more after a scan that showed a gestational sac without a yolk sac
- Absence of embryo with heartbeat 11 days or more after a scan that showed a gestational sac with a yolk sac.

Role of Biomarker
We can create an extremely certain diagnosis using a combination of medical history, physical examination, and USG as these are important biomarkers to make certain diagnosis.

Prehospital Care
- Shift to hospital as early as possible
- Painkiller can be given
- Supportive therapy such as blood transfusion, antibiotic, and evacuation of product of conception in early first trimester miscarriage is needed.
- Additionally in Rh (–ve) pregnancy, anti-D immunoglobulin should be given.

Acute Pelvic Inflammatory Disease (Table 2)
Acute pelvic inflammatory disease (PID) commonly presents as pelvic pain. This pelvic pain may be cyclical or noncyclical. Certain conditions such as pelvic endometriosis

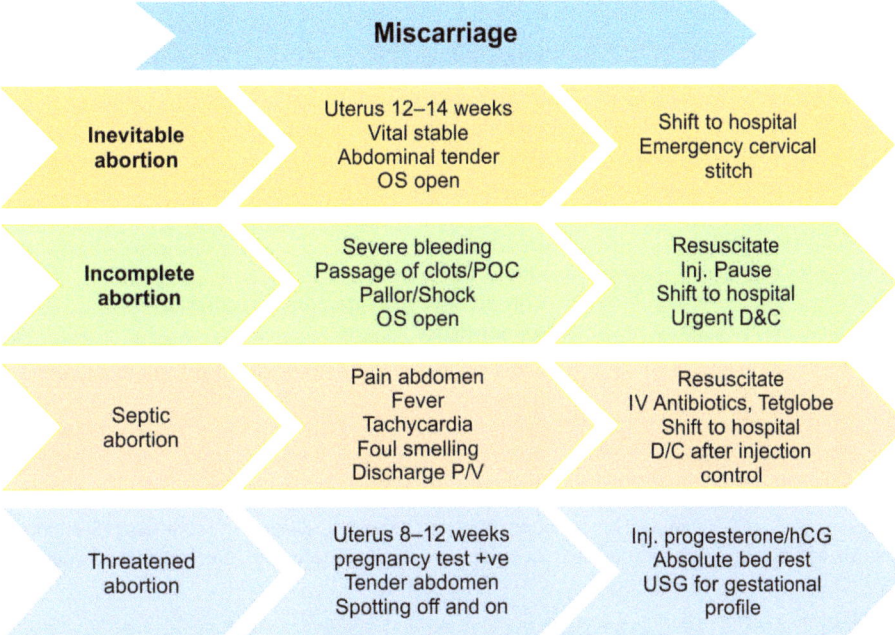

Fig. 4: Types of miscarriage.
(D&C: dilation and curettage; hCG: human chorionic gonadotropin; IV: intravenous; POC: products of conception; USG: ultrasonography)

TABLE 2: Outcome assessment—gynecological emergencies.			
Gynecological emergencies	*Hospital*	*Intervention*	*Outcome*

• Painful ovarian cyst
  – Torsion/Hemorrhagic Ovarian Cyst
	• CBC
	• USG-pelvis + CD
	• ECG/CXR
	• S/CA125
	• S/CEA, S/-hCG
	• RMI
	• Start channel
	• Antibiotic/painkiller
		Laparoscopic/open detorsion + ovarian cystectomy (OC)
		Or
		Laparoscopic/open oophorectomy + toileting (other ovary normal)
		Or
		• Laparotomy:
		  – Detorsion + OC
		  – OC + toileting
			• Relief of symptom
			• Saving ovary + reproductive function

• Painful Myoma
  – Torsion
  – Degeneration
	• CBC, sugar
	• USG-pelvis + CD
	• SDH/LDH
	• Start channel
		• Antibiotic
		• Antispasmodic/paracetamol
		• Open/laparoscopic detorsion + myomectomy
			Relief of symptom + pathology

Acute Pelvic Inflammatory Disease	• CBC, sugar • Urea, creatinine • CRP • USG • CXR/ECG • IV fluids • Vaginal Swab	• IV fluids • Antibiotics	Relief of pain, fever, and infection
Bartholin Cyst/Abscess	• CBC, sugar • USG-pelvis • CRP	• IV antibiotics • Hot compress • Drainage under LA-marsupulization	Relief form symptoms/disease
Sexual Assault	• Police diary • CBC • CRP • X-ray abdomen/chest • Resuscitate • Blood requisition	• Examination under GA • Antibiotic • Repair of injuries • Blood transfusion • Counselling • HIV prophylaxis	• Life saved • Injury repaired • Traumatic experience

Contd...

Contd...

Gynecological emergencies	Hospital	Intervention	Outcome
• Massive Vaginal Bleeding – Puberty Menorrhagia – Heavy Menstrual Bleeding–fibroid/polyp	• CBC/KFT • CXR/ECG • USG-pelvis • Blood requisition • Colposcopy • Urine R/E	Surgery/hysteroscopic polypectomy/myomectomy Or Laparoscopic hysterectomy Or D&C EB Or Conservative management for pubertal menorrhagia	
• Unruptured Hymen/Uterus Septum	• CBC, sugar • CXR/BT, CT, PT • USG-pelvis • Catheterization	Hysteroscopy + hymenotomy by cruciate incision Or Excision of septum	• Bleeding stops • Diagnosis made • Relief from DS • Relief of pain, swelling, and urine retention

(β-hCG: β-human chorionic gonadotropin; CBC: complete blood count; CXR: chest X-ray; D&C: dilation and curettage; EB: endometrial biopsy; ECG: electrocardiogram; HMB: heavy menstrual bleeding; LA: local anesthetic; LDH: lactate dehydrogenase; SDH: succinate dehydrogenase; USG: ultrasonography)

and ovulatory pain present as cyclical pain while pelvic congestion syndrome, appendicitis, diverticulitis, and pelvic tumors are example of noncyclical pain.

Pelvic inflammatory disease often presents as urinary tract infection (UTI), weight loss, foul smelling vaginal discharge, and fever. A general and systemic examination of the patient should be done thoroughly and work for masses in abdomen and genitalia.

Along with blood counts, workup would include USG, abdomen along with pelvic ultrasound, and pelvic swabs.

A growth in the lower genital tract may require a biopsy; and tumor marker screen for cancer antigen 125 (CA-125), carcinoembryonic antigen (CEA), and alpha fetoprotein (AFP) may be required for pelvic tumors. A CBC, C-reactive protein, and urine culture are usually required. Diagnostic laparoscopy, when available, is a positive addition in the management of chronic pelvic pain when there is diagnostic difficulty, but not forgetting idiopathic pain.

Endometriosis

When the tissue characterizes the normal epithelial lining of the uterine cavity and the endometrium is found in ectopic locations, it is known as endometriosis. Most typically, endometriosis is found on or within the ovaries. Absolute incidence is unknown as it is a surgical diagnosis, because surgery and/or histology is required for its diagnosis, but estimates of 3–10% of women in the reproductive age group, and 25–35% of infertile women have been made.[10]

The diagnosis of endometriosis ought to be considered in any reproductive-aged women complaining of any one or combination of the subsequent signs and symptoms: premenstrual pelvic pain, acute adnexal pain, worsening dysmenorrhea, and deep dyspareunia. The foremost serious complication is rupture of an ovarian endometrioma. The approach is that directed at acute adnexal accidents.

Treatment and Patient Disposition

The diagnosis of endometriosis of any extent or variety cannot be created by any combination of historical, laboratory, examination, or radiographic studies. The physician should offer the patient analgesia and refer her to a gynecologist for definitive diagnosis and management.

Hemorrhagic or Corpus Luteum Cyst Rupture (Table 2)

In a normal functioning ovaries, little bleeding is common. Similarly, little bleeding occurs during the vascularization phase of corpus luteum. However, if this bleeding is massive it leads to formation of corpus luteal cyst and hemorrhagic cyst. Rupture of the corpus luteal cyst or hemorrhagic cyst into the abdomen may occur and cause a clinical picture indistinguishable from that of a ruptured ectopic pregnancy, in terms of the patient's menstrual history and physical examination.

If the corpus luteum persists and also the cyst ruptures, the clinical presentation once more might be similar to that of an ectopic pregnancy or spontaneous abortion. β-hCG determinations and USG will be required for differentiation between the possible diagnoses (Fig. 5).

Acute rupture of a corpus luteum cyst with consequent hemoperitoneum, in either a pregnant or nonpregnant state, usually requires surgical intervention and ovarian cystectomy.

Tubo-Ovarian Abscess

Patients suffering from tubo-ovarian abscess also have PID additionally. Fever, blood leukocytosis, and imaging clinch the diagnosis.

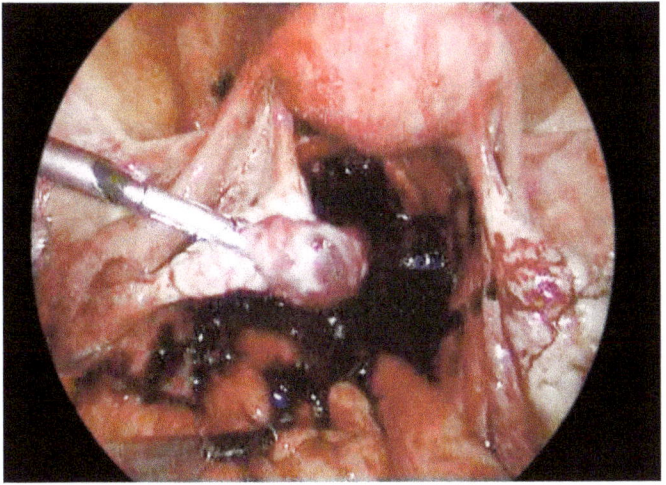

Fig. 5: Ruptured corpus luteum cyst.

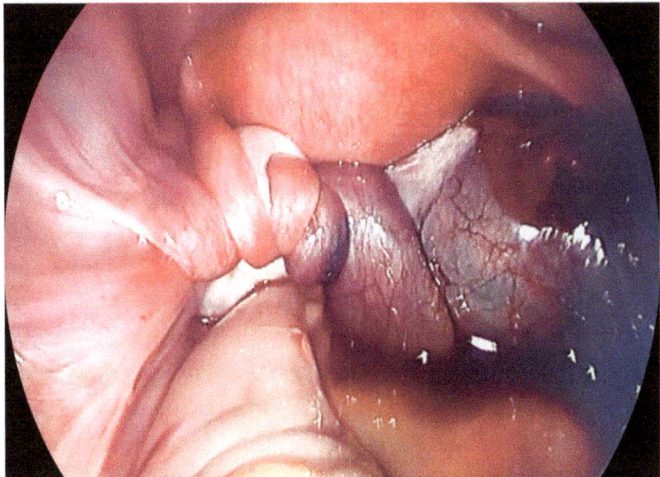

Fig. 6: Torsion of ovarian cyst.

Ultrasound is central to the diagnosis and management of tubo-ovarian abscess. Ultrasound is unable to clearly outline the borders of the ovaries and fallopian tubes; these structures are therefore described as the tubo-ovarian complex. Blood counts can slow leukocytosis with raised erythrocyte sedimentation rate (ESR).

Pain killers, antibiotics, and intravenous fluids should be initiated.

In patients with ruptured tubo-ovarian abscess with features of shock, prompt surgical intervention under anesthesia should be employed. Peritoneal toileting and drainage of pus by laparoscopy usually resolves the septic shock. Alternatively USG-guided transvaginal aspiration has been described in literature but results are not consistent.

Diagnostic laparoscopy and drainage of pus and hemorrhage usually resolves this condition.

Torsion of Ovarian Cyst/Pedunculated Myoma/Paraovarian Cyst (Table 2)

Mature cystic teratoma is the most common tumor of ovary which undergoes torsion (3.5–10% of ovarian torsion). Only 2% of ovarian torsion are due to malignant ovary **(Fig. 6)**.

Acute or subacute abdominal pain, nausea and mild shock, and vomiting may be presenting symptom in ovarian torsion.

Per abdominal examination presents muscle guarding with tender adnexal mass.

In case of unstable torsion, recurrence of pain can occur. Finally the pain becomes continuous because the ovarian blood supply is disrupted and the ovary may become gangrenous.

Special case: Pregnancy with adnexal torsion **(Fig. 7)**.

Ruptured Ovarian Cyst

Ovarian cyst may occasionally rupture spontaneously or due to trauma. Signs and symptoms depend upon size of cyst. Small cyst rupture may be silent but rupture of large mucinous or dermoid cyst may lead to peritonitis or shock **(Fig. 8)**.

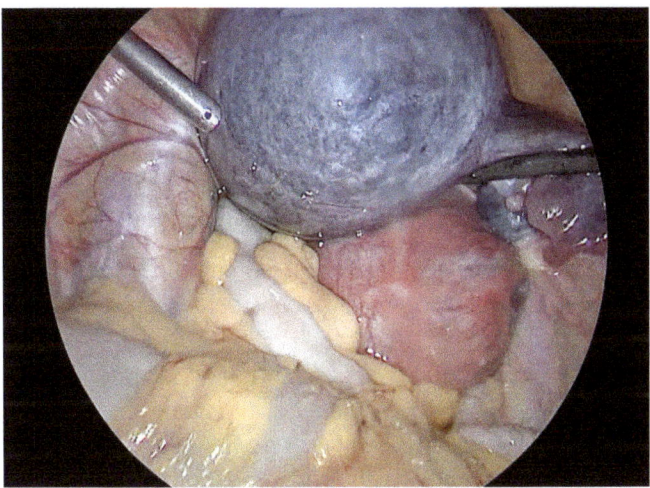

Fig. 7: Pregnancy with adnexal torsion.

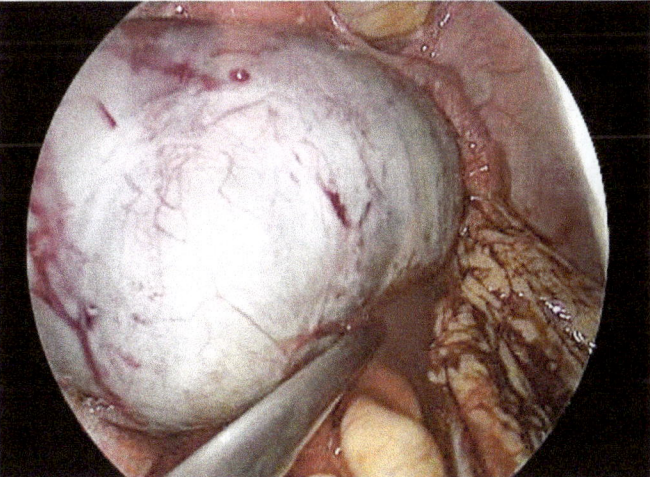

Fig. 8: Ruptured endometrioma.

It causes symptoms such as abdominal pain and shock. Serous cyst rupture does not cause such shock.

Massive Uterine Bleeding[2,11,12] (Table 2)

Usually a menstrual cycle ranges from 21 to 30 days with 5 days of flow. Blood loss up to 80 mL is normal.

PALM-COEIN is a well-accepted acronym to describe the abnormalities of uterine bleeding in reproductive age women. It represents polyp, adenomyosis, leiomyoma, malignancy and hyperplasia, coagulopathy, ovulatory dysfunction, endometrial, iatrogenic, and not-yet-classified. Heavy vaginal bleeding may not always be due to menstrual abnormality. It could be related to fibroids adenomyosis, or uterine malignancy. In case of very heavy flow, other causes like miscarriage or cervical malignancy should be looked for **(Fig. 9)**.

In case of severe anemic with heavy flow, patient should be admitted in hospital and treated. Resuscitation with IV fluids, blood transfusion, and antibiotics should be done. Hemostatic drugs may be used to decrease bleeding. Definitive treatment is done according to suspected diagnosis.

Sexual Assault and Rape (Table 2)

Rape is defined as nonconsensual penetration by penis into vagina or anus of women and is considered as most serious sexual offence.

In case of traumatic genital injury, the victim of sexual assault can present as gynecological emergency.

Any rape or sexual assault patient should be managed by taking comprehensive history, documentation, and treating genital injury. Prophylactic antibiotic and prophylaxis for human immunodeficiency virus (HIV), hepatitis B, and emergency contraception with psychological support with support of forensic experts and police is required.

During the initial assessment, detailed history should be obtained including the date, time, place, and nature of assault. During examination, attention should be focused on the patient's appearance, possible genital injury, and swabs taken from the vulva, vagina, and cervix, perineal, and rectal area as appropriate.

Blood and urine samples may need to be taken for toxicological studies. Detailed documentation of clinical findings and results of investigations are important as these may become vital evidence in subsequent prosecution.

Prophylactic antibiotic should cover for common sexually transmitted infections, and postexposure prophylaxis for HIV should be offered, guided by the risk of acquisition.

CONCLUSION

Acute emergency (obstetric or gynecological) constitutes a significant morbidity among young girls and women. Unsafe abortions and ectopic pregnancy are the most common life-threatening gynecological emergencies. Torsed ovary should be de-twisted and saved even if it appears gangrenous as blue black color is due to venous stasis. Transverse uterus septum should be considered in young girls complaining of pain abdomen and primary amenorrhea. Sexual assault patients to be handled gently and counselled to take them out through mental trauma.

Facilities for prompt diagnostic testing, imaging and laparoscopy equipped operation theatre and anesthetist will be crucial to prevent morbidity and mortality of emergency gynecology.

Take Home Messages

- For diagnosing ectopic pregnancy, a doctor should always be ectopic minded while treating a female with acute abdomen.
- In any women having acute abdomen always elicit correct LMP and cross check with a pregnancy list.
- Right factor assessment is important to anticipate probability of postpartum hemorrhage (PPH) and blood/blood products should be arranged accordingly.
- While managing antepartum hemorrhage (APH), patient should be dealt in a multidisciplinary approach with high-dependency unit (HDU)/ICU facility.
- Timely referral of patient to tertiary care center is crucial but if patient condition is critical hemodynamic stabilization is must.

REFERENCES

1. Ferreira H, Bras R. Acute gynaecological emergencies. In: Mahmood T, Savona-Ventura C, Messinis I, Mukhopadhyay S (Eds). The EBCOG Postgraduate Textbook of Obstetrics and Gynaecology. Cambridge: Cambridge University Press; 2021. pp. 6-14.
2. Abam DS. Overview of gynaecological emergencies. In: Darwish A (Ed). Contemporary Gynecologic Practice [online] Available from: https://www.intechopen.com/chapters/47706. [last accessed January 2023].
3. Fawole A, Awonuga D. Gynaecological emergencies in the tropics: recent advances in management. Ann Ib Postgrad Med. 2007;5(1):12-20.

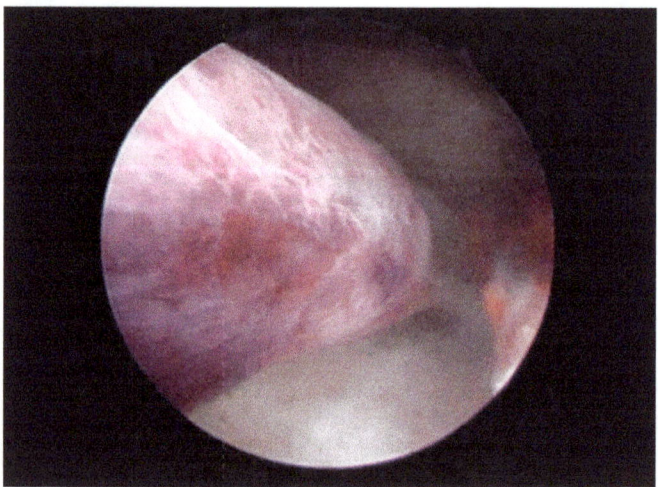

Fig. 9: Endometrial polyp.

4. Olarewaju RS, Ujah IAO, Otubu JAM. Trends in ectopic pregnancy in the Jos University Teaching Hospital, Jos, Nigeria. Nig J Med. 1994;26:57-60.
5. Grimes DA. The morbidity and mortality of pregnancy. Still risky business. Am J Obstet Gynecol. 1994:170:1489-94.
6. Saxena R. Early Pregnancy bleeding due to miscarriage. In: Saxena R. Bedside Obstetrics and Gynaecology, 2nd edition. New Delhi: Jaypee Brothers Medical Publishers (P) Ltd.; 2014. pp. 161-86.
7. World Health Organization. Maternal mortality in 1995. Estimates developed by WHO, UNICEF and UNFPA. WHO/RHR/01.9. Geneva: World Health Organization; 2001.
8. Sedgh G, Henshaw S, Singh S, Ahman E, Shah I. Induced abortion: estimated rates and trends worldwide. Lancet. 2007; 370(9595):1338-45.
9. World Health Organization. Unsafe abortion: global and regional estimates of incidence of unsafe abortion and associated mortality in 2008, 6th edition. Geneva: World Health Organization; 2011.
10. Memarzadeh S, Muse KN, Fox MD. Endometriosis. In: Decherney AH, Nathan L (Eds). Current Obstetrics and Gynaecology Diagnosis and Treatment, 9th edition. New York: Lange/McGraw Hill; 2003. pp. 767-75.
11. Committee on Practice Bulletins-Gynecology. Practice bulletin no. 128: diagnosis of abnormal uterine bleeding in reproductive-aged women. Obstet Gynecol. 2012;120(1): 197-206.
12. Committee on Practice Bulletins-Gynecology. Practice bulletin no. 136: management of abnormal uterine bleeding associated with ovulatory dysfunction. Obstet Gynecol. 2013; 122(1):176-85.

SECTION 8

Trauma

Section Editor: Subhasish Deb

28. **Road Traffic Accidents**
    Subhasish Deb

29. **Household Trauma**
    Subhasish Deb

28. Road Traffic Accidents

Subhasish Deb

EMERGENCY MANAGEMENT BEFORE AND ON REACHING THE HOSPITAL

The causes of road traffic accident (RTA) can range over a very broad spectrum but the common ones include:
- Over speeding
- Drink driving
- Talking on the mobile phone
- Underage driving.

Following figures show different types of accidents **(Figs. 1 to 3)**.

Road traffic accident can happen in a split of a second due to a momentary lapse of concentration while driving.

The following figures from police records give us a more realistic picture of how common RTAs are in Kolkata and in other parts of West Bengal. Following are the records of accidents in year 2021:

Kolkata Police Records
- Total road traffic accidents = 1,405
- Total fatalities = 196

West Bengal Police Records (Except Kolkata)
- Total road traffic accidents = 10,220
- Total fatalities = 5,220.

The principles of advanced trauma life support (ATLS) are always followed in the management of any RTA.
- AIRWAY (including cervical spine)
- Breathing
- Circulation.

By far use commonest vehicles to be involved in RTA on the Indian roads are motorbikes **(Fig. 4)**.

On the road, there are limited resources but the principles of ATLS must always be adhered to.

A salient feature in dealing both motorbike RTAs is the correct technique of removal of helmet.

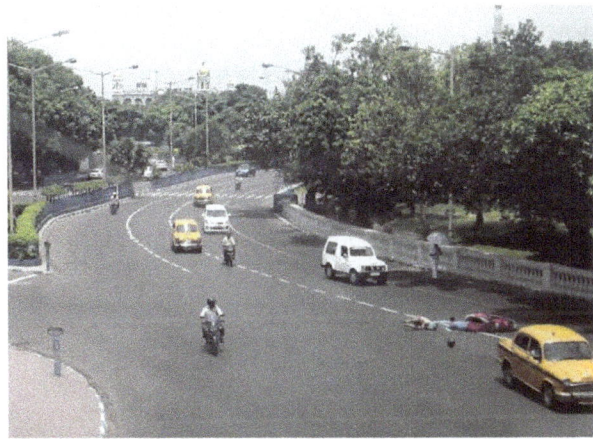

Fig. 2: Rash driving.

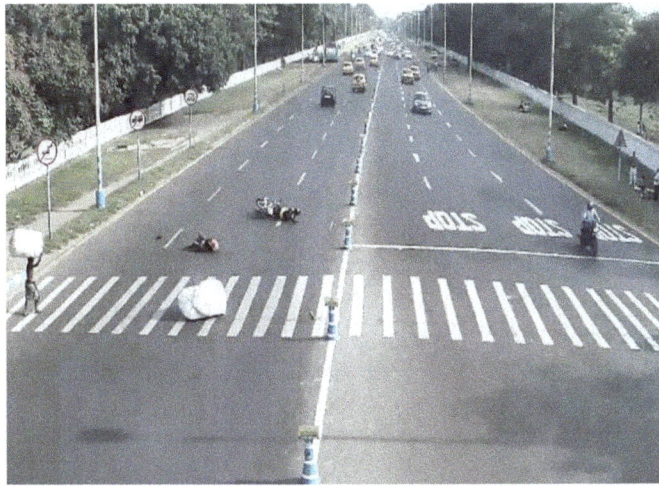

Fig. 1: Over speeding.

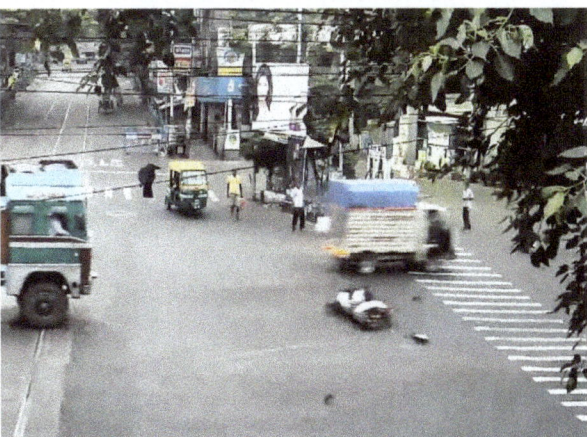

Fig. 3: Drinking and driving.

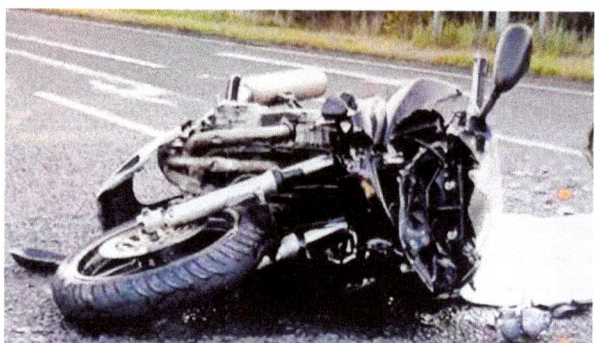

Fig. 4: Motorbike accident.

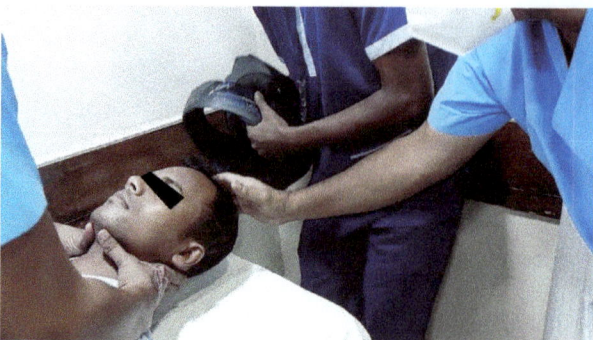

Fig. 6: After helmet removal.

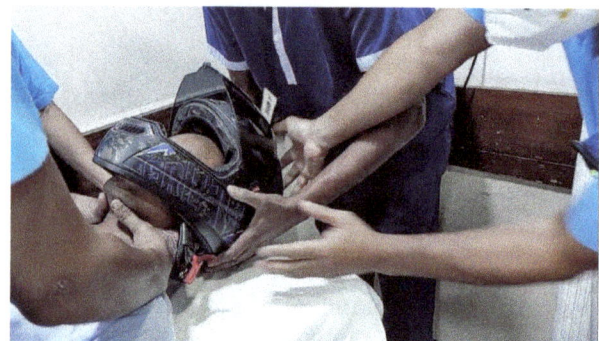

Fig. 5: Before helmet removal.

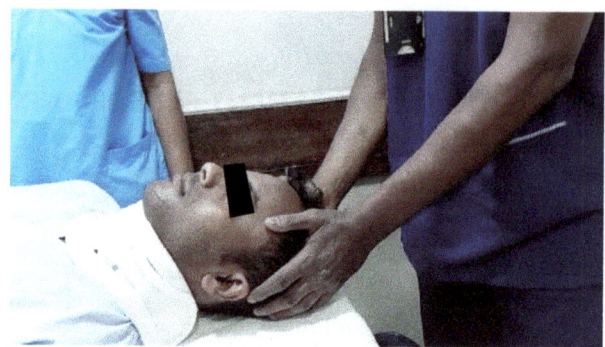

Fig. 7: Trauma collar.

Following are the principles:
- Removal of vizor
- Unclip the helmet
- Stabilize the neck and jaw **(Fig. 5)**

It is important to take the vizor off. One can then communicate with the patient and reassure him/her that help is here.

One can check his/her airway using both hands by one person and then sliding out of helmet from the top end by a second person **(Fig. 6)**.

Then apply the hard cervical collar sliding it under the neck while somebody holds onto the head without moving the head at all.

Once the helmet is safely removed and the neck is stabilized by using a collar **(Fig. 7)**.

Provide oxygen from the cylinder in the ambulance using a mask and at higher flow.

The immediate next step is to identify any active source of bleeding.

The single most cause of preventable death after any RTA is blood loss. Hence, the identification and check control of blood loss and an initial resuscitation are vital steps in the management.

STOP THE BLEED: SAVE A LIFE

Once we have identified a source of bleeding (limb or trunk), use direct pressure on the bleeding area using both your hands and some gauze or cloth whatever is available.

In certain cases of uncontrollable limb bleed, a tourniquet may be used proximal to the bleeding point.

Also start an intravenous (IV) access and start any fluid to initiate the volume replacement and prevention of any hypo volume shock.

Once that is over, we need to get the patient ready to be safely transported from the road to the hospital emergency.

Any suspected lower limb fracture should be stabilized in a Thomas splint OR any other form of splint.

Then using a spinal board, shift the patient from the road to the ambulance. Inform the hospital whilst in the ambulance regarding the status of the patient including all vitals and all injuries which one has been able to assess so far.

The trauma team and the emergency staff should all be ready to receive one's patient with all urgency. The trauma team should ideally include:
- Emergency medical officer
- Anesthetist
- Orthopedic surgeon
- General surgeon
- Neuro surgeon
- Trained nursing staff.

Once in the emergency department of the hospital, once again one should reassess the patient with giving importance to:
- Airway (including cervical spine)
- Breathing
- Circulation.

Airway (including cervical spine):
- Remove the oxygen mask temporarily
- Look at his/her mouth whether there is any obstruction or injury to nose/mouth
- Whether there is any bleeding from nose/mouth and use suction to clear the airway.

Breathing:
- Nasopharyngeal tube
- Oropharyngeal tube
- Intubate if airway cannot be maintained
- Use a bougie in case of difficult intubation
- Listen to his/her chest
- Purcuss his chest
- Chest drain if one is worried about a pneumothorax.

Circulation: Use two thick Venflons (Gray color) one in each upper limb to get venous access. Blood may be taken at the same time for testing, grouping, crossmatching, and saving. It is important to start IV crystalloid/colloid at the same time.

Examine the abdomen for tenderness/guarding/suspected internal hemorrhage in the abdomen, retroperitoneum, long bones, and pelvis.

If required hold the pelvic ring with a towel or sheet in separated pelvis injuries.

Check the patient's limbs for fractures, wounds, and external bleeding points.

STOP THE BLEEDING

If one identifies any limb external bleeding point, use all measures available to:
- Pressure directly on bleeding wound with heel of both hands
- Expose the area (cut off the clothes)
- Use tourniquet
- Pack the wound with gauze.

MAKE SURE ONE STOPS THE BLEEDING

Splintage
Stabilize the affected limb using a splint.

Logroll
Use as many people to logroll to check the spine, look for any step/deformity, look for any puncture, wound, etc.

The relevant investigators at this stage include:
- eFAST USG scan
- Chest X-ray
- X-ray abdomen
- X-ray spine
- X-ray pelvis
- X-ray of affected limb
- CT-scan Brain
- All relevant blood tests and then **REFER TO APPROPRIATE SPECIALTY FOR FURTHER MANAGEMENT**.

Take Home Messages
- Initial Assessment and Management
- Airway and Ventilator Management
- Shock
- Thoracic Trauma
- Abdominal and Pelvic Trauma
- Head Trauma
- Spine and Spinal Cord Trauma
- Musculoskeletal Trauma.

CHAPTER 29: Household Trauma

Subhasish Deb

INTRODUCTION

Household trauma includes a wide range of effects including a mental issue and the physical issue which can be related to domestic violence and accidental physical injuries at home **(Flowchart 1)**.

In this chapter we are dealing with purely the physical injuries arising from:
- Accidental injuries at home
- Others following:
  - Household Chores
  - Tendonitis
  - Rotator cuff pain
  - Trigger finger
  - Tennis elbow
  - Golfer's elbow
  - Carpal tunnel syndrome.

These are injuries, which arise from repetitive motions that can lead to nerve and tendon pain, causing short- and long-term injuries.

"The incidence of domestic accidents was found to be 1.7% .
—DJ Bhandari (2008).[1]

Domestic accidents are more common in extreme age groups and in females. Falls being the most frequent type of accidents.

"Prevalence and pattern of domestic accidents" (T Rehman, 2020)[2] showed the prevalence of domestic accidents at the household level in an urban population of Southern India was found to be 10.2%. The common type of injury was falls injury mostly the upper limbs and took place predominantly in morning hours in the kitchen.

We will now discuss the treatment for the various types of injuries, secondary to fall at home.

- *Head Injury*
  It can occur at any age presenting features could be:
  - Head laceration
  - Headache
  - Dizziness
  - Loss of consciousness (LOC)
  - Vomiting

  Application of ice and pressure to the area for 10–15 min will cause the bleeding to stop.

  Stitches may be required.
  LOC needs to be attended at local hospital.
  Otherwise rest at home under observation for 48 hours.

- *Wrist injury—the most common* **(Fig. 1)**
  Fractures of distal radius account for up to 20% of all fractures treated in emergency department.[3]
  - Being fracture of distal radius (Colles Fracture)
  - Elevate in a sling

Flowchart 1: Types of physical trauma due to household accidents.

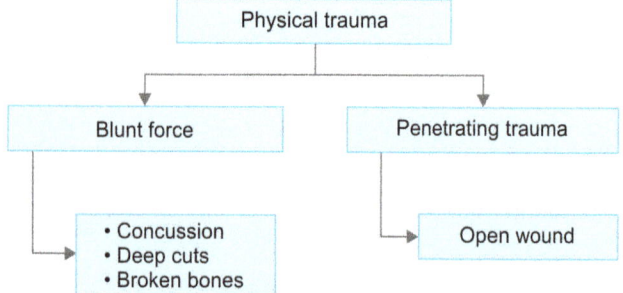

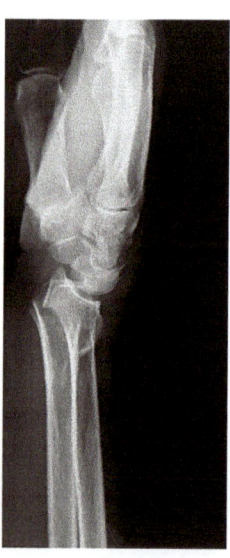

Fig. 1: Wrist Injury.

- Ice compress
- 4" crepe bandage
- Analgesic
- X-ray: Further treatment, plaster/surgery

■ *Elbow injury in a child, suspect supracondylar fracture (Fig. 2)*
Supracondylar humerus fracture is one of the most common fractures encountered in pediatric age group at all levels (both rural and urban).[4]
- Check radial pulse
- Elevate in a sling
- Ice compress
- X-ray

■ *Shoulder injury (Fig. 3)*
- Dislocation
  - Loss of rounded bony contour of the shoulder
  - Reduction of dislocations as early as possible
  - Not comfortable in a sling
  - Check fingers
  - Reduction of dislocation as early as possible
- Fracture
  - Pain and range of movement
  - Sling
  - X-ray and analgesics

■ *Vertebral body compression fracture*
- Severe back pain
- Should be advised rest lying down
- Check of leg movement or power
- Apply brace
- Check for bladder bowel incontinence
- X-ray

■ *Hip injury (Fig. 4)*
Hip fractures are fractures of the proximal femur, common in the elderly population following a fall. It has a high rate of morbidity and mortality. Surgical intervention is often required.[5]
- Common being hip fracture
  - Intracapsular
  - Extracapsular
- Shortening and rotation of affected leg. Reduced rage of movement with pain.
- Portable X-ray should include X-ray pelvic AP view to see both hips and X-ray lateral view of the affected side.
- Admission to hospital
- Less common is fracture of pubic ramus which can be treated with rest lying down.

■ *Knee injury/pain*
- It could be a result of a fracture or exacerbation of preexisting osteoarthritis (OA) or hemarthrosis
- Rest
- Ice compress
- Crepe bandage

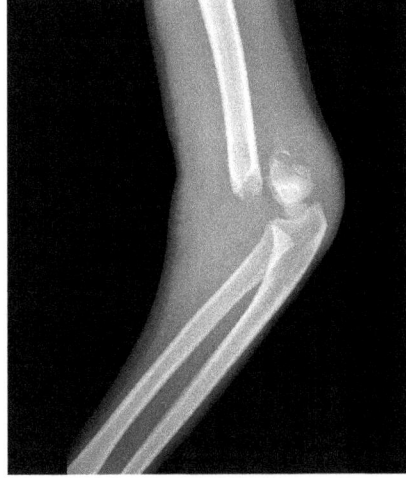

Fig. 2: Elbow injury.

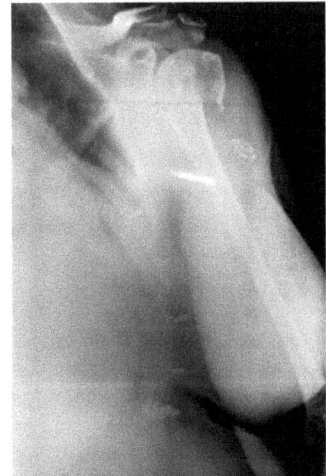

Fig. 3: Shoulder injury.

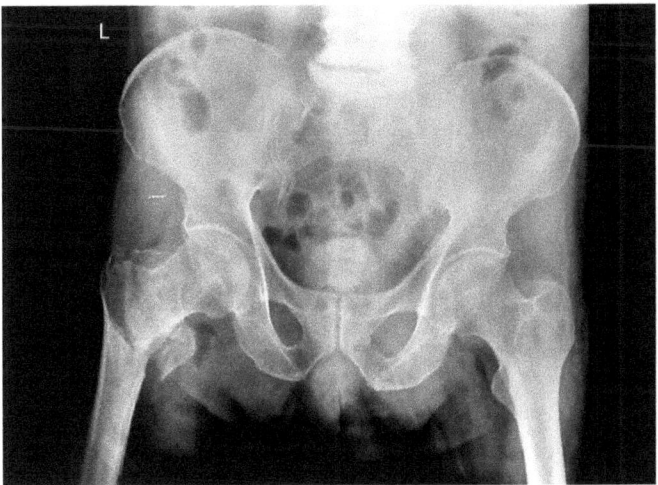

Fig. 4: Hip injury.

- X-ray
- Aspirations, if required

■ *Tibial shaft fracture* can also happen but not so common. They almost always require surgery.

- *Ankle fractures are common.* They quite often require surgery ankle sprain/inversion injury are quite common, requiring
  - Ice compress in the initial 7 days
  - Elevation
  - Crepe bandage
  - Wearing a crepe bandage/ankle support should be continued till 6 weeks
- *Foot injury*
  It is also common resulting in fracture of base of 5th metatarsal (MT). Initial 2–3 days of elevation and ice compress followed by Elastoplast strapping for 6 weeks can heal this injury. Sometimes it may require surgery.

PREVENTION OF FALLS

- Avoid loose electrical wires on the floor
- Always have a corridor/night lamp on
- Avoid keeping carpet on this floor
- Use hip pads
- Avoid wet bathroom floors.

> **Take Home Messages**
> - Household injuries are more common than we think they are.
> - The most common one is due to fall and occurs more in the elderly population.
> - Prevention of falls must be given importance and suggested practical measures must be adhered to.
> - Limb injuries should always have elevation; ice compress and support with crepe bandage or some splintage.

- Joint dislocation should be reduced as soon as possible.
- Cuts and lacerations should have pressure dressing initially and then surgical repair/exploration if there is gaping wound or loss of function.
- Small sized limb burns can be treated at home but larger trunk burns should be treated at hospital.
- Injuries however small, must not be ignored and medical advice should always be taken.
- Being aware of the possible household injuries is important and ways and means to prevent them can go a long way.
- The other aspects of household trauma especially the mental aspect, is outside the perspective of this chapter and hence has not been discussed but they are equally if not more important.

REFERENCES

1. Bhanderi DJ, Choudhary S. A study of occurrence of domestic accidents in semi-urban community. Indian J Community Med. 2008;33(2):104-6.
2. Rehman T, Sulgante S, Sekhar SK. Prevalence and pattern of domestic accidents in the field practice area of Jawaharlal Institute of Urban Health Centre, Puducherry: a cross-sectional analytical study. J Inj Violence Res. 2020;12(1):1-10.
3. Meena S, Sharma P, Sambharia AK, Dawar A. Fractures of distal radius: an overview. J Family Med Prim Care. 2014;3(4):325-32.
4. Kumar V, Singh A. Fracture Supracondylar Humerus: a review. J Clin Diagn Res. 2016;10(12):RE01-RE06.
5. Emmerson BR, Varacallo M, Inman D. Hip Fracture Overview. Treasure Island (FL): StatPearls Publishing; 2022.

SECTION 9
Psychiatric Emergencies

Section Editor: Sanjay Garg

30. **Violence in Mental Health**
    Sanjay Garg

CHAPTER 30: Violence in Mental Health

Sanjay Garg

INTRODUCTION

It is a common misconception in the society that individuals with mental illness have a propensity for violence. Depictions in popular culture of mentally disturbed perpetrators of violent crimes or disproportionate and sensationalized representation of actual news of crimes being committed by mentally ill persons contribute to this opinion.[1] This wrongly held belief further perpetuates the fear and stigma associated with psychiatric disorders, and in turn leads to the marginalization and isolation of persons suffering from such disorders. Due to the vast number of factors, both personal as well as situational, involved, it is difficult to conclude whether there is increased risk of violence amongst individuals with mental illness. A review of literature provides evidences of all three possibilities of mentally ill persons being more, less or equally violent than persons with no history of mental illness.[2] However, an understanding of the varying perspectives regarding the links between mental illness and violence, is instrumental to the risk minimization in health care settings as well as in the community.

ETIOLOGICAL EXPLANATIONS OF VIOLENCE

As is the case in mental illnesses, violent or aggressive behaviors also appear to arise from a combination of biological, psychological, and societal or environmental factors. Naturally, individual differences in behavior imply that the relative preponderance of these factors may be different from person to person.

Amongst biological factors, genetics play a significant role in violence; violent individuals tend to have a family history of aggressive behaviors. Studies indicate that the coordination of multiple genes produces the propensity for violence.[3] However, it is unclear whether a family history of violence leads to violent behaviors by way of genetic transmission, learning of observed behaviors, or a combination of both. Twin studies indicate that a large degree of variance in aggressive behaviors can be explained by genetic factors.[4] On the other hand, adoption studies reveal that a combination of nature and nurture characteristics predicts violent behaviors.[5]

The role of neurotransmitter involvement in violence is well-documented. Several studies have replicated the finding of an inverse relation between 5-hydroxyindoleacetic acid (5-HIAA) in cerebrospinal fluid (CSF) and tendency for aggressive behaviors in mentally ill persons.[6-8]

Neuroimaging studies further provide insights into the areas or circuitry involved in aggressive behaviors. Robust evidence implicates problems in executive functions stemming from deficits in prefrontal or frontal functioning. Disturbances in subcortical structures of the temporal lobe were also found to play a role in violent behaviors amongst the mentally ill.[9]

Lower resting heart[10] and reduced response to anxiety provoking stimuli[11] have also been found to be associated with aggressive behaviors.

Several psychosocial factors have been presented by different schools of thought as the factors behind violence. For instance, the psychodynamic school of thought views aggression as stemming from the thwarting of libidinal impulses or the unhealthy utilization of defense mechanisms such as projection of unwanted characteristics onto the victims of violence.[12]

The cognitive behavioral explanation of violent behaviors is a distorted schema or cognitive distortion which places the blame of all negative events onto others, thereby provoking aggressive reactions.[13]

Learning of observed violent behaviors, direct or vicarious reinforcement of aggressive acts and desensitization to violence due to frequent witnessing of the same in different forms of media, are other factors that may explain violence in individuals. Disturbed home environment or being subject to abuse have also been frequently implicated in violent behaviors.

VIOLENCE AND MENTAL ILLNESS

While violence as a symptom may be a component of any or all mental illnesses, some psychiatric disorders tend to have a greater possibility of manifest violent behavior amongst its symptoms **(Box 1)**. These include:

- *Disorders associated with substance use:* Amongst the link between psychiatric disorders and violence, most evidence exists for substance use disorders. Several studies have indicated that the use of substances, or even withdrawal from it can lead to violent behaviors.[14,15] A 73% increase in probability of aggression was found in persons with dual diagnosis of mental illness and substance use disorders than those without a history of substance abuse, irrespective of the presence of mental illness.[16] A study by Fazel et al., (2009)[17] found that the use of alcohol or drugs significantly accounted for the increased rates of violent crimes committed by persons with schizophrenia (13.2%) as compared to the general population (5.3%).
- *Schizophrenia and psychosis:* Many researches on serious mental illnesses have included persons suffering from schizophrenia or other psychotic disorders. A 2014 study found a four times greater incidence of violent crimes among patients with schizophrenia than the general population.[18] A 2013 study further implicates the presence of a diagnosis of schizophrenia in violent crimes by removing the effect of comorbid substance use and still finding double the likelihood of violence compared to matched community sample.[19] On the other hand, a study by Swanson et al. (1990)[20] concluded that violence for not more prevalent in persons with schizophrenia when compared to those with other mental illness diagnoses. An explanation for violent behaviors associated with schizophrenia may be the finding that roughly 20% of violent offenses by such persons are motivated by their psychotic symptoms such as persecutory delusions or command hallucinations.[21]
- *Other psychiatric disorders:* A wide range of psychiatric conditions have been associated with violence that include mood disorders, personality disorders, delirium and dementia, externalizing disorders of childhood onset, dissociative disorders, and premenstrual dysphoric disorder.[22]
- *Untreated psychiatric conditions:* Many violent offenses appear to be committed by mentally ill persons while they are untreated. Nonadherence to medication and therapy was identified as a major risk factor for violence in a meta-analysis including 110 studies and 45,533 individuals with a diagnosis of schizophrenia and other psychoses.[23] Several other studies have substantiated this finding of increased susceptibility for violent crimes in mentally ill persons not receiving treatment.

MANAGEMENT OF VIOLENCE IN THE MENTALLY ILL

A multipronged approach seems best suited for the management of violence associated with mental illness. Dealing with an aggressive patient requires care, judgment, and self-control.

PSYCHIATRIC EMERGENCIES

Environmental Adaptations

One of the foremost strategies for containment of violence includes awareness of, and training in identifying warning signs leading up to aggression. Features of irritability, psychomotor agitation, and paranoia, liability of affect are some of the salient warning signs of violent behaviors.[26] Mindfulness to these signs of violence and prompt intervention aimed at de-escalation are the keys to management of aggression **(Box 2)**.

A key thing often ignored in the Indian context, is the place of interaction with an acutely unwell patient. Attention needs to be given to the layout and location of the interview room **(Box 3)**.

> **BOX 1:** Mental disorders and violence.
>
> - People with mental disorders are more likely to be violent than community controls
> - Substance misuse greatly increases the risk of violence in people with mental disorders and community controls
> - Gender, age, past violence, and socioeconomic status have a much greater effect on risk of violence than the presence of mental disorder
> - Comorbid personality disorder independently increases the risk of violence
> - The increased risk of violence is mediated in part by active psychotic symptoms
> - "Threat/control override symptoms", i.e., persecutory delusions, delusions of control, and passivity phenomena, seem particularly important
> - The vast majority of people with mental disorder are not violent
>
> *Source:* Davison S. The management of violence in general psychiatry. Adv Psychiatr Treat. 2005;11(5):362-70.[24]

> **BOX 2:** Environmental risk factors that increase the risk of violence.
>
> - Lack of structured activity (there are fewer violent incidents in occupational and other therapy areas)
> - High use of temporary staff
> - Low levels of staff–patient interaction
> - Poor staffing levels
> - Poorly defined staffing roles
> - Unpredictable ward programs
> - Lack of privacy
> - Overcrowding
> - Poor physical facilities
> - Availability of weapons
>
> *Source:* Royal College of Psychiatrists. Management of Imminent Violence: Clinical Practice Guidelines to Support Mental Health Services (Occasional Paper OP41). London: Royal College of Psychiatrists; 1998.[25]

> **BOX 3:** Essentials for interview room safety.
>
> - Easily accessible, functioning alarm systems
> - Clear, unobstructed exits
> - Doors that open outwards, cannot be locked from the inside and allow easy access from the outside in the event of an emergency
> - Location close to staff areas
> - Removal of all potential weapons (these are a particular risk if the room has a dual function)
> - An unobstructed viewing window
> - A furniture layout that minimizes violence
>
> *Source:* 1. Osborn DPJ, Tang S. Effectiveness of audit in improving interview room safety. Psychiatr Bullet. 2001;25:92-4.[27]
> 2. Galloway J. Personal safety when visiting patients in the community. Adv Psychiatr Treat, 2002;8(3):214-22.[28]

De-escalation can be achieved by attention to one's own body language and postures. Polite and calm voice tones, provision of personal space, employment of distraction, and relaxation techniques and the reduction of unpleasant stimuli such as crowds or loud noises, can go a long way to reduce violent tendencies.[26] Calmness and friendliness in behavior is perhaps the single most powerful arrow in the quiver of techniques at the disposal of staff members required to manage agitation. Responding with concern and empathy has also been found to be highly effective in reducing aggressive intent in patients.

Asking open-ended questions, reassuring and acknowledging their grievances, and giving them the opportunity to voice what has angered them may help find a solution. Maintain eye contact—but not for too long, keep an adequate distance, leave the room if necessary and moving the patient away from public view helps in reducing the acute flare up.

A functional analysis of the aggressive behavior and suggestions of alternative approaches to fulfilling the same function can help patients to drop violent approaches of emotional expression.[29]

While restrictive strategies such as the use of physical restraints or isolation are never the preferred mode of containing aggression, sometimes, these techniques have to be utilized when other less intrusive and more benign approaches do not seem to help. It is crucial that while employing the use of restraint or seclusion also, a calming, and soothing body language and speech be adopted by the staff.

Psychotherapeutic Interventions

Environmental adaptations alone may not suffice to minimize the risk associated with violent offenses, especially when the patient has a long history of violent acts. Different modalities of psychotherapy can help approach the problem of agitation from different angles and adopt suitable interventions for the same.

From the behavioral point of view, the use of token economy may be employed to reinforce appropriate nonviolent behavior; from the learning theory point of view, training in more effective forms of communication as opposed to aggressive modes of expression can equip individuals with the necessary tools to express their concerns in a nonconfrontational manner; from the cognitive perspective, disputing and restructuring of the unhelpful schemas that predispose individuals to behave in aggressive ways can provide lasting changes in violent behaviors. Training in relaxation techniques and other strategies of anger and emotional management can pave the way for reduction in agitated behaviors. Couples and family therapy must also be considered when behavior or expressed emotions of significant others are found to be contributory factors in violent behaviors of the patient.

Restraint

This is a mechanism used as a last resort when all other interventions have failed. This includes moving patient to a safe space or seclusion, physical restraint, and chemical restraint or rapid tranquilization.

Physical restraint needs to be done by trained staff using recognized techniques to hold the patient and restrict the movement to reduce the risk of injury to self and others. Consideration for self-respect, dignity, privacy, cultural, and special needs is essential.

Finally, chemical restraint or rapid tranquilization has a very important part to play in the management of acutely violent behavior amongst the mentally ill **(Flowchart 1)**. The necessity of pharmacological interventions is proportional to the risk of harm to self and others that is potentially posed by the violent behavior **(Box 4)**.

> **BOX 4:** Skills of doctors prescribing rapid tranquilization.
>
> - Be familiar with the properties of benzodiazepines and their antagonists, antipsychotics, antimuscarinics, and antihistamines
> - Be able to assess the risks associated with rapid tranquilization, particularly when the patient is highly aroused and may have been misusing drugs, be dehydrated or physically ill
> - Understand the cardiovascular effects of the acute administration of the tranquillizing drugs and the need to titrate the dose
> - Recognize the importance of nursing in the recovery position
> - Recognize the importance of monitoring pulse, blood pressure, and respiration
> - Be familiar and trained in the use of resuscitation equipment
> - Undertake regular resuscitation training
> - Understand the importance of maintaining an unobstructed airway
>
> *Source:* 1. Royal College of Psychiatrists. Management of Imminent Violence: Clinical Practice Guidelines to Support Mental Health Services (Occasional Paper OP41). London: Royal College of Psychiatrists; 1998.
> 2. National Institute for Clinical Excellence. Short-term Management of Violent (Disturbed) Behaviour in Adult Psychiatric In-patient and Accident and Emergency Settings. Second Draft for Consultation. London: NICE; 2004.[25,30]

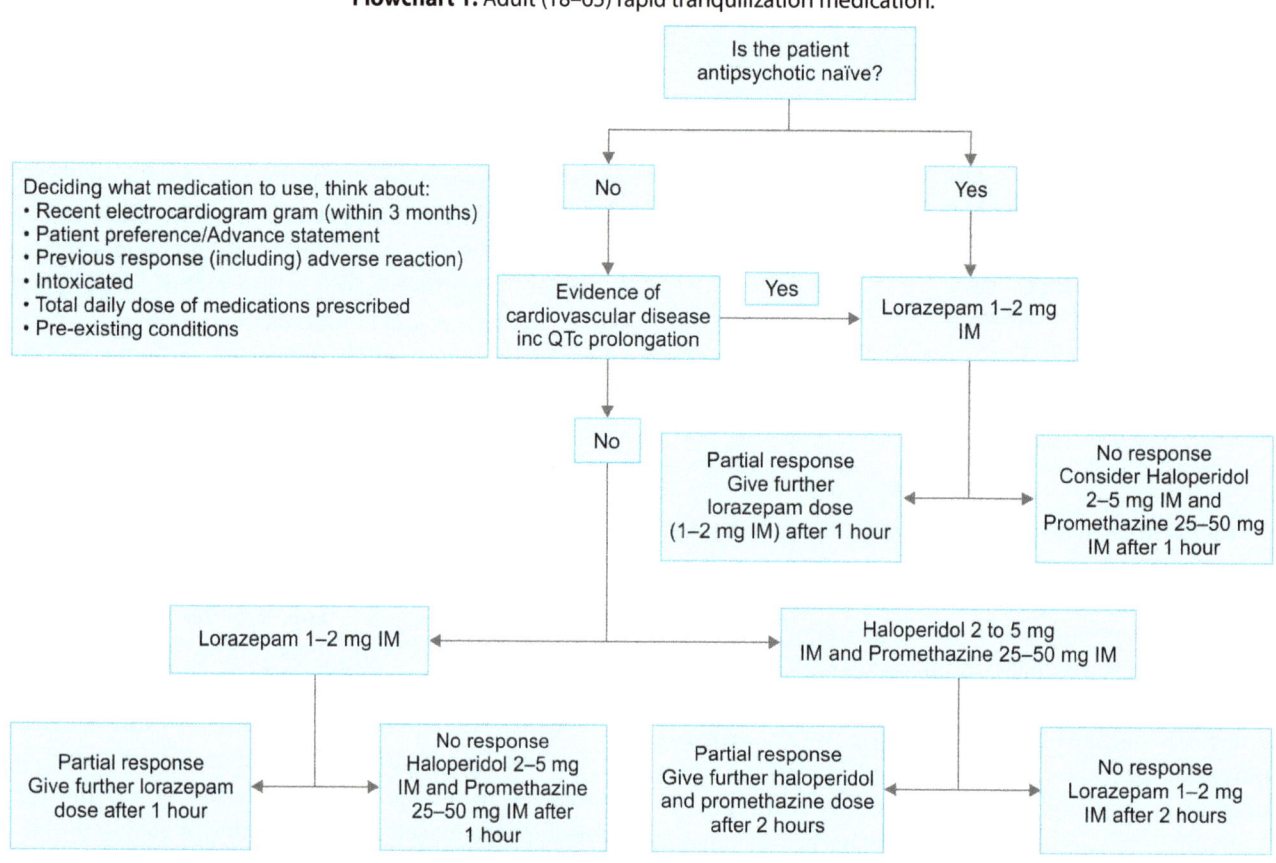

Flowchart 1: Adult (18–65) rapid tranquilization medication.

Source: Sheffield Health and Social Care NHS Foundation Trust. Policy MD 011 - Rapid Tranquilisation Policy and Guidelines for Inpatient Wards.

After rapid tranquilization, the patient should be monitored. The response to medication and any emergent side effects documented in care records. Ensure the patient is observed within eyesight by a trained staff member postrapid tranquilization. The following physical health observations should be monitored and recorded every hour until there are no concerns about their physical health status (physical observations within range or agreed with a doctor).

- Pulse
- Blood pressure
- Respiratory rate/O_2 saturation
- Temperature
- Level of hydration
- Level of consciousness

The focus of long-term medical intervention needs to be also on the alleviation of the underlying psychiatric symptoms associated with the violence rather than the violent behavior itself. As discussed before, nontreatment of psychiatric conditions is one of the biggest risk factors of violent offences.

Training and Support to Frontline Staff

An important aspect in the management of aggression is the awareness, understanding, and training of staff who first come across such patients. A zero-tolerance policy with adequate staff support is essential to provide a safe working environment.

Take Home Messages

Violence among the mentally ill poses significant risks to the individuals themselves as well as their immediate family members, the community at large, and to healthcare professionals. Thus, understanding of the link between psychiatric disorders and aggressive behaviors is crucial to the management of such behaviors and to risk minimization. A complex interplay of etiological factors plays a role in determining whether a mentally ill person is likely to perpetrate violence. Huge individual differences exist and it cannot be concluded definitively that mentally ill persons are more prone to behave violently than the general population or that a large part of violence in the society is attributable to persons with psychiatric diagnosis. However, being mindful that the possibility of aggressive behaviors amongst the mentally ill exists and being cognizant of the warning signs for the same are the primary steps to the containment and reduction of potentially harmful behaviors. A majority of violent behaviors and situations can be de-escalated simply by environmental modifications and adoption of helpful body language and behavioral strategies by the staff. The more chronic or long-term instances of violence or the more complex cases may require pharmacological and psychotherapeutic interventions both for immediate as well as long-term management.

Take home points—the Do's
- Calm, soothing tone of voice with a positive and friendly attitude of helpfulness
- Expressing concern for patient's wellbeing with verbal redirection and limit-setting
- Distraction with a more positive activity and use of relaxation techniques
- Close observation or one-to-one nursing or quiet time or open seclusion
- Removal of potentially dangerous items from the immediate environment
- Physical and/or chemical restraint (rapid tranquilization) with regular monitoring

Take home points—the Don'ts
- Overcrowding patients or unpleasant or polluted surroundings
- Loud and irritating noise
- Intimidating direct eye contact or unnecessary invasion of personal space
- Direct confrontative stance with crossed arms or hands concealed in pockets

REFERENCES

1. Stuart H. Violence and mental illness: an overview. World Psychiatry. 2003;2(2):121-4.
2. Wessely S. Violence and psychosis. In: Thompson C, Cowen P (Eds). Violence: Basic and Clinical Science, London: Butterworth-Heinemann; 1993. pp. 119-34.
3. Cadoret RJ, Leve LD, Devor E. Genetics of aggressive and violent behavior. Anger, Aggression, and Violence. 1997; 20,301-22.
4. O'Connor M, Foch T, Sherry T, Plomin R. A twin study of specific behavioral problems of socialization as viewed by parents. J Abnorm Child Psychol. 1980;8(2):189-99.
5. Cadoret RJ, Yates WR, Troughton E, Woodworth G, Stewart MA. Genetic environmental interaction in the genesis of aggressivity and conduct disorders. Arch Gen Psychiatry. 1995;52:916-24.
6. Van Praag H, Asnis G, Kahn R, Brown S, Korn M, Friedman J, et al. Monoamines and abnormal behaviour a multi-aminergic perspective. Br J Psychiatry, 1990;157(5):723-34.
7. Brown G L, Ebert MH, Goyer PF, Jimerson DC, Klein WJ, Bunney W, et al. Aggression, suicide, and serotonin: relationships to CSF amine metabolites. Am J Psychiatry. 1982;139(6):741-6.
8. Stanley B, Molcho A, Stanley M, Winchel R, Gameroff MJ, Parsons B, et al. Association of aggressive behavior with altered serotonergic function in patients who are not suicidal. Am J Psychiatry. 2000;157(4):609-14.
9. Bufkin JL, Luttrell VR. Neuroimaging studies of aggressive and violent behavior: current findings and implications for criminology and criminal justice. Trauma, Violence Abuse. 2005;6(2):176-91.
10. Scarpa A, Raine A. Psychophysiology of anger and violent behavior. Psychiatr Clin North Am. 1997;20(2):375-94.
11. Patrick CJ, Bradley MM, Lang PJ. Emotion in the criminal psychopath: Startle reflex modulation. J Abnorm Psychol. 1993;102(1):82-92.
12. Blue HC, Griffith EE. Sociocultural and therapeutic perspectives on violence. Psychiatr Clin North Am. 1995;18(3):571-87.
13. Beck AT. Prisoners of Hate: The Cognitive Basis of Anger, Hostility, and Violence. New York: HarperCollins Publishers; 1999.
14. Holcomb WR, Ahr PR. Arrest rates among young adult psychiatric patients treated in inpatient and outpatient settings. Hosp Community Psychiatry. 1988;39(1):52-7.
15. Lindqvist P, Allebeck P. Schizophrenia and assaultive behaviour: the role of alcohol and drug abuse. Acta Psychiatr Scand. 1990;82(3):191-5.
16. Steadman HJ, Mulvey EP, Monahan J, Robbins PC, Appelbaum PS, Grisso T, et al. Violence by people discharged from acute psychiatric inpatient facilities and by others in the same neighborhoods. Arch Gen Psychiatry. 1998;55(5):393-401.
17. Fazel S, Långström N, Hjern A, Grann M, Lichtenstein P. Schizophrenia, substance abuse, and violent crime. J Am Med Assoc. 2009;301:2016-23.
18. Fleischman A, Werbeloff N, Yoffe R, Davidson M, Weiser M. Schizophrenia and violence: a population-based study. Psychol Medicine. 2014;44:3051-7.
19. Short T, Thomas S, Mullen P, Ogloff JR. Comparing violence in schizophrenia patients with and without comorbid substance-use disorders to community controls. Acta Psychiatra Scand, 2013;128:306-13.
20. Swanson JW, Holzer CE 3rd, Ganju VK, Jono RT. Violence and psychiatric disorder in the community: evidence from the Epidemiologic Catchment Area surveys. Hosp Community Psychiatry. 1990;41(7):761-70.
21. Taylor PJ. Motives for offending among violent and psychotic men. Br J Psychiatry. 1985;147:491-8.
22. Petit JR. Management of the acutely violent patient. Psychiatr Clin North Am. 2005;28(3):701-11.
23. Witt K, van Dorn R, Fazel S. Risk factors for violence in psychosis: systematic review and meta-regression analysis of 110 studies. PloS One. 2013;8(2):e55942.
24. Davison S. The management of violence in general psychiatry. Adv Psychiatr Treat. 2005;11(5):362-70.
25. Royal College of Psychiatrists. Management of Imminent Violence: Clinical Practice Guidelines to Support Mental Health Services (Occasional Paper OP41). London: Royal College of Psychiatrists; 1998.
26. Rueve ME, Welton RS. Violence and mental illness. Psychiatry (Edgmont). 2008;5(5):34-48.
27. Osborn DPJ, Tang S. Effectiveness of audit in improving interview room safety. Psychiatr Bullet. 2001;25:92-4.
28. Galloway J. Personal safety when visiting patients in the community. Adv Psychiatr Treat, 2002;8(3):214-22.
29. Buckley PF, Noffsinger SG, Smith DA, Hrouda DR, Knoll JL 4th. Treatment of the psychotic patient who is violent. Psychiatr Clin North Am. 2003;26(1):231-72.
30. National Institute for Clinical Excellence. Short-term Management of Violent (Disturbed) Behaviour in Adult Psychiatric In-patient and Accident and Emergency Settings. Second Draft for Consultation. London: NICE; 2004.

SECTION 10: Ophthalmological Emergencies

Section Editor: *Jitendra Shah*

31. **Ophthalmic Emergencies**
    Jitendra Shah

CHAPTER 31: Ophthalmic Emergencies

Jitendra Shah

INTRODUCTION[1]

"Beautiful eyes look good in others. The heart smiles through the eyes." This phrase tells us the significance of our *eyes*. Sometimes physical or clinical injuries and pathophysiological changes of the eyes may end up in loss of vision if not treated in time.

The World Health Organization (WHO) has reported 55 million eye emergencies causing restriction of daily activities of which 1.6 million become blind everyday. The procedure of ocular trauma to be 2.4% of population in an urban city of India.

Eye emergencies include cuts, scratches, objects in the eye, burns, chemical exposure and blunt injuries to the eye or eyelid. Certain eye infections and other medical conditions, such as blood clots or glaucoma, may also need medicine care straightaway. Since the eye is easily damaged, any of these conditions can lead to vision loss if treated. Eye problems such as painful red eye or vision loss also need urgent medical attention.

DEFINITION

An emergency is defined as a condition requiring prompt medical attention due to sudden change in ocular health or vision.

Ophthalmologic emergencies are like most medical emergencies where there is a rather short window in which if things we have done effectively a lot damage can be controlled.

THE RED EYE

The topic that merits discussion first is the one that is most often seen—*the red eye*.

Upon seeing a red eye, the first thing that one should assess is—the red eye associated with pain and/or discharge, is there photophobia, vomiting, or reduced vision. **Table 1** may be helpful to understand the severity of an eye infection.[2]

While taking the history, it is important to check for trauma, general health, and drugs.

TABLE 1: Types of an eye infection with severity.

	Conjunctivitis	Anterior uveitis	Acute glaucoma
Discharge	++	Watering +	Watery ±
Redness	Throughout the surface	Usually around the cornea (limbal area)	Throughout the surface
Photophobic	±	++	-
Acuity of vision	Normal	Reduced	Reduced to 0 or very hazy
Pain	±	++	++++
Pupil	Normal	Small or irregular	Large, dilated
Intraocular pressure to be assessed digitally	Normal	Normal	+++

If conjunctivitis is suspected, a short regime of tropical antibiotics can be safely prescribed along with advice on ocular hygiene.

Should iritis be suspected then an ophthalmic referral is necessary. If there is a slightest hint a suspicion of acute glaucoma and an immediate ophthalmic referral is warranted, as a delay may result in blindness.

In addition to the above another reasonably common presentation of red eye is due to sub-conjunctival hemorrhage **(Fig. 1)**.

This is usually a self-limiting but alarming looking collection of blood behind the conjunctive from a small bleed. It may occur after a sudden or severe sneeze or cough, may lifting, straining, vomiting or even rubbing over eyes too roughly. It may also occur as a side effect of blood thinners (blood thinners may be stopped temporarily unless it is absolutely essential).

Management includes a detailed history of trauma or taking blood thinners. It is advisable to check blood pressure. If the hemorrhage does not resolve in 2–3 weeks then with ophthalmic opinion is warranted.

Immediate treatment may include reassurance and possibly some ocular lubricants like artificial tears.

Allergic (Vernal) Conjunctivitis

Here in addition to the redness there is often a complaint of intense itching.

The patients usually give a history of persistent itching, discomfort, watering and light sensitivity of the eyes. They are characteristically young and often have a history of additional atopic disease such as hay fever, eczema, and asthma.

Treatment includes typical steroid for the severe cases and sodium cromoglycate 2% and antihistamine eye drops to the less severe cases.

Note: Long-term steroid treatment should never be allowed as they can present later with complications such as cataract and glaucoma.

Keratitis

Acute inflammation of the cornea may present with rapid blurring of vision, redness, pain, photophobic and watering.

Important causes include:
- Adenoviral keratitis (where there may be preceding symptoms of fever, sore throat) and preauricular lymphadenopathy.
- Shingles (or Herpes Zoster ophthalmicus) which is usually associated with a typical painful rash.

■ EYE INJURIES AND IMMEDIATE CARE

Injuries of the eye are dramatic and can cause severe emotional distress to the patient. Some of the items that a clinic should preferably have include eye pad, cotton buds, micropore tape, single dose antibiotic eye drops, normal saline, and a torch for good illumination.

Suspected Foreign Body Injuries (Fig. 2)

When a foreign particle is suspected of being lodged in the eye a single dose of anesthetic eye drop should be instilled and the eye viewed under good illumination. A cotton bud may be used to remove the foreign particle and antibiotic eye drop instilled. No sharp instruments should be used.

If no foreign body is visualized and the patient is complaining of foreign body sensation and watery then the upper lid should be everted in the following manner. Surprisingly, many a time, a foreign body is found to be lodged under the upper eye lid **(Fig. 3)**.

Corneal Abrasion (Fig. 4)

The diagnosis can be easily established by using fluorescein eye drops. Antibiotic eye ointment should be used and eye patched and reviewed after 24 hours.

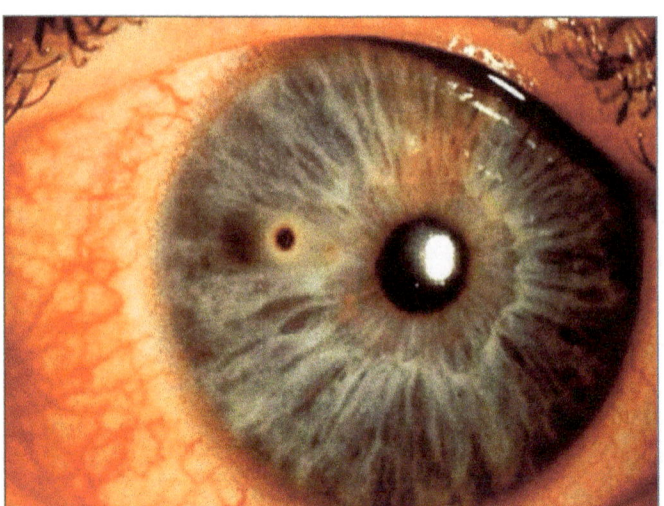

Fig. 1: Subconjunctival hemorrhage.

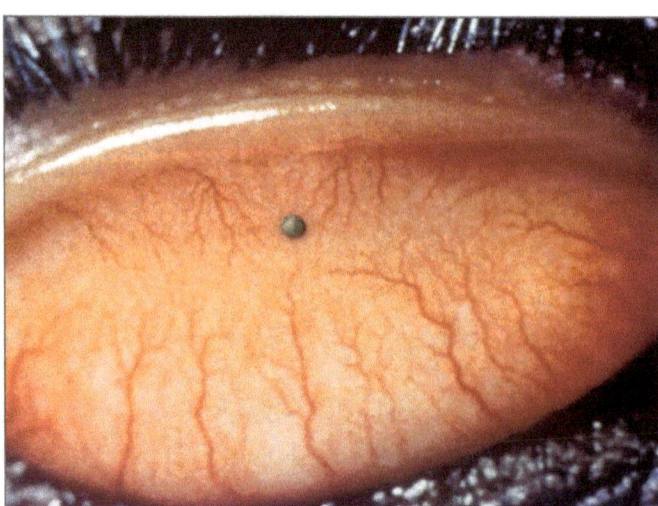

Fig. 2: Foreign body under the eye lid.

CHAPTER 31: Ophthalmic Emergencies

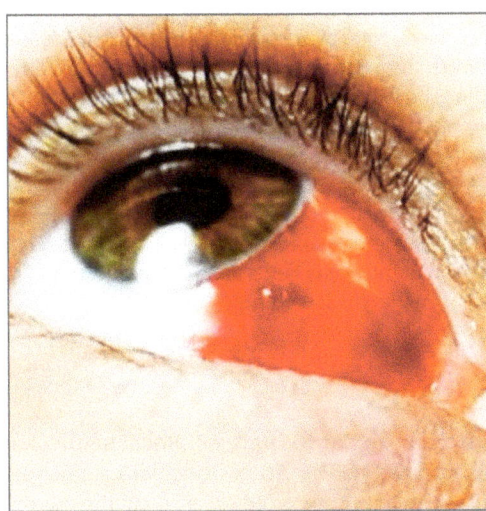

Fig. 3: Corneal foreign body.

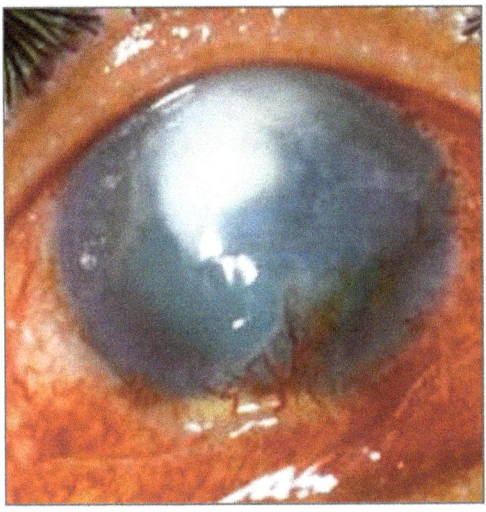

Fig. 5: Chemical injury.

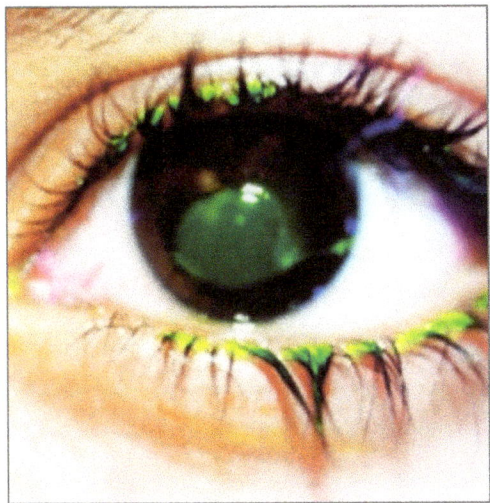

Fig. 4: Corneal abrasion.

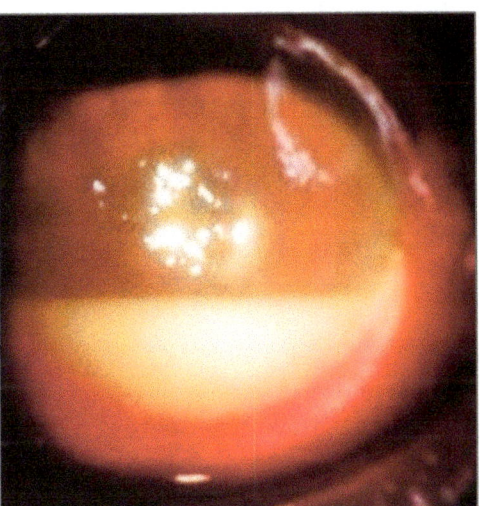

Fig. 6: Hyphema.

Chemical Injuries (Fig. 5)

The immediate management should be to immerse the eye under water and thorough washing of the eyes, preferably in running water for 20 minutes. Following this a specialist referral should be done at once.

Hyphema (Fig. 6)

This can be caused by a concussion injury to the eye from a blow, say a fist or some blunt object or some explosion.

The iris vessels rupture and as a result the blood collects between the cornea and the iris. They usually absorb in a weeks' time with adequate rest but an ophthalmic referral should be sought.

Orbital Injuries

They can result in periorbital hematinic proptosis or enophthalmos (due to blow out fracture of the orbit). One should seek further opinion at the earliest.

Penetrating Injuries

A sharp object may penetrate the eye and cause severe pain, watering, and loss of vision. Objects that may cause such injuries include darts, screw drivers, plant thorns, knives, flying metal pieces, etc. Immediate surgical repair should be initiated.

Take Home Messages

Suspected Foreign Particle in Eye

- *Patient presenting with foreign body sensation. Watering and/or pain. No rubbing of eyes, gentle eye bath. Administer local ocular lubricant and then refer.*
- *Sometimes waking up in the morning with watering and foreign body sensation with or without redness.* This could be due to corneal abrasion. To avoid rubbing of eyes or splashing water, ocular lubricants or antibiotic eye ointments can be used.
- *Sudden onset of redness and discomfort in a contact lens wearer.* Please ensure that the contact lens is out of the eye (in one piece). To commence some ocular lubricants and/or antibiotic eye ointment and to refer to ophthalmologist for further care.

- *Accidental spillage of household detergents in the eye.* Please ensure thorough and persistent eye wash/irritation. This is the single most step that will go long way in preventing further or long-standing damage.
- *Accidental injury due to cooking oils.* Avoid eye rubbing and gentle eye wash. This may be followed by application of ocular lubricants.
- *Injury to the eye by getting pricked by a thorn* or branch or any organic matter (especially during gardening or agricultural work). One must be very cautious about the potential of getting a fungal infection which is very resistant to therapy and needs meticulous management.

Sudden Loss of Vision[3]
The important points to consider are:
- Is it associated with headache (giant cell arteritis in the people aged 55 years and above). Check BP, blood for ESR.
- Are eye movements painful (optic neuritis needs to be considered as the most likely cause). This is usually associated with reduced color vision.
- Was this history of flashing lights that preceded the visual loss? In this case, it is important to rule out retrieval detachment.
- Was there any feeling of a descending curtain in the field of vision preceding the loss? In this case, amaurosis fugax may have been preceding the loss usually from an emboli or giant cell arteritis.
- Last but not the least it may be from a sudden vitreous bleed in a partly managed diabetic patient.
- *Last but not the least*—it is important to find out if the loss of vision is mono-ocular or binocular. One can very easily do a confrontation method of testing to clinically identify if the type of field loss. Hemianopia fields are quite suggestive of CUA and need to be managed accordingly.

REFERENCES

1. Kroesen CF, Snider M, Bailey J, Buchanan A, Karesh JW, La Piana F, et al. The ABCs of ocular trauma: adapting a familiar mnemonic for rapid eye exam in the pre-ophthalmic zone of care. Mil Med. 2020;185(Suppl 1):448-53.
2. Wills Eye Hospital. The Wills Eye Manual. Philadelphia: Lippincott Williams and Wilkins; 2017.
3. Denniston AK, Murray PI. Oxford Handbook of Ophthalmology. New York: Oxford University Press; 2018.

SECTION 11: ENT Emergencies

Section Editor: Ramanuj Sinha

32. **Emergencies in ENT**
    Ramanuj Sinha, Titas Kar, Tanya Panja, Preethi Rubinath

    32.1. **Foreign Bodies in ENT: A Nightmare for Patients and Doctors Alike!**
    Ramanuj Sinha, Titas Kar

    32.2. **Tracheostomy**
    Ramanuj Sinha, Tanya Panja

    32.3. **Otalgia**
    Ramanuj Sinha, Preethi Rubinath

CHAPTER 32

Emergencies in ENT

Ramanuj Sinha, Titas Kar, Tanya Panja, Preethi Rubinath

32.1 Foreign Bodies in ENT: A Nightmare for Patients and Doctors Alike!

Ramanuj Sinha, Titas Kar

INTRODUCTION

Foreign bodies constitute of about 11% otorhinolaryngological emergencies.[1] Children with their inherent tendency to put things into their mouth, nose or ears frequently result in a situation where the foreign body is irretrievable.[2] Parents usually notice about these accidents when the child turns up to them, visibly irritated or disturbed. The common vegetative items that children lay their hands on are peas, gram seeds, peanuts, seeds of various fruits. The nonvegetative items range from coins, earrings, rings, whistles, marbles, button batteries, erasers, pen caps, cotton buds, etc. Apart from these, foreign bodies might also end up involuntarily in the ear canals such as ants, cockroaches or other live insects.

TYPES OF FOREIGN BODIES IN ENT

A patient with ingestion of a coin (**Fig. 1**) or earring (**Fig. 2**) will usually have the foreign body stuck at one of the constrictions of the esophagus. These foreign bodies, being radiopaque are easily seen on a straight X-ray. A foreign body stuck in the esophagus for prolonged time will lead to

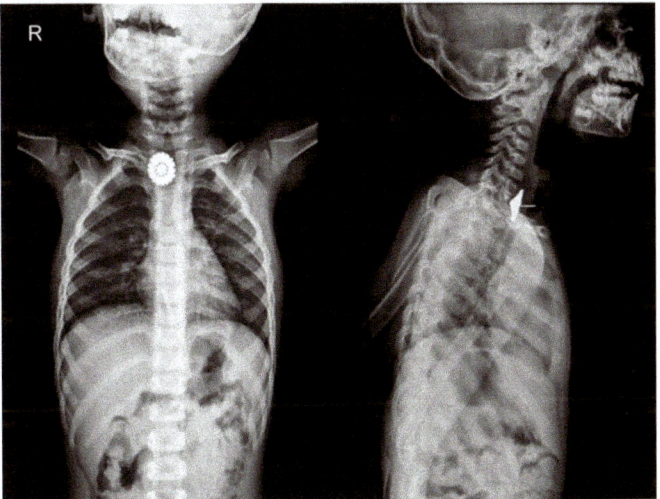

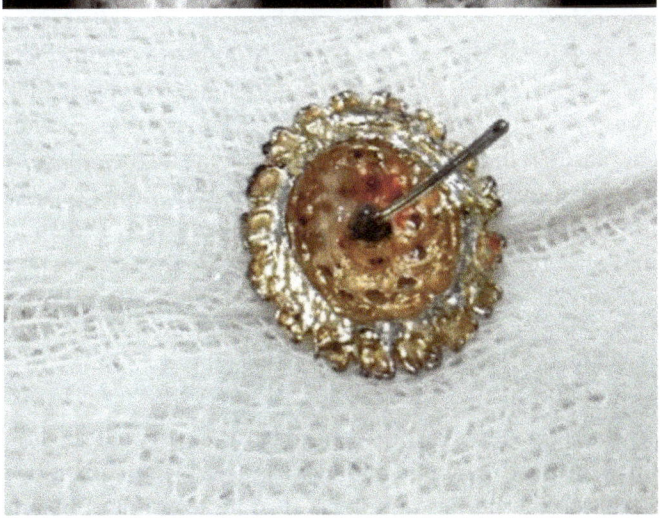

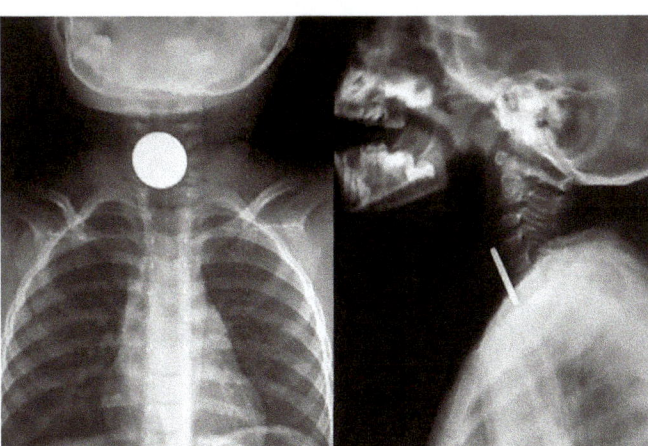

Fig. 1: Coin stuck at cricopharynx.

Fig. 2: Earring stuck at upper esophagus.

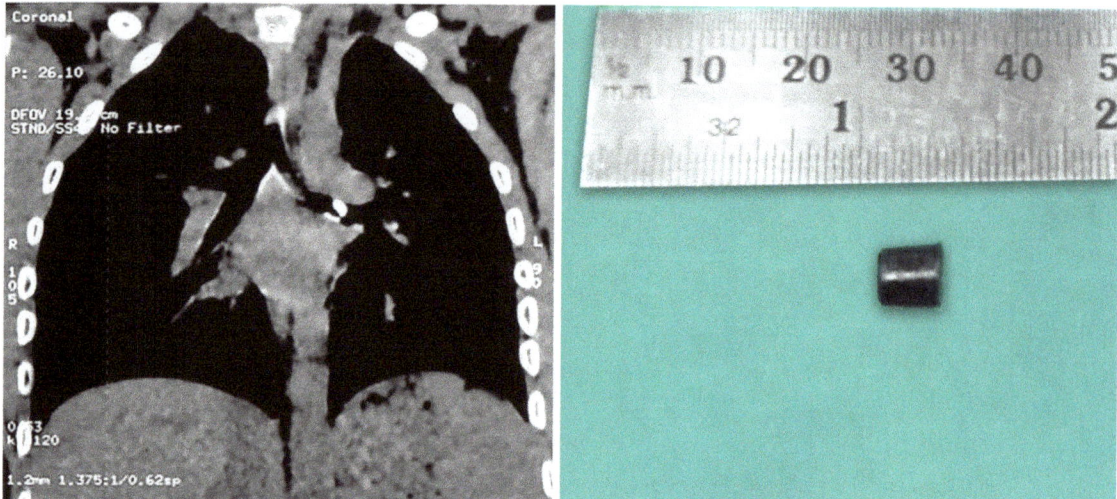

Fig. 3: Foreign body in left bronchus.

dysphagia to both solids and eventually to liquids as well, neck swelling, alteration of voice if they are in the upper esophagus. Such cases need to be brought to the emergency room (ER) with arrangement for esophagoscopic removal under general anesthesia. Under no circumstance should the parents be advised to make the foreign bodies pass by feeding the child bananas or any other fruits. When the foreign body is seen to be in the abdomen already, inspection of the stool of the child till it passes is advisable. Sometimes, removal of fish bones stuck in the throat in children can be difficult as an apprehensive and irritable child might make examination impossible. Even if removal is not possible immediately, the patient is to be put under antibiotic coverage and sent for removal of foreign body under sedation. A retained fish bone can lead to an abscess formation.

Foreign bodies in the bronchus (**Fig. 3**) constitute a dire emergency as such episodes can lead the child to rapidly deteriorate due to lack of ventilation in the lungs. The parents might notice the child suddenly having violent fits or cough after putting something in the mouth, with subsequent cyanosis. These patients are to be brought to the ER as soon as possible as time is of paramount importance in these cases of bronchoscopic removal under general anesthesia. These children often need pediatric ICU support even after successful removal of foreign body from the airway. In cases where there has been a foreign body which has passed on to a bronchus undetected and stayed there, the child may suffer from regular bouts of respiratory tract infection and atelectasis. Unexplained cough and LRTI in children with abnormalities in radiological investigations should raise the suspicion of an old undetected foreign body in a bronchus.

Foreign bodies in the nose can be seen just on lifting the tip of the nose. A foreign body hook is a useful tool to remove nasal foreign bodies if patients turn up to primary health care. The hook is to be introduced along the roof of the nose with the idea to go beyond the foreign body and then pull anteriorly. However, care should be taken so that the foreign body is not pushed backward onto the nasopharynx from where it can rapidly go into the airway. Difficult to localize foreign bodies might be found on X-rays and often, such cases are to be taken up under general anesthesia for removal under endoscopic vision. Of particular importance are the button batteries (**Fig. 4**) that power small electronic devices. Such batteries are dangerous for the chemicals they produce which can destroy the nasal septum causing gross charring and perforation of the septum.

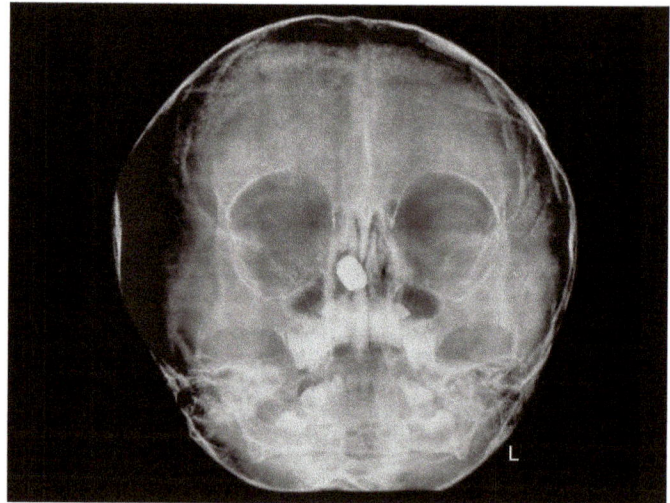

Fig. 4: Button battery seen in the nose which has eroded the nasal septum.

Ear foreign bodies are often quite small in size and can be attempted to be removed by syringing at primary health care facilities. Live insects are another nuisance. In these cases, trying to catch the insect within the ear is not advisable. Rather, instilling drops into the ear to kill the insect first should be the aim following which, the insect can be smoothly removed.

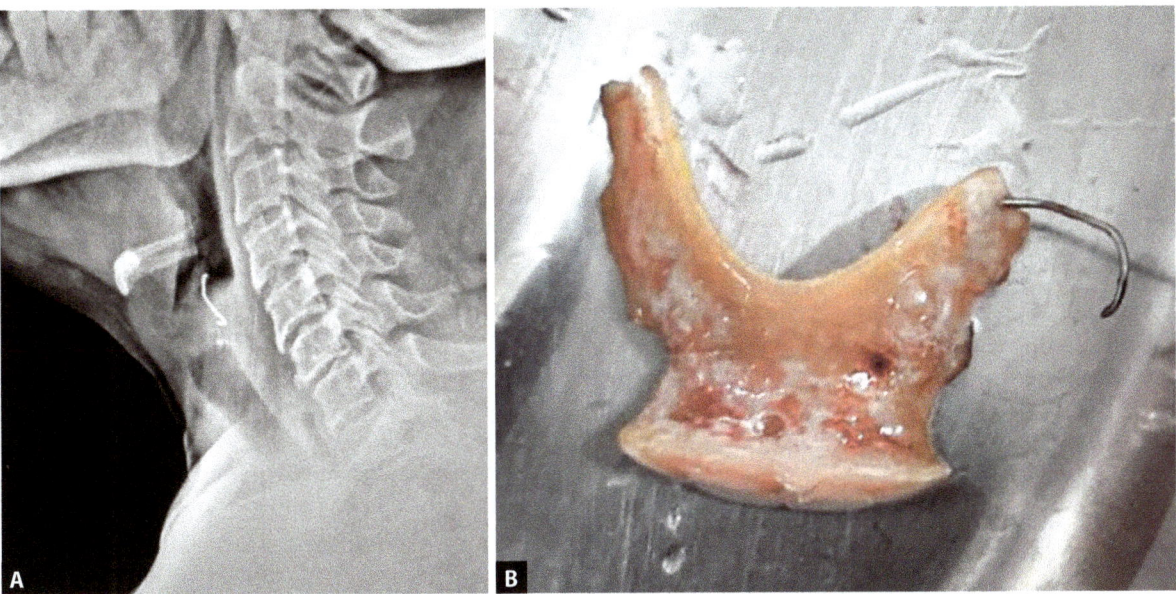

Figs. 5A and B: Wired denture stuck in throat (A); after removal (B)

The best way to avoid emergencies is by keeping small loose objects out of a child's reach[3] as keeping a watch on the child might not always be feasible. These foreign body ingestion cases can happen also in adults, who often swallow their dentures **(Figs. 5A and B)**. These require esophagoscopic removal. Dentures which have metal wires jutting out of them are quite problematic as they can damage the mucosa of the esophagus. Other causes of adult foreign bodies are by meat bones/bolus. Failure to remove such foreign bodies lead to the development of retropharyngeal abscesses.

Take Home Messages

Foreign bodies in the natural orifices of nose, throat and ears constitute one of the most common ENT emergencies. The best way to avoid emergencies is by keeping small loose objects out of a child as keeping a watch on the child might not always be feasible. These foreign body ingestion cases can happen also in adults, who swallow dentures or aspirate peanuts while talking. Most of these procedures require intervention by an ENT surgeon and so, the patient should be brought to the ER as soon as possible.

REFERENCES

1. Ribeiro da Silva BS, Souza LO, Camera MG, Tamiso AG, Castanheira VR. Foreign bodies in otorhinolaryngology: a study of 128 cases. Int Arch Otorhinolaryngol. 2009;13(4): 394-9.
2. Das SK. Aetiological evaluation of foreign bodies in the ear and nose. J Laryngol. Otol. 1984;98:989-91.
3. Ologe FE, Dunmade AD, Afolabi OA. Aural foreign body in children. Ind J Pediatr. 2007;74:755-8.

32.2 Tracheostomy

Ramanuj Sinha, Tanya Panja

BACK TO BASICS: PREOPERATIVE MANAGEMENT OF TRACHEOSTOMY

Otorhinolaryngology has emerged as a separate specialty only in the early 20th century, but since then, especially in the past three decades, it has evolved dramatically with the advent of endoscopy, microscopy, LASER, navigation, and newer anticancer drugs. Regardless of the technical advancements, what makes the otorhinolaryngologists unique and exclusive is the very basic and noble life-saving procedure, and emergency tracheostomy.

Tracheostomy is defined as the procedure for creating an opening in the anterior wall of trachea and converting it into a stoma on the skin surface.[1] It can either be an emergency procedure to alleviate acute upper airway obstruction at bedside or in emergency operation theater (OT) room, or an elective one as an alternative pathway of ventilation in the intensive care units (ICU) or surgical units.

The ancient Egyptian *hieroglyphics* documents the first attempted tracheostomy in 3100 BC.[2] In 4th century BC, Alexander the Great punctured the wall of trachea with sword to relieve a soldier from choking with a foreign body, i.e., meat bone in the battlefield.[3] Trousseau, in 1833 documented almost 200 cases of tracheostomy in patients with diphtheria.[1] Thereafter, huge rate of complication and morbidity demoralized the then physicians for attempting tracheostomy unless in dire emergency; until an article published in the *Laryngoscope* in 1909 in which Chevalier Jackson standardized the indication, surgical steps an precautions, helped in lowering the risk significantly.[4] The modern era started only in the 1960s and has introduced the scope of elective tracheostomy, percutaneous dilatational tracheostomy, and cricothyroidotomy.

Differential diagnosis of airway obstruction is almost always clinical. Wheezes are high pitched, continuous, adventitious sounds, produced mostly due to multiple small airway obstruction and is pathognomonic of bronchial asthma.[5] But, stridor is harsh, low pitched, monomorphic sound, mostly while expiration due to obstruction to larger upper airway, i.e., larynx and trachea with foreign body, malignant lesions, edema, etc.[5] More importantly, stridor signifies existing partial obstruction of upper respiratory tract and impending complete obstruction as well.

Apart from the Otorhinolaryngologists, General Surgeons, Onco-Surgeons, Pediatric Surgeons, Thoracic Surgeons, and Intensivists are specialists who are also qualified for performing a tracheostomy.[6] In elective surgeries, the surgeon team should do the tracheostomy.[6] In principle, any physician or surgeon can perform a tracheostomy, if they are confident enough regarding the anatomy and surgical steps, and willing to take responsibilities.[2]

An informed written consent is necessary from the patient and patient party, for elective and emergency procedure both, after properly explaining the intraoperative risks, postoperative complications and rehabilitation. In potentially lifesaving situations, where it is impossible and impractical to obtain a consent, tracheostomy can be done without consent under the emergency doctrine.[7] Bedside or in an OT, wherever the emergency procedure is performed, if possible, it is always advisable to have a team as backup.[8]

Once the patient comes, a thorough history is taken, including past medical and surgical history, and a thorough examination is done including vitals, i.e., sensorium, pulse, BP, SpO_2, CBG, etc., to assess the cause of upper airway obstruction and to check neck landmarks and extent of neck extension. The preoperative routine investigations are sent, patient and patient party are counseled regarding the absolute requirement of tracheostomy and it is postoperative sequelae. Reassurance and emotional support should be given as much as possible, and a preoperative assessment by a speech therapist is an additional in elective cases. Emergency tracheostomy is done by a vertical incision, whereas we put horizontal incision in the elective procedure, along with creation of a tracheal flap. The postoperative set up is arranged in ward or ICU beforehand, with provision of giving oxygen via T-piece, pulse oximeter, nebulization, back-rest and suction machine, where the patient will be kept along with a bystander for the next few days.

But, in our country, most of the cases turn up with severe stridor, giving time only for the very basic history taking, clinical examination, i.e., vitals, counseling and consent signing. The patients' group in India are mostly smokers, with associated chronic obstructive pulmonary disease and lower respiratory tract infection, and are prone to an acute CO_2 washout just immediate to tracheostomy. That is why in our daily practice, we give routine preoperative oxygenation and nebulization with bronchodilators to candidates for emergency tracheostomy to prevent postoperative apnea to some extent.

Over the last 50 years, the incidence of pediatric tracheostomy has decreased, mostly due to improvement in immunization protocol. The indication has shifted from acute upper airway obstruction in diphtheria or croup to need for prolonged mechanical ventilation due to subglottic stenosis or any neurological disease.[9] The parents need to be thoroughly counseled regarding the postoperative rehabilitation and probable line of definitive management.

Elective tracheostomy should be avoided in coronavirus disease 2019 (COVID-19) positive patients in mechanical ventilation when they are unstable and ventilator-dependent, to avoid aerosol generation and spread of infection;[10] it can be considered after 2-3 weeks of intubation[10] preferably with negative COVID report. During acute upper airway obstruction, a tracheostomy should not be delayed by waiting for the definitive COVID report, rather a negative rapid antigen test performed just prior to OT will suffice.

Elective tracheostomy is considered when there is requirement of endotracheal intubation for 14-21 days[1] for mechanical ventilation. It is difficult to mobilize this type of patients to the OT, leading to advent of bedside percutaneous tracheostomy technique. It was first described by Shelden et al. in 1955[11] which was later modified by Ciaglia et al. using the Seldinger technique.[12] The Ciaglia technique is performed by a Cook Blue Rhino Single Dilator Kit, with a transverse incision just below the cricoid cartilage, under direct visualization via bronchoscopy. In a meta-analysis comparing percutaneous and open procedure, Higgins and Punthakee showed that the complication rate was similar[13] and the trend is favoring the percutaneous tracheostomy.

Cricothyroidotomy is an uncomplicated, safe, rapid but temporary procedure for maintenance of airway, especially in emergencies, and needs to be replaced by a permanent tracheostomy in 24-72 hours.[14] It is done when there is a difficulty in intubation, or when acute emergency airway is required, at bedside only. 32% was due to facial fracture requiring urgent airway, 11% due to intubation failure[15] as per Chang et al. in 1998.

Tracheostomy is one of those very basic yet challenging surgical procedures that gives instant relief to the patients and is very rewarding for the surgeons, too. All the preoperative preparations need to be done very calmly yet promptly, and the preoperative counseling should be thorough. The surgical steps can be performed either skillfully or with hesitancy, either at an ICU set up or in areas with very minimal medical support, either by a renowned Onco-Surgeon or by a postgraduate trainee of otorhinolaryngology, tracheostomy should remain the same noble and dramatic lifesaving procedure.

Take Home Messages

Although having various postoperative morbidities such as inability to phonate, perform any strenuous work or swim, a timely performed tracheostomy, after all, can save a life, and that makes it mandatory for the family members to take patients with acute onset respiratory distress and stridor urgently to nearest hospital facility.

■ REFERENCES

1. Dhingra PL, Dhingra S. Diseases of Ear, Nose, Throat and Head and Neck Surgery, 7th edition. New Delhi: Elsevier Publication; 2017. pp. 359.
2. Pires de Farias T. Tracheostomy A Surgical Guide. Switzerland: Springer International Publishing; 2018.
3. Gordon BL, FA Davis. The Romance of Medicine. Philadelphia: FA Davis; 1947. pp. 461.
4. Jackson C. Tracheostomy. Laryngoscope. 1909;19:285.
5. Hollingsworth HM. Wheezing and stridor. Clin Chest Med. 1987;8(2):231-40.
6. Portal Educação [Education Portal]. Google Analytics. [online] Available from: http:www.portalmedico.org.br/pareceres/2009/15_2009.htm. [Last Accessed January, 2023].
7. Segen's Medical Dictionary. (2011). Emergency doctrine. [online] Available from: https://medical-dictionary.thefreedictionary.com/emergency+doctrine. [Last Accessed January, 2023].
8. Portal Educação [Education Portal]. Google Analytics. [online] Available from: http:www.portalmedico.org.br/pareceres/CFM/2015/12_2015.pdf. [Last Accessed January, 2023].
9. Lewis CW, Carron JD, Perkins JA, Sie KC, Feudtner C. Tracheotomy in pediatric patients: a national perspective. Arch Otolaryngol Head Neck Surg. 2003;129(5): 523-7.
10. Parker NP, Schiff BA, Fritz MA, Rapport SA, Schild S, Altman KW, et al. Tracheotomy Recommendations During the COVID-19 Pandemic. Am Acad Otorhinolaryngol Head Neck Surg. 2021:8.
11. Shelden CH, Pudenz RH, Freshwater DB, Crue BL. A new method for tracheotomy. J Neurosurg. 1955;12:428-31.
12. Ciaglia P, Firsching R, Syniec C. Elective percutaneous dilatational tracheostomy. A new simple bedside procedure; preliminary report. Chest. 1985;87:715-9.
13. Higgins KM, Punthakee X. Meta-analysis comparison of open vs percutaneous tracheostomy. Laryngoscope. 2007;117:447-54.
14. Toon SSH, Stephens RCM, Smith H. The emergency airway. Br J Hosp Med. 2009;70(12):186-8.
15. Chang RS, Hamilton RJ, Carter WA. Declining rate of cricothyroidotomy in trauma patients with an emergency residency: implications for skills training. Acad Emerg Med. 1998;5(3):247-51.

32.3 OTALGIA

Ramanuj Sinha, Preethi Rubinath

■ INTRODUCTION

Otalgia or earache is a debilitating symptom commonly occurring in both children and adults. These patients attend the emergency room in hopes of immediate relief from the pain **(Flowchart 1)**.

The first step is to determine if the pain is primary or referred.

Primary otalgia can be diagnosed by careful examination of the pinna, external auditory canal, and tympanic membrane. In the presence of a normal ear, the source of referred otalgia poses a diagnostic challenge due to the diverse sensory innervation of the ear.

■ PRIMARY CAUSES OF OTALGIA

Perichondritis

The inflammation or infection of the perichondrium of the external ear is termed as perichondritis. It usually follows trauma ranging from piercings to lacerations, or spread of superficial infections of the pinna or external auditory canal to involve the perichondrium. The most common presenting symptom is dull aching pain with increasing severity. Swelling and erythema often accompanies, and may even progress to subperichondrial abscess formation with cartilage destruction. *Pseudomonas aeruginosa, Streptococcus* spp., and *Staphylococcus aureus* are the common organisms implicated.

First line of management would be to use broad-spectrum antibiotics, possibly intravenously, along with antipseudomonal cover. Analgesics are they key to help control the immense pain. Incision drainage with regular dressings is advocated in case of abscess. Resistant cases require extensive workup and surgical excision.[1]

Acute Otitis Externa

A disruption in the lipid/acid balance of the skin of the external auditory canal predisposes to otitis externa which is characterized by edema, erythema and associated pain, itch, and discharge. It may also present with purulent otorrhea and debris within the meatus following secondary bacterial infection. Eczematous skin, macerated skin, and hot and humid conditions are some predisposing factors. Commonly involved organisms include *Pseudomonas aeruginosa*, other gram-negative species and *Staphylococcus aureus*.[2] Aural toileting followed by broad-spectrum systemic (oral) antibiotics, analgesics, and topical therapy using steroid and antibiotics with or without a wick forms the mainstay of the treatment.

Otomycosis

Fungal otitis externa often occurs secondary to prolonged use of topical antibiotics or immunocompromised individuals, like diabetics. *Aspergillus* (80–90%) and *Candida* (10–20%)

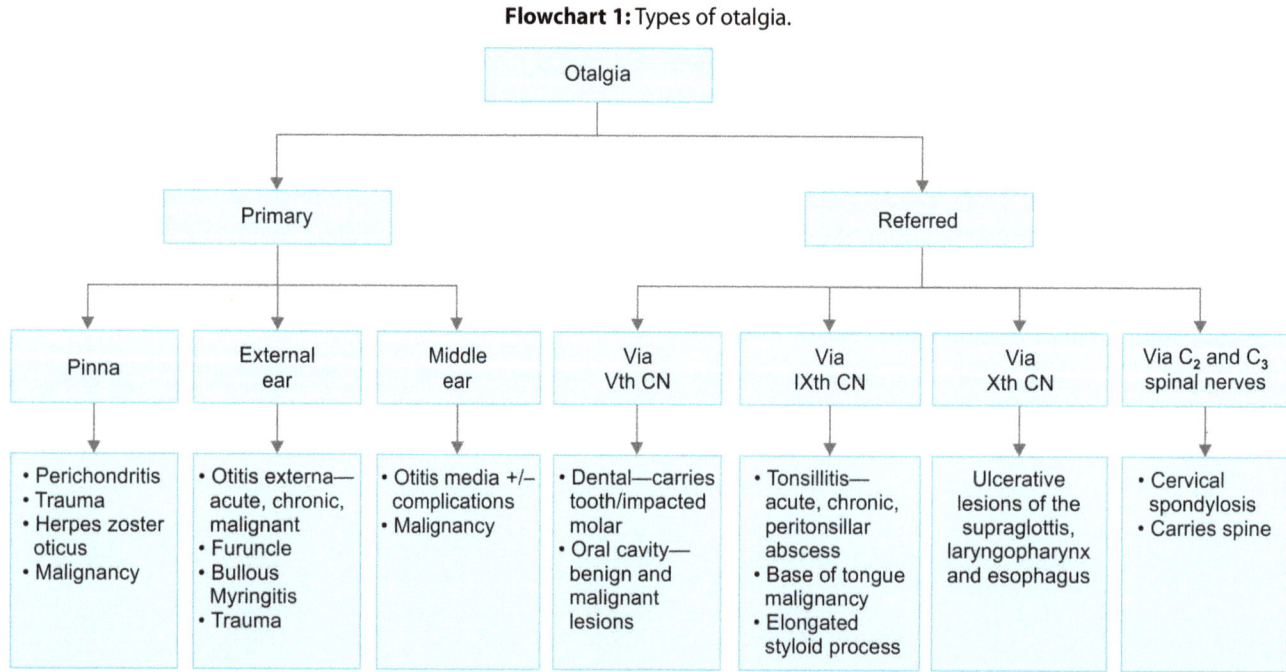

Flowchart 1: Types of otalgia.

(CN: cranial nerve)

are the typically involved species. In addition to pain, the most common finding is black, brown, gray, or white discharge with debris and at times fungal hyphae may also be visible. Aural toilet with removal of debris is the treatment of choice, but topical antifungals are used to expedite the recovery along with analgesics and systemic antibiotics to prevent superadded bacterial infection.

Malignant Otitis Externa

Malignant otitis externa is an invasive infection of the ear canal typically affecting immunocompromised individuals, particularly the elderly, and poorly controlled diabetics. The most common organism implicated is *Pseudomonas*. This aggressive disease can spread to involve the middle ear, lower cranial nerves, and even lead to skull base osteomyelitis. Other than otalgia clinical features include granulation in the middle ear, discharge in the canal, and facial palsy in advanced cases. Ciprofloxacin is the antibiotic of choice, but in resistant cases, ceftazidime, piperacillin, or imipenem can be used. Strong analgesics may be required along with monitoring and control of blood sugar levels.

Furunculosis

Staphylococcal infection of a single hair follicle within the lateral segment of the external auditory canal is called furunculosis. It is characterized by extremely painful and tender ear, with severe edema blocking the canal and scanty serosanguinous discharge. Examination is a challenge due to the immense pain. Optimal treatment combines specific antistaphylococcal antibiotics (macrolide, cephalosporin, clindamycin, and penicillinase-resistant penicillin) with strong analgesia and topical treatment to reduce the swelling (glycerol and icthymol solution on a wick).[3]

Herpes Zoster Oticus

Reactivation of the latent varicella zoster virus in the geniculate ganglion can produce a peripheral facial nerve palsy accompanied by erythematous vesicular rash on the ear and otalgia. The recommended regime of prednisone (1 mg/kg × 5 days followed by 10 days taper) and antiviral (acyclovir—800 mg 5 times/day × 7 days) reduces the associated vertigo, otalgia, and postherpetic neuralgia.

Acute Otitis Media

Acute inflammation of the middle ear cleft with rapid onset and infective origin, more commonly seen in children than adults, generally presents with the cardinal signs of otalgia, hearing loss, and tinnitus. Bacterial infection (*Haemophilus influenzae*) accounts for majority of the adult acute otitis media (AOM) cases whereas respiratory viruses are associated with 60–90% of AOM cases in children.[4] Although otoscopy might be challenging, the most reliable indicator has been found to be the bulging of tympanic membrane. Analgesics and antipyretics form the mainstay of the treatment, but antibiotics like amoxicillin can be used, especially in recurrent cases.

■ CAUSES OF REFERRED OTALGIA

The rich and diverse sensory supply of the ear signifies that the origin of referred otalgia is equally widely distributed throughout the head and neck, perhaps even beyond. It is incumbent upon us to, therefore, examine the peripheral areas and the presence of a normal ear, canal, and tympanic membrane. Any pathology that may involve the sensory divisions of cranial nerves V, VII, IX, X, and cervical nerves C_2 and C_3 can produce referred otalgia.

Dental Disorders

The trigeminal nerve is the most commonly involved and accounts for 5.75% of referred otalgia, specifically due to dental disorders. Dental carries and impacted molar causing pulpitis and periodontitis respectively are the major causes.

Temporomandibular joint (TMJ) dysfunction syndrome produces diffuse pain (around TMJ), crepitus, trismus, and otalgia in 64% of the cases.[5] Bruxism is the major causative factor and tenderness of the masticatory muscles is common finding. Initial treatment should include a nonsteroidal anti-inflammatory analgesic along with soft diets before further management by maxilla-facial surgeons.

Cervical

Cervical otalgia affects the older age groups through the posterior auricular and lesser occipital nerves. Cervical spine degenerative disease may be treated conservatively with analgesia and physiotherapy before referring for expert opinion and management.

Tonsillitis

Otalgia seen in tonsillitis via Jacobson's nerve (CN IX) is common in young children. It may also be seen 5–7 days post-tonsillectomy. Simple analgesics for treating the primary cause should be sufficient.

Malignancy

Otalgia can either be a part or the sole symptom of an oropharyngeal malignancy. The malignancies usually arise from the lateral pharyngeal wall, tonsil, or the base of the tongue. It is therefore essential to subject such patients with high suspicion to full examination of the oral cavity, pharynx, and larynx through flexible nasendoscopy.

Neoplasms of the infratemporal fossa can also cause referred otalgia through the trigeminal nerve, Jacobson's nerve, and Arnold's nerve.

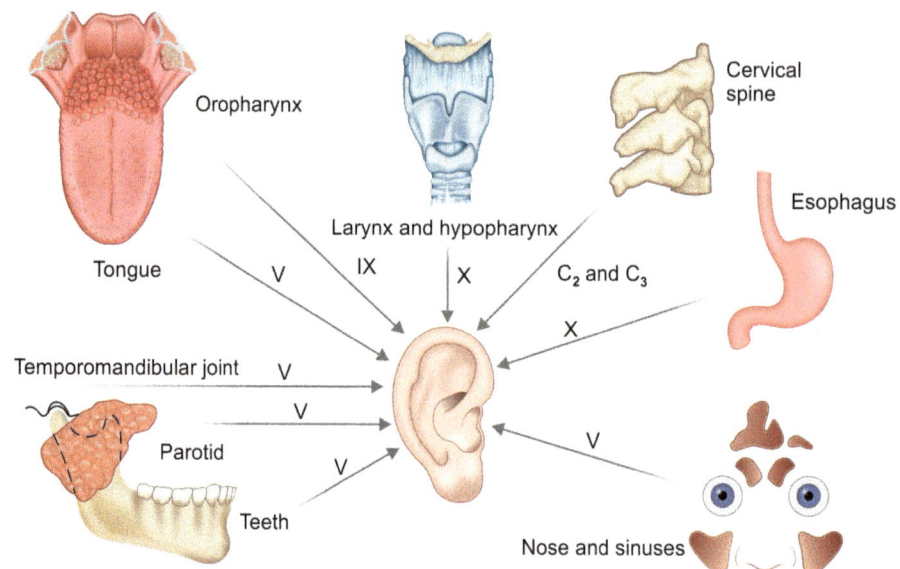

Fig. 1: Various causes of referred otalgia.[6]
(*Source:* Dhillon RS, East CA. Ear, Nose and Throat and Head and Neck Surgery: An Illustrated Colour Text, 3rd edition. London, United Kingdom: Churchill Livingstone; 2006.)

Temporal bone malignancies may present with otalgia in the presence of preauricular swelling and facial nerve weakness.

Neuralgia

Eagle's syndrome or stylohyoid syndrome produces neuralgia via CN IX due to an elongated styloid process or mineralization on stylohyoid ligament. Although surgical management is preferred, initial treatment with steroids and local anesthetic along with carbamazepine has been suggested.

Trigeminal neuralgia and postherpetic neuralgia are the most common forms, but rare forms of glossopharyngeal and geniculate neuralgia have also been encountered.

Miscellaneous

Compression or stretching of the nervus intermedius in case of vestibular schwannoma has been noted to cause otalgia in 4–5% of cases.

Since the mucosa of the upper airway is proposed to be more sensitive to acid exposure, laryngopharyngeal reflux disease is thought to cause otalgia in both adults and children, especially in the absence of other typical symptoms.

Cholesterol granuloma and subdural hematoma are other causes noted.

In all cases of referred otalgia, proper examination, initial conservative management with analgesics, and appropriate referral to experts for further management is indicated **(Fig. 1)**.

Take Home Messages

We must acknowledge that otalgia, though a simple symptom can implicate a wide range of diagnoses; varying from an obvious ear pathology to being the sole clue to an underlying malignancy. Although the incidence of the latter is less commonly encountered in an emergency room, it must nevertheless be kept in mind while managing any patient of otalgia.

■ REFERENCES

1. Pattanaik S. Effective, simple treatment for perichondritis and pinna haematoma. J laryngol Otol. 2009;123:1246-9.
2. Sundström J, Jacobson K, Munck Wikland E, Ringertz S. *Pseudomonas aeruginosa* in otitis externa: A particular variety of the bacteria? Arch Otolaryngol Head Neck Surg. 1996;122(8):833-6.
3. Ahmed K, Roberts ML, Mannion PT. Antimicrobial activity of glycerine-ichthammol in otitis externa. Clin Otolaryngol Allied Sci. 1995;20:201-3.
4. Heikkinen T. The role of respiratory viruses in otitis media. Vaccine. 2001;19:S51-5.
5. Tuz HH, Onder EM, Kisnisci RS. Prevalence of otologic complaints in patients with temporomandibular disorder. Am J Orthod Dentofacial Orthop. 2003;123(6):620-3.
6. Dhillon RS, East CA. Ear, Nose and Throat and Head and Neck Surgery: An Illustrated Colour Text, 3rd edition. London, United Kingdom: Churchill Livingstone; 2006.

SECTION 12

Pediatric Emergencies

Section Editor: Arun Kumar Manglik

33. **Pediatric Emergencies**
    Arun Kumar Manglik, Gautam Ghosh, Mihir Sirkar, Nitin Manglik

CHAPTER 33: Pediatric Emergencies

Arun Kumar Manglik, Gautam Ghosh, Mihir Sirkar, Nitin Manglik

INTRODUCTION

The assessment of a sick child starts from the moment the child is brought to the doctor, either in the OPD or emergency. While the child is being brought in, the doctor gets an immediate visual cue, how sick this child maybe by simply looking at the child. The child's level of alertness, looking toward the mother and surroundings, the breathing pattern and color are enough for the doctor to make a quick assessment in just a few seconds.

ASSESSMENT

Assessment of the patient should follow a pattern. The important clinical assessment and examinations with their description have been described in **Tables 1 and 2**.

After the *First look assessment*, one now goes into further assessing the clinical status of the child in a systematic fashion. The primary assessment follows the A-B-C-D pattern, i.e., airway, breathing circulation and disability **(Table 3)**.

Breathing

Evaluation includes:
- Respiratory rate
- Respiratory effort
- Chest rise/tidal volume
- Airway and lung sounds
- Pulse oximetry.

TABLE 1: Types of clinical assessment in a child.

Clinical assessment	Description
First look assessment	*Visual and auditory* assessment of: Appearance, work of breathing and circulation *(within few seconds of seeing patient)*
Primary assessment	Hands-on ABCD approach to evaluate *(it includes vital signs and pulse oximetry)*
Secondary assessment	• Focused medical history • SAMPLE (Signs/symptoms, Allergies, Medicines, Past illness, Last meal, Events leading to current status) • Complete physical examination: From head to toe
Tertiary assessment	Investigations

TABLE 2: First look Assessment: Using visual and auditory clues in a few seconds.

First look	Assessment
Appearance	*Look/gaze, interaction,* speech/cry or consolability, muscle tone
Work of breathing	How is the respiratory effort, abnormal respiratory sounds
Color	Pink, pale, blue, mottled, bleeding

TABLE 3: Primary assessment: Airway and circulation.

Status	Description
Clear	Open and unobstructed, the child is in comfort
Maintainable	Maintained by simple measures, i.e., simply extending the neck maybe, mostly the child would spontaneously maintain the position of comfort
Not maintainable	Needs advanced measures, e.g., an oropharyngeal airway, herein the child's sensorium is very likely to be on the downside
Cardiovascular function	**Indirect assessment: End-organ function**
• Heart rate • Peripheral and central pulses: regularity, volume (radial/femoral/brachial) • Capillary refill time (CRT) ≤3 seconds • Blood pressure • Minimum: >1 year: 70 + age × 2	• Level of consciousness: Brain perfusion/AVPU • (Awake/response to Voice /Response to Pain/Unresponsive) • Skin perfusion (cool and pale/warm and vivid) • Renal perfusion (urine output) • When last passed urine

TABLE 4: Upper airway obstruction (UAO): Features of some types.

Clinical finding	Croup	Bacterial tracheitis	Retropharyngeal abscess	Epiglottitis
Stridor	+	+	+	+
Voice alteration	Hoarse	Hoarse	Hoarse	Muffled
Dysphagia	–	–	++	+
Postural preference	+	+	+	+
Barking cough	+++	++	+	–
Fever	+	+++	+++	+++
Toxicity	–	++	++	++
Treatment	Nebulized adrenaline/steroid	Antibiotics	Antibiotics/surgical drain	Antibiotic/No X-ray

Disability

Temperature, AVPU/Glasgow Coma scale, Pupils
A = Alert, V = responds to voice, P = responds to Pain, U = Unresponsive

■ APPROACH TO A BREATHLESS CHILD

Categorization and clinical clues: Clinical cues do guide us to the cause and our interventions.

By Rapidity of Onset

- *Hyperacute:* Foreign body (FB), anaphylaxis
- *Acute:* Pneumonia/bronchiolitis
- *Chronic:* Cardiac/chronic lung disease (less common)
- *Intermittent/recurrent:* Asthma/aspiration syndromes.

By Location of Pathology/Etiology

- *Respiratory:* Apart from increased respiratory rate and effort, some added sounds
- *Upper airway obstruction (UAO):* Stridor, suprasternal retractions **(Table 4)**
- *Lower airway obstruction (LAO):* Wheeze, subcostal retractions
- *Lung tissue disease:* Grunt, intercostal retractions
- *Cardiac:* Tachycardia ++/silent tachypnea/rales+
- *Metabolic:* Quiet tachypnea with a clear chest.

Foreign Body: Management Priorities

- *Incomplete obstruction:* Allow position of comfort; allow to continue coughing/O_2
- *If complete obstruction:* Heimlich (>1 year)/back blows and chest thrusts (<1 year)/laryngobronchoscopy to remove FB.

Anaphylaxis

Suspect anaphylaxis if there is acute onset (minutes to hours) of urticaria, flushing, swollen lips/tongue/uvula with any of the following: respiratory distress, stridor hypoxemia, hypotension, syncope, abdominal pain, and vomiting.

TABLE 5: Community-acquired pneumonia.

Age	Common	Less common
Birth to 20 days	E. coli, other Gram 3-ve, GBS, Listeria	Gr B strep, anaerobes
3 weeks to 3 months	S. pneumoniae, Chlamydia	HIB, S. aureus
4 months to 5 years	S. pneumoniae, HiB, viruses, mycoplasma, chlamydia,	Moraxella, S. aureus
Beyond 5 years	S. pneumoniae, mycoplasma, chlamydia	HIB, S. aureus, viruses

Etiology:

- Food (peanut, shellfish, egg, and milk)
- Insect sting
- Medications (e.g., penicillins)
- Exercise
- idiopathic.

Treatment:

- Injectable epinephrine: 0.01 mg/kg (i.e., 0.01 mL/kg of 1:1,000 which is available in India) given IM at anterolateral thigh, repeat every 15 min if required
- Oral/IV diphenhydramine 1–2 mg/kg (maximum 50 mg)
- Oral/IV promethazine 0.5 mg/Kg (maximum 10 mg)
- Transport to emergency facility
- Oxygen and airway management.

Childhood Asthma

Remember the red flag signs **(Table 5)**:

- *Unable to talk or cry:* Cyanosis
- *Feeble chest movements:* Absent breath sound
- *Fatigue/exhausted/agitated:* Altered sensorium
- SpO_2 <92%

Treatment:

- Oxygen
- Nebulized salbutamol (Albuterol) (β_2-agonist)
- Minimum dose is 1.25 mg <6 months, 2.5 mg >6 months and 2.5–5 mg for older children (always dilute in normal

TABLE 6: Blood pressure and circulation time in children.

Age	Systolic BP, 5th cent, minimum	50th cent, i.e., average
Term neonates (0–28 days)	<60	<70
Infants (1–12 months)	<70	<80
Children 1–10 years	70 + (age × 2)	90 + (age × 2)
Children >10 years	<90	110

TABLE 7: Maintenance fluid volume requirement as per Holliday and Segar formula.

Body weight	Energy requirement	Fluid requirement
For the first: 3–10 kg	100 cal/kg/day	100 mL/kg/day
Plus, for next: 11–20 kg	50 cal/kg/day	50 mL/kg/day
Plus, for any weight >20 kg	20 cal/kg/day	20 mL/kg/day

saline only, never distilled water)/may aggravate hypoxemia initially—use O_2 to drive the nebulizer. Repeat salbutamol nebulized x3, every 20 mins.
- Equally effective at home or clinic is salbutamol Inhaler (MDI), with spacer (and add mask if below 6 years). Six puffs with MDI/spacer = one nebulization[1]
- *Steroids:* (oral/parenteral)/All equally efficacious: (Prednisolone/Methylprednisolone/Hydrocortisone)
- Add neb with Ipratropium bromide (no benefit after 24 hours)
- *ICU:* Magnesium sulfate/aminophylline/terbutaline may be used

Acute breathlessness:

Fever ++	Fever +/–	Hepatomegaly
Pneumonia	Bronchiolitis	Cardiac

Danger signs requiring admission:
- Severe respiratory distress
- Hypoxia/cyanosis
- Toxic appearance
- Dehydration
- Significant comorbid disease, e.g., malnutrition
- Parent or caretaker unable to cope or comply
- Immune deficiency.

Acute metabolic breathlessness = metabolic acidosis
- Quiet tachypnea
- Normal chest findings
- Normal cardiovascular findings
- Normal SpO_2.

Approach to Shock
- Clinical state of inadequate tissue perfusion resulting in insufficient metabolic substrate supply especially O_2 to meet metabolic demands
- Shock is *not* defined by blood pressure, rather classified by BP, i.e., compensated or hypotensive **(Table 6)**
- Early signs (in compensated)
- Increased heart rate, thready peripheral pulses, poor systemic perfusion
- Late signs (decompensated)
- Weak central pulses, altered mental status, hypotension.

Management involves taking care of the airway, i.e., positioning the child, 100% O_2 to start with, ideally by non-rebreathing mask or head box, IV fluids, and close monitoring.

Administration of intravenous fluid (IVF) is the most common intervention done in hospitalized children.

Fluid is a drug and we should pay attention regarding dose, side effect and monitoring.

Adequate fluid management involves:
- Resuscitation fluid for shock
- Maintenance requirements
- Repleting deficits
- Compensating ongoing losses.

BASIC FLUID THERAPY

Resuscitation Fluid for Shock

Goal is to restore intravascular volume immediately. 10-20 mL/kg of isotonic fluid: 0.9% NaCl is most commonly used. It is cheap and easily available.

Balanced salt solution such as Ringer's lactate or Plasmalyte, if patient requires high volume of resuscitation fluid >40 mL/kg or hyperchloremia is noted.

Five percent albumin, if patient has severe hypoalbuminemia or requiring high volume of crystalloids.

MAINTENANCE

The goal of maintenance therapy is the accurate replacement of ongoing water and electrolyte losses to maintain zero balance so that *all intakes = all outputs.*

Holliday and Segar (*Pediatrics*, 1957) proposed that **(Table 7)** water requirement was based on the energy expenditure of healthy children, with 1 mL of fluid provided for each kilocalorie (kcal) expended. The resting energy expenditure in healthy children is vastly different in those with an acute disease and/or illness or after surgery (averages 50 to 60 kcal/kg per day). So, Holliday and Segar formula overestimates fluid requirements of sick children.

Electrolytes: The electrolyte concentration of IVFs was estimated to reflect the composition of human and cow milk. The final composition consisted of 3 mEq of sodium and 2 mEq of potassium per 100 kcal metabolized. But most

TABLE 8: Features in different degrees of dehydration and fluid requirements.

Degree of dehydration	% volume of depletion	Signs and symptoms	
Mild	3–5% (30 mL/kg)	Thirst, decrease in urine output, dry mucous membrane	WHO-ORS in case of diarrhea if accepts orally with a volume of 50–60 mL/kg over 4 hours in small aliquots
Moderate	6–10% (60 mL/kg)	Postural changes in BP, heart rate, dry mucous membranes, sunken eyes and fontanel, skin tenting, listlessness, and tachycardia	
Severe	>10% (100 mL/kg)	Poor perfusion, tachycardia, hypotension, lethargy, and coma	100 mL/kg NS or RL IV over 2–3 hours in >1 years of age or 5–6 hours in case of infants or malnourished (SAM) child

Note: No antibiotics, oral Zinc 20 mg/day (10 mg/day in <6 months) for 14 days.

TABLE 9: Composition of different IV fluids used in pediatric ICU.

Fluids	Na⁺ mmol/L	K⁺ mmol/L	Cl⁻ mmol/L	Carbohydrate gm/dl	Bicarbonate mmol/L (converted)	Osmolarity mOsm/L
Normal saline	154	0	154	0	0	308
Ringer lactate	130	4	109	0	28	273
5% dextrose	0	0	0	5	0	252
Plasmalyte*	140	5	98		27	295

*Balanced salt solution

hyponatremia in patients who are hospitalized is hospital acquired and related to the administration of hypotonic IVFs in the setting of elevated AVP concentrations. *Use of 1/5th DNS (Isolyte-P) or so called "pediatric" solutions for maintenance in inpatients is outdated, dangerous and must stop.*

Take home on maintenance fluid: Start with DNS/NS in most settings, and then modify to increase or decrease sodium and dextrose concentration as per serum Na and glucose levels. For sick child frequent evaluation and calculation are needed **(Tables 8)**.

Deficit Fluid Correction

Gastrointestinal (GI)—diarrhea, vomiting or Skin losses - (cystic fibrosis, burns) or renal losses (renal tubular acidosis, diabetes insipidus, acute interstitial nephritis) or 3rd space loss (peritonitis, pancreatitis) **(Tables 9)**.

Ongoing Loss Replacement

All ongoing g losses to be measured and effort is given to replace volume to volume. Losses include patients with chest tubes in place, uncontrolled vomiting, continuing diarrhea, or externalized CSF shunts. Replacement fluid should be of similar composition as the lost fluid **(see Table 10)**.

■ ACUTE ABDOMEN IN CHILDREN

History

- *Pain:* Duration, quality, intensity, location, radiation, Response to position, eating, urinating, defaecating, periods, and sleep

TABLE 10: Electrolytes composition of different body fluids and compatible replacement fluids.

Fluid	Replacement fluid
Gastric	½ NS
Small gut	NS
Bile	NS
Diarrhea	½ NS
Burn	NS or RL

- *Associated features:* Fever, vomiting, bowels (+/–), micturition (+/–), bleeding
- *Recent history:* Weight loss, polyuria, rashes, RTI, recurrent episodes of abdominal pain, trauma
- *Other systemic complaints:* Headaches
- *Visceral pain:* Ill-defined, spasmodic, poorly localized
- *Somatic pain:* Sharp, deep and dull, well localized.

Examination

- *General examination:* Other systems, rashes, lymphadenopathy
- *Inspection of abdomen:* Distended, scaphoid, visible bowel loops, lumps, and hernial sites
- If there is tenderness, but no guarding: observe, reassess
- *If tenderness with guarding:* Surgical cause likely (guarding may not be as marked as in an adult)
- Percussion tenderness, pain on coughing, rebound tenderness

- *Per Rectal examination:* Suspected ovarian pathology/low diffused tenderness suspicious of pelvic appendicitis/long duration of symptoms, bloody mucoid diarrhea suggesting pelvic collection.

Investigations
- CBC, ESR, electrolytes, LFT, amylase/lipase, CRP
- Urine routine/CS, plain X-ray/USG.

Differential Diagnosis
- Acute appendicitis, Meckel's diverticulitis
- Obstructed hernia, intestinal obstruction
- Gall stones, acute pancreatitis
- Tubo-ovarian pathology
- Ectopic pregnancy
- Testicular torsion
- *Acute abdomen:* Nonsurgical conditions
- Acute diarrhea, viral, Shigellosis, Salmonella infections, hepatitis, and UTI
- Tuberculosis, acute pancreatitis, dengue hemorrhagic fever
- Mesenteric adenitis, cholecystitis
- Pneumonia, pleural effusions
- *Toxins:* Lead/mercury
- *Metabolic:* DKA, acute porphyrias
- *Others:* Sickle cell anemia, Henoch-Schonlein Purpura, nephrotic syndrome congestive heart failure, sexual abuse.

■ POISONING IN CHILDREN

Why kids get "poisoned": 1–3 years of age are curious about environment. Older children are often experimenting. Poisoning should be considered whenever there is an acute onset of multiorgan dysfunction with "puzzling complex of signs and symptoms".

Patient may Present with Stable or Unstable Condition

If the Patient is Stable
- Every patient with suspected poisoning needs at least 12 hours observation
- Attempt to elucidate and clearly document: type of substance(s), amount ingested, patient's weight, time of ingestion, clinical manifestations, underlying clinical condition of patient.

Pharmacological poisons: Where even 1–2 tablets that can be lethal to a 10 kg toddler:
- Beta blockers
- Calcium channel blocker: Delayed onset bradycardia, hypotension, conduction block
- Chloroquine/hydroxychloroquine
- Oral hypoglycemic
- Tricyclic antidepressant
- Theophylline.

Small volumes of nonpharmaceuticals than can result in severe toxicity:
- Organophosphates
- Paraquat
- Camphor
- Naphthalene
- Hydrocarbons, solvents, Eucalyptus oil, kerosene
- Corrosive.

They need close monitoring even if a small amount is ingested.

Common household poisons, clinical presentation, and their management are described in **Table 11**.

If the Patient is Unstable
The principle is—"treat the patient not the poison". Approach should be as follows:
- A-Airway
- B-Breathing

TABLE 11: Common household poisons, clinical presentation, and management.

Name	Signs and symptoms	Management
• Mosquito repellant (Pyrethroid) • Prallethrin	If taken in large volume—similar to those of organophosphate poisoning	• Large volume Ingestion—gastrointestinal decontamination if reported within 2–3 hour • Symptomatic management. No atropine
Nail polish (Toluidine, butyl acetate)	Multiorgan dysfunction may occur in high volume ingestion	Symptomatic
Nail polish remover (acetonitrile)	Methemoglobinemia	• Gastric decontamination, • Injection Methylene blue (2 mg/kg)
Rat killer (zinc phosphide and anticoagulant)	Diarrhea, pain abdomen, vomiting, pulmonary edema, bleeding manifestation	• Decontamination: Activated charcoal, • Antidote: Vitamin K, and Supportive
Naphthalene mothballs	Hemolytic anemia and methemoglobinemia	Methylene blue and exchange transfusion, N-acetyl cysteine or ascorbic acid injection if patient is G6PD deficient

- C—Circulation
- D—Dysrhythmias
- D1—Disability
- D2—Decontamination
- D3—Drug antidotes
- E1—Exposure; hyper/hypothermia >38.5°C requires urgent cooling
- E2—Enhanced elimination

Airway
Intubation: Indications
- Cardiorespiratory arrest
- Airway injury
- Corrosive ingestion
- Decreased level of consciousness (GCS <8) or anticipated decrease in GCS
- Prolonged seizures

Breathing
Oxygen/ventilation, if required.

Circulation
- *Treatment of hypotension:*
  - IV fluids (20ml/kg 0.9% NaCl if in shock)
  - Inotropes
- *Treatment of hypertension*
  - Avoid beta-blockers in sympathomimetic toxicity

D-Dysrhythmias
- $NaHCO_3$ if sodium channel blocker ingested
- $MgSO_4$ if potassium channel blocker ingested
- Generally, there is poor response to defibrillation in poisoning

D1-Disability
- *Seizure control:* Not typical conventional treatment
  - Midazolam (0.1–0.2 mg/kg) is most commonly used
  - 2nd choice-phenobarbitone (20 mg/kg IV)
  - *Avoid phenytoin:* Prolongs sodium channel blockade
- Treat hypoglycemia if present
- *Maintain normothermia:* Hyperthermia may precipitate seizure
  - Physical cooling
  - May require intubation and paralysis

D2-Decontamination
Must not distract from resuscitation and supportive care
- Skin
  - Remove all clothes contaminated
  - Wash whole body with copious water, then soap and water
- Eyes
  - Irrigate with 0.9% NaCl until pH is <8.0
  - Use local anesthetic eye drop
- *GI tract decontamination:* Do's and Don'ts
  - Dilution with milk/water is generally not recommended
  - Emesis should never be induced

- *Gastric lavage:* Controversial, maybe done if patient comes within 2–4 hours (contraindicated in corrosive, volatile substances poisoning).

Activated charcoal (AC)
- GL and AC indicated only if ALL of the following are true:
  - Presentation within 2 hour of ingestion
  - Toxin is absorbable by AC – exception ethanol/glycols, alkalis / corrosives, metals, lithium, iron compounds, hydrocarbons
  - Currently maintaining airway and their GCS will remain normal
  - Otherwise only give if airway is protected
  - If the substance has significant toxicity and is not easily treatable.

D3-Drug antidotes…Certain examples are:

Poison	Antidotes
Paracetamol	N-acetylcysteine
Opioids	Naloxone
Benzodiazepines	Flumazenil
Na Channel Blocker	$NaHCO_3$
Iron	Desferrioxamine
Glipizide	Octreotide
Digoxin	Digi-Bind
Organophosphate	Atropine, PAM

Whole bowel irrigation (WBI):
It is very rarely performed.

Indicated if:
- There is ingestion of a slow release/extended release preparation
- Patient presents prior to onset of symptoms
- Ingestion is likely to result in significant toxicity despite supportive care/antidote
- Polyethylene glycol – 30 mL/kg/h until effluent runs clear

Possible indications for WBI:
- Iron (>60 mg/kg elemental iron has been ingested)
- Sustained release diltiazem/verapamil
- Slow release potassium chloride.

SEIZURES IN CHILDREN

The most common cause is febrile convulsions (FC), which usually occur at the onset of fever, the level of which is not important. Fits may occur with fever as low as 99°F only. A positive family history predisposes to FC. Mostly the FC are of typical variety **(Table 12)**, i.e., all the features mentioned for typical are there.

Febrile Status

Convulsions last for over 30 min, 25% of all status epilepticus are febrile status.

TABLE 12: Types of seizures in children.		
Feature	Typical	Atypical (any one of the following)
Type	Generalized, tonic/clonic	Focal
Duration	Less than 15 min	Longer
Recurrence	Does not recur within 24 hours	Recurs in 24 hours

Treatment: At home, turn the face to the side, and give Intranasal Midazolam spray (0.5 mg), given in the dose of 0.2 mg/kg, i.e., 2 puffs/5 kg weight. FC usually cease within 60 sec. May repeat half dose after 2 min if FC do not stop.

Meanwhile rush to hospital. At hospital: Take care of the Airway, breathing and circulation. Give IV Lorazepam (0.05–0.1 mg/kg) or Diazepam (0.1–0.2 mg/kg), followed by fosphenytoin if not controlled.

Prevention: Oral Clobazam (0.5 mg/kg/dose BD for 3days) with the onset of fever. This prevents recurrence in the majority, but as most children have as many episodes of fever per year, the child has to bear this. Alternate method is continuous phenobarbitone or valproate for 2-3 years, something which has its side effects. Current recommendation is no prophylaxis.

Risk of subsequent epilepsy is minimal in typical FC, but more if atypical FC or family history of epilepsy is there.

Caveat: Remember: Pyogenic meningitis is a DD, and must be ruled out.

CONCLUSION

Pediatric emergencies are mostly respiratory or gastrointestinal in origin and must be handled with care and proper expertise. The vast majority of them recover successfully, barring a few. Neurological emergencies are the ones which may end up with long-term handicap, but we need to ensure as intact a survival as possible.

Take Home Message

- A rapid but systematic approach ensures that a really sick child, in need of immediate attention is detected fast and without any loss of valuable time. We always hear of "the golden hour or the golden first few minutes" in emergency situations, a concept which simply braces the fact of minimizing the time lag between arrival of the patient and the initiation of services. The first look thus tells us a lot about the patient.

REFERENCE

1. Dhanani J, Fraser JF, Chan HK, Rello J, Cohen J, Roberts JA et al. Fundamentals of aerosol therapy in Critical Care. Critical Care (2016) 20:269.

SECTION 13: Rheumatological Emergencies

Section Editor: Sukumar Mukherjee

34. **Emergencies in Rheumatological Practice**
    Parthajit Das, Sukumar Mukherjee

CHAPTER 34

Emergencies in Rheumatological Practice

Parthajit Das, Sukumar Mukherjee

INTRODUCTION

Rheumatological emergencies are commonly encountered in clinical practice. Rheumatic diseases are usually of insidious onset and chronic in nature. However, certain disease may present acutely such as crystal arthropathy and with significant organ or life-threatening complications such as connective tissue diseases and systemic vasculitis. Rheumatic patients may present with pharmacotherapy-related medical emergencies such as oral hypoglycemic-agents induced hypoglycemia in diabetic patients, corticosteroid induced hyperglycemia or nonsteroidal anti-inflammatory drugs-related gastrointestinal toxicity, etc. It has been reported that patients with rheumatic diseases may account for around 8% of all emergency department attendances,[1] and around 10–25% of them may require inpatient care.[2,3] Early recognition of ominous signs and prompt initiation of appropriate therapeutic strategy may significantly reduce morbidity and mortality and improve clinical outcome. This chapter is aimed to provide an overview of the organ specific or life-threatening complications of rheumatic diseases which may present as emergency in clinical practice.

Complications of systemic rheumatic diseases frequently have protean manifestations and may present a diagnostic problem. Patients with connective tissue diseases and vasculitides may have dangerous or life-threatening conditions, which must be recognized and treated promptly to prevent rapidly evolving morbidity and mortality. Knowledge of possible emergencies in the context of a defined rheumatic disease may aid in promoting a high index of suspicion and contribute significantly to the timely diagnosis of many potentially dangerous conditions. This review is written for the emergency room physician and discusses the early recognition of selected emergencies in the context of a defined rheumatic disease.

CLASSIFICATION OF EMERGENCIES IN RHEUMATOLOGY

For the better understanding, these emergency presentations have been classified into two categories including: (1) Common but urgent (window period beyond 8–24 hours); and (2) less common but life and organ threatening (window period: 6–8 hours) as depicted in **Table 1**. Life-threatening emergencies in rheumatology can pose a significant mortality risk and require prompt recognition and appropriate management plan to ensure patient survival, whereas apposite treatment plan should be instituted in organ-threatening emergencies to prevent organ damage.

Category 1: Urgent Emergencies

Acute Hot Joint

The major causes of acute monoarthritis are septic arthritis, crystal arthritis (gout, pseudogout), hemarthrosis, reactive arthritis, monoarticular presentation of inflammatory arthritis or traumatic synovitis. It is imperative to exclude

TABLE 1: Classification of emergencies in rheumatological practice.

Category		

Category 1	Urgent	• Acute Hot Joint
		  – Septic arthritis
		  – Acute gouty arthritis
		• Acute low back pain
		• Acute skin failure
		• Osteoporosis and fracture
		• Seizures—recurrent
		• Adverse drug reactions

Category 2	Life- and organ-threatening	• Scleroderma renal crisis • Catastrophic antiphospholipid syndrome • Macrophage activation syndrome (MAS) • Acute lupus flare • Ocular emergencies • Pulmonary renal syndrome (PRS) • CNS emergencies • Cardiovascular emergencies • Respiratory emergencies • Gastrointestinal emergencies • Renal emergencies • Hematological emergencies • Atlantoaxial dislocation syndrome

septic arthritis because it can result in rapid joint destruction and significant morbidity and mortality (up to 18%).

Acute Septic Arthritis

Septic arthritis or acute bacterial arthritis is a rheumatological emergency which can lead to rapid joint destruction. The usual presentation is acute monoarticular or oligoarticular arthritis, however a polyarticular presentation can rarely be found in an immunocompromised patients. Closed needle aspiration and synovial fluid study is the gold standard test to establish the diagnosis. The choice of antibiotic is determined by the synovial fluid culture and antibiotic sensitivity result. The most common inciting pathogen is *Staphylococcus aureus*, followed by gram-negative organisms. The recommended course of antibiotics therapy is parenteral therapy for 2 weeks followed by 4 weeks of oral therapy.[4]

Acute Gouty Arthritis

Gout is a common inflammatory arthritis which is characterized by recurrent episodes of extremely painful and debilitating articular, periarticular and/or soft tissue inflammation induced by monosodium urate crystals. Acute gouty arthritis should be treated with urgency. NSAID, unless contraindicated, should be used at a maximum dose along with a gastroprotective agent and/or colchicine (doses of 0.5 mg BD-QDS). Joint aspiration and intra-articular corticosteroid injection can be effectively used to treat acute monoarticular gout. A single intramuscular corticosteroid injection or a short course of oral corticosteroid may be used as an alternative where NSAIDs or colchicine are not tolerated or contraindicated. IL-1 blockers such as anakinra, canakinumab, should be considered for refractory acute gouty flares. Initiation of urate lowering therapy (ULT) at the first presentation is debatable, however ULT is indicated in all patients with recurrent flare (≥2/year), tophi, urate arthropathy and/or renal stones. Patient education plays an important role in the management of acute gouty flares.

Acute Back Pain

Around 90% of low back pain are mechanical in nature.[5] The common causes of acute low back pain are mentioned in **Table 2**. It is of paramount importance to exclude limb or life-threatening spinal and medical emergencies such as cauda equina syndrome, epidural abscess **(Figs. 1A and B)**, aortic dissection or rupture of aortic aneurysm.

It is also imperative to ascertain the difference between mechanical or inflammatory back pain. According to ASAS criterion,[6] inflammatory back pain fulfills 4 out of 5 parameters including (1) age at onset <40 years, (2) improvement with exercise, (3) pain at night, (4) insidious onset, (5) no improvement with rest.

Relevant investigation including HLAB27, radiographic and MRI screen of spine and sacroiliac joint should

TABLE 2: Causes of Acute back pain.

Mechanical	• Prolapse intervertebral disk • Lumber canal stenosis • Spondylosis/spondylolisthesis
Neoplastic disease	• Multiple myeloma • Metastasis
Infection	• Pott's spine • Epidural abscess **(Figs. 1A and B)**
Metabolic	• Osteoporosis fracture • Paget disease (secondary fracture)
Referred pain	• Pancreatitis • Aortic dissection • Rupture of aortic aneurysm • Pelvic inflammatory disease • Urolithiasis
Inflammatory spondyloarthropathy	• Ankylosing Spondylitis • Psoriatic Spondyloarthropathy • Inflammatory bowel disease • Reactive arthritis

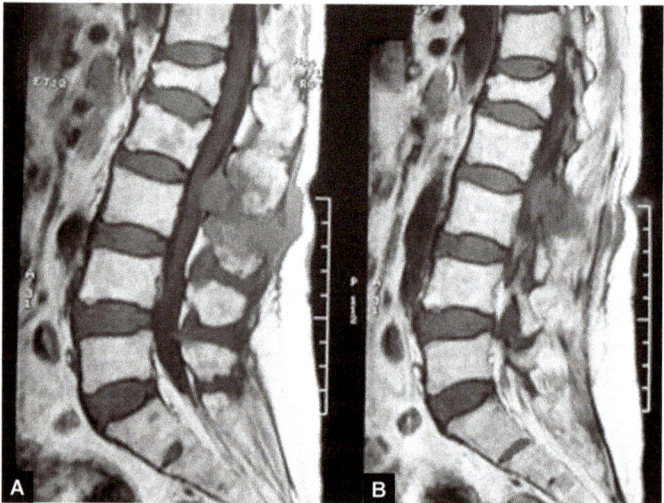

Figs. 1A and B: MRI showing hyperintense shadow of posterior epidural abscess compressing L2 and L3 facet joints and adjoining thecal sac.

enable and/or exclude the diagnosis of inflammatory spondyloarthropathy. Inflammatory spondyloarthropathy should ideally be managed by a rheumatologist with the apposite use of NSAIDs, physiotherapy and biological therapy.

In nonemergency back pain, appropriate analgesics, restricted physical activity for 4–6 weeks, supervised mobilization and physiotherapy is advised. No >2 days of bed rest is advisable. Surgical intervention is needed for patients with compressive myeloradiculopathy, vertebral fractures, epidural abscess, Pott's spine, tumors, etc.

Acute Skin Failure

Skin is commonly affected in rheumatic diseases such as SLE, dermatomyositis, SSC, and rheumatoid arthritis.

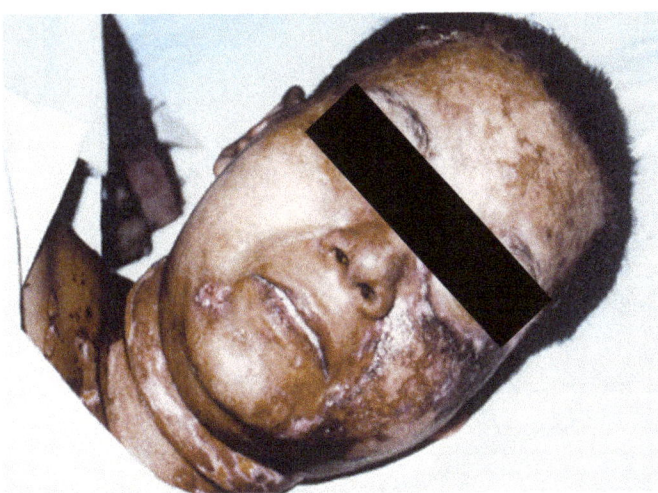

Fig. 2: Toxic epidermal necrolysis in a systemic lupus erythematosus (SLE) patient.

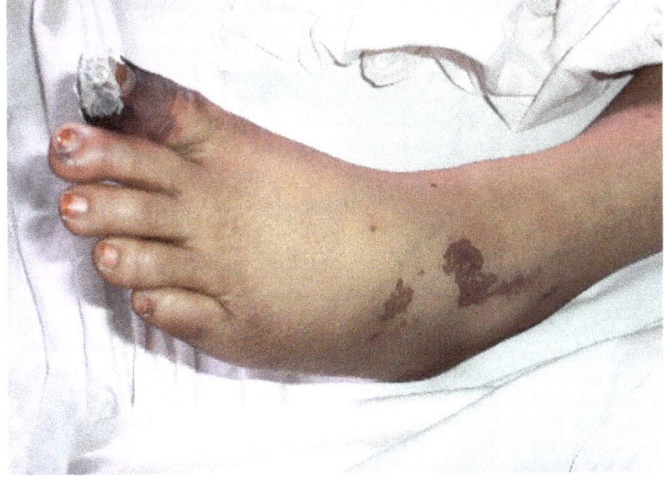

Fig. 4: Digital gangrene in a patient with necrotizing vasculitis.

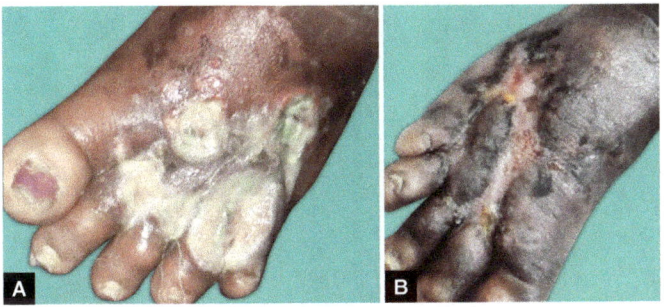

Figs. 3A and B: Rheumatoid vasculitis (before and 9 months after Rituximab infusion).

SLE may present with a wide range of dermatological emergencies such as painful oral or palatal ulcers, Raynaud phenomenon, digital infarct or gangrene, exfoliative skin lesions, cutaneous vasculitis, urticarial vasculitis or toxic epidermal necrolysis (TENS) **(Fig. 2)**. Rheumatoid vasculitis **(Figs. 3A and B)**, necrotizing vasculitis **(Fig. 4)** may present with significant skin necrosis and/or digital ischemia leading to digital gangrene.

Osteoporosis and Spinal Fractures

Vertebral fractures are the most common type of insufficiency fracture related to autoimmune inflammatory condition and corticosteroid therapy. The patients of ankylosing spondylitis with rigid and osteoporotic spine are increasingly vulnerable toward fracture. Prompt recognition, appropriated pain management strategies, spinal immobilization and surgical fixation is essential to avoid catastrophic neurological compromise.

Seizure Disorder

Seizures may be an initial clinical presentation in patients with cerebral sinus venous thrombosis, antiphospholipid syndrome or SLE. Seizures and psychosis can be present in approximately 54% of patients with neuropsychiatric systemic lupus erythematosus (NPSLE).[7] It is essential

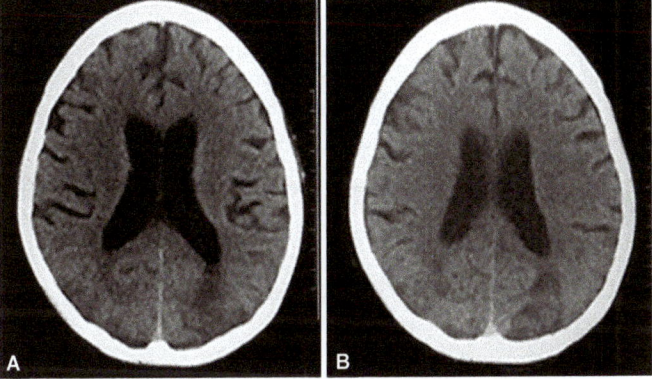

Fig. 5: Occipital infarct in a patient with systemic lupus erythematosus (SLE).

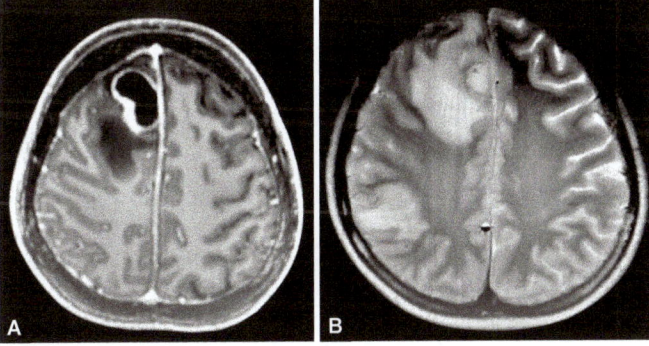

Fig. 6: Multiple tuberculomas in a patient with systemic lupus erythematosus (SLE), presenting with refractory seizures.

to organize appropriate brain imaging and CSF study to exclude other causes of seizures including cerebrovascular event, meningitis, CNS infection **(Fig. 5)**, CNS vasculitis and metabolic causes of seizures. Cerebral infarction occurs in 5% of patients with SLE **(Fig. 6)**.

Adverse Drug Reaction

The adverse drug reactions are depicted in **Table 3 (Figs. 7 and 8)**.

TABLE 3: Treatment-related emergencies in rheumatology.

Drugs	Emergencies
Nonsteroidal anti-inflammatory drugs	• Acute gastritis • Perforated/bleeding peptic ulcer • Analgesic nephropathy • Acute interstitial nephritis • Hypersensitivity reactions • Pancytopenia • Steven Johnson syndrome **(Fig. 7)** • Erythema multiforme **(Fig. 8)** • Toxic epidermal necrolysis
Glucocorticoids	• Psychosis • Acute Addisonian crisis related to withdrawal • High risk of infection
Disease-modifying antirheumatic drugs	• Hypersensitivity reactions • Aplastic anemia • Exfoliative dermatitis • Steven–Johnson syndrome • Bone marrow suppression
Biological drugs	• Colitis (Tocilizumab) • High risk of infection/sepsis • Herpes (JAK inhibitors)
Anticoagulation in antiphospholipid syndrome	Internal or external bleeding

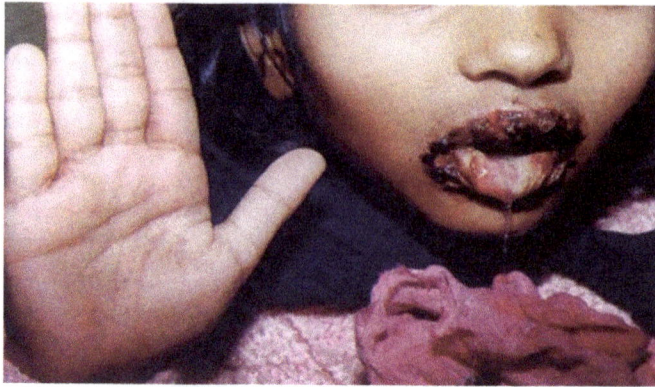

Fig. 7: Steven–Johnson syndrome.

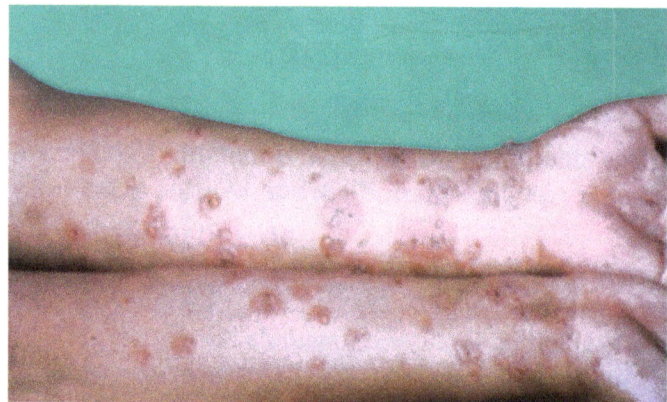

Fig. 8: Erythema multiforme with target lesions and bulla following Sulfasalazine treatment.

Category 2: Life and Organ-threatening Emergencies

Rheumatic diseases are multisystemic autoimmune disease and they often present to various specialties with multifaceted challenges which are nonlife-threatening but organ-threatening in nature. Combined multidisciplinary team effort is often necessary to reduce morbidity and end organ damage.

Scleroderma Renal Crisis

Scleroderma renal crisis (SRC) may be a serious and life-threatening event, with an incidence of 8–10% among limited SSC and 10–20% of patients with diffuse SSC.[8] SRC is characterized by accelerated hypertension, acute renal failure, headache, hypertensive retinopathy, encephalopathy, pulmonary edema, microangiopathic hemolytic anemia, hyperreninemia and thrombocytopenia. Blood pressure is usually abnormal, however normotensive renal crisis has been reported. Several risk factors have been identified including diffuse SSC, high dose corticosteroid therapy, anemia, a new cardiac event such as pericardial effusion or congestive cardiac failure, the presence of anti-RNA polymerase III antibody.[8] The treatment of choice for SRC is therapy with ACE inhibitors (ACEI), e.g., captopril, enalapril, ramipril and quinapril. Additional antihypertensive agents could be used for optimum blood pressure control. Plasmapheresis, corticosteroids and immunosuppressives have no role in the management of scleroderma renal crisis.

Catastrophic Antiphospholipid Syndrome

Antiphospholipid syndrome (APS) is a systemic autoimmune disease characterized by arterial or venous thrombosis and/or obstetric complications in the presence of persistent laboratory evidence of antiphospholipid antibodies including lupus anticoagulant, anticardiolipin antibodies, anti-beta-2-glycoproteins antibodies. APS can be associated with other systemic connective tissue diseases, especially SLE.

The catastrophic antiphospholipid syndrome (CAPS) is a rare and devastating complication of APS resulting in multiorgan failure and high mortality. Clinical criteria of catastrophic antiphospholipid syndrome include:
- History of APS or presence of antiphospholipid antibodies
- Three or more episodes of organ thrombosis, within the last week
- Biopsy confirmation of microthrombi
- Exclusion of other reasons for organ thrombosis and microthrombi

Heparin (LMWH or unfractionated), warfarin and Aspirin are the most frequently used medications to treat APS. Disease-modifying therapy, e.g., hydroxychloroquine may have an important role. The most effective treatment of CAPS include treatment of potential inciting infectious agent and

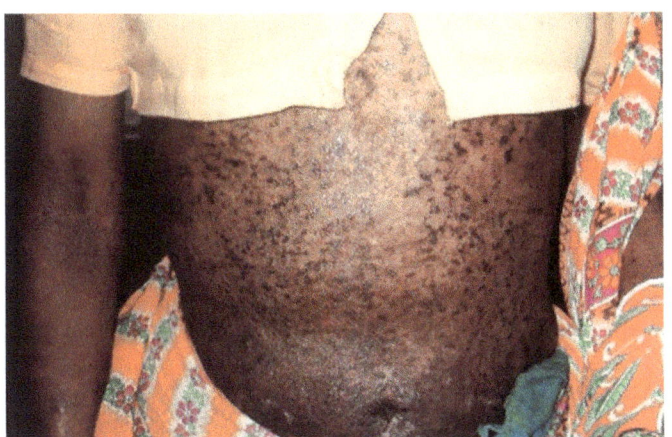

Fig. 9: Macrophage activation syndrome (MAS) with widespread purpura with hepatosplenomegaly and thrombocytopenia.

TABLE 4: Classification criterion for Macrophage activation syndrome (MAS).

2016 EULAR/ACR/PRINTO classification criteria for MAS[9]

Fever and hyperferritinemia (ferritin level >84 ng/mL), and fulfilled more than two of the following four criteria:
- Platelet count >181,000/mL
- Aspartate aminotransferase (AST) level >48 units/L
- Triglyceride level >156 mg/dL
- Fibrinogen level <360 mg/dL

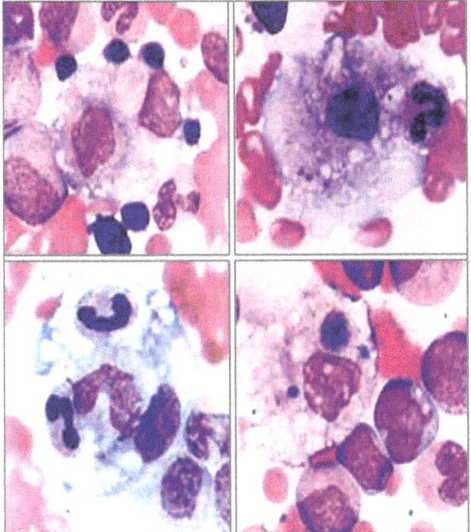

Fig. 10: Bone marrow changes during hyperactive macrophage in a patient of juvenile idiopathic arthritis (JIA).

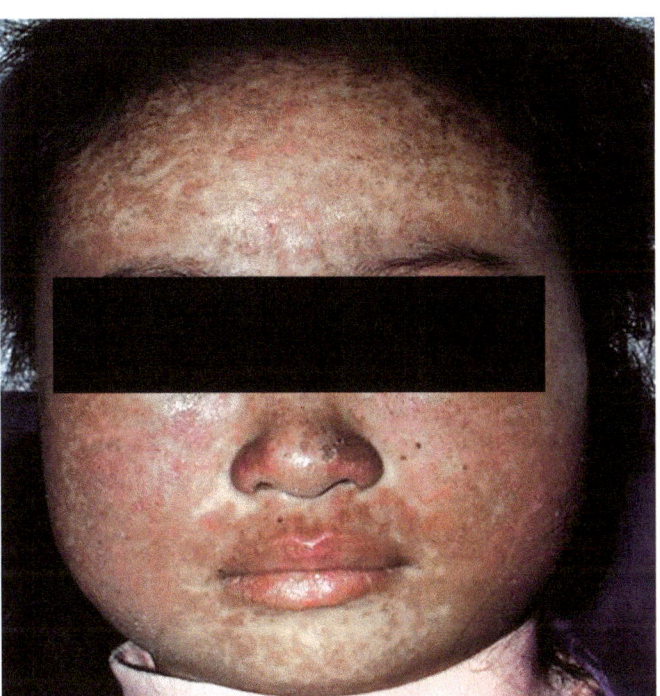

Fig. 11: Acute flare of lupus.

effective combination of anticoagulation, corticosteroids, plasmapheresis and intravenous immunoglobulins.

Macrophage Activation Syndrome

Macrophage activation syndrome (MAS) is an aggressive life threatening condition characterized by fever >39°C (for at least 7 days), skin rash **(Fig. 9)**, jaundice, hepatosplenomegaly, consumption coagulopathy, encephalopathy, bone marrow-activated macrophages with signs of hemophagocytosis **(Fig. 10)**. The 2016 EULAR/ACR/PRINTO classification criterion for MAS is mentioned in **Table 4**.[9] MAS has been associated with autoimmune disease including SLE, juvenile idiopathic arthritis (JIA), adult onset still disease, systemic vasculitis, etc., and is often triggered by systemic infections. The mainstay of MAS treatment is the treatment of cause and/or inciting infection and glucocorticoid therapy (intravenous methylprednisolone 30 mg/kg/dose for 1–3 days). Other effective therapeutic strategies are intravenous immunoglobulins, cyclosporin A, allogeneic transplant of hematopoietic cells therapy.

Acute lupus flare: The SLE flare may be "mild" characterized by mucocutaneous exacerbation **(Fig. 11)** of SLE (SLEDAI 2K score <6 and/or 1 BILAG B score), or "moderate" flare of SLE (SLEDAI-2K score in the range of 6–12 and/or two or more BILAG B scores) or "severe" flare of SLE (SLEDAI2K score of >12 and/or at least one BILAG A score) characterized by neuropsychiatric features, lupus nephritis, myocarditis, thrombocytopenia. Low dose steroids (0.25–0.5 mg/kg) such as prednisolone daily is appropriate in "mild" flare but high dose oral prednisolone 1–2 mg/kg or pulsed methylprednisolone is considered in "severe" flare, along with judicious use of immunosuppressive therapies such as azathioprine, cyclophosphamide, mycophenolate or IV rituximab is recommended in difficult patients.

Ocular Emergencies

Inflammatory eye conditions associated with various autoimmune rheumatic diseases can cause significant visual morbidity including sudden blindness such as anterior ischemic optic neuropathy (AION) related to giant cell arteritis and polyarteritis nodosa, acute hypopyon uveitis and retinal vasculitis related to Behçet's syndrome, retinal vasculitis related to systemic lupus erythematosus and acute vitreous hemorrhage and veno-occlusive disease secondary in antiphospholipid syndrome. Prompt recognition, urgent referral to ophthalmologist and early institution of appropriate immunosuppressive therapy is crucial.

Pulmonary-renal Syndromes

Pulmonary-renal syndromes (PRS) are life-threatening emergency situations characterized by rapidly progressing glomerulonephritis (RPGN) and diffuse alveolar hemorrhage (DAH) secondary to an autoimmune process. The diagnosis of DAH relies on combination of clinical, laboratory, radiological features such as hemoptysis, a drop in hematocrit, diffuse alveolar infiltrates and hypoxemic respiratory failure. The most common cause of PRS in adults is ANCA associated vasculitis (56–77.5 %), followed by anti-GBM Ab disease representing 12.5–17.5% of the patients.[10] Although chest radiograph and computed tomography scans are useful modalities, early bronchoscopy with bronchoalveolar lavage is often advocated to exclude infection and to demonstrate either hemosiderin-laden macrophages or a rising RBC count in sequential BAL aliquots from the same location. Pulsed glucocorticoid therapy remains the mainstay of therapy followed by the maintenance dose of 1 mg/kg/dose. Induction of disease remission has been successful with cyclophosphamide and/ or Rituximab in the management of ANCA associated vasculitis, followed by maintenance of remission immunosuppressive agents such as methotrexate, azathioprine, and mycophenolate mofetil. Plasmapheresis has shown effective results in anti-GBM associated PRS and ANCA associated vasculitis.

CNS Emergencies

Neurological complications are present in 10–20% of ICU admissions.[11] Intracranial hemorrhage has been reported in patients with SLE, CNS vasculitis, GPA. Polymyositis and dermatomyositis patients with the respiratory muscles and the bulbar muscles involvement may require mechanical ventilation. Corticosteroid therapy is the mainstay of therapy with autoimmune rheumatic diseases.

Cardiovascular Emergencies

Hypertension is the most common cardiovascular manifestation of rheumatic diseases. Acute Coronary arteritis may be seen in SLE, systemic vasculitides, APLA and in children with Kawasaki disease. Other serious cardiac manifestations of SLE are acute left ventricular failure secondary to myocarditis, mitral valve regurgitation, and marantic (Libman-Sacks) endocarditis, pericarditis (cardiac tamponade is uncommon). Cardiac arrhythmias may be related to myocarditis.

Respiratory Emergencies

Hypoxic respiratory failure can be attributed to pulmonary parenchymal involvement in SLE, rheumatoid arthritis, scleroderma, and Goodpasture's syndrome. Patients with systemic vasculitis and Goodpasture's syndrome may present with DAH. Stridor reflects involvement of the vocal cords, subglottic area, and/or the trachea and is found in GPA, relapsing polychondritis, or rheumatoid arthritis. Pleuritic chest pain may indicate pleural involvement in SLE or pulmonary embolism. Interstitial lung disease (ILD) is usually associated with rheumatoid arthritis, systemic sclerosis, mixed connective tissue disease and dermatomyositis.

Gastrointestinal Emergencies

Hematemesis is related to erosive gastritis and peptic ulcer disease in patients receiving corticosteroids and NSAIDs. Hematochezia could be found in HSP, SLE, systemic sclerosis, systemic necrotizing vasculitis caused by bleeding from ischemic ulceration of the small intestinal or colonic mucosa or ruptured aneurysms. Bowel ischemia could be found in patients with GPA, RA, Behçet's disease, SLE and PAN. SLE and scleroderma patients may present with visceral smooth muscle myopathy producing intestinal pseudo-obstruction. Acute pancreatitis is a serious gastrointestinal complication of SLE, IgG4 related diseases and Kawasaki disease. Familial Mediterranean fever may present with episodic peritonitis without infection or perforation.

Renal Emergencies

Acute kidney injury and rapidly progressive renal failure are the most common manifestations. Common pathophysiological mechanisms producing renal failure are acute glomerulonephritis (found in SLE), crescentic glomerulonephritis (found in microscopic polyarteritis nodosa, GPA, SLE or Goodpasture's syndrome), renal artery stenosis (found in scleroderma, rheumatoid arthritis with vasculitis, or Sjögren's syndrome) and, rarely, tubulointerstitial nephritis (found in SLE, Sjögren's syndrome, use of NSAIDs).

Hematological Involvement

Rarely, severe autoimmune hemolytic anemia may occur in SLE and microangiopathic hemolytic anemia may be associated with in scleroderma renal crisis. Although thrombocytopenia is commonly associated with SLE and APLA syndrome, it may rarely occur as a part of thrombotic thrombocytopenic purpura in patients with rheumatoid arthritis, overlap syndrome and SLE. Severe leukopenia may be associated with SLE, Felty's syndrome (hypersplenism),

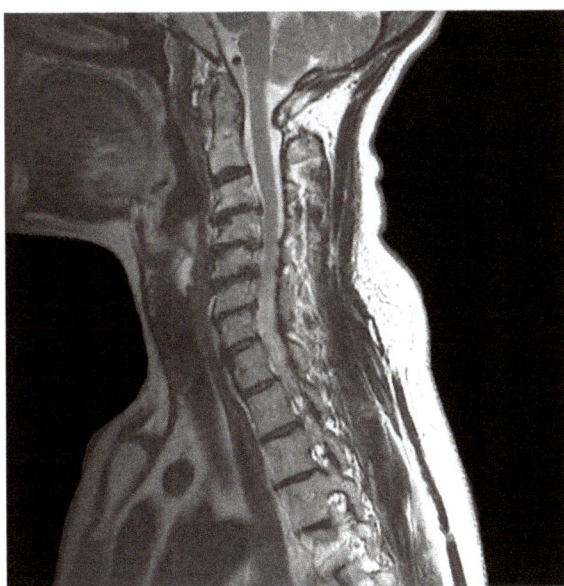

Fig. 12: Rheumatoid arthritis with atlantoaxial dislocation.

bone marrow suppression by immunosuppressive drugs and macrophage activation syndrome.

Atlantoaxial and Subaxial Subluxation

Atlantoaxial subluxation is rarely found among longstanding seropositive erosive rheumatoid arthritis patients **(Fig. 12)** with forward dislocation of C_{1-2} occurring in 43% patients with a mean duration of 12 years. But a vertical dislocation is ominous surgical intervention is often indicated for spinal stabilization.

CONCLUSION

Rheumatic diseases such as rheumatoid arthritis, SLE, systemic vasculitis and scleroderma constitute around 75% of ICU admissions related to rheumatological emergencies. These emergencies should be treated with utmost urgency involving multidisciplinary specialist teams to improve survival. Judicious use of IVIG, plasmapheresis, immunosuppressive therapies, biological therapies such as rituximab may yield success in the special subsets of patients.

Take Home Messages

- More often 50% rheumatological admission result from infection and 25–35% result from disease 'flare' and the mortality risk is 50% with systemic infection.
- Early diagnosis and institution of early treatment is the key towards successful clinical outcome.
- Rheumatological emergencies can be life-threatening and should be treated under the supervision of a specialist multidisciplinary team.
- Newer therapeutic options including biological therapies, IVIG, plasmapheresis, may yield success in the special subsets of patients.

REFERENCES

1. Schlosser G, Doell D, Osterland CK. An analysis of rheumatology cases presenting to the emergency room of a teaching hospital. J Rheumatol. 1988;15:356-8.
2. Rojas-Serrano J, Cardiel MH. Lupus patients in an emergency unit. Causes of consultation, hospitalization and outcome. A cohort study. Lupus. 2000;9:601-6.
3. Sharma M, Leirisalo-Repo M. Arthritis patient as an emergency case at a university hospital. Scand J Rheumatol. 1997;26:30-6.
4. Mathews CJ, Kingsley G, Field M. Management of septic arthritis: a systematic review. Ann Rheum Dis. 2007;66(4): 440-5.
5. Borenstein DG. Epidemiology, etiology, diagnostic evaluation, and treatment of low back pain. Curr Opin Rheum. 1997;9:144-50.
6. Sieper J, van der Heijde D, Landewé R, Brandt J, Burgos-Vagas R, Collantes-Estevez E, et al. New criteria for inflammatory back pain in patients with chronic back pain: a real patient exercise by experts from the Assessment of SpondyloArthritis International Society (ASAS). Ann Rheum Dis. 2009;68:784-788.
7. Sofat N, Malik O, Higgens CS. Neurological involvement in patients with rheumatic disease. QJM Int J Med. 2006; 99(2):69-79.
8. Denton CP, Lapadula G, Mouthon L, Müller-Ladner U. Renal complications and scleroderma renal crisis. Rheumatology (Oxford). 2009;48(Suppl 3):S32-5.
9. Ravelli A, Minoia F, Davi S, Horne A, Bovis F, Pistorio A, et al. 2016 Classification Criteria for Macrophage Activation Syndrome Complicating Systemic Juvenile Idiopathic Arthritis: A European League Against Rheumatism/American College of Rheumatology/Paediatric Rheumatology International Trials Organisation Collaborative Initiative. Ann Rheum Dis. 2016;75(3):481-9.
10. West SC, Arulkumaran N, Philip W, Pusey CD. Pulmonary-renal syndrome: a life threatening but treatable condition. Postgrad Med J. 2013;89:274-83.
11. Kollef MH, Enzenauer RJ. Predicting outcome from intensive care for patients with rheumatologic diseases. J Rheumatol. 1992;19:1260-2.

SECTION 14

Miscellaneous Emergencies-1

Section Editor: ML Saha

35. **Burns**
    Kamal Singh Chhajer

36. **Postoperative Emergencies**
    Prakash K Sasmal, Pankaj Kumar

CHAPTER 35

Burns

Kamal Singh Chhajer

INTRODUCTION

Over the last two decades there has been a significant improvement in the overall care of the burned patient. These advances are reflected in the decreased mortality rate among those sustaining major burns. These improvements are the direct result of a continuously expanding body of knowledge of the pathology of thermal injury and its systematic consequences along with rapid growth of medical technology and improved surgical techniques.

Certain important aspects of burn injuries are:
- Prevention
- Injury Assessment (ABCDE)
- Goal
  - Control Pain
  - Secure Airway
  - Maintain circulation
  - Prevent bacterial proliferation
  - Convert wound status from open to close
  - Healing within minimal period
  - Maintain and preserve body function and appearance
  - Stability of patient (mental, emotional, and Social)
- Financial aspects
- Medico-Legal aspect
- Rehabilitation
- Myth like putting ice or ice-cold water on the burnt area.

DEFINITION

What is Burn?

Heat can cause partial or complete destruction of the skin and underlying tissues. There may be great local and general effects. A large burn is a major illness and can be life-threatening.

Burns injuries can be classified on the basis of the extent or the depth of the injury.

The extent is expressed as a percentage of the total surface area.

Depth is classified as 1st degree, 2nd degree and 3rd degree.

- 1st degree:
  - Involves only the thinner outer epidermal layer, characterized by erythema.
- 2nd degree:
  - Superficial second degree:
    - This involves entire epidermis and variable portion of dermis
    - Deep second degree—Extends well into dermal layer
- 3rd degree:
  - Defined as destruction of entire epidermis and dermis.

Partial thickness: Damage to epidermis but the dermis intact, therefore skin can regenerate. With infection and inappropriate care it can become full thickness.

Full thickness: It involves epidermis as well as dermis and unlikely to regenerate.

Rule of 9's (Fig. 1)

This is a quick way to estimate, the surface area that is affected by burns. In children, the head is >9% and a good way of estimating burns is to say the child's palm is 1% of its surface area.
- Face and scalp 9%
- Back 18%
- Perineum 1%
- Front 18%
- Upper limb each 9%
- Lower limb each 18%

FIRST AID/AIRWAY–BREATHING–CIRCULATION (FIGS. 2 TO 4)

- Ensure your own safety. Remove the person from further danger
- Perform rapid trauma assessment.
- Be alert and treat for **A**irway and **B**reathing-respiratory compromise
- Be alert to treat for shock-**C**irculation.

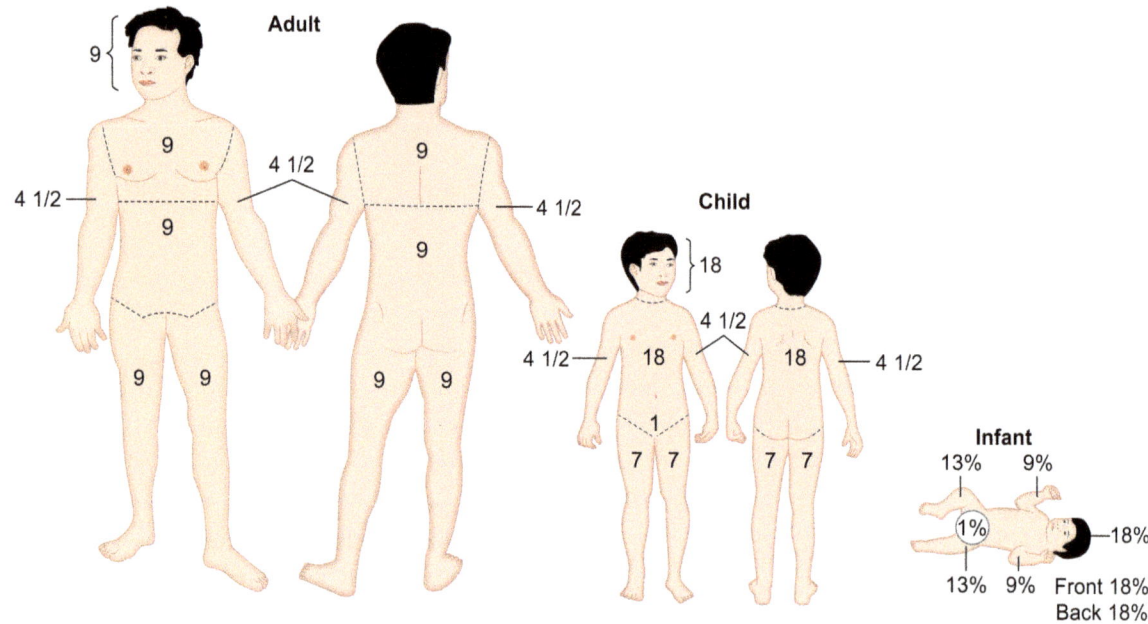

Fig. 1: Rule of nine.

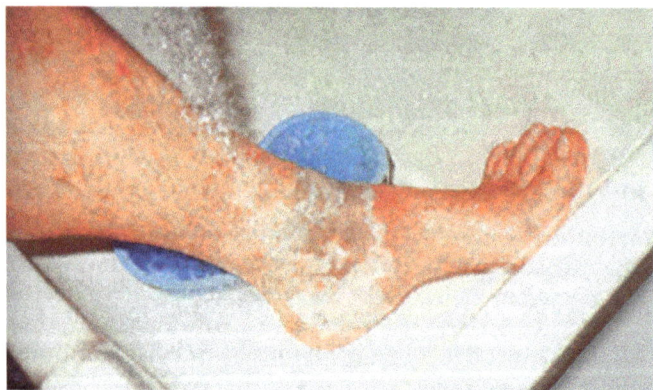

Fig. 2: Wash off the chemical from the skin.

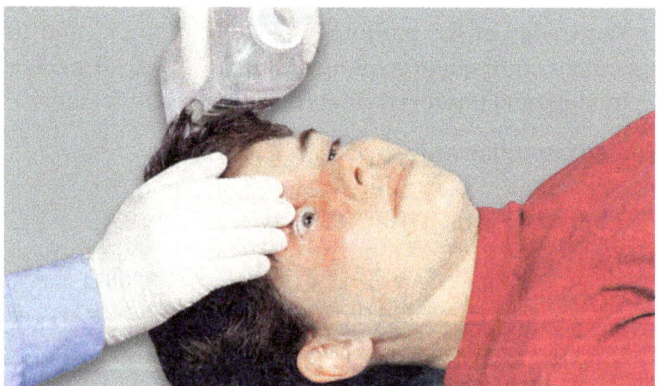

Fig. 4: Wash off the chemicals from the eyes.

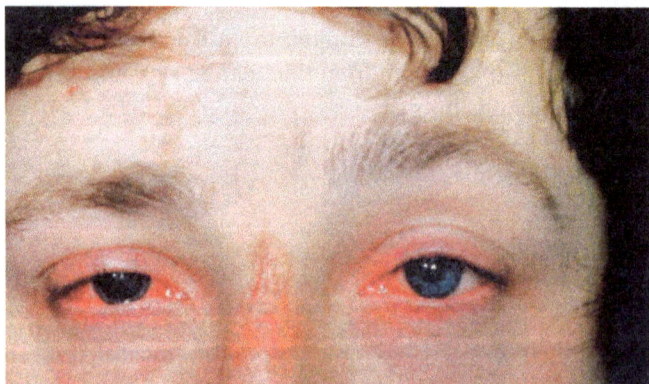

Fig. 3: Chemical burns in eyes.

- Neutralize chemicals—water in copious amount is good
  - *Acid:* 3% sodium bicarbonate
  - *Alkali:* 1% acetic acid (vinegar)
  - *Phosphorus:* Keep wet at all times, then copper sulfate and sodium bicarbonate
  - *Hydrofluoric acid:* Apply calcium gluconate gel
- *Wound:* Cover with a clean wet sheet/towel
- *Fluid:* Major burn nil by mouth, get an intravenous (IV) fluid channel.

GUIDELINES FOR MANAGEMENT

Admission

- Any burn 10% or more in area
- IV fluids for burns over 15%
- Burns in special areas face, neck, hands, feet, perineum **(Fig. 5)**
- Electrical burns any burn with history of smoke inhalation
- Chemical burns.
- Circumferential chest and limb burns.
- Full thickness burns unlikely to regenerate and need skin cover

On Admission

- *Re-evaluation of the airway-breathing-circulation (ABCs)* **(Fig. 6)**

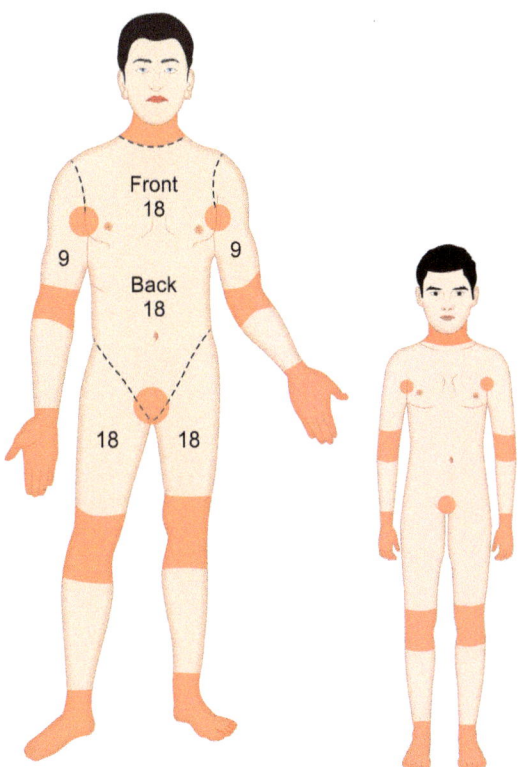

Fig. 5: Red areas show area of special attention and needs admission.

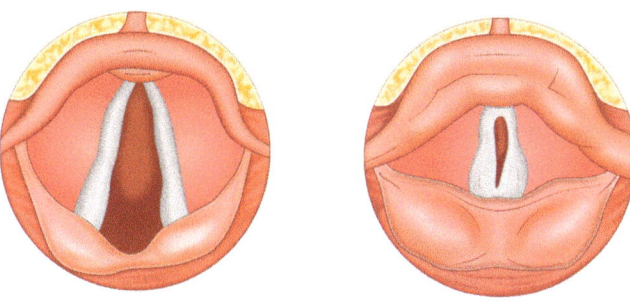

Fig. 6: Inhalation injury with edematous vocal cords and narrowed opening.

- Get a history, include time and place of burn, causing agent, details of the accident (can provide clue to the depth of burn)
- Age of patient, weight, general health (heart, lung, kidney)
- Ask for possibility of inhalation injury
- Look for cofactors that can affect course, e.g., drug addiction, immune or CVS system
- Fluid prior to admission, urine output since injury
- Medication given, check tetanus status
  Life-threatening factors to be stabilized followed by wound case.

Examination
- Estimate area of burn, how much is full thickness
- Look for sign of respiratory burns
- Examine eyes
- Look for circumferential burns on chest, limbs
- Complete full physical examination

Treatment
- IV fluids
- Airway in unconscious patient
- How much and what type of fluid? Work out the requirement from the following formula.

$$\text{Volume} = \text{weight} \times \text{percent burn} \times 4 \text{ mL}$$
(Eg.: 30% burn in a 70 kg patient V = 70 × 30 × 4 = 8400 mL in 24 hours)

This volume is then given at different rates and periods
First 8 hours—give half of total
Next 16 hours—give half of total
Next 24 hours—given half of total

The greatest loss of fluids occurs in first 48 hours.

Ringer lactate or Hartmann's solution is the preferred first line fluid recommendation. It's composition and osmolity closely resemble bodily physiological fluid. If RL is not available one can start with 0.9% sodium chloride (NS) but soon to be replaced by RL. From Day 3 onward the amount of fluid requirement to be calculated according to routine maintenance, replacement and redistribution.

■ PATHOPHYSIOLOGY

The key to any development in burns management lies in a better understanding of burn pathology and its dynamic and reciprocal relationship with fluid management **(Flowchart 1)**. Burn injuries of at least partial-thickness in depth, exceeding 15–20% total body surface area (TBSA) in the adult, and 10–15% TBSA in the child, disrupt homeostasis and lead to a complex series of events that ultimately leads in the release of systemic inflammatory mediators; as a result huge fluid shift occur causing life-threatening electrolyte and hemodynamic changes giving rise to massive edema and burn shock **(Flowchart 2)**.

The postburn vascular changes in volume shift involves four process:
1. Loss of intravascular volume into the interstitium both in burn and nonburn tissue.
2. An increase in burn tissue osmotic pressure leading to further edema in burn tissue.
3. Generalized impairment of cell membrane function leading to extracellular to intracellular water shift.
4. Shift of intravascular water into interstitium in nonburn tissue due to hypoproteinemia.

Antibiotic Policy

Topical Antibiotic: 1% silver sulfadiazine (silverex) cream is the first choice.

Systemic—Start with empiric or broad spectrum followed by presence of sepsis identifying source and organism.

Flowchart 1: Burn pathophysiology and its relationship with fluid management.[18]

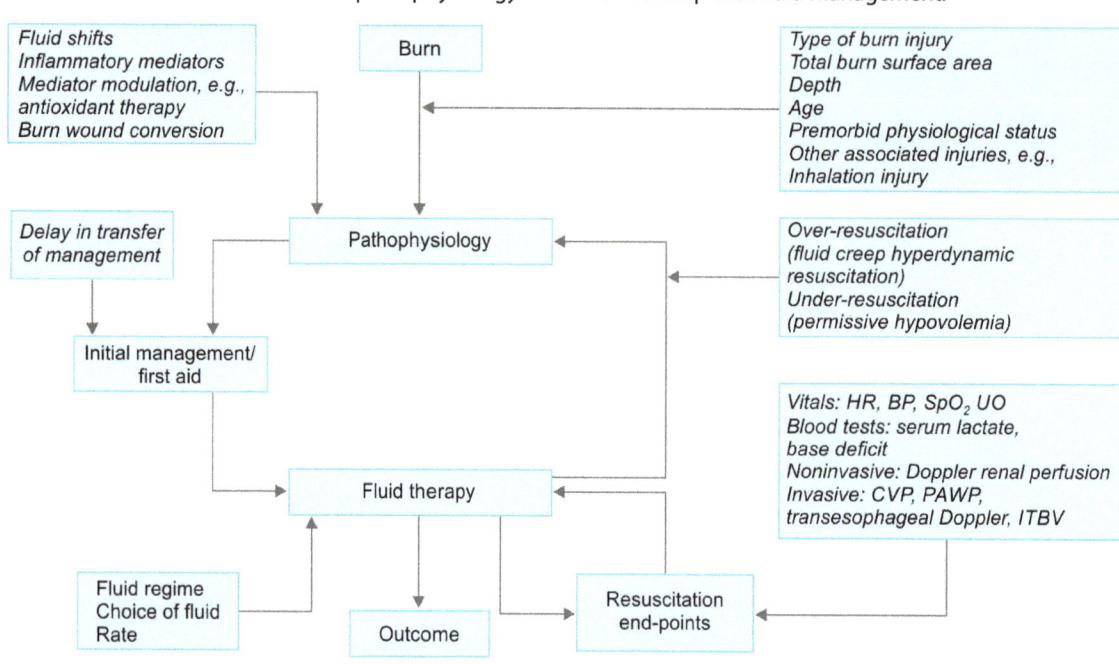

(BP: blood pressure; CVP: central venous pressure; HR: heart rate; ITBV: intrathoracic blood volume; PAWP: pulmonary artery wedge pressure; SpO_2: oxygen saturation; UO: urine output)

Flowchart 2: Events after burn injury.[18]

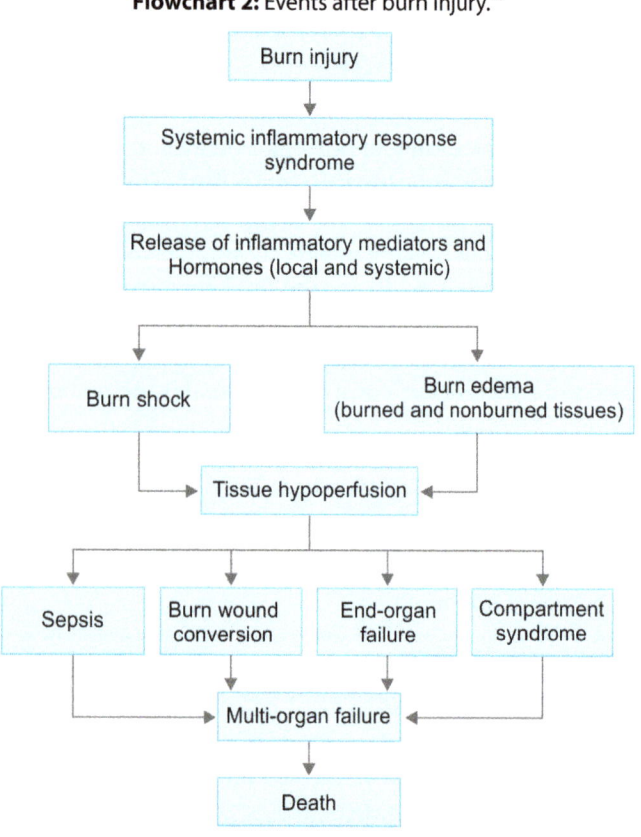

> **BOX 1:** Factors that increase resuscitative fluid needs in burn patients.[18]
>
> - Inhalation injury
> - Delay in resuscitation
> - Crush injury
> - Electrical injury
> - Large full-thickness burn
> - Associated injuries

Patient outcome depends upon patient factors, the nature of the injury and treatment. Patient factors are:
- Preburn physical and mental status some time genetic make-up also play vital rate
- Nature relates to surface area, depth and concomitant injuries as given in **Box 1**.

CARE OF THE BURN WOUNDS

Structure of skin: Stratum corneum is the surface layer composed on nonliving, dry, keratinized cells. Under this is the epidermis. Cell division is limited to the basal layer. Under this is the dermis, the thickness of which varies with age and part of the body. It is composed of collagen fibers and fibroblasts. The blood vessels and nerves run through this layer. Hair follicles and sweat glands originate in the dermis. Under the dermis is fat of varying thickness. The hair layer prevents drying out and to some extent protects from bacterial invasion.

Determination of burn depth can be difficult. Superficial burns tend to blister and skin retains its color (blenches on pressure) is very sensitive to pin prick. As the burn gets

Nutritional Support

- *Enteral Nutrition:* This is preferred route, safe, economical.
- *Parenteral Nutritional support:* nonfunctioning GI tract. Provide adequate calories and protein.

deeper, the pink surface changes to a dry white reticulated surface. Pin prick is less sensitive. Sometimes it takes several days before it is obvious that a burn is superficial. Experience is helpful.

First Aid Care for Different Burns (Algorithm of Burn Care—Flowchart 3)

Thermal Burns

- Stop the burning process and remove burned clothes if charred and adherent like nylon or polyester, don't remove forcefully.
- O_2 per nonrebreather mask at 10-15 L/min
- Do not cool burns with water (Exception—presence of smoldering clothes, or material adhering to skin that could continue burning process)
- Remove external accessories
- For large surface burn, place patient between clean sheets or cover with wet towel/sheets
- Be alert for hypothermia
- Burns affecting <10% of the body may require moist sterile dressing

Chemical Burns

- Chemical on skin
  - Remove clothing and jewelry, pour water for 10 minutes, and wash gently with soap and water, then rinse if possible.
  - If contaminant is dry powder, brush off before flushing
  - Apply sterile dressing or burn sheet
  - Identify contaminant

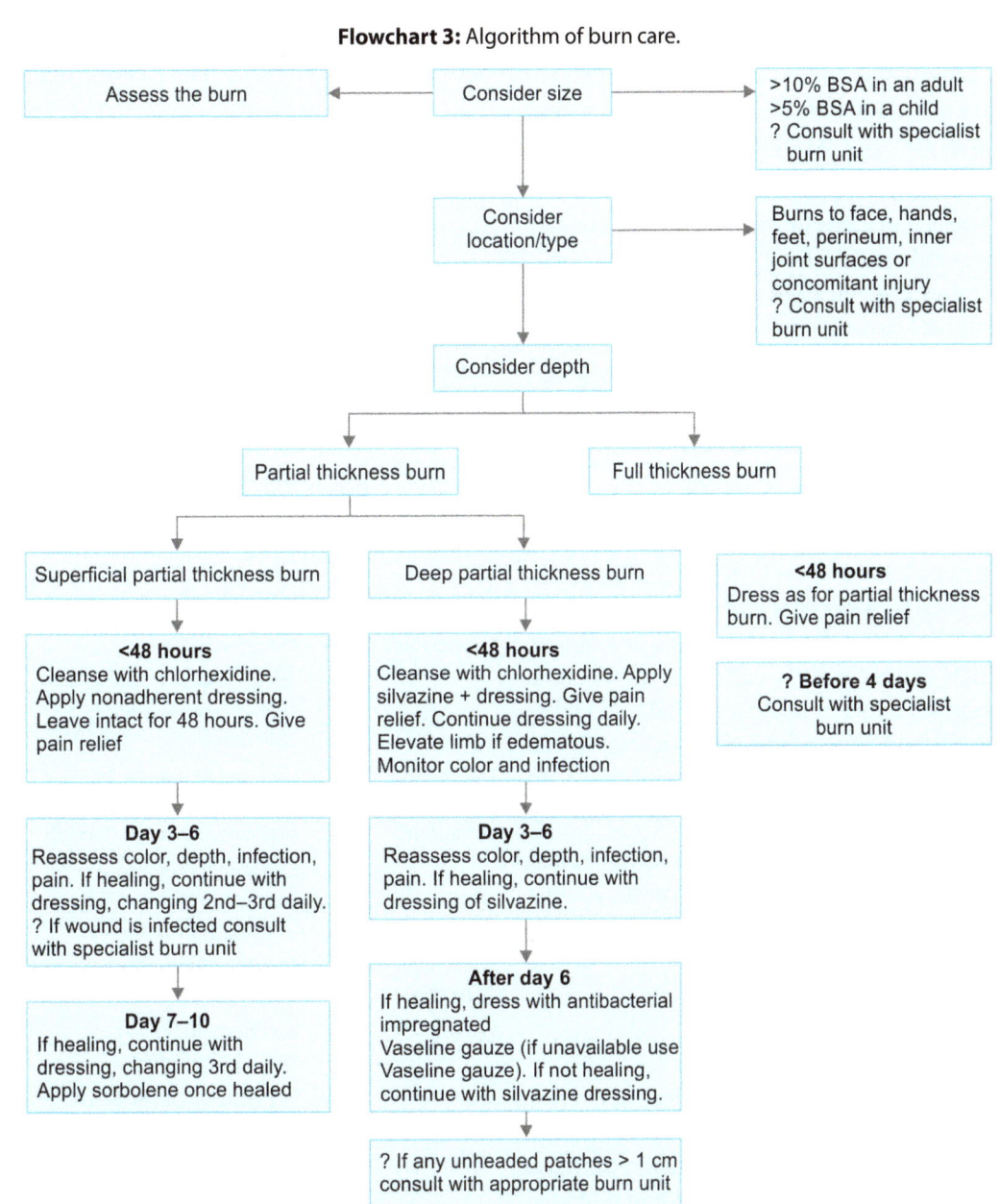

Flowchart 3: Algorithm of burn care.

- Chemical on eye
  - Flood eye(s) with lukewarm water for at least 15 minutes; have patient blink frequently during irrigation.
  - Identify contaminate

Electrical Burns

- Ensure your safety and remove electric source
- O_2 per nonrebreather mask at 10–15 BPM
- Identify both entry and exit wounds. It is necessary to remove all clothing because exit wounds may be on feet, etc.
- Place patient between clean sheets
- Obtain vitals every 5 minutes
- Be prepared for cardiac arrest

Antibacterial Therapy: Silver sulfadiazine (SSD) is the main agent used. The rationale is that by controlling local infection we will prevent systemic infection. Antibiotics given systematically have limited use as they cannot get to the injured site. Topical SSD and bulky dressings which are changed daily are the main methods of local wound care. Daily baths help in the process debridement. SSD slows down eschar separation.

Dressing: There have been many in vogue and new products are coming on the market all the time. Pig skin, potato peels; synthetic membranes have all been used. Simple dressing with Vaseline gauze are cost-effective and work well.

Grafting: Hands should be grafted early to prevent contractures and tearing of extensor tendons.

Eyelids and ears need early intervention to prevent permanent loss.

Areas of motion such as elbows, knees must receive early attention.

Large flat areas should be covered early. General emphasis is on early interference for functional and economic reasons. Donor site—can be anywhere depending on the availability, generally the thigh is used as it is easier to harvest. The abdomen and back are difficult. Using a dermatome makes the process more efficient. When short of skin a mesher can be used to increase the area of coverage. To speed things up in the theater we now use staples to fix the skin **(Flowchart 3)**.

Rehabilitation: An important aspect of care which in detail is beyond the scope of this chapter. However, one must remember that positioning of the limbs and the hands especially is very important. Early involvement of the physiotherapist, splinting is important.

Fluid Therapy

Fluid therapy has played the key role in major burns over the years, it most stated as soon as possible to prevent or reduce the risk of burn shock, electrolyte imbalance, renal shut down and mortality. Due to lack of studies and evidence it has been a constant challenge about type of fluid, rate of infusion and method of monitoring fluid resuscitation.

With advance in understanding and technology, different formulae from time to time have been arrived with many controversies.

Fluid resuscitation aims to support the patient through the initial 24–48 hour period of burn shock by:
- Re-expanding the intravascular volume
- Delivering adequate amounts of sodium to restore cellular transmembrane potential
- Replacing other extracellular electrolytes, thereby preventing life-threatening electrolyte disturbances that can lead to cardiac arrhythmias, and
- Correcting hypoproteinemia and increasing colloid oncotic pressure. The British Burns Association advocates the use of the Parkland formula although numerous other fluid resuscitation formulae are also available **(Table 1)**.

As Muir and Barclay emphasized, any fluid regime must be viewed as guidance rather than rule and fluid administration

TABLE 1: Fluid resuscitation formulae.[18]

Colloid formulae	Electrolyte	Colloid
Evans	Normal saline 1.0 mL/kg/%TBSA	1.0 mL/kg/%TBSA
Brooke	Lactated Ringer's 1.5 mL/kg/%TBSA	0.5 mL/kg/%TBSA
Slater	Lactated Ringer's 2 L/24 hours	
Crystalloid formulae		
Parkland	Lactated Ringer's 4 mL/kg/%TBSA	
Modified Brooke	Lactated Ringer's 2 mL/kg/%TBSA	
Hypertonic saline formulae		
Hypertonic saline solution (Monafo)	Maintain UO at 30 mL/h	
	Fluid contains sodium 250 mmol/L	
Modified hypertonic (Warden)	Lactated Ringer's + 50 mmol/L $NaHCO_3$ for 8 h to maintain UO at 30–50 mL/h	
	Lactated Ringer's to maintain UO at 30–50 mL/h beginning 8 h postburn	
Dextran formula (Demling)	Dextran 40 in saline— 2 mL/kg/h for 8 h	
	Lactated Ringer's— maintain UO at 30 mL/h	
	FFP—0.5 mL/kg/h for 18 h beginning 8 h postburn	

(FFP: fresh frozen plasma; TBSA: total body surface area (burns); UO: urine output)

TABLE 2: Fluid choices.[18]		
Fluid	**Advantages**	**Disadvantages**
Lactated Ringer's	Cheap	Isotonic, only 25% remains intravascularly
	Safe	No plasma expansion properties
	Readily available	No protein replacement
	Lactate buffers metabolic acidosis	Contributes to burn edema
		May require more fluid to maintain physiological parameters compared to other fluids
Hypertonic saline/sodium	Plasma expansion	Hypernatremia and hyperosmolar state
	May decrease burn edema	No protein replacement
	Restore cellular transmembrane potential	Hypertonicity may dehydrate cells
		Progressive burn wound necrosis
		Transient plasma expansion
Albumin (5% or 25%)	Naturally occurring colloid	Expensive
	Strong oncotic properties	May increase interstitial and pulmonary edema if given in first 8 hours postburn
	Decreases edema	Transmissible blood-borne diseases
	Reduced fluid requirements	
Fresh frozen plasma (FFP)	Naturally occurring colloid	Limited availability
	Plasma expansion	Transmissible blood-borne diseases
	Replenishes protein deficiencies	
	Decreases edema	
Dextran and starches	Synthetic colloid of high molecular weight	Risk of allergic reaction
	Decreases edema	May interfere with blood typing
	Plasma expansion	Impair coagulation
	Reduced fluid requirements	Dextran 40 is associated with acute renal failure
	Cheaper than albumin and FFP	Cannot use urine output as guide to resuscitation adequacy
		No protein replacement, may worsen hypoproteinemia
		Volume expansion effect dissipates upon discontinuation of infusion
Starches (pentastarch, pentafraction, hetastarch/Hespan)	Synthetic colloid	Capillary "sealing" effect—inhibits capillary leak
	6% solution (hyperoncotic compared to 5% albumin)	Pentafraction and pentastarch have less effect on coagulation than hetastarch
	Low risk of allergic reaction	No protein replacement
	Improved retention of colloid in intravascular space	May alter coagulation in large doses
	Cheaper than albumin and FFP	

must be carefully titrated against physiological response.[1] Major concern of fluid therapy and resuscitation is to ensure adequate resuscitation and perfusion to end-organs and prevent overload and edema.

Therefore, accurate monitoring of resuscitation endpoints is vital. All types of fluid have been used and to an extent able to restore tissue perfusion but there are certain situations where a particular solution may be more appropriate **(Table 2)**.

Crystalloids

Lactated ringer's solution: A crystalloid is an aqueous solution of mineral salt and other small water-soluble molecules. Most commercially available are isotonic to human plasma. These are capable of diffusion through a semipermeable membrane. These fluids are safe, economical and widely available. Furthermore, it contains no protein and hence exerts no oncotic pressure, which may exacerbate edema formation in states of severe hypoproteinemia as seen in burns. This has been a concern particularly in the context of pulmonary edema, but various studies using the transpulmonary double indicator dilution method (which measures fluid accumulation within the lung) have rejected this.[2,3] Its contribution to edema formation (due to lack of protein) can lead to organ dysfunction, compartment syndrome, ARDS, but so far no better and convincing option to tis is available.

Hypertonic Saline

The use of hypertonic solutions in burn resuscitation was introduced by Monafo.[4] The rationale was to increase intravascular osmolality in order to reverse the fluid shifts, thereby restoring hemodynamics and minimizing burn edema formation. Demling demonstrated that smaller amounts of fluid could be given with an equivalent improvement in intravascular volume.[5] Hypertonic saline (HS) has been shown in one study to reduce the risk for abdominal compartment syndrome whilst maintaining an adequate urine output with lower volumes of resuscitation fluid when compared to the Parkland regime.[6] Furthermore, hypertonic saline may improve myocardial contractility, by quickly restoring cell membrane potential, and also reduce vascular resistance.[7]

Despite these advantages, routine HS use is uncommon. The restoration of hemodynamics is mostly transient (unless colloid is used in addition). A prospective randomized study of patients with 20% TBSA burns evaluating hypertonic sodium lactate versus Lactated Ringer's solution did not demonstrate decreased fluid requirements.[8] Furthermore, serious adverse effects can occur with rapid infusions, including severe hypernatremia and hyperosmolality, leading to renal failure, myocardial fluid overload, brain shrinkage, seizures and intracranial vessel rupture. Despite the lack of evidence, hypertonic crystalloid continues to be popular in infant and elderly patients in whom there is minor risk of hypernatremia.[9,10]

A study by Huang et al.[11] found that HS is associated with a four-fold increase in renal failure and two-fold increase in mortality. It has also been suggested that it causes progressive wound necrosis.[12] Recent systematic reviews[13,14] concluded that there was insufficient data to settle the debate over whether hypertonic was better than isotonic crystalloid for burn resuscitation. However, Brown, in his review of 17 trials, noted that the confidence intervals were wide which meant that clinically important differences might exist.[15] One major problem for comparative analysis is that there is no standardization of hypertonic saline administration, neither in terms of fluid composition nor rate of infusion.

Colloids

Colloids are used in both forms either synthetic (nonprotein) in form such as dextrans and starches or naturally occurring protein solutions, e.g., blood/FFP/albumin. Their plasma expansion property is thought to confer an advantage over crystalloids by exerting an oncotic pressure across the capillary membrane and hence reducing edema formation.[16] The protein-containing solutions are also able to replace serum protein deficiencies.

Albumin

Albumin solution is the most commonly used colloid. It is negatively-charged and therefore repelled by the negatively-charged endothelial glycocalyx, extending its intravascular duration. As well as being an important serum transport protein, it scavenges free radicals and possesses anticoagulant properties. In health, it contributes approximately 80% of the plasma oncotic pressure but in the critically ill, serum albumin correlates poorly with colloid oncotic pressure. It is expensive but has a long shelf-life and there is a risk of disease transmission including prion Creutzfeldt-Jakob disease. Two concentrations 4.5% and 20% from pooled donors are available. The half-life of exogenous albumin in the circulating compartment is 5–10 days, assuming an intact capillary wall membrane. In the critically ill, capillary leak limits its effectiveness, at least during the initial 8 hours post-burn. Demling showed that albumin increased intravascular volume better than Lactated Ringer's solution and reduced edema in uninjured tissue.[15]

Nonprotein Colloid Solutions: Dextran and Starch Resuscitation Solutions

Dextrans consist of high molecular-weight glucose polysaccharides and are designed to restore intravascular oncotic pressure. Dextran designed to restore intravascular oncotic pressure whereas starches possess a sealing property but has short half-life, they also improve micro circulation.

Blood

In severe hemorrhage, blood is the best replacement which increases Hb and improves in O_2 carriage. Furthermore, it is in short supply, expensive, antigenic and requires cross-matching and storage facilities.

Hemoglobin-based Blood Substitutes

Recently, *Diaspirin* cross-linked hemoglobin, hemoglobin-based blood substitutes have been developed. They are incapable of being melted, oxygen-carrying fluids with long shelf-lives without any requirement of refrigeration or cross-matching. They show similar oxygen-dissociation curves to blood and are free from disease transmission. These fluids can be lifesaving but are not free from serious life-threatening complications. So still a long way to go.

Crystalloids versus Colloids

Crystalloids are low cost, salt solution with small molecule which can move around easily. Colloid can be man-made (starch, dextran, gelatin) or naturally occurring (albumin, FFP). These are expensive and bigger in size so stay for a longer period in the blood.

Many investigators advocate the use of colloids when large total fluid volumes are anticipated such as in inhalation injuries or large burns, children and the elderly, or those demonstrating refractory burn shock.[15]

While various trials and systematic reviews, including two Cochrane reviews, have found no evidence that colloids or albumin are associated with an improvement in the survival of critically ill patients, including burn victims,[16,17] some have reported an increased mortality associated with the use of albumin. Unfortunately, these reviews have been filled with procedural errors and restrictions with the use of different end-points and physiological protocols for fluid administration, circulatory and respiratory treatment. Furthermore, there was inappropriate grouping of study treatments. Nevertheless, this does not preclude the possibility that there exists highly-select subgroups of critically ill patients in whom colloids may be beneficial. Despite the lack of robust outcome data, albumin remains the mainstay of colloid therapy in some pediatric intensive care units.

■ CONCLUSION

- The burn patient undergoes a number of dramatic physiologic and metabolic changes over the course of injury state. These changes are so masked that the treating doctor have the feeling of treating a different patient every few days as the process evolves.
- It is essential to have a clear understanding of pathophysiologic differences and necessary treatment modification (especially fluid resuscitation) needed over time following burn.

Take Home Messages

- Safe removal of victim from site with emphasis on safety of the rescuer.
- Proper assessment of the injury (**A**irway, **B**reathing, **C**irculation)
- Fluid therapy as per protocol
- Local management (follow the algorithm).

■ REFERENCES

1. Muir IFK, Barclay TL. Burns and their treatment. London: Lloyd-Luke (Medical books) Ltd., 1962.
2. Holm C, Melcer B, Horbrand F, Worl H, von Donnersmarck GH, Muhlbauer W. Intrathoracic blood volume as an end point in resuscitation of the severely burned: an observational study of 24 patients. J Trauma. 2000;48(4):728-34.
3. Holm C, Mayr M, Tegeler J, Horbrand F, Henckel von Donnersmarck G, Muhlbauer W, et al. A clinical randomized study on the effects of invasive monitoring on burn shock resuscitation. Burns. 2004;30(8):798-807.
4. Monafo WW. The treatment of burn shock by the intravenous and oral administration of hypertonic lactated saline solution. J Trauma. 1970;10(7):575-86.
5. Demling R, Gunther RA, Haines B, Kramer G. Burn edema Part II: complications, prevention, and treatment. J Burn Care Rehabil. 1982;3:199-206.
6. Oda J, Ueyama M, Yamashita K, Inoue T, Noborio M, Ode Y, et al. Hypertonic lactated saline resuscitation reduces the risk of abdominal compartment syndrome in severely burned patients. J Trauma. 2006;60(1):64-71.
7. Kien ND, Reitan JA, White DA, Wu CH, Eisele JH. Cardiac contractility and blood flow distribution following resuscitation with 7.5% hypertonic saline in anesthetized dogs. Circ Shock. 1991;35(2):109-16
8. Gunn ML, Hansbrough JF, Davis JW, Furst SR, Field TO. Prospective, randomized trial of hypertonic sodium lactate versus lactated Ringer's solution for burn shock resuscitation. J Trauma. 1989;29(9):1261-7.
9. Bowser-Wallace BH, Caldwell FT Jr. A prospective analysis of hypertonic lactated saline v. Ringer's lactate colloid for the resuscitation of severely burned children. Burns Incl Therm Inj. 1986;12(6):402-9.
10. Bowser-Wallace BH, Cone JB, Caldwell FT Jr. Hypertonic lactated saline resuscitation of severely burned patients over 60 years of age. J Trauma. 1985;25(1):22-6.
11. Huang PP, Stucky FS, Dimick AR, Treat RC, Bessey PQ, Rue LW. Hypertonic sodium resuscitation is associated with renal failure and death. Ann Surg 1995; 221(5):543-54; discussion 554-7.
12. Kuroda T, Harada T, Tsutsumi H, Kobayashi M. Hypernatremia deepens the demarcating borderline of leukocytic infiltration in the burn wound. Burns. 1997;23(5):432-7.
13. Natanson C, Kern SJ, Lurie P, Banks SM, Wolfe SM. Cell-free hemoglobin-based blood substitutes and risk of myocardial infarction and death: a meta-analysis. JAMA. 2008; 299(19):2304-12.
14. Bunn F, Roberts I, Tasker R, Akpa E. Hypertonic versus near isotonic crystalloid for fluid resuscitation in critically ill patients. Cochrane Database Syst Rev. 2004;(3):CD002045.
15. Brown MD. Evidence-based emergency medicine. Hypertonic versus isotonic crystalloid for fluid resuscitation in critically ill patients. Ann Emerg Med. 2002;40(1):113-4.
16. Perel P, Roberts I. Colloids versus crystalloids for fluid resuscitation in critically ill patients. Cochrane Database Syst Rev. 2007;(4):CD000567.
17. Alderson P, Bunn F, Lefebvre C, Li WP, Li L, Roberts I, et al. Human albumin solution for resuscitation and volume expansion in critically ill patients. Cochrane Database Syst Rev. 2004;(4):CD001208.
18. Chan J, Ghosh S. Fluid Resuscitation in Burns: An Update. Hong Kong Journal of Emergency Medicine. 2009;16(1):51-62. doi:10.1177/102490790901600112.

36 Postoperative Emergencies

Prakash K Sasmal, Pankaj Kumar

INTRODUCTION

The care of a patient with a surgical disease does not end up with a surgical procedure itself. Every surgeon wishes to watch the patients recover completely before leaving the hospital. Unfortunately, unexpected events can cause some patients to stay in the hospital longer than necessary. The postoperative complications requiring emergency attention may be, at times, life-threatening. It is possible to foresee postoperative complications and optimize in elective instances to reduce these complications. However, occasionally these complications are unexpected and necessitate quick action to save the patient. These unexpected occurrences are known as postoperative emergencies and, if ignored for a while, can lead to multiorgan involvement and be lethal for the patient.

Postoperative emergencies may not be limited to the organ or system operated upon. In emergency procedures, postoperative outcomes are mostly related to the underlying pathology for which the surgery was done. Depending on the situation, the postoperative complications may be related to the underlying factors.

POSTOPERATIVE COMPLICATIONS

- General
    - Cardiovascular and respiratory complications
- Anesthetic
    - Local/regional/general
- Surgical
    - General/specific
    - Immediate/delayed.

The common postoperative emergencies are discussed here in detail.

CARDIOVASCULAR COMPLICATIONS

Deep Vein Thrombosis and Thromboembolism

In the postoperative period, especially after a prolonged surgery or immobilization, one has a higher chance of developing a deep vein thrombosis (DVT). Immobilization for >48 hours is a potential risk factor for developing DVT.[1] DVT can develop in the legs (most commonly), arms or other deep veins. When a piece of thrombus dislodges and travels to the pulmonary circulation, the patient becomes symptomatic and needs emergency care. About two-thirds of venous thromboembolism (VTE) episodes manifest as DVT and one-third as pulmonary embolism (PE) with or without DVT.[2] Various series involving the Western populations, the prevalence of DVT from 15 to 40% among patients undergoing major general surgical procedures.[3] PE carries high mortality (2.8–12%). The most commonly used noninvasive investigation is venous ultrasonography. However, it is less sensitive in asymptomatic individuals, as most thrombi are small and nonocclusive. So, it is not advisable to screen all individuals. Prevention of VTE is the best approach. Early ambulation and mechanical or pharmacologic interventions can lower the risk of VTE. Mechanical prophylaxis such as compression stockings and sequential compression device (SCD) or intermittent pneumatic compression (IPC), can be uncomfortable and cannot be used for prolonged periods due to pressure-related complications. Pharmacologic prophylaxis is preferred unless the risk of bleeding is too high. Recent studies support using Low Molecular Weight heparin (LMWH) and low-dose direct oral anticoagulants to prevent VTE. The most accepted tool to assess the risk of VTE is the CAPRINI score. The CAPRINI score can guide the healthcare provider to initiate pharmacologic prophylaxis after surgery and continue for an extended period.[4]

Myocardial Infarction, Hypotension, Arrhythmia, Cardiogenic Pulmonary Edema and Shock

Cardiac complications are not uncommon after major noncardiac surgery. The 30-day mortality rate after a major adverse cardiac event (MACE) in the postoperative period is estimated to be around 0.5–2%, with perioperative myocardial infarction (MI) being the leading culprit.[5] Asymptomatic troponin rise and its association with high mortality, especially in high-risk patients aged 65 and

85 years or younger with a significant cardiovascular risk, is reported.[5] Myocardial injury after noncardiac surgery (MINS) is a term commonly used nowadays to label a cardiac event in the postoperative period. Paroxysmal atrial fibrillation (AF) and other arrhythmia occur in 3% of the postoperative patients. Most resolve spontaneously, but persistent AF increases the risk of stroke, heart failure, MI and cardiac arrest. Persistent AF warrants chemical or electrical cardioversion to restore sinus rhythm. Daily normal sensitivity troponin-I as a screening tool for postoperative MI seems encouraging but needs further research. Since perioperative hypotension increases the risk of myocardial ischemia, daily troponin level measurements could be of some benefit in this group of patients. The use of perioperative beta-blockers and calcium channel blockers has shown some benefit in recent trials but is controversial.[6]

Preoperative diastolic dysfunction has decreased tolerance of hypovolemia, as well as hypervolemia, with exaggerated increases in left atrial pressure, leading to pulmonary edema. They should be monitored closely in an ICU setup under the guidance of a cardiologist.

RESPIRATORY COMPLICATIONS

Postoperative pulmonary complications (PPCs) can be any lung abnormality occurring in the postoperative period that produces an identifiable disease or dysfunction that is clinically significant and adversely affects the clinical course **(Fig. 1)**. PPCs occur in 5–10% of patients undergoing nonthoracic surgery and 22% of high-risk patients, with atelectasis occurring most commonly.[7] As many as 25% of deaths occurring within a week of surgery are related to pulmonary complications, thus making it the second most common serious morbidity after the cardiovascular event.[8]

The common PPCs in order of frequency are:[7]
- Atelectasis
- Pneumonia, bronchitis

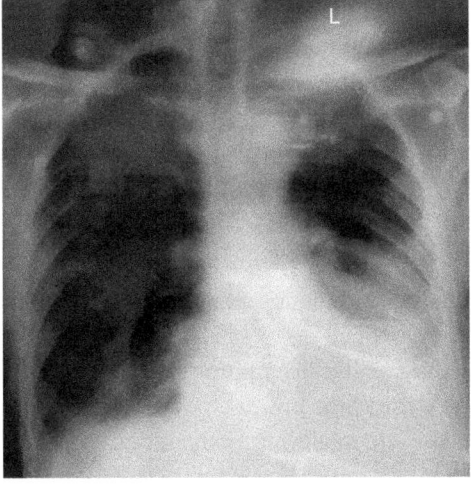

Fig. 1: Postoperative chest X-ray showing left-sided pleural effusion.

- Bronchospasm
- Exacerbation of previous lung disease
- Pulmonary collapse due to mucus plugging the airways
- Respiratory failure with ventilatory support >48 h
- Acute lung injury (ALI), including aspiration pneumonitis, transfusion-related ALI (TRALI) and acute respiratory distress syndrome (ARDS)
- Pulmonary embolism.

The peculiarity of pulmonary complications is that they are preventable or modifiable to a considerable extent. The preoperative patient-related risk factors associated with PPCs include elderly age >65 years, smoking, known chronic obstructive pulmonary disease (COPD), obesity, and obstructive sleep apnea.

Development of postoperative hypoxemia in the immediate postoperative period can result from the residual depressant effect of the anesthetic agents resulting in hypoventilation, airway obstruction, depressed CO_2 responsiveness of the respiratory center, residual neuromuscular blocking agent (NMBA) action, and splinting of the diaphragm due to pain, especially in the upper abdominal surgeries are few of the causes. Due to pain in the immediate postoperative period, the patient tends to underventilate, avoiding deep breathing, there is an inadequate cough with the retention of secretions, all leading to increased chances of infection. Respiratory support in the form of continuous positive airway pressure (CPAP)/ noninvasive ventilation (NIV) till adequate spontaneous respiration is established will correct this hypoxemia.

Atelectasis, mostly affecting the basal segments, can be due to compressive effects on the lung due to recumbent and Trendelenburg's patient position and increased intra-abdominal pressure (like in laparoscopic surgery). The postoperative measures to prevent atelectasis include good postoperative analgesia, lung expansion techniques, that is, incentive spirometry, deep breathing exercises and lung hyperinflation by CPAP along with early mobilization and ambulation. The atelectatic area acts as a nidus for infection, and the patient may suffer from postoperative pneumonia (PP).

Respiratory failure associated with ALI is one of the most important contributors to postoperative mortality. The ALI is a hypoxemic respiratory failure caused by diffuse lung injury, characterized by decreased lung compliance and noncardiogenic pulmonary edema resulting from widespread capillary leakage. When the causative agent of ALI is a transfusion of blood/blood products, it is termed TRALI. It is defined as the acute onset of respiratory distress and noncardiogenic pulmonary edema developing during or within 6 hours of transfusion.[9]

If the risk factors for PPCs are identified preoperatively, lung expansion techniques in the preoperative period and proper anesthetic planning can reduce the incidence of complications. In the presence of risk factors, the duration of surgery should be minimized along with the application of minimal access surgery and regional techniques.

SURGICAL COMPLICATIONS

Hemorrhage

Postoperative bleeding or hemorrhage can be divided into primary, reactive or secondary hemorrhage.

Primary bleeding refers to bleeding that occurs during the surgical procedure.

Reactive bleeding refers to bleeding within 24 hours of the operation in the postoperative period, as blood pressure rises and vasodilatation occurs, a damaged blood vessel may subsequently begin to bleed.

Secondary bleeding occurs within 7–10 days after the operation **(Fig. 2)**. Secondary bleeding is often associated with wound infection. Typical clinical signs associated with postoperative bleeding include tachycardia, hypotension, tachypnea, cold, clammy extremities, and syncope. The best way to reduce the risk of hemorrhage is to identify and correct potential causes of coagulopathy both pre- and postoperatively. Every effort should be made preoperatively to identify patients who have an elevated risk for bleeding related to abnormalities of platelet function and coagulation and address them. In patients with known hemostatic disorders, proper evaluation and preparation are mandatory to minimize the risk of surgical bleeding.

Perhaps the most important aspect of managing postoperative hemorrhage is the early recognition of this potentially devastating complication. The decision to return to the operating room should be judiciously made on whether the patient's estimated postoperative blood loss exceeds the expectations of the operative surgeon. Postoperative hemorrhage can occur from arteries, veins or capillaries. The control of hemorrhage from arteries or veins is to be done by meticulous ligation. In contrast, diffuse bleeding from raw surfaces is often the most challenging mode to control. Applying surgical hemostatic agents such as oxidized regenerated cellulose (surgical snow) or abdominal packing is an option if adequate hemostasis cannot be achieved.

Gastrointestinal

Postoperative Nausea and Vomiting

Along with pain, postoperative nausea and vomiting (PONV) is the second most frequent complaint and has a complex etiology.[10] Females, nonsmokers, abdominal surgeries, diabetes mellitus, hypothyroidism, pregnancy, elevated intracranial tension and incomplete bowel preparation have increased incidence of PONV.[10] A significant incidence of PONV is linked to cholecystectomy, gynecological and laparoscopic procedures and longer operative procedures. Nitrous oxide, ether, ketamine, and cyclopropane increase the prevalence of PONV. Halothane, desflurane, enflurane, and sevoflurane are linked to PONV to a lesser extent. Postoperative opioids increase the risk for PONV in a dose-dependent manner. Various drugs used to treat PONV are 5-hydroxytryptamine subtype 3 receptor antagonists, anticholinergic/antimuscarinic drugs, transdermal scopolamine, histamine receptor antagonists such as Dimenhydrinate and Promethazine, and dopamine antagonist-metoclopramide.[11,12] Other antiemetics utilized include butyrophenones, droperidol, phenothiazines-perphenazine, and chlorpromazine, with fewer side effects.[13] It is better to use combination therapy and avoid opioids for PONV prevention. An organized multimodal strategy beginning in the preoperative stage can drastically lower the incidence of PONV.

Ileus

An aberrant pattern of sluggish or absent gastrointestinal motility following surgery is known as postoperative ileus. Clinically, abdominal distension and obstipation are commonly present, along with sluggish bowel sounds **(Fig. 3)**. It can result in extended hospital stays, higher healthcare costs, and discomfort for the patient. Colonic motility usually returns within 72 hours postoperatively. Therefore, the ileus that persists past this point is frequently regarded as pathologic. The causes of prolonged ileus can be broadly divided into three groups: (1) pharmacologic, (2) neurogenic, and (3) inflammatory.[14,15]

High correlation with ileus was identified with the following conditions:[14]

- Interruption of the GI continuity (in cases of resection) or manipulation of the bowel
- Anesthetic and analgesic medications
- Immobility
- Electrolytes imbalance, especially hypokalemia

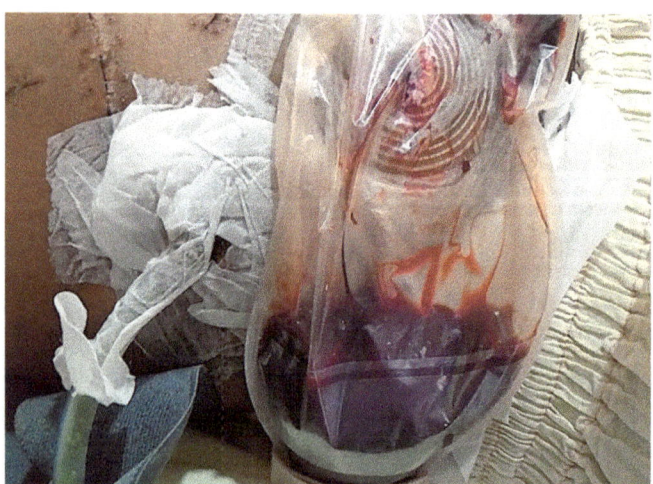

Fig. 2: Secondary hemorrhage on day 9 following excision of insulinoma in the head of the pancreas.

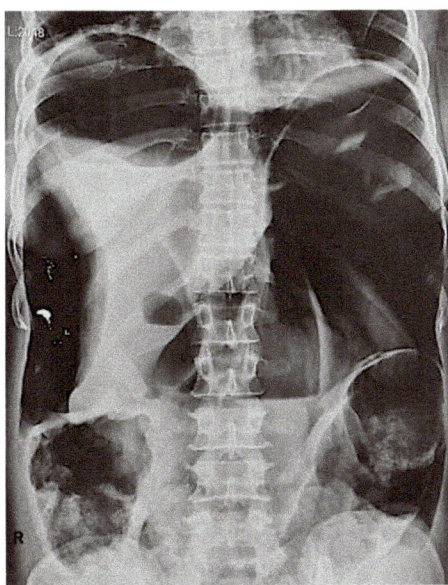

Fig. 3: Postoperative abdomen with ileus.

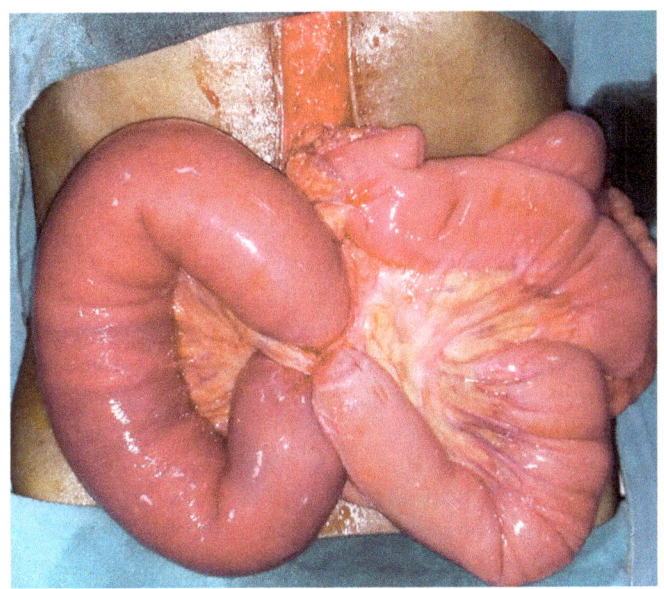

Fig. 4: Intestinal obstruction due to postoperative band and adhesions.

- Intra-abdominal hematoma
- Intra-abdominal severe infection or sepsis
- Chronic medical conditions such as diabetes mellitus (DM)
- Local or generalized abdominal inflammation such as pancreatitis
- Severe pain
- Cardiopulmonary failure.

It is important to differentiate this condition from peritonitis and mechanical obstruction. Peritonitis invariably requires surgical care and could be differentiated by tenderness, guarding and rigidity. Similarly, mechanical obstruction mostly presents with abdominal distension, colicky abdominal pain, and bilious vomiting. A transition point with dilated proximal and collapsed distal small bowel is seen in mechanical bowel obstruction, while ileus exhibits diffuse air-fluid levels and bowel distention on radiological (X-rays and computed tomography) scans. Supportive care, electrolyte correction and drainage of collections invariably result in the resolution of the ileus if major or treatable diseases have been ruled out. Other measures include early ambulation, intravenous fluid replacement, and sometimes the insertion of a nasogastric tube.

Acute Bowel Obstruction

Early small bowel obstruction occurs in 1–12% of abdominal operations.[16] Postoperative acute bowel obstruction, mechanical or functional, is associated with increased morbidity and mortality if not diagnosed and treated early. Bowel obstruction can occur in the early postoperative period within the first 30 days.

Postoperative adhesion, bands and internal hernias are the common causes (**Fig. 4**). Other causes are volvulus, intussusception, and anastomotic leaks.[16]

As explained earlier, clinically, patients present with abdominal distension, colicky abdominal pain and bilious vomiting. Most patients fail to pass flatus and feces, but the passage of stool should not exclude intestinal obstruction. Sometimes patients with intestinal obstruction can still pass stool for a few days from the bowel distal to the obstruction. Increased bowel sound is a constant feature. The disappearance of bowel sounds with the appearance of tenderness is a dangerous scenario. It suggests bowel ischemia or perforation and must be treated urgently. Four compounds have been studied to prevent postoperative adhesion formation: hyaluronate-carboxymethyl cellulose (HA-CMC), polyethylene glycol, oxidized regenerative cellulose and icodextrin.[17] Only HA-CMC and Icodextrin have shown some benefit in reducing postoperative SBO.[17] In the evaluation of adhesive SBO, a water-soluble contrast study may aid in predicting the need for operative intervention.[18] In patients with early postoperative small bowel obstruction (ESBO) that is not relenting, a water-soluble contrast study confirming nonpassage of contrast into the colon may be useful if reoperation is contemplated. Most cases of ESBO can be safely treated nonoperatively without clinical deterioration and signs of strangulation. However, a substantial proportion of patients (14–58%) with ESBO will still require reoperation.[19] There is no consensus as to an acceptable period of nonoperative management before deciding to operate. However, reoperation is thought to be hazardous after 2 weeks due to the maturation of adhesions.[20]

Anastomotic Leak

Anastomotic leak is a communication between the intra- and extraluminal compartments owing to a defect of the integrity of the intestinal wall at the anastomosis (proposed by the International Study Group of Rectal Cancer).[21]

Detailed criteria are as follows: (1) apparent discharge of gas/pus/feces from abdominal or pelvic drainage tube; (2) anastomotic defect confirmed by proctoscopy, CT scan using contrast medium or rectal examination (only for lower rectal anastomosis); (3) confirmed during relaparotomy.

The clinical presentation varies on the anastomotic site, intraperitoneal or extraperitoneal anastomosis, and the contents leaking into the peritoneal cavity.

The cause of the anastomotic leak may be multifactorial, including faulty technique, ischemic change of the intestine at the suture line, excessive tension across anastomosis and mesentery, local sepsis, and the presence of obstruction distal to the anastomosis.

The lowest leak rates are found with ileocolic anastomoses (1–3%), and the highest occur with coloanal (10–20%). Leaks usually become apparent between 5 and 7 days postoperatively.[22] Late leaks, often after a month postoperatively, present insidiously with low-grade fever, prolonged ileus, and nonspecific symptoms attributable.[23] Small leaks often result in a localized collection, detected radiologically and often requiring drainage.

Early diagnosis is crucial as the delay may result in poor outcomes. The laboratory markers often deranged are leukocytosis, serum procalcitonin (PCT) and C-reactive protein (CRP), which may help in early diagnosis. Most often, small leaks are detected by contrast-enhanced computerized axial scans showing extravasation or collections. The outcome of the complication depends upon the early diagnosis and treatment. The common surgical procedure done to salvage the patient is a defunctioning stoma.

Peritonitis

Postoperative peritonitis (PP) is a life-threatening hospital-acquired intra-abdominal infection after abdominal surgery with high mortality rates.

The most frequent causes of postoperative peritonitis are intraabdominal abscesses and the anastomotic leakage or breakdown of the digestive suture from enteric, bilioenteric or pancreatoenteric anastomosis **(Fig. 5)**.

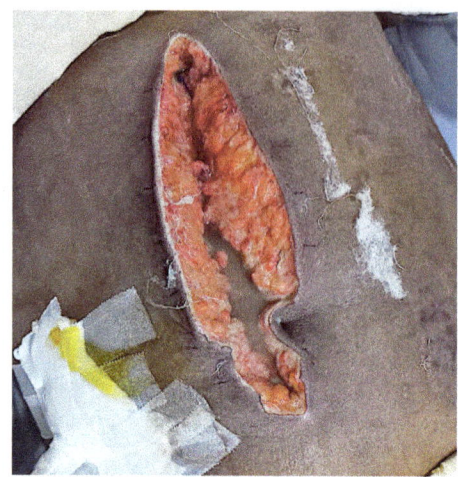

Fig. 5: Postoperative case of Whipple's procedure with wound dehiscence and pancreatic fistula.

The peritoneal lining, on contact with the intestinal contents, including bile and pancreatic enzymes, becomes inflamed, resulting in diffuse abdominal pain, guarding and systemic signs of sepsis.

The treatment of postoperative peritonitis is based on three principles: (1) focus elimination, (2) intensive care management, and (3) broad-spectrum antibiotic therapy. Bile or pancreatic enzymes leak after a biliary tract, or pancreatic surgery is a surgical emergency. Unless prompt drainage of the contents is done with the control of infection, the patient may deteriorate suddenly due to sepsis.

Hepatic Dysfunction

Mild liver dysfunction sometimes occurs after major surgery, even without preexisting liver disorders. This dysfunction usually results from hepatic ischemia or poorly understood effects of anesthesia.[24]

Postoperative hepatic dysfunction is seen more often with upper abdominal surgeries that may significantly reduce total hepatic blood flow. Resection of hepatocellular carcinoma poses a significant risk of liver failure from insufficient hepatic reserve following the operation.[24]

Jaundice secondary to excessive hemolysis is characterized by anemia and indirect (unconjugated) hyperbilirubinemia with preservation of normal serum alkaline phosphatase and alanine transaminase (ALT). Various causes include the breakdown of transfused erythrocytes from multiple blood transfusions, reabsorption of extravasated blood (e.g., retroperitoneal or intra-abdominal hematomas from trauma or ruptured aortic aneurysms), ABO incompatibility, hemolytic anemia, glucose-6-phosphate dehydrogenase deficiency, malaria, sickle cell anemia, and kidney diseases leading to hemolytic uremic syndrome.

The other condition is ischemic hepatitis due to cardiogenic shock or accidental ligation of the hepatic artery during cholecystectomy and after major hepatectomies.[25]

Pancreatitis

Postoperative pancreatitis is a well-described complication and usually follows surgery involving the abdomen or the use of cardiopulmonary bypass, including transurethral resection of the prostate.[26,27] Acute pancreatitis following cholecystectomy in the early postoperative period can result from the passage or slippage of a stone or biliary sludge and microliths along the ampulla of Vater. Although the association between pancreatitis related to propofol use remains unproven, there are still anecdotal reports on the same.[28]

Stoma-related Complications

Among all stoma types, the incidence of peristomal skin problems is as high as 40% **(Fig. 6)**.

Parastomal hernia is the second most common complication, mostly with colostomy. Stoma dehiscence,

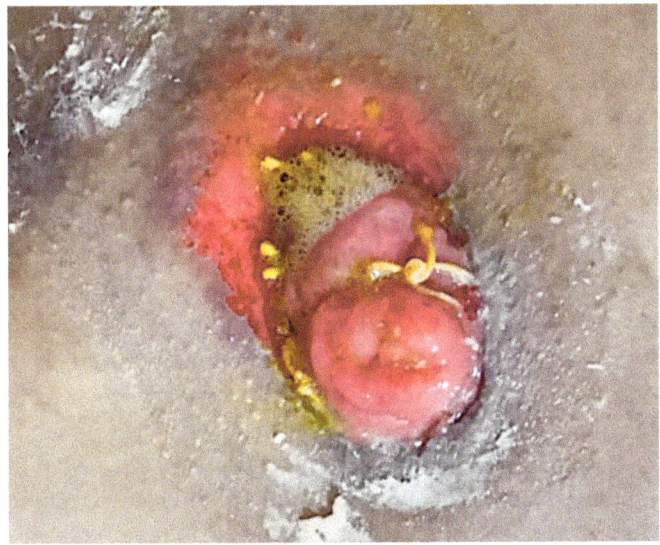

Fig. 6: Stomal retraction with skin excoriation.

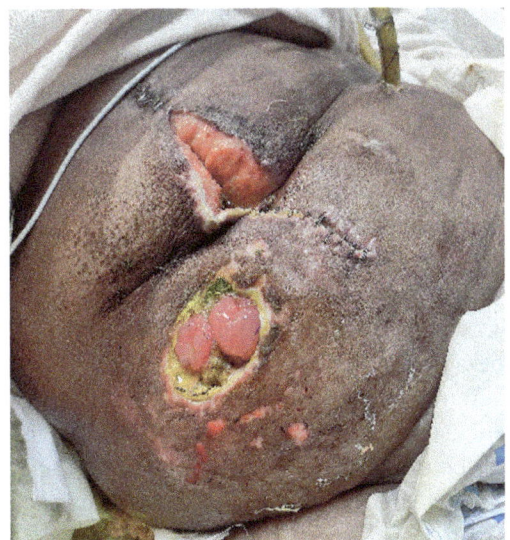

Fig. 7: Stoma retraction with fecal peritonitis.

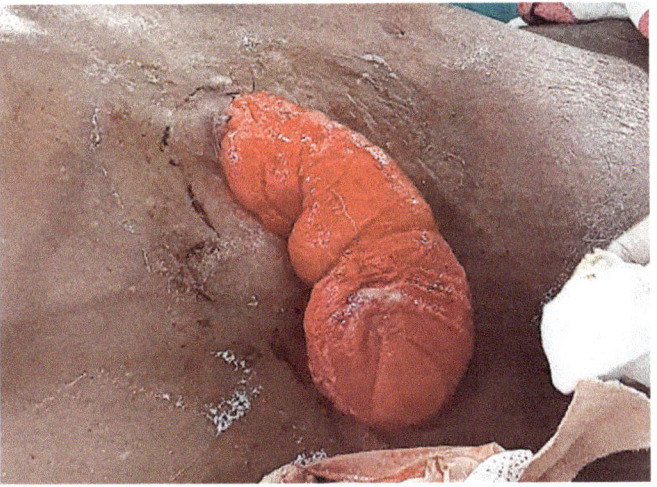

Fig. 8: Stomal prolapse.

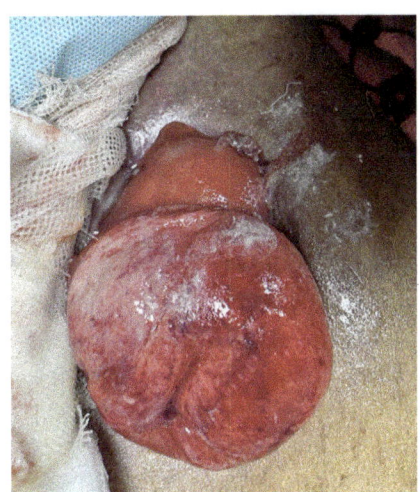

Fig. 9: Stomal prolapse with edema.

stoma obstruction, stoma infection, and stoma stenosis occur in 2–5% of cases. High output stoma (1–18%), stoma ischemia (2–7%), stoma prolapse (2–10%), and stoma retraction (1–5%) requires immediate attention. Unless treated urgently, it carries high morbidity and mortality. The stoma may retract **(Fig. 7)**, or prolapse **(Figs. 8 and 9)**, resulting in intestinal obstruction and requiring emergency care.[29] Most complications are avoidable with proper preoperative planning, good surgical technique and early identification of the complication. The stoma should be evaluated daily by an experienced surgeon and a stoma care nurse. Many times, the patient with a stoma may present with high output or nil output in the emergency and need to be managed accordingly.

Enterocutaneous Fistula

Enterocutaneous fistulas are iatrogenic in about 75–85% of cases. The mortality rate often is high (10–30%).[30,31] Missed perforations, enterotomy, an anastomotic leak and ischemia are frequently the cause of enterocutaneous fistulas. Other causes could be erosion by the foreign body and trauma.

The main goal of treatment is to avoid intra-abdominal collection and encourage spontaneous fistula closure. If this is not possible, the fistula tract is resected, and if possible, the continuity of the bowel is restored after the patient's clinical conditions have been improved.

Serial measurement of the transferrin and serum albumin levels can guide the optimal timing of the surgery. Proximal small bowel fistulas are less likely to close spontaneously.

Octreotide, proton pump inhibitors, and loperamide can be used to reduce fluid and electrolyte loss from high-output fistulas. Dehydration and electrolyte imbalance are frequent with enterocutaneous fistulas with high output. Daily weighing, central venous pressure monitoring and measurement of the urinary output is highly recommended.

Peristomal skin protection using snugly fit colostomy bags, and skin barrier creams should be a top priority.

Sepsis is the leading cause of death; hence quick and aggressive treatment is needed. Any collection must be drained immediately.

A fistula will typically close on its own within 6 weeks unless the bowel is diseased or has an ongoing disease at the site of the fistula (such as Crohn's disease, cancer, or radiation damage; involves >50% of the bowel's circumference and a very short tract. A fistula is unlikely to close if it has not been by 12 weeks.

To determine the amount of intestinal disease, the site of the fistula's origin, rule out any obstructive lesions, and describe the anatomy of fistulous tracts, radiographic contrast tests, small bowel follow-through investigations, enemas, and fistulogram can be performed. CT scan is extremely useful for identifying the anatomy, undrained collections, and the pathology site. It is recommended to wait for at least 6 weeks for the patient to be nutritionally-replete (i.e., in positive nitrogen balance) or for the surgical site to have matured sufficiently to attempt a cure.

Surgical Site Infections

Postoperative wound infections are a common problem, often unduly increasing the morbidity and mortality of a patient. As per the Centers for Disease Control and Prevention (CDC), surgical wound infections are classified as superficial or deep incisional infections and organ-specific infections.

Most surgical site infections are due to the endogenous flora that is usually present on the mucous membranes, skin, or hollow viscera. The most common endogenous causative organisms are *S. aureus*, coagulase-negative staphylococci, Enterococcus and Escherichia coli. Exogenous flora may come from the theater room, including air, instruments, materials, and staff members.

The most common exogenous organisms are staphylococci and streptococci.[32]

Clinical features of surgical site infections are similar to the classical five signs of inflammation, but some small details set them apart. These include erythema, localized pain, unexplained persistent pyrexia, discharge from the wound (often purulent), wound dehiscence, and problems with wound healing **(Figs. 10 and 11)**. When suspecting wound infection, the occlusive dressings should be removed. The wound blisters, gray or black tissue will alert the clinician that there is ischemia and/or necrosis, therefore, increased risk of wound infection. If there is discharge, a microbiology swab at this point needs to be taken, and treatment commenced. A serous or sanguineous discharge does not indicate infection, but a purulent discharge does **(Fig. 12)**.

For prophylaxis, a safe, narrow-spectrum agent should be administered 30–60 minutes before knife-to-skin time to allow tissue concentrations to reach therapeutic levels at the time of operation with coverage for the expected microorganisms and should be prescribed for the shortest effective period.

Wound-related Complications, Including Dehiscence/Burst Abdomen

Common wound complications include flap necrosis **(Fig. 13)**, surgical-site infections (SSIs), wound dehiscence, and burst abdomen. Abdominal wound dehiscence is the disruption or breakdown of a wound after abdominal surgery. It may be partial when one or more layers have separated, but the skin or the peritoneum is intact. Complete wound dehiscence occurs when all layers of the abdominal wall have opened apart, and this may or may not be associated with the evisceration of the viscus **(Fig. 14)**. Every surgeon will face complications or emergencies in the postoperative period. Although postoperative complications are inevitable, some can be prevented or avoided through vigilant care immediately after surgery and throughout the healing period. However, prevention is better than cure. One need to adequately prepare a patient planned for

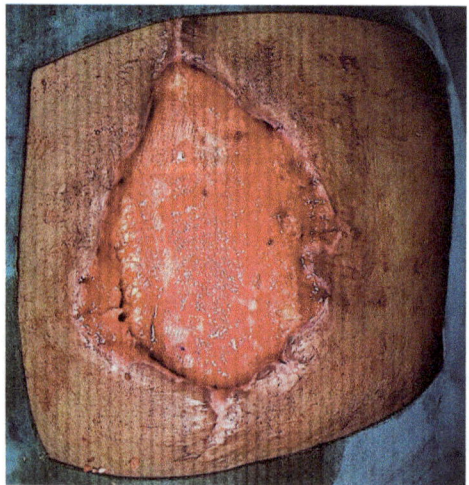

Fig. 10: Wound dehiscence.

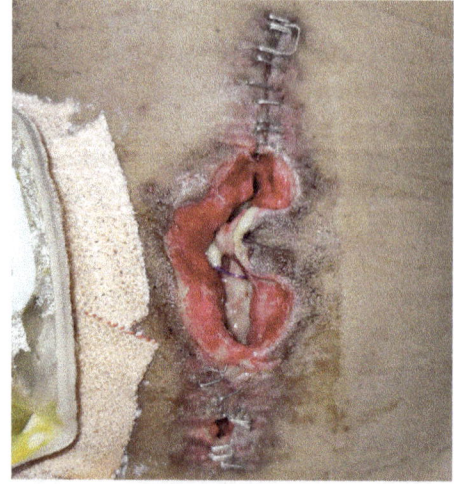

Fig. 11: Wound surgical-site infections with partial dehiscence.

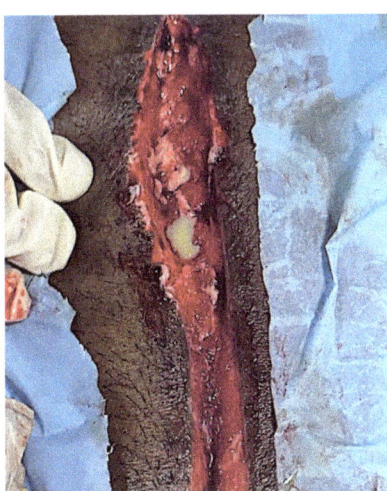

Fig. 12: Deep surgical-site infections with purulent discharge from the incision site.

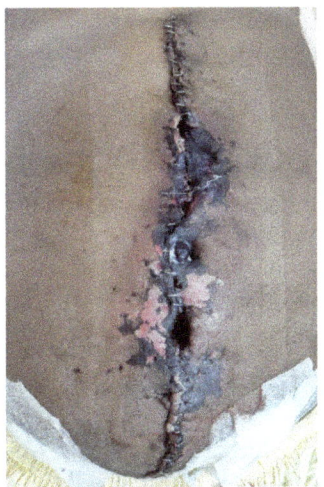

Fig. 13: Skin flap necrosis.

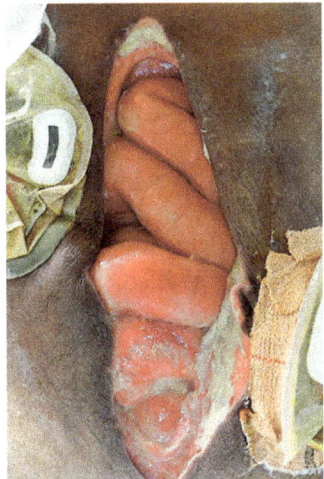

Fig. 14: Burst abdomen.

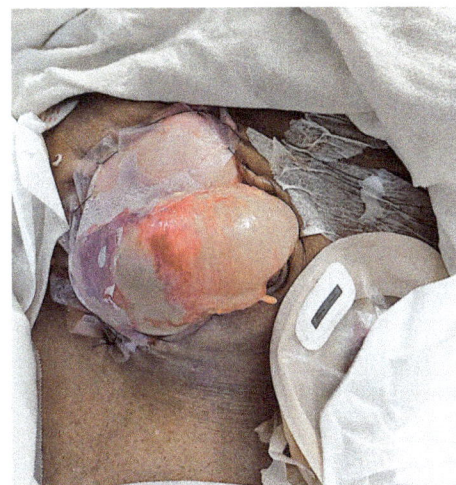

Fig. 15: Burst abdomen with gangrene of the exposed colon.

elective surgery keeping all the systems into purview. In case of emergency surgery the postoperative course will be highly unpredictable as the patient was not physically or mentally prepared for the surgery. Hence strict vigilance is recommended in the postoperative recovery period. Also, adequate patient and their relative education is mandated to handle themselves the postoperative care at home after discharge and informs any untoward problem early. Disruption can take place at any time in the postoperative period but most often occurs between the 5th and 12th postoperative day **(Fig. 15)**.

In about half the cases, disruption becomes evident by the appearance of a serosanguinous discharge on the dressing. Some factors that may be related to a burst abdomen include elderly age, in patients operated on for peritonitis due to hollow viscus perforation, malignancy, increased bilirubin levels, hypoproteinemia, and altered liver function tests. The burst abdomen is defined as the separation of all layers of an incision **(Fig. 15)**. Appropriate treatment at the

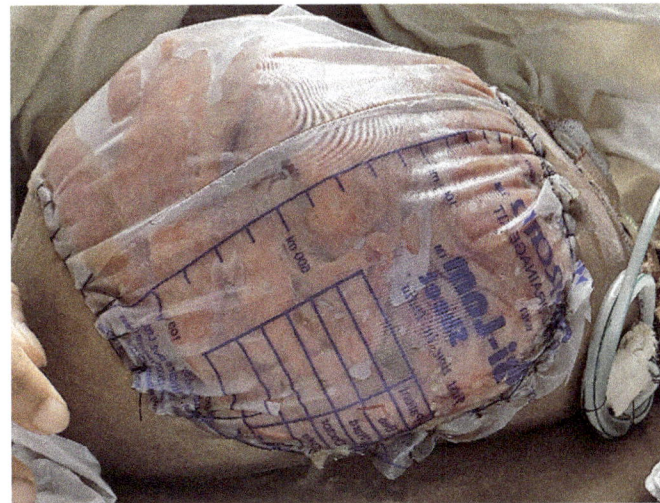

Fig. 16: Burst abdomen managed by Bogota bag closure.

bedside includes protecting the intestines with sterile towels and shifting the patient to the operating room soon **(Fig.16)**.

A meticulous suturing technique, with appropriate suture material, is recommended to prevent the dreaded postoperative complication.

NEUROLOGICAL COMPLICATIONS

Postoperative neurological disorders such as postoperative delirium (POD), postoperative cognitive dysfunction (POCD), postoperative covert ischemic stroke, and hemorrhagic stroke cause cognition declines and poor long-term functional outcomes in the elderly especially. This complication can cause significant financial loss to the family, including increased mortality.

Postoperative delirium, frequently linked to anesthesia, is defined as the acute emergence of confusion, disorientation, perceptual disturbances, emotional dysregulation, or sleep disturbances manifesting within a certain time.[33] Blood pressure fluctuation in the postoperative period is an important risk factor for postoperative stroke.[34] Early prevention is likely to be more effective than prognosis treatment. Significantly, dexmedetomidine may be an effective medication for preventing POD or POCD.

RENAL COMPLICATIONS

Postoperative acute kidney injury (PO-AKI) is a common complication of major surgery, which can result in substantial long-term morbidity and mortality. PO-AKI is best defined as AKI occurring within 7 days of an operative intervention using the Kidney Disease Improving Global Outcomes (KDIGO) definition of AKI.[35]

Commonly implicated mechanisms for PO-AKI include ischemia–reperfusion injury, endogenous or exogenous nephrotoxins, physical causes such as obstruction, inflammatory factors, vasoconstriction, and oxidative stress.[36] Most commonly, a combination of preoperative risk factors like elderly, diabetes, and preexisting kidney dysfunction along with intraoperative and postoperative events leads to the development of AKI.

The important intraoperative factors include hypovolemia caused by bleeding, increased intra-abdominal pressure, anesthetic-induced decreased cardiac output and vasodilatation.

Postoperative factors attributed to PO-AKI include hypovolemia, kidney inflammation, exposure to nephrotoxins, urinary obstruction and mechanical ventilation.

As a general principle, treatment of AKI should be initiated as early as possible. The 2012 KDIGO clinical practice guideline for AKI consists of supportive measures, including volume management, maintenance of adequate blood pressure and judicious avoidance of nephrotoxins. As postoperative hyperglycemia is strongly associated with AKI, avoidance of perioperative hyperglycemia (>180 mg/dL) is recommended.[37]

Preoperative Care

- *Pulmonary exercises:* Pulmonary exercises including incentive spirometry before surgery and continuing it postoperative will help to regulate breathing by recruiting more alveoli, thus ensuring adequate oxygenation for healing. These exercises can also clear the lungs and lower the risk of pneumonia especially after surgery.
- *Good control of comorbidities:* Needless to stress upon, good control of diabetes and hypertension is essential before any elective surgery. Other factors to ensure should be good hydration, electrolytes balance and nutrition.

Intraoperative Care

- *Proper hand washing to avoid cross-contamination:* Appropriate hand hygiene is the single most effective strategy to protect patients from health care–associated infections, including SSIs.
- *Strict adherence to aseptic surgical and sterilization techniques:* Recommended sterilization techniques, preoperative, and intraoperative skin preparation of the patient, and general techniques for working in a sterile field can minimize microbial contamination and reduce SSIs and other wound related complications.
- *Tissue respect and meticulous surgical techniques:* Judicious use of energy sources will limit unnecessary normal tissue damage. Also, the vessels need to be securely tied to prevent a postoperative catastrophe. Point to reiterate, vigilant postoperative clinical observation of the patient for early detection of emergencies.
- *Good hydration:* Dehydration can contribute to poor oxygen perfusion and prevent essential nutrients from being delivered to the wound, thereby delaying wound healing. Additionally, adequate hydration can help to prevent complications such as deep vein thrombosis and pulmonary embolism.

Postoperative Care

- *Early ambulation:* Walking and exercising the legs as soon as possible after surgery promote the delivery of oxygen throughout the body and prevent stagnation of blood to decrease the potential development of blood clots. In order to reduce postoperative difficulties, we finally recommend implementing the ICOUGH regimen (registered trademark of Boston University).[38]
- *Early start of enteral nutrition:* Balanced and healthy nutrition definitely helps in tissue healing and prevents intestinal anastomotic complications.

Take Home Messages

- Postoperative complications requiring emergency attention may be life-threatening.
- VTE after major surgery carries a significant mortality and is better prevented by early mobilization and pharmacoprophylaxis by LMWH.

- Major adverse cardiac event should be carefully monitored to avoid mortality. Sensitivity Troponin-I is a good screening tool.
- Atelectasis, Pneumonia and Pulmonary Embolism are risk in elderly patients. Risk factors should be identified preobtained and patient should be prepared accordingly by spirometry, breathing exercise and use CPAP.
- Risk of hemorrhage is reduced by identification and correction of coagulopathy both pre- and postoperatively.
- Low threshold for re-exploration often save life in post-operative hemorrhage.
- Postoperatively, ileus should be differentiated from mechanical obstruction or peritonitis with usual requirement of urgent re-exploration.
- Disappearance of tenderness is dangerous sign and may suggest bowel ischemia or perforation.
- Early detection of a bowel leak by contrast CT may change the approach.
- Urgent drainage and control of sepsis is lifesaving in peritonitis.
- Enterocutaneous fistula should be treated conservatively for at least before surgical intervention/is undertaken.

REFERENCES

1. Ahmed MM, Akbar DH, Al-Shaikh AR. Deep vein thrombosis at King Abdul Aziz University Hospital. Saudi Med J. 2000; 21(8):762-4.
2. Bergqvist D, Lindblad B. A 30-year survey of pulmonary embolism verified at autopsy: an analysis of 1274 surgical patients. Br J Surg. 1985;72(2):105-8.
3. Hirsh J, Hoak J. Management of deep vein thrombosis and pulmonary embolism: a statement for healthcare professionals from the council on thrombosis (in consultation with the council on cardiovascular radiology). Am Heart Assoc Circ. 1996;93:2212-45.
4. Lobastov K, Barinov V, Schastlivtsev I, Laberko L, Rodoman G, Boyarintsev V. Validation of the Caprini risk assessment model for venous thromboembolism in high-risk surgical patients in the background of standard prophylaxis. J Vasc Surg Venous Lymphat Disord. 2016;4(2):153-60.
5. Sazgary L, Puelacher C, Lurati Buse G, Glarner N, Lampart A, Bolliger D, et al; BASEL-PMI Investigators. Incidence of major adverse cardiac events following noncardiac surgery. Eur Heart J Acute Cardiovasc Care. 2020;10(5):550-8.
6. POISE Study Group, Devereaux PJ, Yang H, Yusuf S, Guyatt G, Leslie K, Villar JC, et al. Effects of extended-release metoprolol succinate in patients undergoing noncardiac surgery (POISE trial): a randomised controlled trial. Lancet. 2008;371(9627):1839-47.
7. Kelkar KV. Post-operative pulmonary complications after non-cardiothoracic surgery. Indian J Anaesth. 2015;59(9):599-605.
8. Fischer SP, Bader AM, Sweitzer BJ. Preoperative evaluation. In: Miller RD, Eriksson LI, Fleisher LA, Wiener-Kronish JP, Young WL (Eds). Miller's Anesthesia, 7th edition. New York: Churchill Livingstone; 2010.; pp. 1019-22.
9. Dave MH, Frotzler A, Spielmann N, Madjdpour C, Weiss M. Effect of tracheal tube cuff shape on fluid leakage across the cuff: an in vitro study. Br J Anaesth. 2010;105:538-43.
10. Shaikh SI, Nagarekha D, Hegade G, Marutheesh M. Postoperative nausea and vomiting: a simple yet complex problem. Anesth Essays Res. 2016;10:388-96.
11. Swaika S, Pal A, Chatterjee S, Saha D, Dawar N. Ondansetron, ramosetron, or palonosetron: which is a better choice of antiemetic to prevent postoperative nausea and vomiting in patients undergoing laparoscopic cholecystectomy? Anesth Essays Res. 2011;5:182-6.
12. Diemunsch P, Gan TJ, Philip BK, Girao MJ, Eberhart L, Irwin MG, et al. Single-dose aprepitant vs ondansetron for the prevention of postoperative nausea and vomiting: a randomized, double-blind phase III trial in patients undergoing open abdominal surgery. Br J Anaesth. 2007;99:202-11.
13. Storrar J, Hitchens M, Platt T, Dorman S. Droperidol for treatment of nausea and vomiting in palliative care patients. Cochrane Database Syst Rev. 2014;2014(11):CD006938.
14. Khawaja ZH, Gendia A, Adnan N, Ahmed J. Prevention and Management of Postoperative Ileus: A Review of Current Practice. Cureus. 2022;14(2):e22652.
15. Lee MJ, Vaughan-Shaw P, Vimalachandran D; ACPGBI GI Recovery Group. A systematic review and meta-analysis of baseline risk factors for the development of postoperative ileus in patients undergoing gastrointestinal surgery. Ann R Coll Surg Engl. 2020;102(3):194-203.
16. Stewart RM, Page CP, Brender J, Schwesinger W, Eisenhut D. The incidence and risk of early postoperative small bowel obstruction. A cohort study. Am J Surg. 1987;154(6):643-7.
17. Waldron MG, Judge C, Farina L, O'Shaughnessy A, O'Halloran M. Barrier materials for prevention of surgical adhesions: systematic review. BJS Open. 2022;6(3):zrac075.
18. Koh A, Adiamah A, Chowdhury A, Mohiuddin MK, Bharathan B. Therapeutic Role of Water-Soluble Contrast Media in Adhesive Small Bowel Obstruction: a Systematic Review and Meta-Analysis. J Gastrointest Surg. 2020;24(2): 473-83.
19. Goussous N, Kemp KM, Bannon MP, Kendrick ML, Srvantstyan B, Khasawneh MA, Zielinski MD. Early post-operative small bowel obstruction: open vs laparoscopic. Am J Surg. 2015;209(2):385-90.
20. Ong AW, Myers SR. Early postoperative small bowel obstruction: a review. Am J Surg. 2020;219:535-9.
21. Rahbari NN, Weitz J, Hohenberger W, Heald RJ, Moran B, Ulrich A, et al. Definition and grading of anastomotic leakage following anterior resection of the rectum: a proposal by the International Study Group of Rectal Cancer. Surgery. 2010;147(3):339-51.
22. Li YW, Lian P, Huang B, Zheng HT, Wang MH, Gu WL, et al. Very Early Colorectal Anastomotic Leakage within 5 Post-operative Days: a More Severe Subtype Needs Relaparotomy. Sci Rep. 2017;7:39936.
23. Lim SB, Yu CS, Kim CW, Yoon YS, Park IJ, Kim JC. Late anastomotic leakage after low anterior resection in rectal cancer patients: clinical characteristics and predisposing factors. Colorectal Dis. 2016;18(4):O135-40.
24. Huang J, Hwang GC. Postoperative Hepatic Dysfunction. In: Freeman BS, Berger JS (Eds). Anesthesiology Core Review: Part Two Advanced Exam. New York: McGraw Hill; 2016.
25. Kauffmann R, Fong Y. Post-hepatectomy liver failure. Hepatobiliary Surg Nutr. 2014;3(5):238-46.
26. White TT, Morgan A, Hopton D. Postoperative pancreatitis: a study of 70 cases. Am J Surg 1970;132:120-3.

27. Lee MH, Chen KK, Lin ATL, Lee YH, Chen MT, Chang LS. Acute pancreatitis following transurethral resection of the prostate. Eur Urol. 1993;23:419-22.
28. Leisure GS, O'Flaherty J, Green L, Jones DR. Jones. Propofol and Postoperative Pancreatitis. Anesthesiology. 199684:224-7.
29. Babakhanlou R, Larkin K, Hita AG, Stroh J, Yeung SC. Stoma-related complications and emergencies. Int J Emerg Med. 2022;15(1):17.
30. Gefen R, Garoufalia Z, Zhou P, Watson K, Emile SH, Wexner SD. Treatment of enterocutaneous fistula: a systematic review and meta-analysis. Tech Coloproctol. 2022;26(11):863-74.
31. Noori IF. Postoperative enterocutaneous fistulas: Management outcomes in 23 consecutive patients. Ann Med Surg. 2021;66:102413.
32. Zabaglo M, Sharman T. Postoperative Wound Infection. Treasure Island (FL): StatPearls Publishing; 2022.
33. Liu B, Huang D, Guo Y, Sun X, Chen C, Zhai X, et al. Recent advances and perspectives of postoperative neurological disorders in the elderly surgical patients. CNS Neurosci Ther. 2022;28(4):470-83.
34. Lin MH, Kamel H, Singer DE, Wu YL, Lee M, Ovbiagele B. Perioperative/postoperative atrial fibrillation and risk of subsequent stroke and/or mortality. Stroke. 2019;50: 1364-71.
35. Prowle R., Forni LG, Bell M, Chew MS, Edwards M, Grams ME, et al. Postoperative acute kidney injury in adult noncardiac surgery: joint consensus report of the Acute Disease Quality Initiative and PeriOperative Quality Initiative. Nat Rev Nephrol. 2021;17(9):605-18.
36. Chronopoulos A, Cruz DN, Ronco C. Hospital-acquired acute kidney injury in the elderly. Nat. Rev Nephrol. 2010;6: 141-9.
37. Frisch A, Chandra P, Smiley D, Peng L, Rizzo M, Gatcliffe C, et al. Prevalence and clinical outcome of hyperglycemia in the perioperative period in noncardiac surgery. Diabetes Care. 2010;33:1783-8.
38. Cassidy MR, Rosenkranz P, McCabe K, Rosen JE, McAneny D. I COUGH: reducing postoperative pulmonary complications with a multidisciplinary patient care program. JAMA Surg. 2013;148(8):740-5.

SECTION 15: Miscellaneous Emergencies-2

Section Editor: Dipashri Bhattacharya

37. **Code Blue and Crash Cart**
    Namrata Biswas

38. **Anesthetic Emergencies**
    Dipasri Bhattacharya

CHAPTER 37

Code Blue and Crash Cart

Namrata Biswas

INTRODUCTION

Hospitals use emergency codes to make the staff aware of various emergency situations without causing panic among visitors and other patients worldwide. Each code is specific for a particular situation which needs immediate tackling from the different categories of staff and every employee needs to be aware of the policies and the disaster plan.

When a patient requires resuscitation or is otherwise needs of immediate medical attention, "Code Blue" is announced, most often it indicates a respiratory or cardiac arrest. Theoretically, any medical professional may respond to a code but in practice policies are made for specific units to provide personnel for code coverage.[1] Commonly anesthesiologists, emergency medicine and internal medicine physicians are in the team. To "run the code" a rapid response team leader or a physician is responsible for directing the resuscitation.

After ensuring the safety of the patient, staff and bystanders, the management of the collapsed patient involves the following:[2]

- Calling for help and asking for a "crash trolley"
- Moving the patient to a safe place
- Check the response to verbal and tactile stimuli
- Care of circulation, airway and breathing
- Stop bleeding if present
- Maintenance of normal body temperature
- Reassurance and continued observation of the collapsed patient.

RESPONSIBILITIES OF A CODE BLUE TEAM

- *Team Leader*
  The anesthesiologist/intensivist/emergency medicine specialist is usually the team leader:
  - Designates roles to other members and instructs their actions
  - Starts the resuscitation according to the ACLS protocol
  - Decides appropriate further action once the patient is stabilized
  - Brief the patient's attendant and family members after resuscitation
  - Makes sure that one member (nursing) is designated to record events in the *code blue* flow sheet and get it verified
- *Physician or Anesthesiologist*
  - Manages the airway and circulation
- *One Nurse*
  - Assists doctor in managing the airway
  - Assists in obtaining IV access and administer the drugs as per team leader's instructions
  - Assists in managing code as requested
  - Will remain with the patient until the transfer
- *Other Nurse*
  - Get the crash trolley
  - AED/defibrillator switched on
  - Fill *code blue* flowsheet and attach to the patient's medical record after showing it to team leader.
- *Security Personnel*
  - Directs team members toward code location
  - Ensuring the safety of the scene before proceeding with their response
  - Keep the crowd and any extra personnel away from the *code blue* site.
- *Hospital Attendant*
  - Help nursing staff in pushing "crash cart" near the patient
  - Assists in various other activities.

CRASH TROLLEY

Recommended Equipment

As per updated guidelines of 2020 published by American Heart Association (AHA):

- Airway (oral and nasal) of all sizes
- McGill forceps, large and small
- Laryngoscope with all three sizes of blades
- Endotracheal tubes of various sizes with bougie
- Bag valve mask (both adult and pediatric)
- Adult and pediatric nasal cannula

- At least three sizes of nonrebreather oxygen face masks
- Intravenous (IV) start packs
- Normal saline solution (1,000 mL bags)
- Intravenous catheters of various sizes
- Three normal saline flush 10 mL syringes
- Gauze and antiseptic solutions
- Monitor with a defibrillator or automated external defibrillator (AED)
- Syringe nasal adaptor and a nasal atomizer
- A checklist hung on the cart.

Recommended Medication

- Aspirin: 81 mg tablets (4)
- Nitroglycerin (NTG) 0.4 mg sublingual tablets (3) or spray
- 25% or 50% Dextrose IV fluid
- Naloxone 1 mg/mL (6)
- Epinephrine 1:10,000 (auto injector preferable) (10)
- Atropine (3)
- Amiodarone 150 mg vial (3)
- Epinephrine 1:1,000 (2)
- Methyl prednisolone 125 mg (1)
- Diphenhydramine 50 mg vial (2)
- Adenosine 6 mg (3)
- Metoprolol 10 mg (2)
- Diltiazem 20 mg vial (2)
- Procainamide 1 g (1)
- Xylocaine 100 mg and xylocard (3)
- Hydrocortisone 100 mg (10).

Arrangement of Crash Trolley

- The defibrillator at the top of the emergency cart should be ready for use as soon as needed and checked daily to ensure it is in good working order.
- Medical personnel should also store a cardiopulmonary resuscitation (CPR) backboard and a resuscitation tape for pediatric patients outside the cart.
- Emergency cart medications are typically in the top drawers. Medications used for treating cardiac arrest are typically kept nearer to the front for faster access. One might store the standard crash cart medical emergency drugs in the first drawer and the pediatric medications in the second.
- Intubation equipment must be easy to access, sorted by size, and, if applicable, separated into adult and pediatric categories.[3]
- It is common to store the equipment needed for medical procedures in the bottom drawer, often the fifth drawer, of the medical cart set.

Top Shelf

- Defibrillator with pads, and adult and pediatric paddles
- Lubricating jelly
- Ambu bag with reservoir (adult and pediatric with mask size 00 to 5)
- Stethoscope
- Gloves of all sizes
- Oxygen key
- Torch and Hammer
- Scissors
- Surgical blade #11
- Kidney dish
- Knife dish with gauge pieces.

First Drawer

- Laryngoscope adult and pediatric and blade size 00 to 4
- Endotracheal tube in different sizes 1.5 to 8 with bougie
- Magill forceps for both children and adults
- Disposable oropharyngeal airways: 00, 0, 1, 2, 3, 4
- Syringes of various sizes (3 each)
- Tube fixation
- LMA of different sizes
- Tracheostomy tube size 2.5–10
- Suction Catheter #6–18
- Oxygen mask adult and pediatric
- High flow nasal cannula.

Second Drawer

- Inj. Adenosine
- Inj. Amiodarone
- Inj. Atropine
- Inj. Dopamine
- Inj. Epinephrine
- Inj. Naloxone
- Inj. Magnesium sulfate
- Inj. Sodium bicarbonate
- Inj. Calcium gluconate
- Inj. Xylocard 2%
- Inj. Digoxin
- Inj. Dobutamine
- Inj. Noradrenaline
- Inj. Aminophylline
- Inj. KCl
- Inj. Dextrose 25% and 50%
- Inj. Furosemide
- Inj. Hydrocortisone
- Inj. Mannitol
- Inj. Dexamethasone
- Inj. Phenytoin
- Inj. Labetalol
- Inj. NTG
- Inj. Pheniramine
- Inj. Metoprolol
- Inj. Midazolam.

Third Drawer

- Syringes 1 mL, 2 mL, 5 mL, 10 mL, 20 mL, 50 ml, and insulin
- Needles gauge 18–26
- IV catheters of different gauges (3 each 16–24 G)
- 3-way connector

- 3-way extension
- Central venous access set
- BT set
- Pedia drip set
- PM line
- Ryles tube #6, 8, 10, 12, 14, 16, 18
- Y-Connector
- Distilled water 10 mL (10)
- NaCl prefilled syringes 10 ml
- Alco swabs
- Tourniquet.

IV Fluids

Colloid and crystalloids.

Additional Requirement
- Full oxygen cylinder at the side of the crash cart
- Portable suction machine
- Sterile suturing set.

Location of Crash Cart

Medical crash trolleys typically have specific locations that allow access to many hospital settings. The most common places to put them are in an operating room, an emergency department, or an outpatient surgery center. They are stationed near areas that might require immediate access to emergency medications or life-saving medical equipment.

Inventory and Maintenance

The following is a maintenance routine that should be completed at least monthly:
- Expiration dates on medications should be checked on the first day of the month
- Expired medications should be promptly removed and replaced
- The defibrillation pads on the AED or the defibrillator should be checked for the expiration date
- The battery charge on the monitor and/or AED should be checked and documented
- Ensure specific schedule for inventories checks on each crash cart with a log of who performed the task. There should also be a record of what was replaced and the date on which it was done. Keeping a record can avoid potential medication mistakes, as well as dangerous situations such as empty oxygen tanks being left unfilled.

HOW CAN TECHNOLOGY HELP IMPROVE A CRASH CART?

Having computer technology available on the cart will allow those using it to access electronic records. When the crash cart is mobilized in an emergency situation, it is still a part of the patient's broader care and helps prevent errors. Easy access to patient files, allergies or additional information on the procedure or treatment at hand, can significantly speed up the activities of the medical staff. Nurses and other medical professionals may input patient data using the crash cart, which can help improve the accuracy and patient communication.

POSTRESUSCITATION CARE

Once the patient is resuscitated, proper post resuscitation care helps to preserve the neurological and cognitive functions. A coordinated multidisciplinary team effort is needed.[4]

The key steps include:
- Assessment and stabilization of cardiopulmonary status
- The etiology of the collapse needs to be determined
- Precautions regarding restoring and protecting neurological functions
- Prevention of a second arrest
- Manage the patient in a tertiary care center where hypothermia, advanced cardiovascular facilities are available[5].

CONCLUSION

Life is fragile. A medical team is dispatched as soon as the code blue is declared to provide resuscitation makes the odds of survival higher. A well equipped crash cart and proper training is mandatory for any hospital. All these will help in reducing immediate mortality of the patients.

Take Home Message

- Continuous training and mock drills need to be carried out at regular intervals for the code blue team. The crash cart has to be checked at regular predefined time interval and awareness campaign carried out among all staffs. All these will help in reducing mortality and the morbidity of patients.

REFERENCES

1. yumpu.com. Postgraduate programme international medicine–health crisis management. Code blue teams in general hospital. Guidelines and best practices postgraduate student. [online] Available from: https://www.yumpu.com/en/document/read/5416242/code-blue-teams-in-general-hospital-guidelines-and-best-practices. [Last Accessed January, 2023].
2. Bhoi, Sanjeev & Sharma, DK & Singh, Sheetal & Ramani Sardana, Sapna & Chauhan, Sonia. (2015). Code Blue Policy for a Tertiary Care Trauma Hospital in India. International Journal of Research Foundation of Hospital and Healthcare Administration. 3. 114-122. 10.5005/jp-journals-10035-47.
3. Ruiz, Josephine N, "In Situ Pediatric Mock Codes: The First Five Minutes" (2019). Doctoral Projects. 95. DOI: https://doi.org/10.31979/etd.7mff-jqss
4. Cobbe SM, Dalziel K, Ford I, Marsden a K. Survival of 1476 patients initially resuscitated from out of hospital cardiac arrest. BMJ. 1996;312(7047):1633-7.
5. Winslow R. Therapeutic hypothermia: can protect the brain in the aftermath of cardiac arrest. Wall Street J. 2009;1-4.

CHAPTER 38

Anesthetic Emergencies

Dipasri Bhattacharya

■ INTRODUCTION

The word *emergency* is borrowed from classical Latin ēmergere (to rise out or up) means unforeseen occurrence requiring immediate attention.

Anesthetic emergencies develop suddenly and require a teamwork for effective management. A clear understanding of the appropriate steps of management will help tackling the problems when emergency situation arises. The goal of crisis resource management (CRM) is to minimize the errors of complex tasks at the level of individual and team, and thereby to improve performance. The CRM team comprises leader, team member, communication, assessment, and resources support.

■ COMMON ANESTHETIC EMERGENCIES

The common anesthetic emergencies are:
- Airway emergencies
- Cardiovascular emergencies
- Respiratory emergencies
- Surgical emergencies
- Metabolic and endocrine emergencies
- Neurological and neurosurgical emergencies
- Obstetric emergencies
- Pediatric emergencies
- Regional anesthesia complications
- Anaphylaxis
- Malignant hyperthermia
- Trauma and disaster emergencies
- Perivascular/intravascular Injection
- Human error
- Ethical consideration.

■ AIRWAY EMERGENCIES

Airway emergencies arising due to difficult mask ventilation, difficult laryngoscopy, difficult or failed intubation and "cannot intubate cannot ventilate" situation, a nightmare for an anesthesiologist.

Difficult Mask Ventilation

This situation arises when it is not possible to provide adequate ventilation [*e.g.*, confirmed by end-tidal carbon dioxide (EtCO$_2$) detection], owing to one or more of the following reasons such as, inadequate seal of face mask, inappropriate leak of fresh gas, or excess resistance to the ingress or egress of gas.[1]

Prevalence: 0.4% of 176,679 adult cases.

Approach to Problem[1]

When mask ventilation is not adequate, the supraglottic airway devices (SADs) is considered for ventilation or as a conduit for intubation. If SADs are inadequate for ventilation, then it leads to "emergency pathway" where emergency invasive airway is indicated.

Difficult Laryngoscopy[1]

Difficult laryngoscopy is a situation when it is not possible to visualize any parts of the vocal cords with multiple attempts of laryngoscopy.

Prevalence: 0.4% of 176,679 adult cases.

Difficult Intubation[1]

Definition: Tracheal intubation requiring multiple attempts or tracheal intubation fails after multiple attempts.

Failed Intubation[1]

Prevalence: 0.1–10.1%

It may be anticipated or unanticipated.

Approach to Problem

Anticipated difficult intubation may be managed by awake fiberoptic intubation using airway block.

Unanticipated difficult airway

Use videolaryngoscope, McCoy laryngoscope, extra-large blade to visualize laryngeal aperture. If unable → try to ventilate to maintain adequate oxygenation

Unable

- *Call for help*
- Ensure that the FiO$_2$ is 100%.
- Call for the difficult airway cart.
- Reposition the patient's head and jaw.
- When laryngospasm is suspected, it is treated with propofol 0.25–0.8 mg/kg or succinylcholine 0.1–2 mg/kg intravenously.
- Insert an oropharyngeal or nasopharyngeal airway or place a laryngeal mask airway. In many such situations, the airway can be secured with insertion of a supraglottic airway.
- Consider two-person ventilation
  ↓ if not

Cannot intubate cannot ventilate situation[1]
↓
- Continue nasal oxygen and ensure adequate muscle relaxation
↓
- Adequate positioning with neck extended
↓
- Identify the cricothyroid membrane
↓
- Use high-pressure jet ventilation with needle cricothyroidotomy[1]

Other Airway Emergencies

Difficult or Failed Tracheal Extubation[1]

The loss of airway patency and adequate ventilation after removal of a tracheal tube or supraglottic airway from a patient with a known or suspected difficult airway.[1]

Approach to problem: Use Bougie, tube exchanger or LMA for extubation.

Aspiration

Aspiration of gastric contents into lungs remains to be a serious complication.

That occur *1 in every 2–3,000 operations.*

Causes:
- Improper cricoid pressure during rapid sequence induction
- Full stomach case, when gastric pH is <2.5 and gastric residual volume is >25 mL, the risk is more[2]
- Neuromuscular blocking agents
- A reduced conscious level from any cause
- Central nervous system disorders, e.g., stroke, bulbar palsy
- General anesthesia obtunds airway reflexes that normally function to protect the respiratory tract from soiling by regurgitated vomitus.[3]

Approach to problem is mainly preventive: Proper fasting guideline (international fasting guideline) should be followed to prevent aspiration.[4]

Recently, the gastric contents and volume is measured in fasting patients prior to elective surgery by using bedside ultrasound.[5]

Aspiration prophylaxis in full stomach:[6]
- Injection ranitidine 50 mg 30 minutes before surgery.
- Injection metoclopramide 10 mg 30 minutes before surgery.

CARDIOVASCULAR EMERGENCIES

Different arrhythmias and cardiac arrest remain to be the most serious emergencies.

Prevalence of perioperative cardiac events is 1% for a general *surgery*.

Common Emergency Cardiovascular Events

Bradycardia

Heart rates <60 beats per min (**Fig. 1**).[7]

Causes:
- Deep anesthesia (inhalant anesthetic overdose)
- Increased vagal tone
- Occulocardiac reflex.

Approach to treatment:
- Identify cause and manage accordingly
- *Atropine:* In adult 1 mg every 3–5 min (3 mg maximum), if no response isoprenaline 2–10 µg/min IV, titrated to desired effect infusion or epinephrine 0.02 µg/min IV infusion.

Tachycardia

Heart rates >100 beats per min (**Fig. 2**).[7]

Causes:
- Light anesthesia
- Sympathetic stimulation
- Blood loss or hypovolemia.

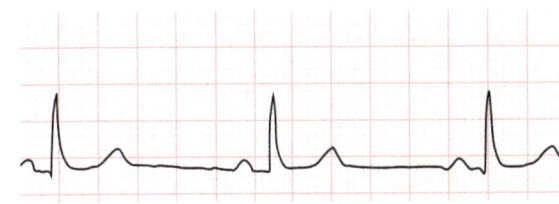

Fig. 1: Bradycardia.

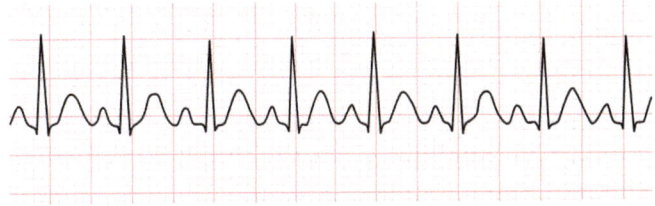

Fig. 2: Tachycardia.

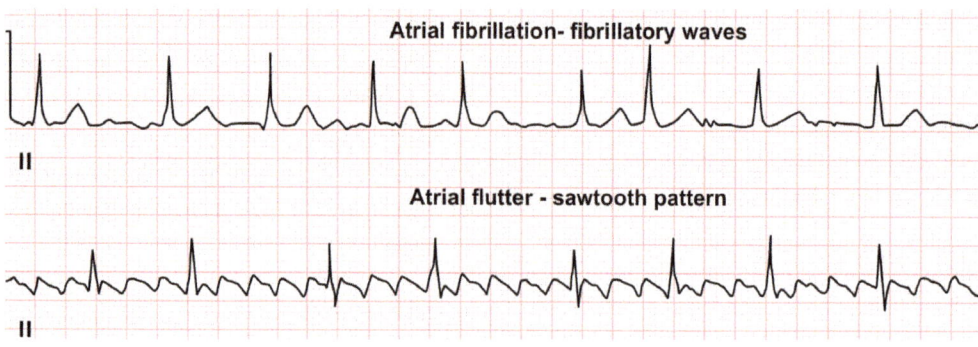

Fig. 3: Atrial arrythmia.

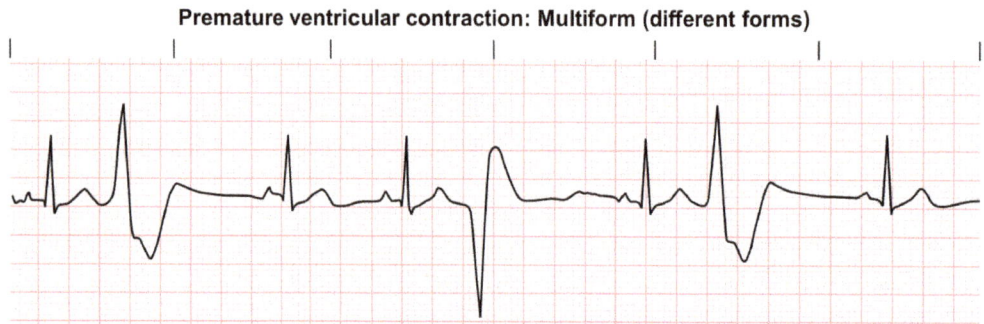

Fig. 4: Premature ventricular contraction.

Approach to treatment
- Identify the cause
- Deepen the plane of anesthesia
- Infusion of balanced salt solution/blood transfusion
- Ultrashort acting β-blocker esmolol 0.5 mg/kg, over 1 min followed by 0.05 mg/kg/min infusion.

Atrial Fibrillation

Atrial fibrillation (AF) is characterized by an irregular and rapid heartbeat. Ischemia, stress, sympathetic stimulation, and hemodynamic instability predispose to AF **(Fig. 3)**.[7]

Approach to treatment: Stop all anesthetics. Administer 100% oxygen and beta blocker. Atrial fibrillation of old onset requires anticoagulant, digoxin.

Ventricular Ectopic Beats

During a premature ventricular contraction (PVC), the heartbeat is initiated by the Purkinje fibers rather than the SA node **(Fig. 4)**. A PVC occurs before a regular heartbeat, there is a pause.[8]

Causes:
- Pain
- Usually acidemia, hypoxia or hypercapnia
- Sympathetic imbalance
- Drug induced – inhalation agent.

If not timely treated may lead to ventricular fibrillation (VF).

Approach to treatment: No treatment required for isolated VPCs. However, VPCs >5/min, multifocal or R on T vulnerable period VPCs or VPCs with hemodynamic instability needs treatment.

Stop all anesthetics. 100% oxygen, amiodarone, cardioversion if unstable.

Lignocaine (preservative free) Xylocard initial bolus dose of 1.5 mg/kg followed by 1–4 mg/min can be given.

The "R-on-T phenomenon" occurs when R wave (ventricular depolarization) of an ectopic beat gets superimposed on the T wave of the preceding beat.[8]

Ventricular Tachycardia

Abnormal rhythm at a rate faster than 100 beats/min.

Ventricular tachycardia lasting <30 seconds is termed as *non-sustained* VT, whereas if it is >30 seconds it is *sustained VT*. VT may be monomorphic (if the QRS morphology is fixed) or *polymorphic* (if QRS morphology is variable) **(Fig. 5)**.[8]

Treatment:
- If there is evidence of hemodynamic compromise, electrical cardioversion is the appropriate intervention, regardless of whether the rhythm is VT or SVT with aberrant conduction. The shocks should be synchronized

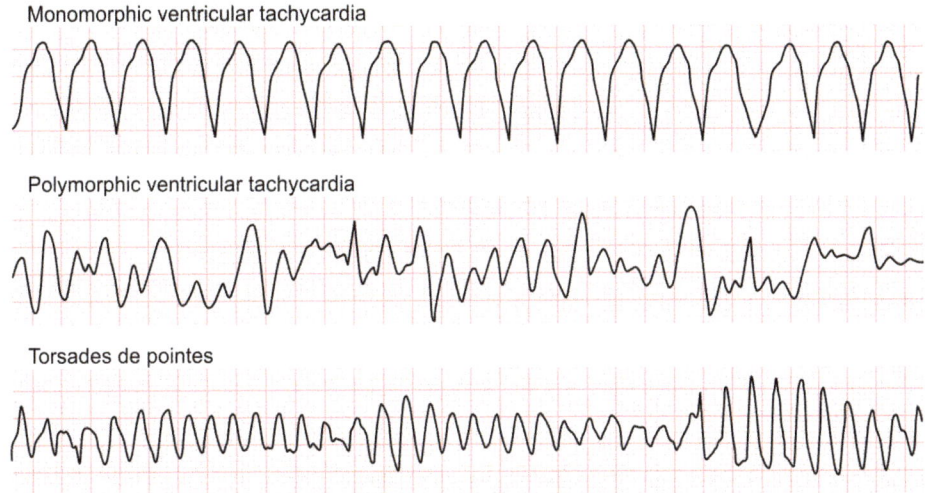

Fig. 5: Monomorphic and polymorphic ventricular tachycardia (VT).

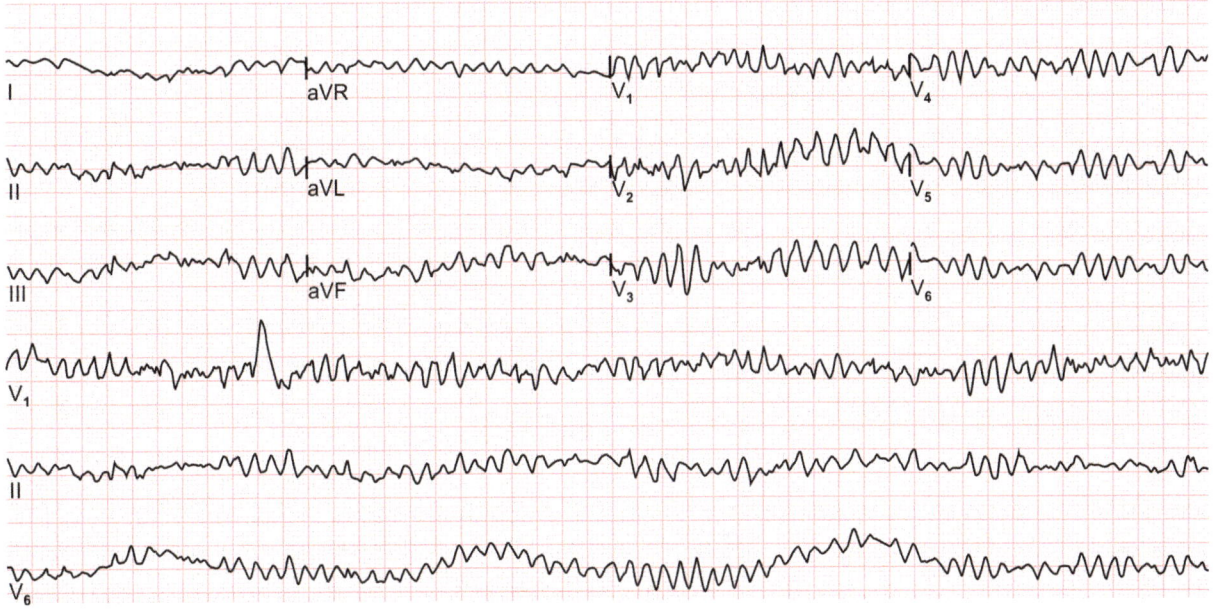

Fig. 6: Ventricular fibrillation.

(timed with the QRS complex), with an initial shock of 100 J (biphasic or monophasic shocks). This should terminate most of monomorphic VT, but, if necessary, shock can be given up to 360 J.[8]
- If patient is hemodynamically stable and the diagnosis of VT is certain, IV amiodarone should be used to terminate arrythmia.
- If the patient is hemodynamically stable and the diagnosis of VT is uncertain, IV adenosine can terminate most cases of paroxysmal SVT. If the likely diagnosis is VT, IV amiodarone and other antiarrhythmics should be opted as choice of treatment.
- Other options:[8]
  - Implantable cardioverter defibrillator
  - Catheter ablation for VT.

Ventricular Fibrillation
It can be defined as continuous irregular activation with no discrete QRS complexes caused by disordered electrical ventricular activation **(Fig. 6)**. Cardiac ischemia is the most common cause of VF.[8]

Treatment
For pulseless VT and VF, AHA guidelines for cardiac arrest to be followed.

Hypotension[7,8]
Causes:
- Anesthetic overdose
- Hypovolemia

Treatment:
- Lighten anesthetic depth
- To reduce volatile anesthetic requirements
- Fluid therapy
- Inotropes dopamine, dobutamine, adrenaline noradrenaline.

Hypertension[9]

Acute rise of blood pressure >20% of baseline during intraoperative period is considered as hypertensive emergencies.

Hypertension that occurs in relation to tracheal intubation, surgical incision, and emergence from anesthesia may be treated with short-acting β-blockers, angiotensin-converting enzyme (ACE) inhibitors, calcium channel blockers, or vasodilators.[9]

Acute Coronary Syndrome[9]

Acute coronary syndrome is of three types:
- Unstable angina
- Non-ST segment elevation myocardial infarction or heart attack (NSTEMI)
- ST-segment elevation myocardial infarction or heart attack (STEMI).

Medications include:
- Nitroglycerine
- Antiplatelet drugs
- Beta blockers
- Angiotensin-converting enzyme (ACE) inhibitors
- Angiotensin receptor blockers (ARBs)
- Statins.

Cardiac Arrest[9,10]

Common causes:
- Hypoxemia
- Respiratory arrest
- Cardiac cause: VF.

Approach to problem:
- Identify arrest
- Start cardiopulmonary resuscitation (CPR)
- Early use of defibrillator
- Use drugs
- Monitor $EtCO_2$ and diastolic BP.

High quality CPR should be applied according to 2020 guidelines. EtCO2 ≥15–20 mm Hg and diastolic BP ≥25 mm Hg correlate with effective return of spontaneous circulation (ROSC). Defibrillators guide the efficacy of chest compressions and ensure adequacy of resuscitation.[11]

■ RESPIRATORY EMERGENCIES

- Bronchospasm, laryngospasm, hypoxemia, and pulmonary embolism.
- Prevalence is 3–7.9% in general anesthesia.

Intractable Bronchospasm

It can occur during intubation, extubation, and intraoperatively.

Predisposing factors: Reactive airway or chronic obstructive airway disease.

Approach to Problem[11]

- 100% O_2
- Add inhalation agent
- IV 200 mg of hydrocortisone
- Nebulization with salbutamol 2.5–5 mg every 15 minutes, ipratropium bromide 0.25–0.5 mg 4/6 hourly when fail, adrenaline IV bolus 0.1 mL, 1 in 1,000.
- Chest X-ray to detect pneumothorax and endotracheal tube position
- Check ABGs and electrolytes
- Refer to ICU.

Laryngospasm

Laryngospasm is a condition in which vocal cords suddenly undergo spasm. As a result, airway becomes temporarily blocked, making it difficult to breathe.

Laryngospasm can occur during general anesthesia. This happens when the anesthesia or extubation irritates vocal cords due to secretion, blood, and foreign body. *Laryngospasm is more common in children, surgery of larynx or pharynx and patient with reactive airway.*

Approach to Problem

Hundred percent oxygen, followed by deepening of anesthesia with propofol, and/or paralyzing with succinylcholine.

Hypoxia[12]

Hypoxia is low oxygen level in tissues. Hypoxemia is low oxygen level in blood.

Causes of hypoxemia: Ventilation-perfusion (V/Q) mismatch, diffusion impairment, hypoventilation, low environmental oxygen, and right-to-left shunting.

An intraoperative hypoxemic event is defined as a reduction in peripheral oxygen saturation (SpO_2) to <90% or arterial partial pressure of oxygen (PaO_2) to <70 mm Hg, measured through pulse oximetry analysis or arterial blood gas, with 100% oxygen during pulmonary ventilation.[12]

Pulmonary Embolism[13]

All perioperative patients, but especially trauma victims and those undergoing prostate or orthopedic surgery, are at increased risk of venous thromboembolism. *Malignancy, immobility, and obesity, smoking, patient taking oral contraceptives, hormone replacement therapy, or antipsychotic medications are important risk factors.* Dyspnea, anxiety, and tachypnea are the most common presenting symptoms in awake patients, and hypotension, tachycardia, hypoxemia, and decreased end-tidal CO_2 are the most common findings in patients receiving general anesthesia. *Shock and right ventricular failure lead to adverse outcomes.* Helical computed tomographic scanning is the preferred definitive diagnostic study.[13]

Pulmonary Edema[14]

Causes according to pathophysiology: Either due to increase in hydrostatic pressure or increase in capillary permeability and decrease in colloidal oncotic pressure.

Management

Intermittent positive pressure ventilation (IPPV) with positive end-expiratory pressure (PEEP) with 100% oxygen, head up position.

Diuretic, morphine, nitroglycerine[14] may be given.

SURGICAL EMERGENCIES

Common general surgical emergencies are:
- Incarcerated and strangulated hernia
- Appendicitis
- Acute intestinal obstruction
- Peptic perforation
- Bleeding esophageal varices
- Abscess
- Acute obstructive uropathy
- Gall bladder and bile duct diseases
- Surgical infections of the skin, muscles, bones, and joints
- Gunshot injury and stab injury
- Blunt trauma abdomen.

Approach to Problem

The important part of management is assessment and treatment of dehydration, electrolyte imbalance, blood loss, fluid loss and pain management.

Usually, general anesthesia is administered after resuscitation. Rapid sequence induction is used.

METABOLIC AND ENDOCRINE EMERGENCIES

Diabetes Management

Diabetic ketoacidosis (DKA) is an emergency condition, characterized by hyperglycemia, the presence of ketone bodies and acidosis. *Plasma glucose is >13.9 mmol/L (250 mg/dL).* However, a wide range of plasma glucose levels can be present, which is independent of the severity of DKA, managed by IV normal saline, glucose insulin potassium regime and sodibicarb.[15]

NEUROLOGICAL AND NEUROSURGICAL EMERGENCY

Tonsillar herniation is a life-threatening and time-critical pathology that may be reversible with emergent surgical intervention and medical management.

The most common cause is traumatic brain injury (TBI). Other causes include intracerebral hemorrhage and subarachnoid hemorrhage.

PEDIATRIC EMERGENCIES[16]

The most common emergency is cardiac arrest and respiratory arrest.

The most common cause of cardiac arrest is bradycardia.

Approach to Problem

- Atropine 0.1–0.2 mg/kg IV
- Cardiac compression ratio 15:2, 100–200 compression/min, 10–12 breath/min, when no vascular access is present immediate intraosseous access is recommended.

Neonatal Resuscitation[16]

Cause: Neonatal asphyxia

Approach to Problem

Dry, wrap, warm the baby, keep the theater warm. Bag mask ventilation and oxygenation, if required intubate and ventilate the patient.

OBSTETRIC EMERGENCIES

Massive obstetric hemorrhage: >1.5 liter blood loss[17] in one sitting.

Causes:
- *Vasa previa, placental abruption, uterine rupture, postpartum, hemorrhage*
- *Sudden collapse:* Amniotic fluid embolism, pulmonary embolism
- Disseminated intravascular coagulation (DIC)
- Prolapsed Cord.

In massive obstetric hemorrhage, massive transfusion protocol to be generated.[17]

REGIONAL ANESTHESIA COMPLICATIONS

Collapse following Spinal Anesthesia

Prevalence is 1.3–18 in 10,000 patients during spinal anesthesia.

Occasionally, unexpected bradycardia and asystole may develop during the administration of spinal anesthesia in apparently healthy and young patients.[1] Cardiac arrests during spinal anesthesia are described as "very rare". Reduced blood pressure is commonly seen associated to spinal anesthesia for cesarean section and efforts to reduce its occurrence and its magnitude is common practice.[18]

In the literature, the reported incidence of cardiac arrest is 6.4 ± 1.2 in 10,000 patients.[19,20]

Approach to Problem

The patient usually recovers after prompt (CPR).[21,22]

Local Anesthetic Systemic Toxicity

The three pillars of *local anesthetic systemic toxicity (LAST) treatment consist of seizure management, advanced cardiac life support (ACLS), and prompt administration of a 20% lipid emulsion.* For hemodynamically stable patients with isolated seizure activity, intravenous (IV) benzodiazepines may be used.[23]

ANAPHYLAXIS

Incidence: 1 in 4,000 to 1 in 25,000.[24]

Approach to Problem

Anaphylactic reaction are life-threatening emergencies due to allergen.[25] Various organ are involved, as evident by flushing, urticaria, angioedema, conjunctivitis, rhinitis, bronchoconstriction with wheezing dyspnea, abdominal pain, nausea, vomiting, diarrhea, tachycardia, hypotension and shock, even can lead to cardiovascular collapse and death.

Recognition of anaphylaxis during general anaesthesia:[26] The common findings of intraoperative reactions are pulselessness, increased peak inspiratory pressure, desaturation[27] and decrease EtCO$_2$.

Discontinue drug administration:
- Maintain airway, provide 100% oxygen, intubation if indicated.
- *Epinephrine* (1:1,000) 0.5 mg IM, to be repeated every 10 minutes until improvement occurs. Alternatively, 50–100 μg IV (1:10,000) over 1 minute has been recommended.[27]
- Start rapid IV administration of crystalloids.
- Give antihistamines:
  - Injection Diphenhydramine 50–75 mg IV
  - Injection Ranitidine 150 mg IV
- *Corticosteroids:* Injection Hydrocortisone 100–500 mg slow IV
- Bronchodilators for persistent bronchospasm
- Vasopressors to maintain hemodynamics
- Extracorporeal life support for anaphylaxis followed by cardiac arrest.

MALIGNANT HYPERTHERMIA[28]

Malignant hyperthermia (MH) is a dire emergency situation due to disorder of muscle induced by exposure to suxamethonium and all the volatile anesthetic agents characterized by hypermetabolism, muscle rigidity and muscle injury. Undiagnosed malignant hyperthermia is a nightmare to an anesthesiologist.

Epidemiology

Incidence is approximately 1:10,000.

Approach to Problem[29]

- Stop all triggering anesthetics, use IV induction agent, nondepolarizing muscle relaxant.
- Dantrolene 2, 5 mg/kg IV to a total dose of 10 mg every 5–10 min until initial symptoms subside.
- Control fever by cold IV fluid infusion, cooling the body surface.
- Monitor and treat metabolic acidosis and arrhythmias.
- Further treatment is guided by arterial blood gas, electrolytes, CK.

TRAUMA AND DISASTER MANAGEMENT[30]

Trauma is injury to living tissue due to an external factor.

Incidence: One million people die and 20 million are hospitalized every year due to injuries in India.

Approach to the Problem[30]

Triage: It is used to prioritize the emergency treatment.
- Triage Level I: Resuscitation
- Triage Level II: Emergent
- Triage Level III: Urgent
- Triage Level IV: Less urgent
- Triage Level V: Nonurgent.

The role of the triage nurse is to make acuity determinations and set priorities **(Fig. 7)**.[30]

Primary advance trauma life support (ATLS) survey should be followed as steps "A-B-C-D-E" [A: Airway, B: Breathing, C: Circulation, D: Disability/neurologic assessment, and E: exposure].

Focused Assessment with Sonography for Trauma (FAST) is used to detect injury early. Golden hour for survival is the first hour after injury.

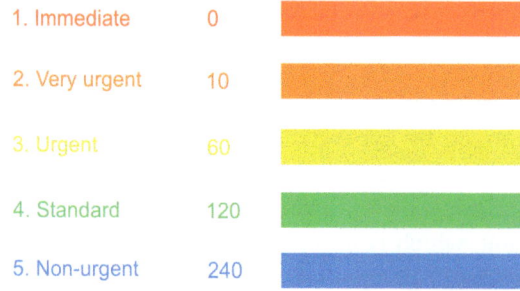

Fig. 7: Levels of triage system.

PERIVASCULAR/INTRAVASCULAR INJECTION

Causes: Use of irritant agents such as thiopental intra-arterial injection

Problem: Causes pain, abscesses, necrosis, thrombosis

Treatment:
- Needle kept in situ
- Dilute with saline
- IV lignocaine
- IV heparin
- Brachial plexus block/Stellate ganglia block.

HUMAN ERROR
- Drug dose is not calculated properly
- Faulty labeling of syringe
- Failure of equipment not checked before
- Double checking can prevent these problems.

ETHICAL CONSIDERATION

Documentation of any emergency event, every aspect of the patient's history and details of the procedures during anesthesia should be done in proper proforma. Informed consent is mandatory before any anesthetic procedure. The approach for getting consent will differ depending on patient and procedure. *Every anesthesiologist should have knowledge to avoid litigation.*

LABORATORY ASSESSMENT

Laboratory studies frequently include blood group type and crossmatching, hemoglobin and hematocrit, electrolyte, blood sugar, ABG, drug screen, blood alcohol, prothrombin time (PT), partial thromboplastin time, and pregnancy test if applicable.

ROLE OF BIOMARKERS (PREDICTIVE AND PROGNOSTIC)[31]

- Identification
- Risk stratification
- Monitoring
- Prognostication of the patients in the critical- and acute-care settings.
  In emergency medical practice, majority of biomarkers work has been focused on cardiology, renal failure, sepsis. also on hepatic diseases, traumatic brain injury, venous thromboembolism.
- Acute Coronary Syndrome
  - CK MB fraction (gold standard)
  - Troponin "I" and Troponin "t"
  - Myoglobin (Mb) P
  - D-Dimer
  - High sensitivity C-reactive protein (Hs CRP)
  - Myeloperoxidase (MPO)
- Cardiac Failure
  - BNP and NT-proBNP
- Pulmonary Embolism
  - D-dimer.
  - Ischemia modified albumin (IMA)
- Sepsis
  - C-reactive protein
  - Procalcitonin
  - Serum lactate
  - Mid-regional pro-adrenomedullin (MR-proADM)
  - Cytokines such as TNF, IL-1 beta, IL-6
  - Lipopolysaccharide-binding protein (LBS).

NEWER MODALITIES ON HORIZON

Most important is *point of care testing (POCT).*

Prehospital Care[32]

Prehospital care is emergency medical care given to patients before arrival in hospital after activation of emergency medical services.

New Concepts of Care[32]
- Community paramedicine
- Emergency care practitioners
- Physician delivered prehospital emergency medicine.

Salient Points in Emergency Anesthesia

All emergency patients should be considered as full stomach case so aspiration prophylaxis is mandatory.
- Preoperative plan[33,34]
  - Clear diagnostic and management plan
  - Early identification of comorbidities and preoperative risk assessment.
  - Adequate emergency investigation facility
  - Triage for trauma victim
  - Informed consent
- Intraoperative plan
  - Documentation of any intraoperative event is very important
- Postoperative plan[35]
  - Proper analgesic therapy
  - Recognize sepsis early that may need
  - Multidisciplinary team approach

Monitoring

The American Society of Anesthesiologists (ASA) standard monitoring should be used in operation theater.

CONCLUSION

Prevention, mitigation, preparedness, response and recovery are the five steps of emergency management. Prevention is always better than cure. But in spite of adequate prevention, Anesthesia Emergency can occur any time during preoperative period. Thorough understanding of the problem, prompt judicious management and proper perioperative care always lead to a successful outcome.

ACKNOWLEDGMENTS

Professor (Dr) Mohan Chandra Mandal, Professor, Department of Anesthesiology, IPGMEandR/SSKM Hospital, Kolkata and Dr Indradeep Sanyal, Department of Anesthesiology, RG Kar Medical College and Hospital.

> **Take Home Messages**
>
> We should follow the Ten Golden Rules[36] as mentioned below for catering safe anesthesia care.
>
> *Ten Golden Rules:*
> 1. Assess and prepare patient adequately
> 2. Follow fasting guidelines
> 3. Use a tipping table
> 4. Check drugs and equipment
> 5. Keep a sucker instantly ready
> 6. Secure airway
> 7. Control ventilation
> 8. Have a vein open
> 9. Standard monitoring
> 10. Have someone in room who can give cricoid pressure effectively and will be useful in emergency (i.e., one trained assistant).

REFERENCES

1. Apfelbaum JL, Hagberg CA, Connis RT, Abdelmalak BB, Agarkar M, Dutton RP, et al. 2022 American Society of Anesthesiologists Practice Guidelines for Management of the Difficult Airway. Anesthesiology. 2022;136(1):31-81.
2. Neelakanta G, Chikyarappa A. A review of patients with pulmonary aspiration of gastric contents during anesthesia reported to the Departmental Quality Assurance Committee. J ClinAnesth. 2006;18(2):102-7.
3. Green SM, Krauss B. Pulmonary aspiration risk during emergency department procedural sedation—an examination of the role of fasting and sedation depth. Acad Emerg Med. 2002;9(1):35-42.
4. Lienhart A, Auroy Y, Péquignot F, Benhamou D, Warszawski J, Bovet M, et al. Survey of anesthesia-related mortality in France. Anesthesiology. 2006;105(6):1087-97.
5. Sharma G, Jacob R, Mahankali S, Ravindra MN. Preoperative assessment of gastric contents and volume using bedside ultrasound in adult patients: a prospective, observational, correlation study. Indian J Anaesth. 2018;62(10):753-8.
6. Draghici AE, Taylor JA. The physiological basis and measurement of heart rate variability in humans. J Physiol Anthropol. 2016;35(1):22.
7. Soar J, Böttiger BW, Carli P, Couper K, Deakin CD, Djärv T, et al. European Resuscitation Council Guidelines 2021: Adult advanced life support. Resuscitation. 2021;161:115-51.
8. Soar J, Berg KM, Andersen LW, Böttiger BW, Cacciola S, Callaway CW, et al; Adult Advanced Life Support Collaborators. Adult Advanced Life Support: 2020 International Consensus on Cardiopulmonary Resuscitation and Emergency Cardiovascular Care Science with Treatment Recommendations. Resuscitation. 2020;156:A80-A119.
9. Varon J, Marik PE. Perioperative hypertension management. Vasc Health Risk Manag. 2008;4(3):615-27.
10. Fister N, Syed A, Tobias JD. Intraoperative cardiac arrest: immediate treatment and diagnostic evaluation. J Med Cases. 2021;12(1):18-22.
11. NICE. Asthma: diagnosis, monitoring and chronic asthma management. London: National Institute for Health and Care Excellence (NICE); 2021.
12. Yao HY, Liu TJ, Lai HC. Risk factors for intraoperative hypoxemia during monopulmonary ventilation: an observational study. Braz J Anesthesiol. 2019;69(4):390-5.
13. Tapson VF. Acute pulmonary embolism. N Engl J Med. 2008;358(10):1037-52.
14. Purvey M, Allen G. Managing acute pulmonary oedema. Aust Prescr. 2017;40(2):59-63.
15. Eledrisi MS, Elzouki AN. Management of diabetic ketoacidosis in adults: a narrative review. Saudi J Med Med Sci. 2020;8(3):165-73.
16. Mehra B, Gupta S. Common pediatric medical emergencies in office practice. Indian J Pediatr. 2018;85(1):35-43.
17. Guasch E, Gilsanz F. Massive obstetric hemorrhage: Current approach to management. Med Intensiva. 2016;40(5):298-310.
18. Limongi JA, Lins RS. Cardiopulmonary arrest in spinal anesthesia. Rev Bras Anestesiol. 2011;61(1):110-20.
19. Jeejeebhoy FM, Zelop CM, Lipman S, Carvalho B, Joglar J, Mhyre JM, et al; American Heart Association Emergency Cardiovascular Care Committee, Council on Cardiopulmonary, Critical Care, Perioperative and Resuscitation, Council on Cardiovascular Diseases in the Young, and Council on Clinical Cardiology. Cardiac Arrest in Pregnancy: a Scientific Statement from the American Heart Association. Circulation. 2015;132(18):1747-73.
20. Auroy Y, Narchi P, Messiah A, Litt L, Rouvier B, Samii K. Serious complications related to regional anesthesia: results of a prospective survey in France. Anesthesiology. 1997;87(3):479-86.
21. Mali S. Anaphylaxis during the perioperative period. Anesth Essays Res. 2012;6(2):124-33.
22. Oddby E, Hein A, Jakobsson JG. Circulatory collapse following epidural bolus for Caesarean section a profound vasovagal reaction? A case report. Int J Surg Case Rep. 2016;23:74-6.
23. Brown V, Brandner B, Brook J, Adiseshiah M. Cardiac arrest after administration of Omnipaque radiocontrast medium during endoluminal repair of abdominal aortic aneurysm. Br J Anaesth. 2002;88(1):133-5.
24. Fisher MM, Baldo BA. The incidence and clinical features of anaphylactic reactions during anesthesia in Australia. Ann Fr Anesth Reanim. 1993;12(2):97-104.
25. Levy JH. New concepts in the treatment of anaphylactoid reactions in anesthesia. Ann Fr Anesth Reanim 1993;12: 223-7.
26. Lagopoulos V, Gigi E. Anaphylactic and anaphylactoid reactions during the perioperative period. Hippokratia. 2011;15(2):138-40.
27. Whittington T, Fisher MM. Anaphylactic and anaphylactoid reactions. Baillière's Clinical Anaesthesiology. 1998;12(2): 301-23.

28. Rosenberg H, Pollock N, Schiemann A, Bulger T, Stowell K. Malignant hyperthermia: a review. Orphanet J Rare Dis. 2015;10:93.
29. Royal College of Anaesthetists. Guidelines for the Provision of Emergency Anaesthesia Services 2022. London: RCOG; 2022.
30. World Health Organization. WHO-ICRC Basic Emergency Care: approach to the acutely ill and injured. [online] Available from: https://www.who.int/publications/i/item/basic-emergency-care-approach-to-the-acutely-ill-and-injured. [Last Accessed January, 2023].
31. Chakrapani AT. Biomarkers of Diseases: Their Role in Emergency Medicine. In: Tunalı NE (Ed). Neurodegenerative Diseases - Molecular Mechanisms and Current Therapeutic Approaches [Internet]. London: IntechOpen; 2020.
32. Wilson MH, Habig K, Wright C, Hughes A, Davies G, Imray CH. Prehospital emergency medicine. Lancet. 2015;386(10012):2526-34.
33. Western University. Anesthetic Emergencies and Accidents (Lee L). [online] Available from: https://www.westernu.edu/mediafiles/veterinary/vet-anesthesia-analgesia/anesthesia-emergencies-accidents.pdf. [Last Accessed January, 2023].
34. Chand M, Armstrong T, Britton G, Nash GF. How and why do we measure surgical risk? J R Soc Med. 2007;100(11):508-12.
35. Romero CS, Afshari A, Kranke P. Adapt or perish: Introducing focused guidelines. Eur J Anaesthesiol. 2021;38(8):803-5.
36. King MH. Primary anaesthesia. Oxford: Oxford University Press; 1986.

SECTION 16: Miscellaneous Emergencies-3

Section Editor: Om Tantia

39. **Unknown Poisoning**
    Nandini Chatterjee

40. **Snakebite: Initial Management, Myths, and Reality**
    Dayal Bandhu Majumdar

41. **Anaphylaxis**
    Shambo Samrat Samajdar, Sougata Sarkar, Saibal Moitra, Santanu K Tripathi

42. **Emergencies in Medical Practice: Common Drugs**
    Lopamudra Chowdhury

43. **Emergency Management of Drowning**
    Sarbajit Ray

CHAPTER 39

Unknown Poisoning

Nandini Chatterjee

INTRODUCTION

Unknown poisoning is a medical emergency that needs urgent recognition and prompt intervention to avoid morbidity and mortality. The easy accessibility of drugs and chemicals in our country is an important cause of huge number of poisoning cases. Industrialization and agricultural modernization has made pesticides abundant in the market, exposure to which leads to severe toxicity.

As per World Health Organization (WHO) data 0.3 million people die every year due to poisoning. In India, mortality due to poisoning is 0.26 per 100,000 people (WHO 2019). Poisoning may be attributed to deliberate or accidental introduction of harmful substance into the body. It has been reported more in the younger age group, with males having greater propensity to deteriorate than females.

In order to holistically deal with poison-related mortality and morbidity, poison information centers have been set up in countries, for providing emergency advice on the management of poisoning cases. They also compile data on toxic exposures and on toxic substances and contribute to chemical safety and public health. As of January 1st, 2021, only 47% of WHO Member States had a poison information center. In India, first such poison information center was set up in AIIMS, New Delhi, the National Poison Information Centre (NPIC) a part of Poison Control Program. It provides assistance and information to physicians via telephone. This has been followed by seven more centers in the country now.

When to Suspect Poisoning?

Some clinical presentations may alert the physician to suspect poisoning:[1]

- Sudden changes in behavior pattern
- History from relatives/friends
- Discovery of pills
- Sudden onset of vomiting altered sensorium, breathlessness, diarrhea
- Cardiac dysrhythmia, hyper or hypothermia

Various factors influence the presentation of unknown poisoning such as:

- *Type of poison:* The common types of poisons encountered in clinical practice are pesticides sedatives, antidepressants, antipsychotics, cardiovascular drugs, analgesic, antibiotics, household materials, and illicit drugs.
- *Quantity:* The amount of poison consumed affects clinical features. The lethal oral dose of various toxins is variable. A term is in vogue "LD50" which is the amount of toxin given at a time that causes the death of 50% of the test animals.
- Duration of exposure to poison
  - *Acute:* When a large amount is introduced at a time with rapid onset of symptoms. Also the time elapsed after exposure to poison is very important for determination of prognosis and outcome.
  - *Chronic:* When a person is exposed to small amounts over a period of time with insidious onset of symptoms
- *Route of entry:* Ingestion, inhalation or injection.

ASSESSMENT OF PATIENT

There are three groups of clues[2]

1. *Visual clues:* The normal pupillary size is 3–4 mm, alteration of size of pupil is to be noted.
2. *Olfactory clues:* Distinct odor of some poisons can be recognized.
3. *Dermal clues:* Often found in chronic poisoning.

Two aspects of manifestations are to be looked for:

1. *Toxic vital signs* that are important clinical pointers are abnormal pulse blood pressure, body temperature respiratory variability, sensorium body odor, cyanosis, pupillary size **(Table 1)**.
2. *Toxidromes:* The substances in a specific class of toxin produce characteristic combinations of symptoms and signs, which is called toxic syndrome (toxidromes). The recognition of a toxidrome may reveal the type of poison involved.

TABLE 1: Abnormalities in vital signs in various poisons.

Poisons	Vital signs
Hypertension	Cocaine, sympathomimetics, caffeine, anticholinergic, nicotine, thyroxine
Hypotension	Antihypertensive, rodenticide, antidepressants, sedatives, opioids, heroin
Tachypnea	Organophosphate (OP) poisoning, chemical pneumonitis, salicylate, toxin-included metabolism acidosis and nerve agents, paraquat
Slow respiration	Marijuana, sedatives, alcohol, and opioids
Hyperthermia	Anticholinergics, antidepressants, antipsychotics, antihistaminics, salicylate, and alcohol withdrawal
Hypothermia	Alcohol, sedatives, and hypnotics, hypoglycemic agent, opioids, carbon monoxide
Tachycardia	Anticholinergic, antihistaminics, antipsychotics, sympathomimetics (cocaine, caffeine, amphetamine) theophylline, and thyroxine, tricyclic antidepressant (TCA)
Bradycardia	Oleander, organophosphorus, anticholinesterase drugs, beta blockers, clonidine, calcium channel blocker antiarrhythmics, alcohol, and opioids
Coma	OP poisoning, alcohol, ethylene glycol, tricyclic antidepressant, anticonvulsants, antipsychotics, antidepressants, antihistaminics, hypoglycemic agents, and isoniazid
Seizure	Organophosphorus poisoning, hypoglycemic agent, isoniazid, salicylate, tricyclic antidepressant, and ethanol withdrawal
Mydriasis	Anticholinergic (datura, atropine), sympathomimetics
Miosis	Organophosphorus compound and other cholinergic agents, carbamates, opioids, clonidine, phenothiazine, and sedatives
Diaphoresis	OP poisoning, salicylates, and sympathomimetics
Dry skin	Antihistamines, anticholinergics like datura
Cyanosis	Dapsone, aniline dyes, nitrate, and ergotamines
Odor	Garlic—OP compound, gasoline—petroleum products. Fruit-like—alcohol, smokey—carbon monoxide

TABLE 2: Toxidromes in different poisonings.

Toxidrome	Features	Poisons
Cholinergic toxidrome muscarinic	Bradycardia, bronchorrhea, miosis, salivation, wheezing, diarrhea, and diaphoresis	Organophosphorus, physostigmine, and pyridostigmine
Nicotinic toxidrome	Abdominal pain, fasciculation, hypertension, paresis, and seizure	Organophosphorus compounds, nicotine
Opioid toxidrome	Miosis, sedation, hypotension, hypoventilation, coma, and bradycardia	Opioids
Sympathomimetic toxidrome	Mydriasis, tachycardia, hypertension, seizure, and hyperthermia	Cocaine, amphetamine, ephedrine, and theophylline
Anticholinergic toxidrome	Delirium, mydriasis, tachycardia, hyperthermia, dry skin, and urinary retention	Antihistaminics, atropine, and tricyclic antidepressants, and psychoactive drugs

The toxidromes are cholinergic, anticholinergic, sympathomimetic, and opioid **(Table 2)**.

■ INVESTIGATIONS

Certain basic investigations are to be readily performed such as:
- Complete blood count
- Serum electrolytes and serum lactate levels
- Blood urea nitrogen (BUN) and creatinine
- Liver function test
- Arterial blood gas
- Electrocardiogram
- Urine pregnancy test universally for women of fertile age group.

The findings depend upon the predilection of involvement of a particular toxin.

Measurement of drug or toxin concentrations in body fluids is riddled with many impediments.

It may not be available in many centers and not mandatory in most poisonings. The enzyme immunoassays detect specific drugs within a class and may take days to weeks to be detected after exposure. Cross-reactivity among different groups of drugs occur. A negative drug screen test may be due to erroneous sample collection or there can be a false negative result. Drugs whose concentration in blood is associated with specific treatment recommendations include acetaminophen, salicylate, theophylline, lithium, lead, iron, carbon monoxide, methemoglobin, toxic alcohol, anticonvulsant, and digoxin. These may be measured when suspected.

MANAGEMENT[3,4]

The resuscitation [airway, breathing, circulation (ABC)] with basic life support takes priority.

The loss of airway-protective reflexes and concern for aspiration or the presence of respiratory failure dictates the need to secure the airway. As many toxins (cyanide, hydrogen sulfide and abnormal hemoglobins) compromise ventilation and oxygenation, this is the first step in management.

Orotracheal intubation, if possible, is preferred over nasotracheal intubation which is technically more difficult. Nasotracheal intubation increases the incidence of sinusitis, purulent and serous otitis, ventilator-associated pneumonia.

The next priority is assessment of the circulatory status as various cardiovascular abnormalities can be seen in poisoned patients. Myocardial depression, arrhythmias, and conduction abnormalities may cause shock from impaired cardiac contractility. An electrocardiogram should be obtained in all such patients.

Initially, administration of intravenous crystalloid fluid is to be started if hypovolemic shock is suspected but it is to be remembered that in a distributive shock or cardiogenic shock, administration of vasopressors or inotropes (noradrenaline) is more appropriate than fluids. Extracorporeal membrane oxygenation (ECMO) is indicated in poisoned patients in refractory shock who fail conventional treatment.

The treatment of hypertension is decided by its underlying etiology which is elusive in unknown poisoning. When hypertension is caused by overdoses of drugs with direct adrenergic activity, direct vasodilators such as nitroprusside is helpful. If withdrawal is suspected, sedation with benzodiazepines should be considered.[3]

Elimination of Unabsorbed Poison

Decontamination: This should depend on route of exposure if it can be suspected.

Skin decontamination: To remove clothing and rinsing with water thoroughly. This retards absorption.

Decontamination of eye: To rinse with water/normal saline for 15-20 minutes. Local anesthetic drop may be given.

Gastrointestinal (GI) decontamination: There are conflicting reports regarding the beneficial role of induced vomiting and gastric lavage.

If GI decontamination is attempted, it should be done within 1 hour of ingestion.

One has to keep in mind the contraindication to gastric lavage in corrosive poisoning and volatile hydrocarbons such as kerosene. Also, to be avoided in restless and unconscious patients.

Activated charcoal and cathartics in decontaminating gastrointestinal tract.

Activated charcoal has not been shown to have significant survival benefits unless used within 1 hour of ingestion.

There are many substances that are not absorbed by activated charcoal such as pesticides, potassium hydrocarbon, acid, alkali, alcohol, iron, insecticide, and lithium solvent.

Substances that are absorbed by activated charcoal are antimalarial, barbiturate, carbamazepine and dapsone.

Whole bowel irrigation—It is done by pouring 1-2 liters of polyethylene glycol through a nasogastric tube. Evidence of improvement has been reported only for enteric coated sustained release drug overdose.

Thus the role of GI decontamination is limited in unknown poisoning and only recommended if patient presents early and there is strong suspicion of any particular toxidrome and no obvious contraindication.

Elimination of Absorbed Poison

Alkaline urine causes ionization of acidotic drugs preventing reabsorption of the ionized drug across the renal tubular epithelium and enhancing elimination through the urine. Urine alkalinization is most effective for weak acids such as salicylate, phenobarbital toxicities. Fluid overload, renal impairment, and hypokalemia are contraindications to this process.

Extracorporeal Removal

Extracorporeal removal techniques, including hemodialysis, hemofiltration, and continuous renal replacement therapies may be useful if a toxin has a low volume of distribution (VD <1 L/kg), low molecular weight, low protein-binding capacity, and a low endogenous clearance.

Hemodialysis is effective in poisoning with salicylates, alcohol, barbiturates, lithium while hemofiltration is useful in theophylline barbiturates as well as carbamazepine. Paraquat poisoning may respond if done in the early phase. The lipid emulsion therapy (LET) is a recent advance in the care of the critically ill patient. LET is said to reverse the toxicity of calcium channel antagonists, tricyclic antidepressants, benzodiazepines, anticonvulsants, and β-adrenergic blocking agents.

Anticonvulsant Therapy

For toxin-induced seizures and alcohol or sedative withdrawal, phenytoin is not generally effective. Benzodiazepines, barbiturates and valproic acid are considered as first and second-line therapy.

Coma Cocktail

In unknown poisoning with unconsciousness a trial with IV glucose can be given to control hypoglycemia. However, availability of blood glucose monitoring device will avoid empirical therapy. It will be indicated in hypoglycemic state.

Naloxone is an opioid antagonist which may be used in suspected cases of opioid overdose if there is circumstantial evidence by history or examination.

Antidotes

There should not be indiscriminate use of antidotes. The number of effective antidotes are few. With the exception of naloxone, antidote therapy is limited in unknown poisoning. Most poisoning patients can have uneventful recovery with routine supportive care.[4]

Ancillary support: It is important to provide adequate nutrition. Protective measures against thromboembolism, aspiration and gastrointestinal (GI) bleeding should be undertaken. Attention should be given to prevention of pressure sores and exposure keratitis.

Psychological support: This is very important if self-harm is suspected and has profound effect on acute and long-term outcomes.

MEDICOLEGAL ASPECT

For all suspected cases of poisoning police information is mandatory. Documentation and notes are to be meticulous. Immediate management is the doctor's foremost duty, but preservation of stomach wash sample, vomitus, urine or stool is desirable in case of suspected unknown poisoning for possible identification.

CONCLUSION

Unknown poisoning is a challenge to the physician. It is of prime importance to suspect and diagnose it promptly for early intervention through various visual, olfactory dermal and vital sign clues. The management relies on resuscitation, elimination of the unabsorbed poison and if possible to identify the poison, administer antidotes.

Take Home Messages

- The first step is to stabilize airway, breathing, and circulation as with any critically ill patient.
- Identifying the poison, either through history, toxidrome or laboratory tests may direct the physicians in the right track.
- A toxidrome is a set of signs and symptoms that specifically indicate a group of toxins.
- Gastric lavage is contraindicated in corrosive and kerosene poisoning and effective only if done by the first hour of ingestion.
- Empirical dextrose infusion may be undertaken in any unconscious patient.
- Antidotes can be used in instances where the exact poison agent is detected.
- The case must be booked as a medicolegal case.
- Detailed documentation of signs and symptoms should be kept recorded.
- It is desirable to preserve vomitus, excreta and other samples for future evidence.
- Psychological or psychiatric assessment and support is mandatory.

REFERENCES

1. Erickson TB, Thompson TM. The approach to the patient with an unknown poisoning. Emerg Med Clin Am. 2007;25:249-81.
2. Frithgen VL, William M, Simpson JR. Recognition and management acute medication poisoning. Am Fam Physician. 2010;81:316-23.
3. Van Hoving DJ, Veala DGH, Muller GF. Emergency management of acute poisoning. African J Emerg Med. 2011;1:69-78.
4. Muller D, Degel H. Common causes of poisoning, etiology, diagnosis and treatment. DTSCH Arztebl Int. 2013;110: 690-700.

CHAPTER 40

Snakebite: Initial Management, Myths, and Reality

Dayal Bandhu Majumdar

INTRODUCTION

Snakebite is marked as a "neglected tropical disease" by World Health Organization.[1] More than 58,000 people die every year in India due to snakebite.[2] Snakebite is a medical emergency; each and every medical graduate should know primary management of a venomous snakebite. Most of the time one doctor may not get enough time to consult an expert to treat a venomous snakebite and save a life. Just timely infusion of the first dose of antisnake venom serum (ASV) can save thousands of lives.

Though there are >250 species of snakes in India only about 60 species are venomous.[3] Out of these 60 species about 50 are sea snakes. Sea snakes cause just a few bites per year. Out of about ten land venomous snakes 4–5 species cause >99% venomous bites. It is estimated that, only four venomous snakes are involved in 99% of the fatal bites; these are called "Big fours." Big fours are Indian Spectacled cobra, Russell's viper, saw-scaled viper, and common krait[3] **(Figs. 1 to 5)**. Indian polyvalent ASV is prepared to treat bites from these big fours only.[4] Bites from other venomous snakes in India are managed symptomatically, current Indian ASV has no role in those bites.[5]

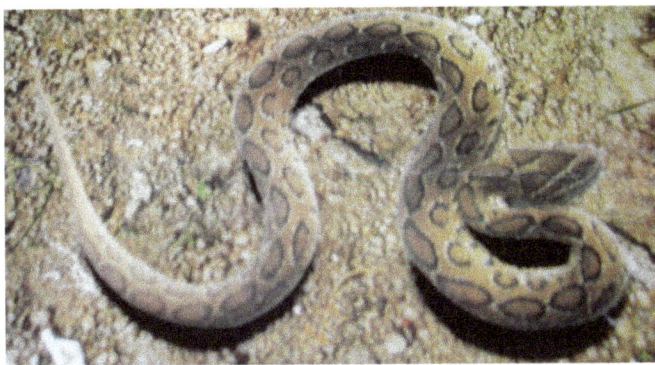

Fig. 2: Russell's viper.

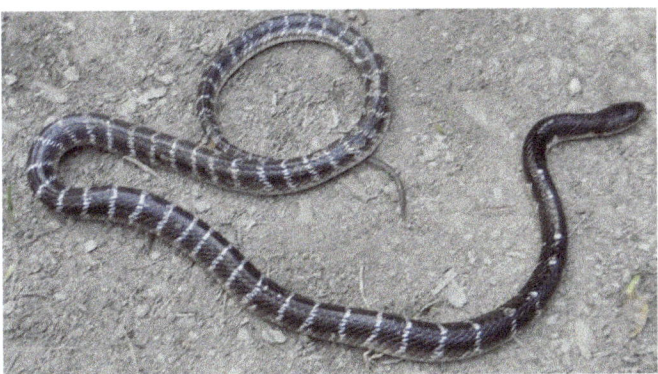

Fig. 3: Common krait.

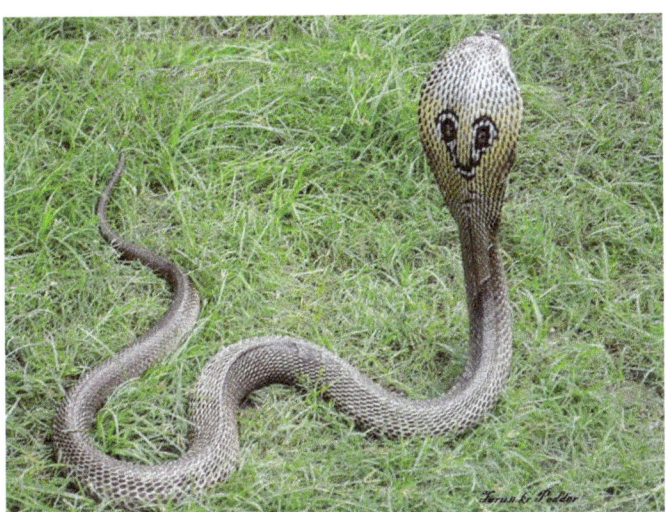

Fig. 1: Spectacled cobra.

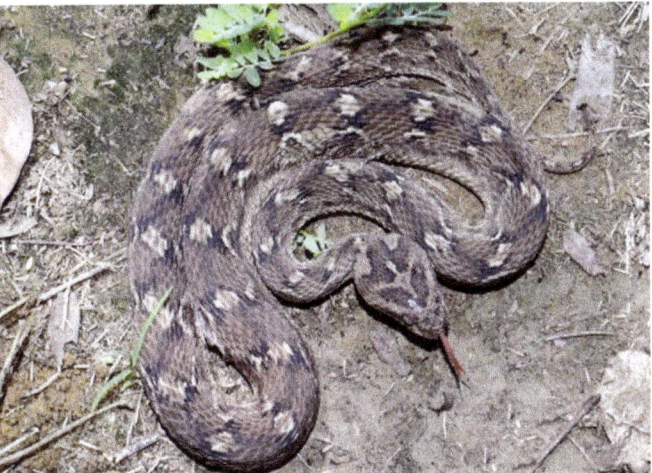

Fig. 4: Saw-scaled viper.

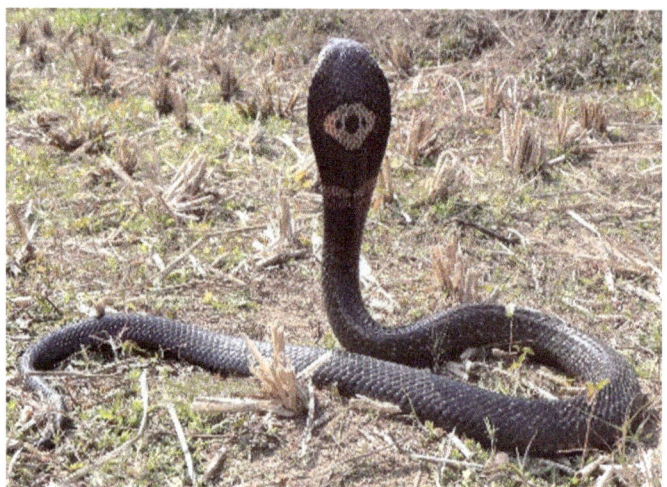

Fig. 5: Monocled cobra.

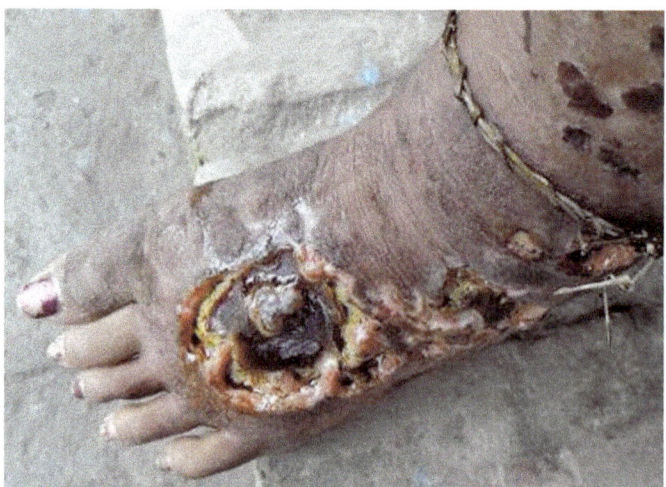

Fig. 6: Gangrene for ligature.

■ PREHOSPITAL MANAGEMENT[6-8]

What should be done and what should not be done?
- Call someone nearby and report the matter. If it is dark, ask them to bring a torch as soon as possible.
- Whoever is bitten, he or she must sit still. Others will try to see if there is any snake in the vicinity for a minute or two.
- Don't waste time looking for or killing snakes.[7]

In the current treatment method, there is no need to recognize snakes for the treatment of snake bites. The doctor who treats snakebite cases, sees the signs and symptoms of the disease.[9] Therefore, it is better not to waste time searching for the snake. If a snake is found, try to have the correct identity of it from an expert but never kill or catch a snake, never bring it to the hospital. If at all, one mobile phone photograph of the snake may be taken to show it to the doctor.[7]

- There is no need to "ligate", a procedure which has been going on for ages. Binding or putting a tourniquet does not prevent spread of venom. A tight tourniquet had done damage to the ligated limb many a times.[6i] **(Figure 6)**
- Do not try to remove the venom by cutting or sucking.
- Do not apply any stains or plant extract on the bite site.
- Do not take any Herbal or totka medicine.[6i,ii,iii,iv,v,vi]
- Do not waste a single minute by taking advice of a faith healer.
- Do not listen to anyone's advice except the hospital doctor. Even non-medical staff at the hospital can increase the risk by misleading you.

The bite site does not need to be washed or cleaned with any medication. This is in contrast to the dog bite area which is to be thoroughly washed with soap and water. It has given rise to the misconception that even a snake bite must be washed; this is a completely wrong idea. Venom spreads more quickly when washed or rubbed. If the hand is bitten, quickly remove the ring, bangle, bracelet, etc. After a while,

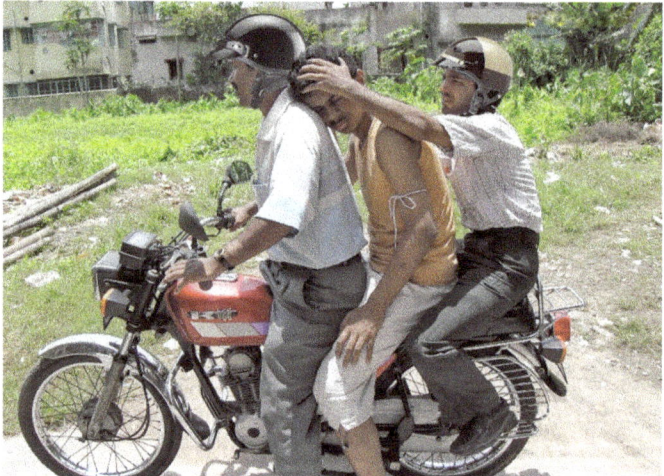

Fig. 7: Motorbike ambulance.

if the hand or finger becomes swollen, all the jewelry can be dangerous.
- Transport the patient immediately to the nearest hospital. If possible, let someone in the hospital know over the phone that a snakebite patient is arriving there.
- If there is an ambulance nearby, call but do not delay for an ambulance, put the injured person on any vehicle, even on a motorbike and drive to the nearest primary health center **(Figure 7)**.

Every patient of snake bite should be admitted at the nearest healthcare facility with availability of round the clock medical personnel.

Every minute is important in case of snake bites. If it takes more than fifteen minutes to get to the big hospital in the city, that can be fatal.

It is very important to be careful that under no circumstances should an injured person ride a bicycle or motorbike himself. In the first case, the body is subdued, but after the bite of some snakes, the limbs will become numb within 15–20 minutes. In that case serious accidents can happen. Exercise, such as cycling, speeds up the blood circulation in the body and spreads toxins (venom).

What is the primary treatment (first aid) for snake bites? The answer is, in the conventional sense, there is no first aid for snake bites. After the bite, the only thing to do is to rush the injured to the hospital without panic.

Reassurance—Talk to the patient to reassure him to boost his morale while going on the road. What the patient was talking about, or how long ago he was talking, is also important for proper treatment. Often the patient loses the ability to speak before reaching the hospital; In that case the doctor has to listen to the accompanying people and treat accordingly.

IV infusion and anti-snake venom (ASV) are the initial line of treatment.

The patient may be referred to higher center, should a situation arise for further treatment. A proper referral letter with sequence of events should accompany the patient.

It should be made sure that the patient does not move much. Walking or running will be dangerous.[6iii]

Take a good look at what has changed in the bite site; for treatment, the doctor will want to know those things. For example, whether there was bleeding from the bite site, whether the area was gradually swollen, or whether the skin around the bite site changed color.

What to do if a snake bites? In a word, the answer is to *take the patient to the nearest health center as soon as possible*.

■ TREATMENT AT PRIMARY HOSPITAL[6-8]

- Always admit the patient.
- Do a prompt assessment of the patient, for any crisis like shock and airway obstruction. Manage crisis first. If the patient is in respiratory failure, immediate intubation and mechanical ventilation is to be started.
- Reassure—Each and every Snakebite patient will be anxious; try to assure the patient. Counsel the patient that, 80% of the snakebites are by non-venomous snakes. Even nearly 40% bites by venomous snakes are "Dry bites"; that means though a venomous snake had bitten, enough venom may not be injected by the snake.[6iv] Just verbal assurance may not be enough. Starting a plain drip and a tetanus toxoid injection are more assuring.
- Though ligatures are being discouraged for years, all the bite patients will come with multiple ligatures. Never remove the final ligature at the emergency room, as it may cause rapid dissemination of the venom.[6v]
- Follow the Syndromic approach to manage a snakebite case. Just identifying the brought snake as a venomous snake and/or presence of bite marks are not diagnostic for envenomation.
- Follow the snakebite treatment flow chart for management **(Figure 8)** of any snake or unknown bite case attending a Hospital.
- Cobra Bite—Bite marks (singe, two or multiple) with severe pain and progressive swelling are diagnostic for cobra bite. In case of cobra bites never wait for neurological signs to appear. The Patient may collapse in few seconds after the first neurological sign is noted.
- Russell's viper and Saw scaled viper bites may not present with much pain and swelling. Confirmation can be done by 20WBCT test (hourly for first four hour–if earlier tests show clotting) which is a bed side test.[6vi] 2-3ml of venous blood is kept in a Glass Test Tube (never plastic) for twenty minutes. Gently tilted after 20 minutes; if blood is not clotted presence of hemotoxic venom is confirmed. This test is also done to monitor the hemotoxic bite cases.
- If 20WBCT remains not clotted six hours after the first loading dose of ASV, more ASV is to be infused. Hemotoxic envenomation is diagnosed much earlier by 20WBCT than any Urine test **(Figure 9)**.
- 7c. Managing Common Krait (CK) bite cases are always challenging. As CK snakes usually bites in sleep in the mid night, and bites are painless almost all the CK bite cases are not noticed by the victims.[10,12] Moreover very fine bite marks of CK bites are almost invisible. Usually CK bite patients attend any hospital, not for any bite but with other symptoms like pain abdomen, pain in throat, joint pains, back aches or just fainting attacks. High degree of suspicion with a history of floor bed without bed net is the road to a diagnosis of CK bite. Sudden onset of bilateral Ptosis without any history of previous suggestive illness is the hall mark to diagnose a CK bite case **(Figure 10)**.

■ SYNDROMIC APPROACH IN SNAKEBITE MANAGEMENT[6-9]

In India, snakebite is managed in a syndromic approach. There are two main reasons for syndromic approach in snakebite management. First reason is nonavailability of any venom detection testing kit. In developed countries such as Australia, highly sensitive venom detection kits are available. Snake species involved in the bite are promptly identified by ELISA test kits. As the snake species is identified perfectly, monovalent antisnake venom serums (ASV) are used. As in India snake species specific monovalent antivenoms are not available, clinicians are trained to treat snakebite by polyvalent antivenoms only; this is the second reason for syndromic management.

Polyvalent ASV are prepared against big four snakes of India, and claimed to cover 99% of the venomous snake bites in India.[4]

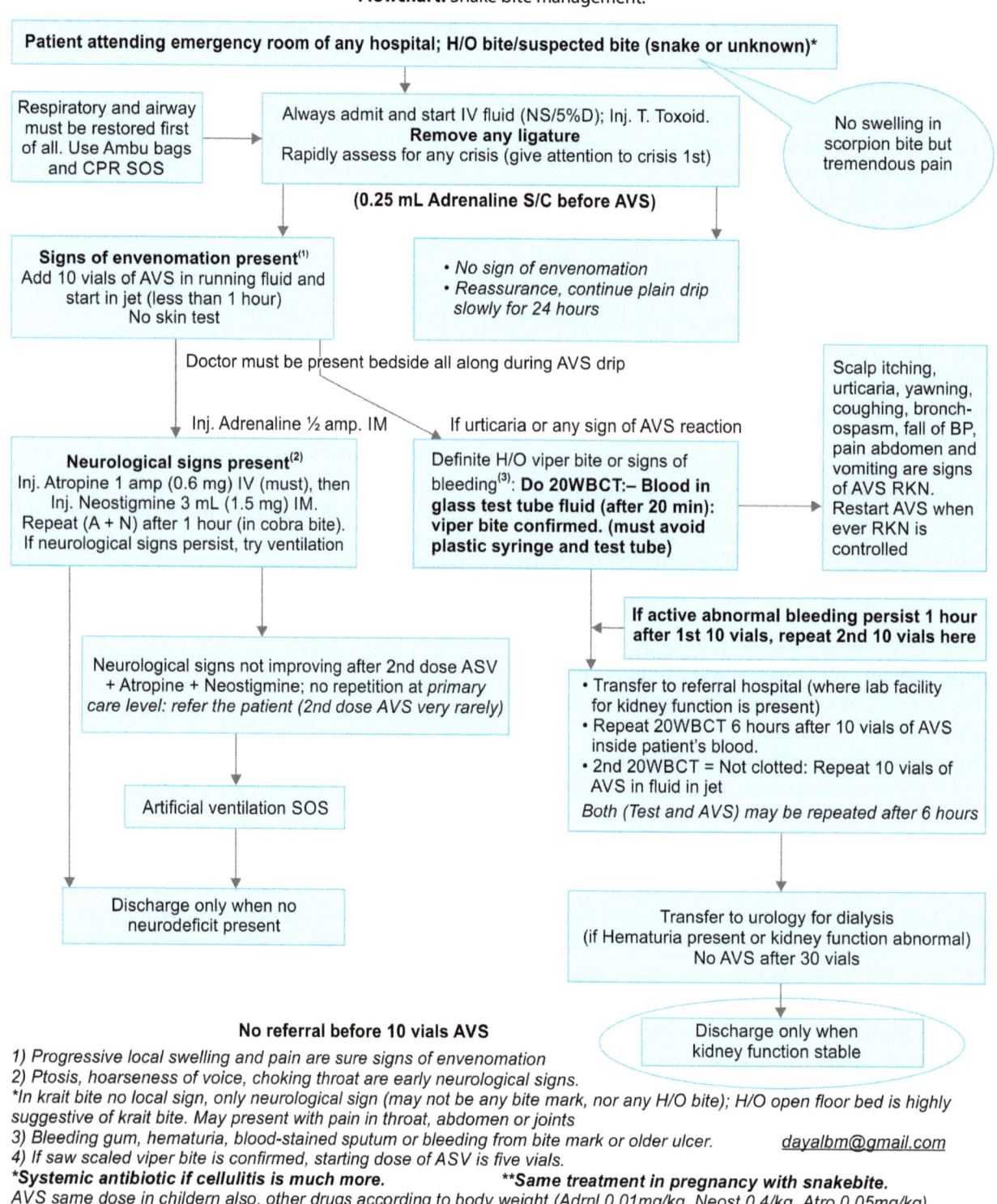

Flowchart: Snake bite management.

No referral before 10 vials AVS

1) Progressive local swelling and pain are sure signs of envenomation
2) Ptosis, hoarseness of voice, choking throat are early neurological signs.
*In krait bite no local sign, only neurological sign (may not be any bite mark, nor any H/O bite); H/O open floor bed is highly suggestive of krait bite. May present with pain in throat, abdomen or joints
3) Bleeding gum, hematuria, blood-stained sputum or bleeding from bite mark or older ulcer.   dayalbm@gmail.com
4) If saw scaled viper bite is confirmed, starting dose of ASV is five vials.
*Systemic antibiotic if cellulitis is much more.   **Same treatment in pregnancy with snakebite.
AVS same dose in childern also. other drugs according to body weight (Adrnl 0.01mg/kg, Neost 0.4/kg, Atro 0.05mg/kg).
      Adequate hydration should be maintained.   Keep attention to avoid fluid overload in childern

In syndromic approach of snakebite management, the protocol is almost same all over India. Only difference is in the dosage of ASV; in SS viper bite cases, less ASV is required; only five vials may be enough. In all other snakes, ten vials of ASV are minimum.

As per our National Standard Treatment Guidelines, all the snakebite and suspected snakebite cases must be admitted in a hospital, for minimum 24 hours. If after 24 hours of observation, no sign of envenomation is observed, the patient may be discharged.

The treatment protocol of any suspected snake bite is explained in **Figure 8**.[8] Whenever one patient (snakebite/unknown bite) is admitted, one plain normal saline drip is slowly started. One tetanus toxoid injection is also given,

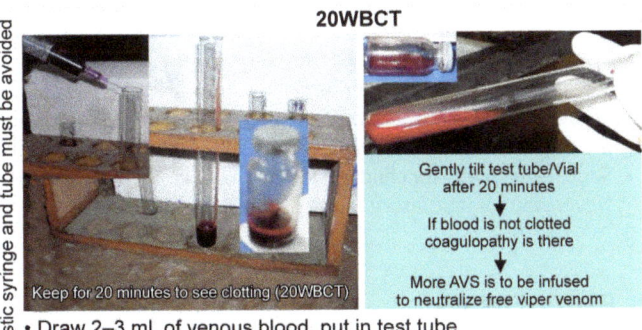

Fig. 8: The 20-minute whole blood clotting test (20WBCT).

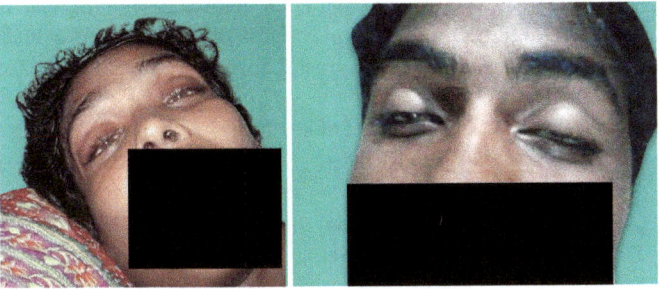

Figs. 9A and B: Cases of ptosis.

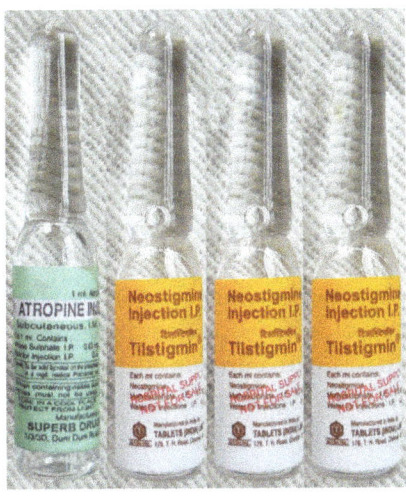

Fig. 10: Atropine and Neostigmine (AN) injection.

if not taken recently. First of all, the patient is assessed and managed for any crisis like airway and shock. If any one or more sign of envenomation is detected, ten vials of ASV is added to the running bottle of NS, and infused in jet. No skin test is required for ASV. If there is no absolute contraindication, 1/4th mL of injection Adrenaline (one in thousand as available) SC is used as a premedication.

If any sign of neurotoxicity such as bilateral ptosis is noted, one loading dose of Atropine and Neostigmine (AN injection) is tried in all cases.[10-12] Adult dose of Atropine is 0.6 mg IV in shot. Adult dose of Neostigmine is 1.5 mg slowly IV or intramuscularly (to be decided according to the stage of neurotoxicity). Atropine must always be given before Neostigmine. In case of cobra bites, ptosis will definitely improve in half an hour following AN injection. If no improvement of ptosis after loading dose of AN injection, further use of AN injection is of no value.

Krait and Russell's viper neurotoxicity will not respond to AN injection.

In case of cobra bites, AN injection can be repeated in two ways. Same loading dose can be repeated after 1 hour. Alternatively, one ampoule of Atropine is to be mixed in one bottle of NS and infused slowly over 8 hours. Injection Neostigmine is to be repeated half hurly 0.5 mg IM, for 4–5 hours till the cobra bite ptosis cures totally. Neostigmine overdose is diagnosed by bradycardia and/or muscle twitching; in that case one ampoule Atropine is to be given IV **(Fig. 11)**.

Severe pain and progressive swelling of bitten part are the early signs of cobra envenomation. If AN injection and ASV are infused in this stage, patient may not progress to the stage of neuroparalysis. But most of the time cobra bite patients reach a hospital in the stage of respiratory distress or even respiratory failure. In these cases, supported respiration and even tracheal intubation may be needed.[11] After infusion of first dose of ASV and AN injection, the patient should be closely monitored. If after initial improvement the patient looks deteriorating, second dose of ten vials of ASV is to be repeated promptly. Usually, 20 vials of ASV are enough to cure neurotoxic bites.

Krait bite patients are always difficult to diagnose as usually there would be no history of any bite. Painless bite and almost invisible bite marks in krait bites makes the diagnosis challenging. Appearance of acute bilateral ptosis is the most important finding to diagnose a case of krait bite.[13-15] As soon as ptosis is noted, first dose of ASV and AN injection should be given. If no clinical improvement of the presenting symptoms after 1 hour of initial dose, second dose of ten vials of ASV to be repeated promptly.

Russell's viper and SS viper bites are usually diagnosed by abnormal bleeding from anywhere.[16,17] In case of doubt 20WBCT to be done bed side.[18] If initial 20WBCT results are clotting, the test is to be repeated hourly for four times minimum. Usually, abnormal bleeding stops in 1 hour following initial ten vials of ASV. If abnormal bleeding continues second dose of ASV should be repeated after 1 hour. If abnormal bleeding or coagulation defect is not corrected by 30 vials of ASV, no more ASV would be effective. Fresh frozen plasma may be tried.

After initial infusion of required ASV and AN injection, cellulitis and local swelling may be attended. Broad spectrum systemic antibiotics, antihistaminics and even steroids may be tried. For persistent swelling of limbs, magnesium sulfate compress, thrice daily in wet bandages may be tried for 3–4 days. For long standing fibrosis and other surgical complications, surgical intervention may be required.

Delay in infusion of adequate volume of ASV, and low efficiency of ASV usually leads to acute kidney injury in Russell's viper bite cases.[17] In those cases oliguria, then anuria leads to accumulation of urea, creatinine and potassium. These patients must be managed by skilled nephrologists. These patients need dialysis.

ASV reactions are usually not life threatening.[17,19,20] Yet the treating doctor must be present near the patient when ASV drip is running. Stop the drip on slightest suspicion of any adverse reaction. Promptly give IM injection of half ampoule of Adrenaline injection, wait for 5–7 minutes. Restart the ASV drip as soon as the adverse reaction is over. Dose of ASV is same in children and in pregnant ladies also.

SOME MYTHS AND REALITY

- All snakes are venomous. No, only few snakes are venomous. 80% of snakebites are from nonvenomous snakes.
- Snake identification is essential for snakebite management. Not at all, syndromic approach of snakebite management needs no snake identification.
- Only specialist physicians can treat snakebites. No, any doctor can treat snakebite patients.
- Snakebite can be managed in medical colleges and tertiary care hospitals only. No, even a bedded primary health center can treat a venomous snakebite patient.
- Two bite marks are essential to diagnose venomous snakebite. One, two or multiple bite marks may be venomous. Even no bite marks may be venomous in common krait bite.
- ASV infusion is dangerous as it may lead to life-threatening reaction. Severe ASV reaction is very rare. ASD reaction can be managed at any hospital.
- Laboratory tests are essential to manage snakebites. For primary management of snakebite, no laboratory tests are needed.
- All neurotoxic bites need ICU for ventilation. Only very few cases need ventilation.
- All viper bites need dialysis. Less than 40% Russell's viper bites ultimately need dialysis.
- Snakebite death is a natural death. No, all snakebite cases are medicolegal cases, and police must be informed.

Take Home Messages

- Do not waste time. Hospitalize the patient immediately.
- Never diagnose envenomation looking toward the snake brought along with. Many a times a wrong snake was brought.
- Bite marks are of no clue to assess envenomation.
- Final ligature must never be removed at the emergency examination room; patient must be admitted and an IV fluid started before removal of the final ligature.
- Never start ASV infusion if Adrenaline injection is not seen by the treating doctor.
- Give AN (Atropine and Neostigmine) injection as early as possible to a cobra bite patient (painful bite with progressive swelling). ASV infusion may be started after AN injection.
- Whatever new sign and symptom is noted after the ASV infusion is started, consider it as ASV reaction.
- Same dose of ASV for children and pregnant ladies is prescribed.
- Never wait for laboratory reports, start ASV early.

REFERENCES

1. World Health Organization. Snakebite envenoming: A strategy for prevention and control. [online] Available from: https://www.who.int/publications/i/item/9789241515641. [Last Accessed January, 2023].
2. Suraweera W, Warrell D, Whitaker R, Menon G, Rodrigues R, Fu SH, et al. Trends in snakebite deaths in India from 2000 to 2019 in a nationally representative mortality study. Elife. 2020;9:e54076.
3. Whitaker R, Captain A. Snakes of India: The Field Guide. Chennai: Draco Books; 2004.
4. Mukherjee AK, Mackessy SP. Prevention and improvement of clinical management of snakebite in Southern Asian countries: A proposed road map. Toxicon. 2021;200: 140-52.
5. Warrell DA, Gutiérrez JM, Calvete JJ, Williams D. New approaches and technologies of venomics to meet the challenge of human envenoming by snakebites in India. Indian J Med Res. 2013;138(1):38-59.
6. WHO-SEARO guideline (2016).
    i. Page 94 and 107
    ii. page 94
    iii. page 116
    iv. page 69
    v. page 107 and 117
    vi. page 108
7. National Health Mission. (2017). Indian National Standard Treatment Guidelines. [online] Available from: https://nhm.gov.in/images/pdf/guidelines/nrhm-guidelines/stg/Snakebite_Full.pdf. [Last Accessed January, 2023].
8. Government of West Bengal. (2018). Training Module for Management of Snakebite and Common Poisons. [online] Available from: https://www.wbhealth.gov.in/uploaded_files/IDSP/Training_Module_For_Management_of_Snake_Bite_Common_Poisons_(2018).pdf. [Last Accessed January, 2023].
9. Ariaratnam CA, Sheriff MH, Arambepola C, Theakston RD, Warrell DA. Syndromic approach to treatment of snake bite in Sri Lanka based on results of a prospective national hospital-based survey of patients envenomed by identified snakes. Am J Trop Med Hyg. 2009;81(4):725-31.
10. Bawaskar HS, Bawaskar PH. Envenoming by the Common Krait (*Bungarus caeruleus*) and Asian Cobra (*Naja naja*): Clinical Manifestations and Their Management in a Rural Setting. Wilderness Environ Med. 2004;15(4):257-66.
11. Bawaskar HS. Snake bite poisoning: A neglected life-threatening occupational hazard. Indian J Crit Care Med. 2014;18(3):9.
12. Bawaskar HS, Bawaskar PH, Punde DP, Inamdar MK, Dongare RB, Bhoite RR. Profile of snakebite envenoming in

rural Maharashtra. India. J Assoc Physicians India. 2008;56: 88-95.
13. Agarwal R, Singh N, Gupta D. Is the patient brain-dead? Emerg Med J. 2006; 23(1):e5.
14. Kohli U, Sreedhar V. Snake Bite: An unusual cause of acute abdominal pain. Indian Pediatr. 2007;44:852-853
15. Meenakshisundaram R. Severe hypertension in elapid envenomation. J Cardiovasc Dis Res. 2013;4:65-7.
16. Bawaskar HS, Bawaskar PH. Diagnosis of envenomation by Russell's and Echis carinatus viper: a clinical study at rural Maharashtra state of India. J Family Med Prim Care. 2019; 8(4):1386-90.
17. Alirol E, Sharma SK, Bawaskar HS, Kuch U, Chappuis F. Snake Bite in South Asia: a Review. PLoS Negl Trop Dis. 2010; 4(1):e603.
18. Warrell DA. WHO Guidelines for the clinical management of snake bites in the South East Asia region. SE Asian J Trop Med Publ Hlth. 1999;30:1-83.
19. Premawardhena AP, de Silva CE, Fonseka MM, Gunatilake SB, de Silva HJ. Low dose subcutaneous adrenaline to prevent acute adverse reactions to antivenom serum in people bitten by snakes: randomised, placebo controlled trial. BMJ. 1999;318(7190):1041-3.
20. de Silva HA, Pathmeswaran A, Ranasinha CD, Jayamanne S, Samarakoon SB, Hittharage A, et al. Low-Dose Adrenaline, Promethazine, and Hydrocortisone in the Prevention of Acute Adverse Reactions to Antivenom following Snakebite: a Randomised, Double-Blind, Placebo-Controlled Trial. PLoS Med. 2011;8(5):e1000435.

CHAPTER 41: Anaphylaxis

Shambo Samrat Samajdar, Sougata Sarkar, Saibal Moitra, Santanu K Tripathi

■ INTRODUCTION

Anaphylaxis is a medical emergency, irrespective of primary discipline of healthcare professionals everyone should know how to manage it. Timely identification followed by prompt therapy initiation could prevent fatalities related to anaphylaxis as it is a poorly recognized and often underdiagnosed entity. Variable symptoms starting from skin and mucosal involvement (90% of cases) to respiratory and cardiovascular systemic manifestations (50% of cases) are experienced by patients. Most commonly food, drug and venom are responsible for anaphylaxis. Peanut, hazelnut, milk, and egg are responsible for most of the pediatric food-induced anaphylaxis cases whereas wheat, celery and shellfish are major causes of adult food-induced anaphylaxis. Drugs such as antibiotics (most commonly beta lactams) and nonsteroidal anti-inflammatory drugs (NSAIDs) are leading causes of drug-induced anaphylaxis. Wasp, fire ant and bee venom are major contributors of venom anaphylaxis. The most common cause of fatal anaphylaxis is drug whereas most common contributors of nonfatal anaphylaxis are foods. There are a few important cofactors such as exercise, stress, infection, NSAIDs and alcohol which could aggravate anaphylaxis.[1-3]

■ DEFINITION

A serious, rapid in onset, systemic hypersensitivity reaction, characterized by life-threatening compromise in airway, breathing or circulation with presence or absence of dermatological features or circulatory shock is defined as anaphylaxis.

■ CLINICAL FEATURES

Rapid development of symptoms following exposure to allergen suggests anaphylaxis. Symptoms such as flushing, pruritus, hives, swelling, morbilliform rashes, swelling and or pruritus of lips/tongue/uvula/palate, periorbital pruritus associated with or without erythema and swelling, conjunctival erythema, tearing, pruritus of external auditory canal/genitalia/palms/soles, laryngeal edema leading to difficulty in speaking or development of stridor, pharyngeal swelling leading to swallowing difficulty, abdominal cramps, nausea, vomiting, altered sensorium, collapse, unconsciousness and feeling of impending doom (patient usually describes like "I felt I was dying") are observed in patients experiencing anaphylaxis. **Box 1** depicted symptomatology of anaphylaxis[4] and **Box 2** had described the criteria to diagnose anaphylaxis[5] in clinical settings as per World Allergy Organization (WAO) 2019 guidelines.

BOX 1: Symptomatology of anaphylaxis.[4]

Sudden onset of following symptoms and signs are features of anaphylaxis:
- *Skin/soft tissue/mucosal involvement*
  - Flushing, pruritus, hives, swelling, morbilliform rashes, piloerection
  - Swelling and or pruritus of lips/tongue/uvula/palate
  - Periorbital pruritus associated with or without erythema and swelling, conjunctival erythema, tearing pruritus of external auditory canal/genitalia/palms/soles
- *Upper and lower respiratory tract*
  - Pruritus and congestion in nose, rhinorrhea, sneezing
  - Larynx involvement leading to throat tightness, pruritus in throat, hoarseness, dry staccato cough, stridor, difficulty in swallowing and dysphonia
  - Pulmonary involvement leading to breathlessness, chest tightness, deep cough, wheeze, bronchospasm leading to decreased peak expiratory flow
  - Cyanosis
- *Gastrointestinal tract*
  - Nausea, vomiting with stringy mucous, diarrhea, cramping pain in abdomen
- *Cardiovascular system*
  - Chest pain, palpitations, arrhythmia
  - Fainting attacks, syncope, fall in blood pressure, mental status alteration, urinary or fecal incontinence, shock, cardiac arrest
- *Nervous system*
  - Impending doom, aura, uneasiness, headache (throbbing in nature), dizziness, tunnel vision, confusion, sudden behavioral changes in infants and children (irritability, cessation of play and clinging to parents)
- *Miscellaneous*
  - Metallic taste
  - Dysphagia
  - Uterine contractions in postpubertal females

BOX 2: Criteria for the diagnosis of anaphylaxis [World Allergy Organization (WAO) 2019].[5]

Anaphylaxis is highly likely when any one of the following two criteria are fulfilled:

1. Acute onset of an illness (minutes to several hours) with involvement of the skin, mucosal tissue, or both (e.g., generalized hives, pruritus or flushing, swollen lips-tongue-uvula)
   - And at least one of the following:
     – Respiratory compromise (e.g., dyspnea, wheeze-bronchospasm, stridor, reduced PEF, hypoxemia)
     – Reduced BP or associated symptoms of end-organ dysfunction [e.g., hypotonia (collapse), syncope, incontinence]
     – Severe gastrointestinal symptoms (e.g., severe crampy abdominal pain, repetitive vomiting), especially after exposure to nonfood allergens
2. Acute onset of hypotension[a] or bronchospasm or laryngeal involvement[b] after exposure to a known or highly probable allergen[c] for that patient (minutes to several hours[d]), even in the absence of typical skin involvement.

[a]Hypotension defined as a decrease in systolic BP >30% from that person's baseline, or
  - Infants and children under 10 years: Systolic BP less than (70 mm Hg + [2 × age in years])
  - Adults: Systolic BP << 90 mmHg.

[b]Laryngeal symptoms include stridor, vocal changes, odynophagia.
[c]An allergen is a substance (usually a protein) capable of triggering an immune response that can result in an allergic reaction. Most allergens act through an IgE-mediated pathway, but some nonallergen triggers can act independent of IgE (for example, via direct activation of mast cells).
[d]The majority of allergic reactions occur within 1–2 hours of exposure, and usually much quicker. Reactions may be delayed for some food allergens (e.g., alpha-gal) or in the context of immunotherapy, occurring up to 10 hours after ingestion.

■ CAUSES[6]

There are multiple potential triggers for anaphylaxis. Foods such as milk, egg, peanut, tree nuts, wheat, soy, fish, shellfish, and sesame and food additives such as spices, colorants as carmine, vegetable gums or gelatin can cause anaphylaxis by IgE-dependent mechanism. Delayed anaphylaxis to red meats, known as alpha-gal syndrome is also IgE mediated. Other causes of IgE-dependent anaphylaxis are venoms from stinging insects like wasps, bees or red ants, drugs including beta lactam antibiotics, NSAIDs, monoclonal antibodies, neuromuscular blockers, local anesthetics, etc., vaccines (generally due to an excipient than microbial component), allergen immunotherapy, latex, and occupational allergen exposures. Rarely inhalants such as horse/dog/cat dander, grass pollen and human seminal fluid containing prostate specific antigen cause IgE-mediated anaphylaxis. IgE independent immunological triggers may cause anaphylaxis. High molecular weight dextran, monoclonal antibodies like infliximab can cause anaphylaxis where IgG plays critical role. Heparin contaminated with over sulfated chondroitin sulfate activates coagulation system leading to IgE-independent anaphylaxis. There are a few nonimmunologic triggers such as medications including opioids/NSAIDs, physical stimulus as cold/heat/UV radiation/exercise, radiocontrast media and alcohol which cause anaphylaxis by direct activation of mast cells and basophils. In case of idiopathic anaphylaxis need to consider possibility of a hidden or previously unrecognized trigger and presence of mast cell activation syndrome or monoclonal mast cell disorder.

■ RISK FACTORS AND COFACTORS[7]

Atopy is an important risk factor for anaphylaxis development. Food, latex, exercise, radiocontrast media and idiopathic anaphylaxis are strongly correlated with presence of atopy. Adolescents and geriatric population are at greater risk for severe anaphylaxis. Preexisting diseases such as asthma, chronic obstructive pulmonary disease (COPD), interstitial lung disease, mastocytosis, mast cell activation syndrome, depression, psychotic disorders, cardiovascular diseases such as ischemic heart disease, hypertensive vascular disease and cardiomyopathy are associated with severe anaphylaxis risk. Fever, upper respiratory infection, emotional stress, and menstruation can play the role of cofactors in developing anaphylaxis. Exercise, alcohol intake and medications like beta blockers, alpha blockers, angiotensin-converting enzyme (ACE) inhibitors, tricyclic antidepressants, monoamine oxidase inhibitors, attention-deficit hyperactivity disorder (ADHD) drugs, etc., can increase severity of anaphylaxis. These medications also interfere with treatment of anaphylaxis. These medicines also prevent compensatory physiological mechanisms and compromise cardiovascular states. Sedatives, hypnotics, antidepressants, recreational drugs, and alcohol affect diagnosis of anaphylaxis leading to delayed recognition. While diagnosing anaphylaxis it is extremely important to search for causes and cofactors behind that to educate patients to prevent future occurrences.

■ PATHOPHYSIOLOGY[7]

There are immunological or nonimmunological mechanisms which play role in development of anaphylaxis. Immunological reactions can be IgE-dependent or independent (immune complex or complement mediated reactions). Without involvement of IgE or other antibodies and immune complex, mast cells and basophils are stimulated and lead to degranulation in case of nonimmunological anaphylaxis. On the surface of blood basophils and tissue mast cells IgE bound FcERI receptors are occupied by IgE in sensitized state. In case of allergy, allergen enters into the circulation and interacts with surface bound FcERI-IgE and cross-links two IgE antibodies on the mast cell or basophil, which initiates intracellular signaling leading to degranulation and release of preformed mediators, enzymes and cytokines and inducing de novo synthesis of inflammatory mediators which directly act on tissues and produce symptoms as described. Preformed intracellular granular substances such as histamine, tryptase, chymase and heparin and lipid-derived mediators such as prostaglandin D2 (PGD_2), leukotriene B_4 (LTB_4), platelet-activating factor (PAF) and leukotrienes (LTC_4, LTD_4 and LTE_4) have played the role of primary chemical mediators in anaphylaxis. Releasing from activated mast cells and basophils histamine is an important chemical mediator of allergic reactions. Cutaneous release of histamine produces urticaria and systemic exposure to histamine leads to flushing, headache, bronchoconstriction, tachycardia, and hypotension. Histamine in systemic circulation can influence coronary vessels, atrial and ventricular contractility. Tryptase, a protease-derived majorly from mast cells and smaller amounts from basophils, activates complement pathways involving $C3_a$ and $C5_a$, coagulation cascade and kallikrein-kinin contact system. Except food-induced anaphylaxis, increased tryptase level is highly correlated with severe form of anaphylaxis. LTC_4, LTD_4 and LTE_4 increase vascular permeability and bronchoconstriction. PGD_2 is responsible for bronchoconstriction, vasodilation and increase in vascular permeability. PAF and platelet-activating factor acetylhydrolase (PAF-AH) activity have increased in anaphylaxis. PAF-AH activity and severity of anaphylaxis have an inverse correlation. In **Figure 1**, we are describing the pathophysiology of type I hypersensitivity reaction and development of anaphylaxis.

IgE-independent anaphylaxis is generally associated with IgG and drugs such as radiocontrast media directly interact with F_c portion of IgG which is already bound to basophils and mast cells. Their direct cross-linking leads to activation of cells and production of cytokine release syndrome (CRS) such as reactions as chills, fever, hypoxemia, hypotension, and cardiovascular collapse. Monoclonal antibodies and chemotherapy can produce similar reactions. Proinflammatory cytokines such as TNF-alpha, IL-1B and IL 6 play critical role in developing CRS.

In case of nonimmune anaphylaxis, drugs such as vancomycin, NSAIDs and opiates directly activate mast cells and or basophils bypassing IgE and release histamine leading to development of symptoms of anaphylaxis such as flushing, urticaria and hypotension.

DIFFERENTIAL DIAGNOSIS[8]

Early diagnosis is extremely crucial for prompt and optimal management of anaphylaxis. Chronological evaluation with emphasis on exposure history, presenting clinical features and ruling out other acute disease conditions is necessary. Acute urticaria or angioedema, acute asthma, vasovagal syncope, panic attacks, and acute anxiety are different most common disorders which can mimic anaphylaxis. Other differentials such as foreign body aspiration, myocardial infarction, pulmonary embolism, pollen-food syndrome, scombroidosis, monosodium glutamate or sulfite additive allergy, basophilic leukemia, mastocytosis, vancomycin flushing syndrome, shock of different etiologies, hereditary angioedema, urticarial vasculitis, pheochromocytoma, progesterone anaphylaxis, hyper-IgE urticarial syndrome

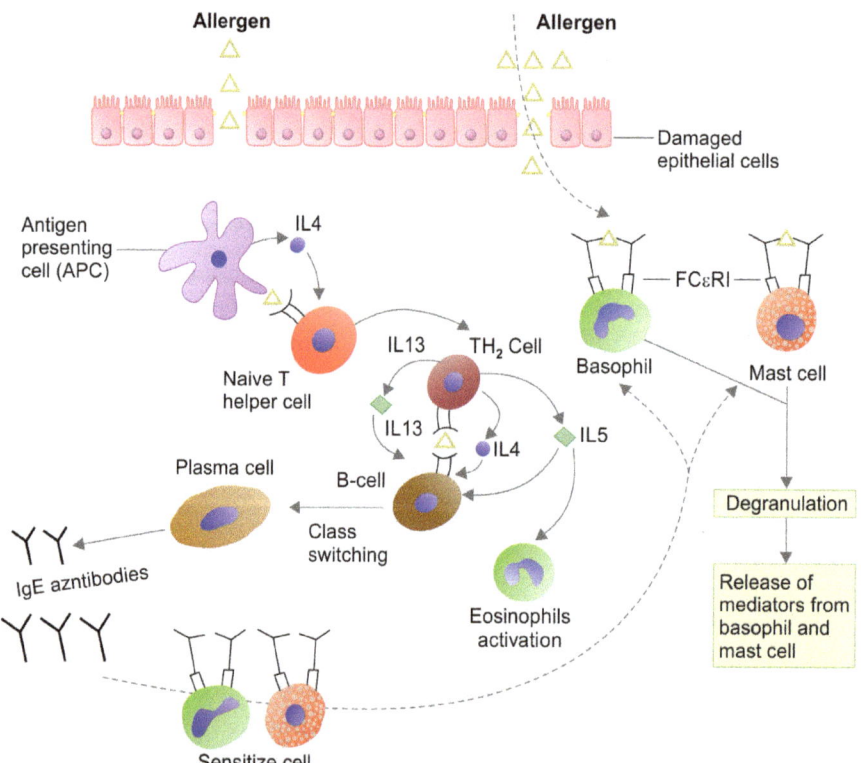

Fig. 1: Mechanism of type I hypersensitivity reaction and anaphylaxis.

and idiopathic systemic capillary leak syndrome need to be considered as other relatively rare conditions which cause similar signs and symptoms like anaphylaxis.

LABORATORY TESTS IN DIAGNOSING ANAPHYLAXIS[8]

Clinical diagnosis should be made in cases of anaphylaxis. Signs, symptoms, and temporal history should guide for prompt diagnosis. Appropriate medical management should not be delayed for confirmation by laboratory tests. Though most laboratory investigations to detect anaphylaxis are not sensitive or specific enough, but samples obtained at the time of presentation of anaphylaxis can be utilized to rule out other differentials and confirm diagnosis of anaphylaxis. If serum tryptase can be measured within 15 min to 3 hours of the onset of anaphylaxis and value more than 11.4 ng/mL (or increased by ≥20% of baseline tryptase value + 2 ng/mL), which returns to normal level after event; diagnosis of anaphylaxis would be confirmed. In case of food induced anaphylaxis tryptase level is not elevated. Urinary histamine, methyl-histamine, LTE_4, LTC_4, PGD_2 and PGF_2 have been elevated for prolonged duration followed by anaphylaxis, which can be measured by collection of 24-hour urine. Logistics involved for testing and timing make these tests not feasible.

Plasma free metanephrine and urinary vanillylmandelic acid assay may be required in a subset of clinically suspected patients to rule out pheochromocytoma. To rule out carcinoid syndrome measurement of serum serotonin and urinary 5-hydroxy indole acetic acid can be considered. Vasointestinal polypeptide (VIP) panel can be considered to exclude VIP secreting tumors.

EVALUATION FOR ETIOLOGY[8]

Identifying the cause of anaphylaxis is extremely important to prevent future exposure of the offending agent. Detailed clinical history guide physician to understand the likely trigger and thorough temporal evaluation of exposure (drug, insects, food or exercise) would often identify the cause. Prior to the onset of event what is the different activities patient was involved, need careful exploration. For IgE mediated allergic reaction, skin prick test with allergen or allergen specific IgE measurements can establish sensitization status of patient. Considering history, temporal relationship with probable trigger exposure and allergy report showcasing sensitization status, probable culprit can be identified and future exposure could be prohibited. Basophil activation test (BAT) is an emerging laboratory tool which is not presently commercially available and clinical utility need to be explored further. Food, insect venom and drug allergen can be identified by using this test. In cases where history and further evaluation fail to understand the trigger, physician needs to re-explore the possibility of other differential diagnosis. Uncommon hidden triggers such as exercise, delayed anaphylaxis to mammalian meats or reaction to stimulus like cold exposure or heat could be responsible for anaphylaxis and need cautious evaluation considering these factors. Patients with recurrent anaphylaxis or anaphylaxis-like symptoms, physicians must exclude systemic mastocytosis, monoclonal mast cell activation disorder, mast cell activation disorder and cutaneous mastocytosis. **Flowchart 1** describes the evaluation of anaphylaxis.

MANAGEMENT[8]

- Earliest introduction of intramuscular (IM) adrenaline is extremely important. The dose of adrenaline is 0.01 mg/kg (maximum dose of 0.5 mg). It could be repeated if required every 5–15 minutes interval.
- High flow oxygen supplementation via high flow oxygen mask, nonrebreather mask or endotracheal tube needs to be administered in presence of hypoxemia. Inhaled short acting beta-2 agonist like salbutamol can be given for bronchospasm. Beta-2 agonist can be used as an adjunctive agent and should not be considered as replacement of adrenaline. In presence of compromised airway (as in some cases of angioedema) intubation should be done immediately.
- Patient should be placed in a recumbent or supine position. Legs can be elevated if patient can tolerate that. If patient is vomiting or having respiratory distress, supine positioning should be avoided.
- Severe anaphylaxis is associated with increase in vascular permeability, causing redistribution of intravascular volume rapidly and development of distributive shock. In presence of hypotension and orthostasis which are not responding to IM adrenaline, large IV bolus of normal saline is required immediately.
- Vasopressors may be required in cases of refractory anaphylaxis where adrenaline and IV bolus fluid therapy fail to manage hypotension.
- Anaphylaxis patients who were on beta blocker face challenges due to their hypotension and bronchospasm become refractory to adrenaline response. They require administration of IV glucagon (1–5 mg over 5 minutes). As glucagon causes vomiting, need to make position change for the patient to lateral decubitus.
- Other adjunctive therapies such as H1 antihistamine (IV diphenhydramine 25–50 mg for relief of pruritus only), H2 antihistamine (IV ranitidine 50 mg), and glucocorticoid (IV methylprednisolone 125 mg) are used in anaphylaxis. Glucocorticoid has a slow onset of action but it can address anaphylaxis by preventing biphasic reactions and attenuating protracted symptoms in patients requiring hospitalization.
- Postanaphylaxis 4–6 hours observation is well enough except those cases with severe anaphylaxis where

Flowchart 1: Evaluation of anaphylaxis.

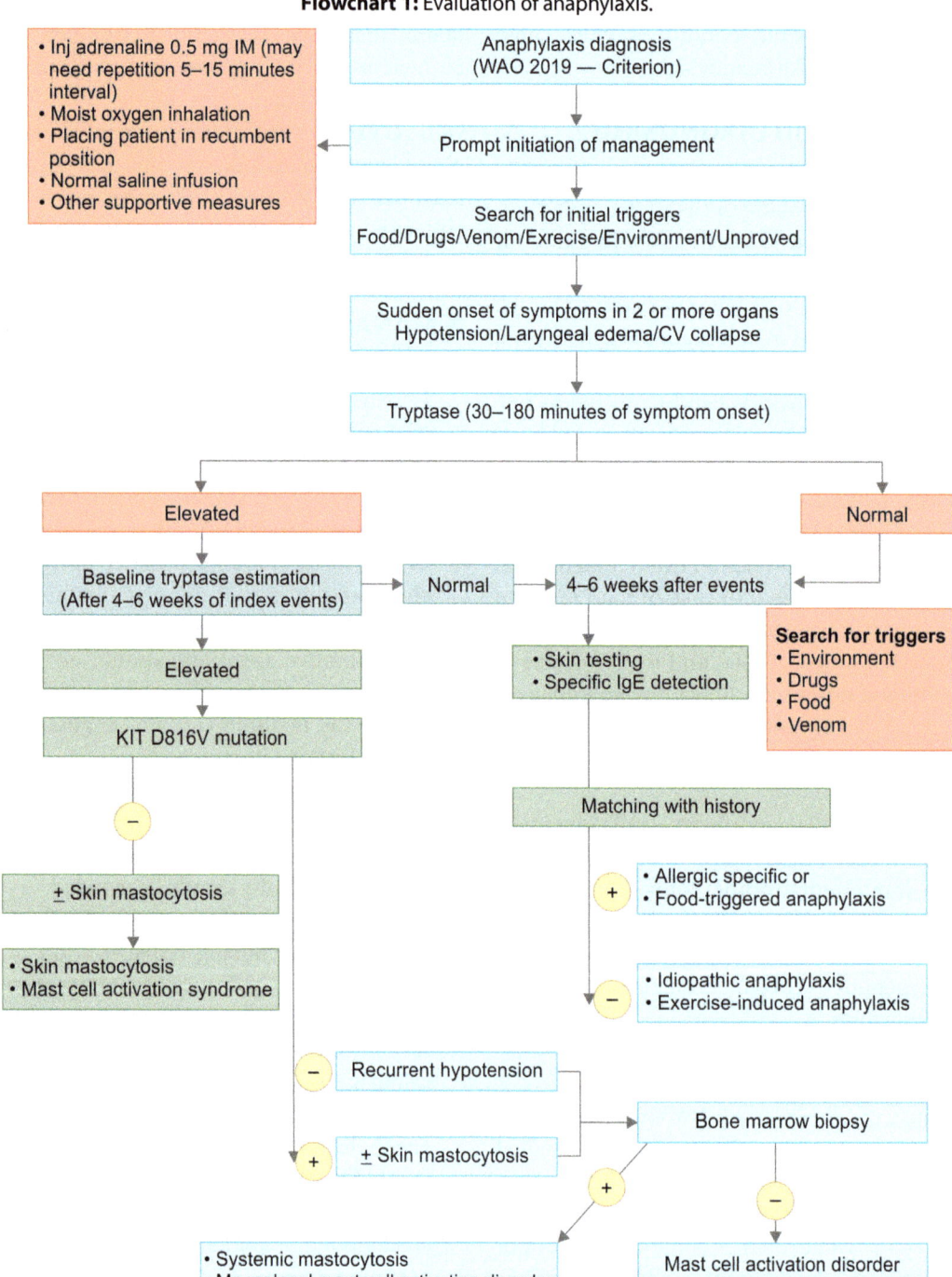

symptoms do not reverse promptly with adrenaline. This subset of patients requires hospitalization for further management and prolonged observation.

- While discharging patients with anaphylaxis need to clarify them regarding identification and avoidance of further exposures to potential triggers. Adrenaline autoinjector is unavailable in our country, which is very unfortunate for our anaphylaxis patients. Clear information on dose and IM injection technique of adrenaline should be disseminated to the patient. An emergency anaphylaxis action plan should be written in patient's understandable language and given to the patient. Patient suffered from anaphylaxis needs referral to an allergist for follow-up. A patient with a history suggestive of drug allergy requires follow-up by a clinical pharmacologist.

CONCLUSION

Anaphylaxis can occur in patients of all ages leading to fatal outcome if not recognize it early. Prompt management with IM adrenaline is lifesaving. Physicians need to be familiar with pathogenesis, clinical features, triggers, and risk factors of anaphylaxis so that they can promptly recognize it and initiate treatment immediately. Physicians across all subspecialties should undergo detailed training of different aspects of anaphylaxis management.

Take Home Messages

- Anaphylaxis is an absolute medical emergency; delay in recognition can lead to fatal outcome.
- Clinical diagnosis is most important.
- Laboratory diagnosis has no role in deciding treatment initiation.
- Early recognition and presumptive treatment with adrenaline which is a physiological antagonist of histamine are two crucial steps.

REFERENCES

1. Greenhawt M, Gupta RS, Meadows JA, Pistiner M, Spergel JM, Camargo CA Jr, et al. Guiding Principles for the Recognition, Diagnosis, and Management of Infants with Anaphylaxis: An Expert Panel Consensus. J Allergy Clin Immunol Pract. 2019;7(4):1148-56.e1145.
2. Aurich S, Dölle-Bierke S, Francuzik W, Bilo MB, Christoff G, Fernandez-Rivas M, et al. Anaphylaxis in elderly patients—data from the European Anaphylaxis Registry. Front Immunol. 2019;10:750.
3. Christensen MJ, Eller E, Mortz CG, Brockow K, Bindslev-Jensen C. Wheat-Dependent Cofactor -Augmented Anaphylaxis: a Prospective Study of Exercise, Aspirin, and Alcohol Efficacy as Cofactors. J Allergy Clin Immunol Pract. 2019;7(1):114-21.
4. Simons FE. Anaphylaxis. J Allergy Clin Immunol. 2010;125(2 Suppl 2):S161-81.
5. Turner PJ, Worm M, Ansotegui IJ, El-Gamal Y, Rivas MF, Fineman S, WAO Anaphylaxis Committee, et al. Time to revisit the definition and clinical criteria for anaphylaxis? World Allergy Organ J. 2019;12(10):100066.
6. Lieberman P. Epidemiology of anaphylaxis. Curr Opin Allergy Clin Immunol. 2008;8(4):316-20.
7. Peavy RD, Metcalfe DD. Understanding the mechanisms of anaphylaxis. Curr Opin Allergy Clin Immunol. 2008;8:310-15.
8. Castells M. Diagnosis and management of anaphylaxis in precision medicine. J Allergy Clin Immunol. 2017;140(2):321-3.

CHAPTER 42

Emergencies in Medical Practice: Common Drugs

Lopamudra Chowdhury

INTRODUCTION

Emergency in medicine can occur anywhere and anytime, be it in the ward, the OPD or in the operation theater. It is particularly common with elderly patients, patients with comorbidities, critically ill patients or due to iatrogenic causes such as surgery done in lighter plane of anesthesia, irrational drug therapy, which again calls for precaution against drug-drug interactions. Here we will discuss the salient features of some commonly used emergency drugs, which should always be available at hand in the emergency drug tray.

ADRENALINE

Adrenaline is one such drug which is indispensable in various emergency situations, at the same time inappropriate use of the drug itself can create an emergency situation. Adrenaline is a sympathomimetic drug used parenterally, the preferred routes are subcutaneous (SC) or intramuscular (IM), if administered intravenous (IV), should always be done slowly, in diluted form and preferably under cardiac monitoring. It acts on α- and β-receptors producing increased cardiac contractility, increased cardiac output, tachycardia, vasoconstriction, increase in BP, bronchodilation, and inhibition of mast cell degranulation.

It is available in preparations of 1 mg/mL injection; used in 1:1,000, 1:10,000, 1:100,000 dilution. The various routes of administration are SC, IM, intracardiac in dire emergency, aerosol for inhalation and as 2% eye solution used in glaucoma.

It is used in *anaphylactic shock*—0.5 mL of 1 in 1,000 dilution IM, repeated every 5 minutes.

Cardiac arrest—10 mL of 1 in 10,000 dilution slowly IV, in *septic shock* or *cardiogenic shock* when other sympathomimetics fail to act. Adrenaline can also be used as compress *epistaxis* or *trauma-related surgical bleeding* from skin or mucous membrane—1 in 10,000 dilution. In *glaucoma*, the prodrug dipivefrine is used topically in eye as 2% solution.

The adverse effects and precautions to be undertaken should also be kept in mind. Adverse effects include palpitation, restlessness, headache, acute rise in BP, precipitation of angina in susceptible patients, arrhythmia, tremor, subarachnoid hemorrhage, and development of acute pulmonary edema. As a precautionary method, adrenaline use should be restricted for emergency use only and in correct dilution. Also, IV use should be under cardiac monitoring. Contraindications are severe hypertension. Moreover, it should not be used along with halothane during anesthesia or along with beta blockers to avoid arrhythmia.

ADENOSINE

Adenosine is used in emergency setting of arrhythmia, which if left untreated may lead to dire consequences. It is an ultrashort acting purinergic agent acting as antagonist at cardiac adenosine receptor type 1 and peripheral adenosine receptor type 2. It acts by producing vasodilation, negative ionotropic and chronotropic action.

It is available in preparations of 3 mg/mL of drug in 2 mL and 10 mL ampoule. The method of administration is 3 mg/6 mg given in IV bolus, may be repeated after 1–2 hours to a maximum of 12 mg.

It is used in *termination of supraventricular tachycardia* (to be done under cardiac monitoring) and also *to distinguish between supraventricular tachycardia and ventricular tachycardia.*

The important adverse effects include flushing, headache, bronchospasm. Patient may complain about "a thump" in the chest. It should be used with caution in 2nd and 3rd degree heart block, asthma, atrial flutter, and hepatic/renal insufficiency.

ATROPINE

Atropine is another important emergency drug to be available at hand for emergency purposes such as severe bradycardia, heart block, cardiac arrest, acute secretory states as in organophosphorus poisoning or mushroom poisoning, sudden precipitation of bradyarrhythmias. Atropine is an anticholinergic drug with antagonistic action at muscarinic receptors.

Its actions are mainly as antisecretory, cardiac vagolytic, mydriatic and cycloplegic.

Preparations available are atropine sulfate 0.6 mg/mL injection, 1% eye drop/5% ointment. It is administered as 0.6–2 mg IM or IV; 10 µg/kg in children.

It is used in *bradyarrhythmias, cardiac arrest, partial heart block*, hypersecretory states, *organophosphorus poisoning, early mushroom poisoning*, as premedication and during reversal from muscle relaxants.

The adverse effects to be kept in mind are tachycardia, palpitation, dryness of mouth, blurring of vision, urinary retention and constipation or precipitation of glaucoma especially in the elderly. It should be used with caution in elderly patients with benign hypertrophy of prostate, narrow angle glaucoma.

■ AMIODARONE

Amiodarone is an iodine containing long-acting and broad spectrum antiarrhythmic. It acts by blocking the myocardial delayed rectifier K^+ channels, the Na^+ channels in the inactivated state as well as the myocardial Ca^{2+} channels; hence useful in a broad range of arrhythmias.

It is available as oral tablets 100 mg, 200 mg and as injection 150 mg/3 mL. Orally it is used as 400–600 mg/day for a few weeks, followed by maintenance dose of 100–300 mg/5 mg/kg body weight especially in post-myocardial period. In case of emergency, it is used as slow IV injection of 5 mg/kg body weight over 30–60 minutes.

It is used in *ventricular tachycardia (VT), paroxysmal supraventricular tachycardia, resistant VT, recurrent VT, atrial flutter, atrial fibrillation and WPW tachyarrhythmias.*

Adverse effects of amiodarone depend on the dose and duration of therapy. Hypotension, bradycardia, nausea, and vomiting are noted on acute therapy. On prolonged therapy, goiter, hypothyroidism, corneal deposits, sun burn like phototoxicity, peripheral neuropathy and even pulmonary fibrosis can occur. Amiodarone should not be co-administered with beta blockers or calcium channel antagonists.

■ ESMOLOL

It is an ultrashort acting beta blocker used parenterally. It has quick onset of action and of short duration, acting as β1- selective blocker.

The preparations available are 100 mg/10 mL, 250 mg/10 mL injection. It is used IV as a loading dose of 500 µg then by slow IV infusion at the rate of 100–200 µg/kg/min action starts in 8–10 minutes and lasts for about 20 minutes.

It is used in *arrhythmias associated with anesthesia, hypertensive emergency, aortic dissection, perioperative and postoperative hypertension, emergency control of ventricular rate in atrial flutter and in atrial fibrillation.*

The adverse effects noted are hypotension, bradycardia or cardiac failure in critically ill patients. It should be used with caution in decompensated heart failure, bradyarrhythmia and heart block.

■ LABETALOL

It is a beta blocker with additional α1-blocking action. Labetalol reduces total peripheral resistance. Its onset of action is faster than other beta blockers, its action on beta receptor is five times more potent than α-blocking action. High doses decrease both total peripheral resistance as well as cardiac output, heart rate may be slightly decreased.

It is used in hypertensive crisis, in pheochromocytoma, following clonidine withdrawal, in essential hypertension. In hypertensive emergency, it is administered as 20–40 mg IV every 10 minutes till desired response is attained or as 50 mg BD, increased to 100–200 mg TDS orally.

It is available as 50, 100, 200 mg tablets or 20 mg/4 mL injection, administered IV or orally.

Adverse effects include postural hypotension and rashes. Precaution should be undertaken if hypotension occurs.

■ ISOPRENALINE

It is a sympathomimetic drug with only β-agonistic action. It acts on β1-receptors to increase cardiac contractility and acts on β2-receptors to cause bronchodilation.

Isoprenaline has limited use. It is used occasionally to *maintain idioventricular rhythm until pacemaker is implanted*. For bronchial asthma β2-selective agonists are preferred.

Preparations available are 4 mg/2 mL injection and 20 mg sublingual tablet.

Isoprenaline is administered as 20 mg tablet sublingually or 1–2 mg IM or as 50–10 µg/min IV infusion.

Adverse effects noted are restlessness, palpitation, and headache. It should be used cautiously in patients with arrhythmia or severe hypertension.

■ ASPIRIN

Aspirin is a nonsteroidal anti-inflammatory agent or cyclo-oxygenase inhibitor used mainly as antiplatelet aggregatory agent. Though it has antipyretic, anti-inflammatory, analgesic, uricosuric actions in higher doses, it is mainly used in low dose as antiplatelet aggregatory agent.

The preparations available are oral tablets of 75 mg, 150 mg, 325 mg, 350 mg as well as injection. Route of administration is oral, as antiplatelet 100–150 mg/day or as analgesic/antipyretic 0.3–0.6 g 6–8 hourly, in acute rheumatoid arthritis as 3–5 g/day and in rheumatic fever in children in the dose of 1 g/4–6 hourly.

It is used for various emergency and nonemergency situations as analgesic or antipyretic (maximum dose 4 g), in *myocardial infarction (MI), acute coronary syndromes, thromboembolic disorders and peripheral vascular disease.*

Adverse effects include hypersensitivity reactions, GI bleeding, including bleeding peptic ulcer, increased clotting time, peptic ulcer formation and Reye syndrome when given in children with viral fever. Necessary precautions should be undertaken in pregnancy, history of asthma or acute febrile illness in children. It should be avoided in patients with history of hypersensitivity, GI bleeding and peptic ulcer.

GLYCERYL TRINITRATE

It is a nitrate available as a volatile liquid adsorbed on the inert matrix of the tablet. Glyceryl trinitrate (GTN) acts by vasodilation, dilates veins more than arteries, decreases both preload and afterload. It decreases systolic BP more than diastolic BP and causes redistribution of coronary blood flow.

It is used in *angina pectoris, acute coronary syndrome, acute LVF with MI, CHF, esophageal spasm, biliary colic.* As it has high first pass metabolism, it is administered sublingually or parenterally in emergency situations. Transdermal patch, intranasal spray or ointment are also used. It is available as sublingual tablets, 5 mg/mL injection, 5–10 mg transdermal patch, transmucosal spray and ointment.

It is administered by IV infusion at the rate of 5 µg/min titrated till 20 µg/min or as 0.4–0.8 mg sublingual/mucosal spray or 5–15 mg tablet sublingually.

Adverse effects are throbbing headache, flushing and palpitation. On chronic use tolerance may develop, calling for a nitrate free interval. It should be used cautiously in hypotensive states.

DOBUTAMINE

Dobutamine is a sympathomimetic drug with structural resemblance to Dopamine and with direct action on both α- and β-receptors but with more potent β-agonistic action.

It has more prominent ionotropic than chronotropic action on the heart, causes modest increase in automaticity of the SA node of the heart and improves oxygen supply to the myocardium. Increase in peripheral resistance and BP is minimum. Lowering of pulmonary artery capillary pressure is an added advantage over other ionotropic drugs.

Preparations available are as injections of 50 mg in 4 mL ampoule, 250 mg in 20 mL ampoule or 250 mg/vial. Dobutamine is used as infusion at the rate of 2–10 µg/kg/min. rate and duration of infusion is determined by the clinical state of the patient. Pharmacological tolerance may obliterate the clinical response if used for >4 days.

Dobutamine is indicated in *cardiogenic shock,* all low flow states including *cardiac decompensation states following cardiac surgery, acute myocardial infarction (AMI), and congestive heart failure.*

Dobutamine increases cardiac output and stroke volume in such patients.

Associated adverse effects are tachycardia, supraventricular or ventricular arrhythmias. As a precautionary method, development of arrhythmias may require reduction of dose. Concurrent use of beta blockers should be avoided as this will result in blunting of response.

DOPAMINE

Dopamine is a catecholamine producing variable response according to variation in dose and acts on D1, D2 as well as α- and β1-adrenergic receptors. At low doses ≤2 µg/kg/min, it causes vasodilation due to action on D2-receptors on sympathetic nerves, reduces stimulation of peripheral α1 receptors by inhibition of NE release and causes vasodilation of renal and mesenteric blood vessels due to action on D1-receptors, thereby increases GFR. In moderately high dose of dopamine in the rate of µg/kg/min, dopamine directly stimulates the heart by acting on the cardiac β1-receptors in addition to the other actions of "low dose dopamine", so enhanced cardiac contractility, is of added advantage. In higher doses, 5–15 µg/kg/min, dopamine causes peripheral vasoconstriction due to stimulation of α1-receptors and is not preferable.

Dopamine is available as 200 mg in 5 mL ampoule. It is administered as IV infusion of 0.2–1 µg/kg/min, with monitoring of BP and rate of urine output.

It is used in *cardiogenic shock, septic shock, and severe CHF.*

The various adverse effects are tachycardia, rise in BP, arrhythmias, nausea and vomiting. It is preferable to use dopamine in low dose or moderate dose depending on the clinical condition. It should not be coadministered with other adrenergic or antiadrenergic drugs.

MEPHENTERMINE

It is a sympathomimetic drug acting on both α- and β-receptors, also indirectly by increasing release of NA. It causes increased cardiac contraction, increased cardiac output, peripheral vasoconstriction, increased systolic and diastolic BP.

Mephentermine is used in *hypotension during spinal anesthesia, cardiogenic shock, and acute hypotensive states.*

Preparations used are 10 mg oral tablet, 15 mg/mL in 1 mL ampoule or 30 mg/mL 10 mL vial for injection. It is used orally or IV in titrated amount.

The adverse effects are BP rise, arrhythmia, and CNS stimulation. Mephentermine crosses blood brain barrier and may cause CNS stimulation.

DIGOXIN

Digoxin is a cardiac glycoside with ionotropic action but narrow therapeutic window so there is chance of easy toxicity. As better and safer drugs are available now, Digoxin is used only when really indicated such as refractory heart failure.

It causes a dose-dependent increase in cardiac contractility, systole is shortened and diastole is prolonged and is especially effective in the failing heart, produces decrease in sympathetic overactivity, decrease in heart rate, with no significant effect on BP.

Preparations available are 0.25 mg tablet, 0.05 mg/mL injection, 0.5 mg/2 mL injection.

It is usually administered as loading dose of 0.05–1 mg followed by 0.05–0.5 mg/day either oral or IV.

Used in *CHF refractory to other drugs, in atrial fibrillation, atrial flutter and paroxysmal supraventricular tachycardia.*

Adverse effects are nausea, vomiting, anorexia, fatigue, headache, visual disturbances, and arrhythmias.

As it is a drug with narrow margin of safety, it should be used cautiously in hypokalemia or deranged renal/hepatic function which might precipitate toxicity as well as in partial AV block and ventricular tachycardia.

■ FUROSEMIDE

It is a high ceiling or loop diuretic. It is a highly efficacious diuretic and its diuretic response increases with increase in dose. It acts by inhibiting Na^+K^+2Cl symporter in the ascending loop of Henle and inhibits the cotransport of Na, K, Cl with excretion of water. Onset of action is 15–20 minutes when given parenterally and 20–30 minutes when given orally.

The preparations available are 20–80 mg tablet and as 20 mg/2 mL injection. It can be used IV or orally in acute LVF, pulmonary edema, cerebral edema, hypertensive crisis, hepatic and renal edema.

It may cause electrolyte imbalance and metabolic adverse effects such as hyponatremia, hypokalemia, hypocalcemia, hypomagnesemia, hyperglycemia, hyperlipidemia, hyperuricemia.

Precaution should be undertaken in history of hypersensitivity to sulfonamides and hypotensive states. Also, resistance is seen in advanced cases of chronic renal failure, CHF, nephrotic syndrome. It should not be coadministered with ototoxic drugs such as amikacin, amphotericin B or vancomycin.

■ DEXAMETHASONE

It is a potent, highly selective, and longest acting glucocorticoid with high anti-inflammatory action. Dexamethasone produces anti-inflammatory action with minimal sodium and water retention.

The preparations available are 0.5 mg tablets, as 4 mg/mL injection and 0.5 mg/mL oral drop. It can be administered 0.5–5 mg /day orally or 4–20 mg IM/IV daily as well as topically.

Dexamethasone is used in *allergic and inflammatory conditions, bronchial asthma, cerebral edema, as an antiemetic in widespread cancer, in acute adrenal insufficiency associated states or in preterm delivery (24–34 weeks).*

The adverse effects are development of hypertension, hyperglycemia or peptic ulcer, fluid and electrolyte imbalance as well as increased susceptibility to infection. Acute adrenal insufficiency can occur due to abrupt withdrawal after prolonged therapy due to suppression of the HPA axis, so the drug should be tapered off before complete withdrawal.

■ HYDROCORTISONE

It is a short-acting glucocorticoid used parenterally. Onset of action requires about 30–60 minutes. It inhibits production of inflammatory cytokines, suppresses bronchial hyperreactivity and inhibits the activation of inflammatory cells, macrophages, mast cells, eosinophils, etc., thereby preventing remodeling and disease progression.

Preparations available are as 25 mg/mL, 100 mg/2 mL, 100, 200, 400 mg injection and 10 mg, 20 mg tablet. It is administered by IV bolus or IV infusion and topically as enema in ulcerative colitis.

Hydrocortisone administration is necessary in *shock, adrenal insufficiency, thyroid storm, and status asthmaticus.*

Adverse effects are development of hypertension, hyperglycemia or secondary infection. Any patient receiving ≥ 20–25 mg/day of hydrocortisone for >2–3 weeks should be gradually withdrawn with tapering of daily dose. It should be used cautiously in active TB/other infection, CHF, renal failure, epilepsy, peptic ulcer.

■ DOXAPRAM

It is a respiratory stimulant and acts by stimulating the carotid chemoreceptors or the medullary respiratory center. At low dose, it stimulates the carotid chemoreceptors and at high dose it stimulates the medullary respiratory centers and promotes excitability of central neurons.

It is available as 20 mg/mL in 5 mL ampoule injection and is administered as IV infusion at the rate of 0.5–2 mg/kg/h.

It is used in *respiratory arrest or until mechanical ventilation is initiated, apnea in premature infant, hypnotic poisoning, and acute respiratory insufficiency.*

The adverse effects of doxapram are overstimulation which can lead to convulsion. As margin of safety of Doxapram is narrow, it should never be used beyond 2 hours.

■ DICYCLOMINE

It is an atropine substitute having direct smooth muscle relaxant activity. It has specific antispasmodic action by relaxation of GI smooth muscles, has additional antiemetic action. Other anticholinergic actions such as dryness of mouth or tachycardia is minimum.

The preparations are available as 20 mg oral tablet and 10 mg/mL of 2 mL/10 mL/30 mL ampoule for injection. It can be administered orally, IM or IV.

It is used in *acute pain abdomen, severe dysmenorrhea, morning sickness, motion sickness and diarrhea predominant IBS.*

Adverse effects of dicyclomine include dryness of mouth and constipation. The use of the drug should be avoided in infants below 6 months of age.

ONDANSETRON

It is a prototype 5HT3 receptor antagonist acting primarily in gastrointestinal tract (GIT) and used as antiemetic. It acts by blocking the 5HT3 receptors of GIT as well as the NTS and CTZ; and prevents nausea and vomiting and reduces gut motility.

It is used in *postoperative nausea and vomiting, drug induced vomiting, vomiting due to uremia or neurological injuries, hyperemesis gravidarum, diabetic ketoacidosis, chemotherapy or radiation induced vomiting.*

It is used in preparations of 4, 8 mg tablet, 2 mg/mL 2 mL, 4 mL injection. It is administered either orally, IV or IM; 4-8 mg IV can be repeated every 4 hours.

The adverse effects are dizziness, headache, allergic reaction and hypotension. Bradycardia may rarely occur on IV administration. Ondansetron should be avoided in pregnancy except hyperemesis gravidarum.

DIAZEPAM

Diazepam is a benzodiazepine with anxiolytic, sedative, hypnotic and anticonvulsant activity. It acts on the benzodiazepine receptor of the gamma-aminobutyric acid type A (GABAA) receptor - chloride channel complex and have GABA facilitatory action, producing anxiolytic, hypnotic, muscle relaxing and anticonvulsant effects.

The preparations available are 2 mg, 5 mg, 10 mg oral tablets, 10 mg/2 mL injection, 2 mg/5 mL syrup. The route of administration is orally as 5 mg/10 mg tablet, 5 mg IM/slow IV injection and as rectal suppository in children.

It is used as *hypnotic, sedative,* anticonvulsant, pre medicant, inducing agent in anesthesia, and in the *control of seizures, febrile convulsion, in status epilepticus.*

The adverse effects are pain on IV injection, dizziness, vertigo, and impairment of psychomotor skills. Tolerance may develop on prolonged use as sedative/hypnotic, paradoxical restlessness and irritability is observed in some. Diazepam should not be co administered with alcohol or other CNS depressant drugs and concurrent use of valproic acid may provoke psychotic symptoms.

FLUMAZENIL

Flumazenil is an imidazobenzodiazepine that binds to benzodiazepine binding site of GABAA receptor with high affinity and acts as a competitive antagonist. Flumazenil reverses the electrophysiological and behavioral effects of benzodiazepines, zolpidem and β-carbolines in overdose.

It is available in preparation of 0.2 mg/mL, 2 mL injection. The route of administration is IV 0.2 mg/min, can be repeated to a maximum of 1 mg over 1-3 minutes and is sufficient to abolish the effects of benzodiazepine overdose. Additional dose may be necessary after 20-30 minutes, should sedation reappear.

It is used in *management of benzodiazepine overdose, reversal of sedative effects of benzodiazepines during anesthesia* but it is not effective in drug overdose due to barbiturates or tricyclic antidepressants.

The adverse effects are dizziness and headache. Administration of Flumazenil in conditions not indicated (e.g., Barbiturate overdose) may cause precipitation of seizures.

MORPHINE

It is a prototype opioid, alkaloid derived from opium with central analgesic action. Morphine produces intensive analgesia, sedation, elevation of mood with the ability to produce tolerance and dependence on prolonged use.

It is used in *acute LVF, MI, pulmonary edema, cancer pain, postoperative pain.*

It is available in preparations of oral tablet and injection. It is administered as 0.1-0.2 mg/kg SC, 2-6 mg IV, 10-15 mg IM, 10-50 mg orally, 3-4 hourly.

The adverse actions are respiratory depression, sedation, hypotension, hypersensitivity reactions, bronchospasm, dependence, and tolerance on prolonged use. Special precaution should be undertaken in elderly, children, history of allergy or bronchospasm and in pregnancy.

LOW MOLECULAR WEIGHT HEPARIN

Low molecular weight heparins (LMWH) are derived after chemical depolymerization of unfractionated heparin. It is a parenteral anticoagulant with better bioavailability, longer duration of action and lesser adverse effects compared to unfractionated heparin.

It is used in *the treatment and prophylaxis of deep vein thrombosis, pulmonary embolism, MI, acute coronary syndrome, or if perioperative anticoagulation is necessary.*

The preparations available are Dalteparin 2,500/5,000 IU in prefilled syringe, Enoxaparin 20 mg in 0.2 mL, 40 mg in 0.4 mL prefilled syringe, Ardeparin 2,500/5,000 IU in prefilled syringe. Route of administration is SC or IV.

Adverse effects are bleeding due to overdose. Hypersensitivity reactions, osteoporosis and thrombocytopenia are less common. Precautions to be undertaken are bleeding disorders, thrombocytopenia, neurosurgery, lumbar puncture, coadministration of antiplatelet drugs and severe hypertension.

MANNITOL

It is a low molecular weight, pharmacologically inert, and nonelectrolyte osmotic diuretic.

It acts by limiting reabsorption of electrolytes and water from the tubules by a variety of ways and enhances diuresis. Major sites of action are the proximal tubule and descending loop of Henle.

Used in *increased intracranial tension, cerebral edema, acute renal failure, dialysis disequilibrium syndrome and increased intraocular tension.*

The preparations used are 10% or 20% solution of 100, 350 and 500 mL vial. It is administered as test dose of 12.5–25 g/IV to maintain a GFR of 100 mL/h. IV infusion at the rate of 1–2 g/kg is used in increased intracranial tension.

The adverse effects of mannitol include headache, nausea, vomiting and hypersensitivity reactions. Mannitol should not be used in dehydration, anuria, pulmonary edema, LVF or cerebral hemorrhage.

PROMETHAZINE

It is a first generation antihistaminic with sedative and anticholinergic actions. It produces antiallergic, antiemetic, cough suppressant and sedative action. It reduces tremor, rigidity and sialorrhea associated with Parkinsonism.

Promethazine has a myriad of uses. It is used as *antiallergic in hypersensitivity reactions, in vomiting of pregnancy, transfusion reactions, suppression of nocturnal cough, tremor, as preanesthetic medication. It is also used in intractable cough, intractable vomiting, and pruritus.*

It is used in preparations as 25–50 mg oral tablet, 15 mg/5 mL syrup and 25 mg/mL injection. The route of administration is either oral, IV or IM.

The adverse effects are mainly sedation, dizziness, loss of alertness and dryness of mouth.

Though there are many other drugs used in emergency, these drugs discussed above need special mention. The need of availability of IV fluids such as 5% Dextrose, DNS, Ringer's Lactate, normal saline, bicarbonate solution, Dextran, facility for provision of blood and blood products are also essential in dealing with emergency situations.

Take Home Messages

- Though there are many drugs used in emergency, drugs discussed should find a place in emergency kit of any physician.
- Some IV fluids like 5% Dextrose, DNS, Ringer's Lactate, normal saline, bicarbonate solution, Dextran should also be readily available.
- Facility for provision of blood and blood products are also essential in dealing with emergency situations

BIBLIOGRAPHY

1. Brunton LL, Dandan RH, Knollmann BC, Goodman and Gilman's The Pharmacological Basis of Therapeutics, 13th edition. New York: McGraw Hill Medical Education; 2018.
2. Chowdhury L. Handbook of Pharmacology for the Anesthesiologists, 1st edition. New Delhi: Jaypee Brothers Medical Publishers (P) Ltd.; 2019.
3. Katzung BG, Masters SB, Trevor AJ. Basic and Clinical Pharmacology, 14th edition. New York: Tata McGraw Hill Publishing Division; 2015.
4. Tripathy KD. Essentials of Medical Pharmacology, 8th edition. New Delhi: Jaypee Brothers Medical Publishers (P) Ltd.; 2018
5. Udwadia FE. Principles of Critical Care, 3rd edition. New Delhi: Jaypee Brothers Medical Publishers (P) Ltd.; 2014.

CHAPTER 43

Emergency Management of Drowning

Sarbajit Ray

■ INTRODUCTION

Drowning as a subject is neglected at the undergraduate as well as postgraduate level of medical education. Worldwide drowning cause many fatalities which is seldom recorded except in cases of boat or shipping accidents. Drowning occurs frequently as a result of leisure activity, e.g., swimming pool accidents or while bathing in river, stream or in the sea. Drowning may also occur in bathtubs. Drowning may occur in very small volume of water as immersion of the face is sufficient enough to cause death of the hapless victim. Many of these deaths occur in young individuals. Timely appropriate intervention can definitely reduce these preventable deaths.

Over the years various terminologies have been used to describe drowning, such as near drowning, dry drowning, active or passive drowning, secondary and silent drowning.

Near drowning: Near drowning is when the subject is rescued before the point of death or the subject has a temporary survival.

Dry drowning: Approximately 10% of drownings are dry drowning. In a dry drowning, the person sinks in fluid and is deeply unconscious but the stimulus for breathing is still present. On attempting to breathe, water enters the pharynx. This water entry reflexly closes the larynx and epiglottis and thus diverts the water to stomach. The airway is sealed and the patient suffocates.

Freshwater drowning: When fresh water enters lungs, water is absorbed in the blood leading to hemodilution. This hemodilution distorts the blood platelets. The body can rectify small changes in pH but changes associated with significant hemodilution may result in cardiac arrest. Fatality can occur as fast as in 2–3 minutes.

Saltwater drowning: Drowning in the sea is called saltwater drowning. Salt water has the opposite effect of fresh water. As salt water is hyperosmolar, water is drawn from the blood into the lungs. This increases the blood viscosity resulting in sluggishness in blood circulation. This may lead to cardiac arrest.

Secondary drowning: A victim of drowning is rescued and resuscitated. The victim appropriately recovers but dies later on. If water has entered the body, rapid absorption from the stomach to bloodstream causing pulmonary edema or "shock lung syndrome" which may occur after many hours of the event.

It was previously thought that patients undergo "wet drowning" or "dry drowning".
- Wet drowning—due to aspiration of water into lungs (85% of causes)
- Dry drowning-hypoxic due to laryngospasm (15% of cause).

Autopsy studies show at least some level of increased fluid in lungs in over 98% of victims, suggesting aspiration occurs in all cases.

Most deaths in hospital are due to hypoxic brain injury rather than from pulmonary edema or lung injury for the initial drowning incident.
- *Submersion:* The act of being completely covered by liquid.
- *Immersion:* Being partly covered by liquid (medically includes the face which causes impairment in breathing).
- Previously the term "near drowning" was used in medical literature to indicate patients who survived for more than 24 hours following an event. Though the term is still in vogue, it has been replaced by "nonfatal drowning".

To bring an end to the confusion arising from different nomenclatures World Health Organization defined it as "drowning is the process of experiencing respiratory impairment from submersion or immersion in liquid".[1,2] Approach to drowning has been simplified by classifying outcomes to three domains: death, morbidity, and no morbidity.

■ EPIDEMIOLOGY

Drowning is an unseen public disaster in India with 83 fatalities occurring every day according to report on Accidental Deaths and Suicides in India (ADSI) 2020.

Most of these deaths involve children and young adults. Males outnumber female by 1:5. Concurrent alcohol consumption is a high-risk factor leading to increased morbidity and mortality.

Almost half of the cases of drowning require hospitalization. Permanent neurologic sequelae ranging from quadriplegia to vegetative state occur in 5–10% of childhood drowning.

■ PATHOPHYSIOLOGY

At the onset of drowning fluid enters the oropharynx and it is attempted to be cleared by the victim. If clearing is not possible, it is followed by breath holding which eventually leads to insurmountable central drive to inspire, resulting in fluid entering the airways. This leads to cough or laryngospasm. If the drowning process continues, this process repeats resulting in fluid and electrolyte shifts, alveolar dysfunctions, and hypoxia. Hypoxia is again aggravated by pulmonary edema, reduced lung compliance and bronchospasm. Cardiac functioning can be compromised within seconds to minutes of hypoxia manifested by tachycardia to bradycardia, pulseless electrical activity and asystole.[3-5]

■ MYTH BUSTER

In nonfatal drowning the complications are due to laryngospasm/asphyxia and or aspiration. Both salt and fresh water wash out lung surfactant leading to noncardiogenic pulmonary edema and acute respiratory distress syndrome.

Heimlich maneuver or other postural drainage techniques to remove water from lungs or stomach are of no value, rather could be detrimental.[6-8]

■ INITIAL MANAGEMENT

In drowning the priority is in the order of *ABC—airway, breathing, compression* in contrast to the usual CAB because hypoxic injury is the root cause including cardiac arrhythmias.[9]

Most of the cases can be managed by only ensuring adequate air delivery to the lungs. The first step is to rescue the victim and place the victim on a dry hard surface. A person trained in cardiopulmonary resuscitation (CPR) would be the best help. At least mouth to mouth ventilation can give the patient a new lease of life **(Figs. 1A and B)**. If oxygen cylinder is available, it will be of immense value to give supplemental oxygen. During transportation, if noninvasive ventilation is available it should be used. Even oxygen delivery by bag and mask will ensure adequate ventilation. Cardiac compression should be started in case of cardiac arrest **(Figs. 2A to C)**.

Ensure the patient is kept warm. Wet clothes should be taken off and the victim wrapped in a blanket. Hypothermia should be prevented. If drowning occurs in cold water, gradual rewarming should be done. This can be achieved by various means, viz. warm saline infusion, warm blankets, etc.

A victim with glasgow coma scale (GCS) <8 needs to be intubated and given ventilator support.

Salient Points in Management (Flowchart 1)

- Prompt correction of hypoxemia and acidosis—Degree of hypoxemia is under-recognized
- Patient should receive 100% oxygen—monitored by pulse oximetry or blood gas analysis
- Electrolyte imbalance generally does not occur in nonfatal drowning.
- Ventricular dysthymias (VT or VF), bradycardia and asystole may occur as result of acidosis and hypoxemia rather than electrolyte imbalance.
- Prevent aspiration
- *Stabilize body temperature. Hypothermia:* Common occurrence
    - Remove wet clothes, dry the victim

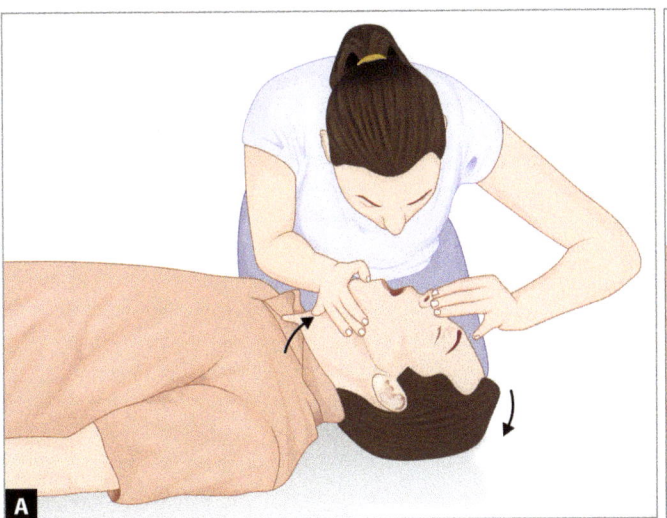
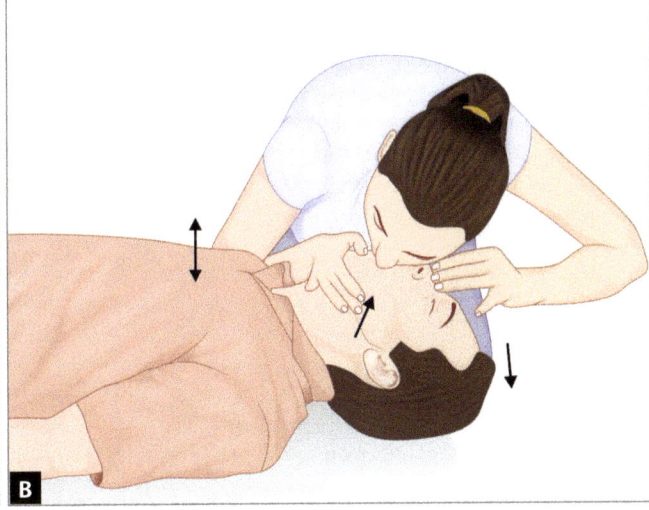

Figs. 1A and B: Mouth-to-mouth respiration.

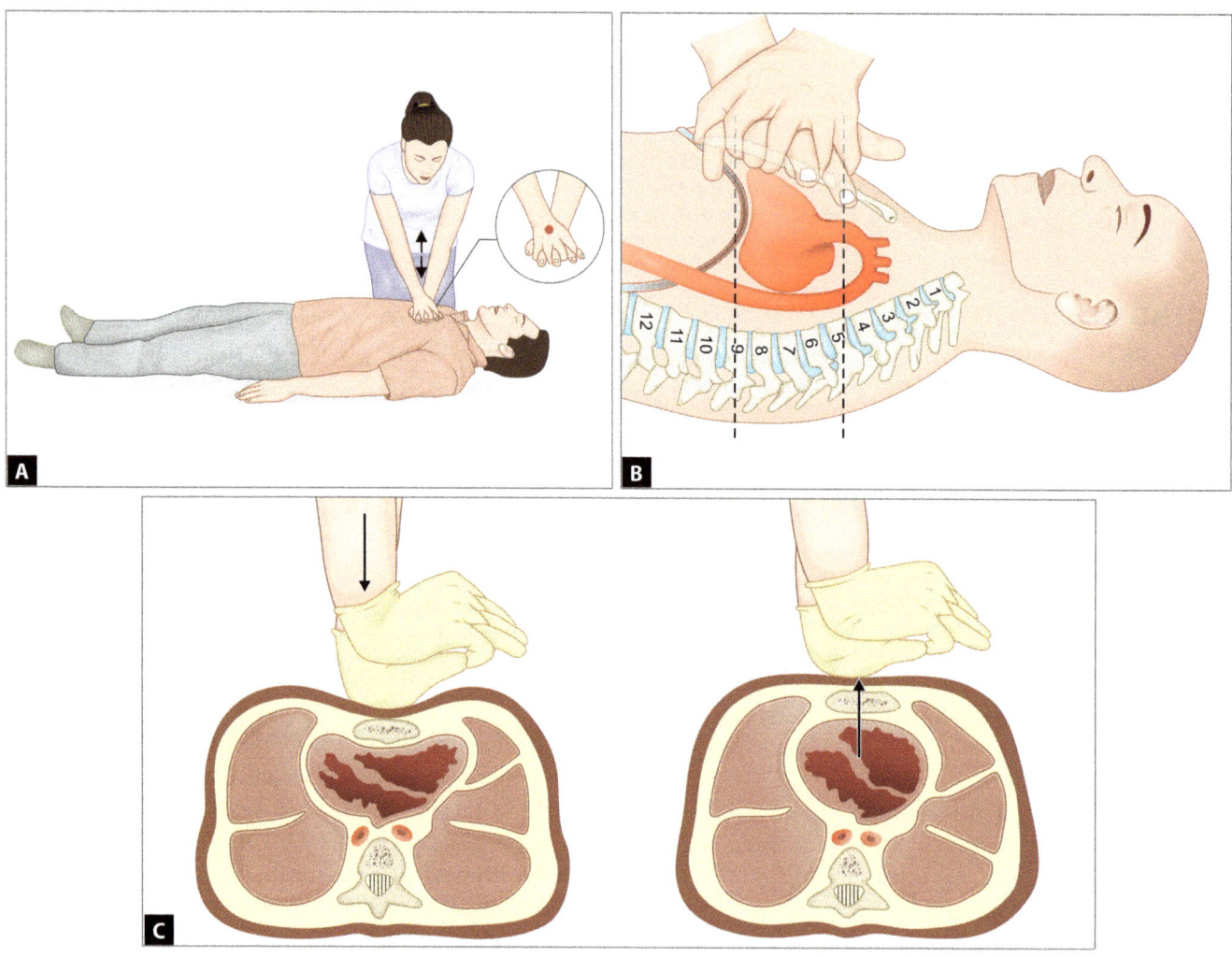

Figs. 2A to C: Techniques of cardiac compression.

Flowchart 1: Treatment approach for a drowning patient.

```
Cardiorespiratory arrest ──Yes──▶ CPR          Rescue breathing is of utmost
                                                importance (Figs. 1 and 2)
         │No                                    Bag mask ventilation with 100% O₂
         ▼
Inadequate respiration
• Hypoxia despite increased O₂ flow  ──Yes──▶  Provide respiratory     Check for airway obstruction —
• Increased respiratory effort                  support – Airway/       foreign material/vomitus (debris)
• Decreased consciousness                       Intubation ± PEEP
         │No
         ▼
Dyspnea
• Increased respiratory effort  ──Yes──▶  Admit
• Abnormal lung sounds                     Maintain SpO₂ >95%
• SpO₂ <95%                                Investigations
         │No
         ▼
Observe for 8 hours from time
       of drowning
```

(CPR: cardiopulmonary resuscitation; PEEP: positive end-expiratory pressure)

- Active warming if core temperature <34°C
  - Warmed IV fluids
  - Warm blankets
  - Humidified O_2
- Cervical spine injury should be ruled out especially in cases of diving
- Consider medical causes:
  - Seizures
  - Hypoglycemia
  - Arrhythmia or long QT syndrome
  - Intoxication.

ADVERSE PROGNOSTIC INDICATORS

- Submersion time >5 minutes
- Time to basic life support >10 minutes
- Cardiopulmonary resuscitation
- GCS <5
- Rectal temperature <30°C
- Arterial pH <7.1 on arrival.

Consider Discharge

- After observation for 8 hours
- Asymptomatic
- Normal respiration
- Education about precautionary measures.

Take Home Messages

- Rescue the victim of drowning
- Time is of utmost essence
- Priority is in the order of ABC—airway, breathing, compression
- Ensure oxygen delivery as early as possible by whatever means one can muster
- Dry the patient
- Keep the patient warm
- Intubation & ventilation whenever needed be.

REFERENCES

1. Van Beeck EF, Branche CM, Szpilman D, Modell JH, Bierens JJ. A new definition of drowning: towards documentation and prevention of a global public health problem. Bull World Health Organ. 2005;83(11):853-6.
2. Weiss J. American Academy of Pediatrics Committee on Injury, Violence and poison prevention technical report: prevention of drowning. Paediatics. 2010;126(1) e253-62.
3. Orlowski JP, Abulleil MM, Phillips JM. The hemodynamic and cardiovascular effects of near-drowning in hypotonic, isotonic, or hypertonic solutions. Ann Emerg Med. 1989; 18(10):1044-9.
4. Grmec S, Strnad M, Podgorsek D. Comparison of the characteristics and outcome among patients suffering from out-of-hospital primary cardiac arrest and drowning victims in cardiac arrest. Int J Emerg Med. 2009;2(1):7-12. doi: 10.1007/s12245-009-0084-0.
5. Rosen P, Stoto M, Harley J. Theme of Heimlich manoeuvre in near drowning. Institute of Medicine report. J Emergency Med. 1995;13:397.
6. Szpilman D, Bierens JJ, Handley AJ, Orlowski JP. Drowning. N Engl J Med. 2012;366(22):2102-10.
7. Lavonas EJ, Drennam IR, Grabrielli A, Heffner AC, Hoyte CO, Orkin AM, et al. Part 10: special circumstances of Resuscitation: 2015 American Heart Association Guidelines Update for Cardiopulmonary Resuscitation and Emergency Cardiovascular Care. Circulation. 2015;132:S501.
8. Schmidt AC, Sempsrott JR, Hawkins SC, Arastu AS, Cushing TA, Auerbach PS. Wilderness Medical Society Practice guidelines to the prevention and treatment of drowning. Wilderness Environ Med. 2016;27:236.
9. Vanden Hoek TL, Morrison LJ, Shuster M, Donnino M, Sinz E, Lavonas EJ, et al. Part 12: cardiac arrest in special situations: 2010 American Heart Association Guidelines for Cardiopulmonary Resuscitation and Emergency Cardiovascular Care. Circulation. 2010;122(18 Suppl 3): S829-61.

Index

Page numbers followed by *b* refer to box, *f* refer to figure, *fc* refer to flowchart, and *t* refer to table

A

Abdomen 137
  acute 137, 250
  postoperative 279*f*
Abdominal compartment syndrome 147
Abscess
  epidural 258
  tubo-ovarian 208
Absorbed poison, elimination of 307
Accidental deaths 328
Acetaminophen 132
Acetone 97
Acetylsalicylic acid 114
Acid 268
Acidosis 166
Acksonian 105
Acquired immunodeficiency syndrome 124, 178
Actinomyces 121
Acute asthma
  management of 89*fc*
  rapid primary assessment of 88*fc*
Acute back pain 258
  causes of 258*t*
Acute bacterial meningitis 118-121
  outcome of 121
Acute coronary syndrome 29, 296, 324, 326
Acute dialysis quality initiative group 157
Acute endovascular thrombectomy treatment 113
Acute hypoglycemia
  clinical classification of 193
  management of 198*fc*
Acute ischemic stroke 111, 112
  management of 111
Acute kidney injury 157, 158, 158*f*, 158*t*, 161, 162, 162*t*, 163*f*, 164*f*, 172*t*
  biomarkers for 164*f*
  causes of 159*f*
  diagnosis of 158
  disease-modifying 171
  drug excretion in 173
  epidemiological consideration of 158
  etiology of 159*fc*
  management of 164
  network 157, 171
  novel biomarkers in 163
  prevention of 165
  Rifle criteria for 158*f*
  spectrum of 163*f*

Acute liver failure 150, 151, 151*t*
  care of 150
  causes of 150
  monitoring of 150
Acute pancreatitis 146
  outcome of 148*fc*
Acute pelvic inflammatory disease 203, 206, 207
Acute renal failure, prerenal 159
Acute respiratory distress syndrome 34, 147, 277
Adefovir 172
Adenoma, adrenal 183
Adenosine 290, 322
  deaminase 65
Adjunctive therapy 121
Adnexal torsion 203, 209*f*
Adrenal insufficiency 325
Adrenaline 322
Adrenocorticotropic hormone stimulation test 151
Adult advance cardiac arrest algorithm 7*fc*
Adult basic life support 4, 6*fc*
Adult postcardiac arrest care 8*fc*
Advanced cardiac life support 10
  principles of 215
Adverse drug reaction 259
Airway 11, 13, 14, , 50, 72, 106, 139, 247*t*, 267
  emergencies 292, 293
  foreign bodies of 87
  management 52*fc*, 55*fc*, 98*fc*
  obstruction 14*f*, 51
    foreign body 10
    partial 51
Alberta Stroke Program 114
Albumin 273, 274, 275
  solution 274
Albuterol 248
Alcohol ingestion 193
Alkali 268
Alkalosis 87, 181
Allergic bronchopulmonary aspergillosis 85, 87
Allergic reaction 317
Almotriptan 132
Alteplase 31
  intravenous 113
Ambu bag 290
American Heart Association 3, 95
American Thoracic Society 66
Amino acids 173
Aminoglycoside antibiotics 172
Aminophylline 290
Amiodarone 290, 323

Amnesia 18
Amphotericin B 172
Amylase concentrations 147
Analgesics 147
Anaphylaxis 248, 292, 298, 316, 318*f*, 319
  diagnosis of 317*b*
  evaluation of 320*fc*
  symptomatology of 316*b*
Anastomotic leak 279
Anemia 166
Anesthesia
  regional 292, 297
  spinal 297
Aneurysm 114
  rupture of 71*f*
Angina
  pectoris 324
  unstable 29, 30
Angioedema, hereditary 318
Angiography, interventional 75
Angiotensin
  converting enzyme inhibitors 38, 317
  receptor blockers 38
Anion gap calculation 187
Ankle fractures 220
Antibiotics 73, 144, 147
  policy 269
  regimens 66*t*
  therapy, selection of 121
Antibody, monoclonal 317
Anticholinergic
  short-acting 61
  toxidrome 306
Anticoagulation treatment 68
Anticonvulsant therapy 308
Antidotes 252, 308
Antiepileptic drug 106, 107, 109, 114
  therapy 106
Antiepileptic medication 108*t*
  first-line 106
  second-line 106
Anti-glomerular basement membrane 160
Anti-hepatitis
  C virus 150
  E virus 150
Antineutrophil cytoplasmic antibody 160, 162
Antinuclear antibody 150
Antiphospholipid syndrome 260
Antiplatelet therapy 114
Antirheumatic drugs, disease-modifying 260
Antismooth muscle antibody 150
Antisnake venom 311

Aortic aneurysm
   abdominal 139
   ruptured 140f
Aortic dissection 44, 98, 258
Apnea 325
Appendicitis 139, 140, 147
Ardeparin 326
Arrhythmia 276
Arsenic 97
Arterial blood 89
   gas 58, 78, 86, 150, 152, 183
Arterial occlusion 111f
Arterial oxygen, partial pressure of 146
Arteriovenous malfunction 114
Arthritis
   juvenile idiopathic 261f
   septic 258
Aspirant, appearance of 65fc
Aspiration 293, 318
   pneumonitis 277
   syndromes 87
Aspirin 290, 323
Asplenia 118
Asthma 89t, 317
   acute exacerbation of 62, 85, 86
   acute severe 85
   bronchial 325
   childhood 248
   life-threatening 86
   management, stepwise 87
Atelectasis 277
Atlantoaxial dislocation 263f
Atlantoaxial subluxation 263
Atrial arrhythmia 294f
Atrial fibrillation 7, 19, 41, 294, 325
Atrial flutter 325
Atropine 9, 290, 313f, 322
Attention-deficit hyperactivity disorder drugs 317
Automated external defibrillator 4, 6, 9, 49, 290
Autonomic neuropathy 193
Azotemia 125

B

Bacteria 120
   intestinal 142
Balanced salt solution 250
Balloon mitral valvotomy 41
Bartholin abscess 207
Bartholin bladder 178
Bartholin cyst 207
Bartholin endometrium 178
Bartholin prostate 178
Basic life support 9, 10, 95
Beck's triad 42
Behçet syndrome 41
Benzodiazepine 107, 109, 252
   short-acting 106
Beta-adrenergic stimulation 181
Beta-agonist therapy 85
Beta-blockers 38, 277
Beta-human chorionic gonadotropin 205, 206, 208
Beta-lactams 316
Bickerstaff migraine 25
Bi-level positive airway pressure 59
Biomarker, role of 35, 206, 299

Biopsy, endometrial 208
Black eye 96
Blood 274
   glucose 112
   investigations 101t
   pressure 34, 40, 67, 69, 82, 151, 249t, 270
      high 112
      management 112
      systolic 17, 35, 146, 317
   transfusion 143
   urea nitrogen 147, 160
   workup 162
Bogota bag closure 283f
Bone marrow 261f
Bowel obstruction, acute 279
Brachytherapy 74
Bradyarrhythmias 323
Bradycardia 9, 293, 293f
   adult 14fc
   pediatric 11fc
Brain
   abscess 118
   disease, metastatic 119
   edema 152
   natriuretic peptide 37
   swelling 114
Brainstem
   compression 116
   encephalitis 125
Breath, shortness of 98
Breathing 11, 13, 14, 50, 58, 72, 106, 139, 216, 247, 267
   circulation 247
   smoothly 50
Breathlessness, acute 249
British Thoracic Society 66
Brittle asthma 86
Brivaracetam 108
Bronchial angiography 72
Bronchial artery 75f
   embolization 73, 75
Bronchiectasis 70, 87
Bronchiolitis 87
   obliterans 87
Bronchitis 87, 277
Bronchoscopy 73
Bronchospasm 322
   intractable 296
Bronchus, foreign bodies in 238
Bundle branch blocks 31
Burn 267, 272
   care of 267, 271, 271fc
   dressing 272
   electrical 272
   grafting 272
   injury 267, 270fc
   pathophysiology 270fc
   thermal 271
   wounds, care of 270
Burst abdomen 282, 283f

C

Calcium
   channel blockers 277
   gluconate 290
Cancer pain 326
Caput medusae 143

Carbon dioxide, partial pressure of 57, 89
Carboplatin 172
Carcinoma 114
   bronchogenic 71
   lung 178
   oropharynx 178
Cardiac arrest 3, 5, 10fc, 296, 323
   situations 6
Cardiac compression, technique of 330f
Cardiac high sensitivity troponins 30
Cardiac output 34, 35
Cardiac tamponade 29, 40, 41f
   acute 41
   subacute 41
Cardiomyopathy 317
Cardiopulmonary resuscitation 3, 6, 7, 9-12, 67, 330
   steps of 4, 4f
Cardiotocography 205
Cardiovascular complications 276
Cardiovascular disease 143, 317
Cardiovascular emergencies 262, 292, 293
Cardiovascular function 247
Cardiovascular monitoring 151
Cardiovascular syncope 19
   diagnosis of 25
Cardiovascular system 52
Carotid artery, pulsations of 49f
Carotid sinus massage 23
Catastrophic antiphospholipid syndrome 260
Catheter directed treatment 81
Cell
   activation of 318
   division 270
   surface antibody mediated encephalitis 127
Central nervous system 119, 131
   emergencies 262
   examination 99
Central venous pressure 165, 270
Cephalosporin 243
Cerebral edema 189, 325
Cerebral venous sinus thrombosis 131
Cerebrospinal fluid 101, 125, 126, 131
   examination 101t
Cerebrovascular accident 119
Cervical 243
   spine 215
      injury 50, 331
Chemical
   burns 268f, 271
   injury 233, 233f
Chest 86
   compressions 49, 50f
   computed tomography of 74
   drain 217
   pain 30, 98
   silent 86
   tube placement 91
   X-ray 42, 64, 205, 208
      postoperative 277f
Choking 10, 51
Cholecystitis 147
Cholesterol granuloma 244
Chronic kidney disease, preexisting 157
Chronic obstructive pulmonary disease 34, 57, 61, 87, 277, 317
   acute exacerbation of 61

Chronology 137
Churg-Strauss syndrome 87
Cidofovir 172
Circulation 11, 13, 14, 58, 72, 106, 139, 247*t*, 267
Circulatory proteins 168
Cisplatin 172
Clindamycin 243
Clopidogrel 31
Coagulation 115
Coagulopathy 113
Cobra bite 311, 313
Cochlear implant 118
Colles fracture 218
Colloids 274, 275
    formulae 272
Coma 96
    cocktail 308
Combitube placement 54*f*
Common krait 309*f*
Complete blood count 205, 208
Compression ultrasonography 67, 79
Computed tomography 42, 65, 74, 139
    noncontrast 101
    pulmonary angiogram 67, 68, 77, 78
Conception, products of 204, 207
Conjunctivitis
    allergic 232
    vernal 232
Conn's syndrome 179
Consciousness 95
    anatomy of 95*t*
    disorders of 95*t*
    level of 95*t*, 226
    loss of 218
    states after coma 96*fc*
    transient loss of 18*fc*
Constrictive pericarditis 40
Continuous positive airway pressure 59, 277
Continuous renal replacement therapy 170
Continuous venovenous
    hemodiafiltration 170
    hemofiltration 170
Convulsive movements 98
Corneal abrasion 232, 233*f*
Coronary artery 31, 31*t*
Coronavirus disease-2019 (COVID-19) 55*fc*, 57, 181
    impact of 6
    resuscitation of 8*b*
Corpus luteum cyst rupture 208, 209*f*
Corticosteroids 89*t*, 116
Cortisol 178
Cranial nerve 242
Cricopharynx 237*f*
Cricothyrotomy 54*f*
Crisis resource management 292
Crystalloids 273, 275
    formulae 272
Cushing's disease 179, 183
Cyanide 97
Cyclooxygenase inhibitor 323
Cyclophosphamide 127
Cyclosporine 172
Cystic fibrosis 87
Cytokine release syndrome, production of 318
Cytomegalovirus 126, 150

D

Danger signs 249
Dawn phenomenon 195
D-dimer 78
De novo heart failure, acute 36
Deep brain stimulation 109
Deep surgical site infections 283*f*
Deep vein thrombosis 67, 276
    prophylaxis 114, 116, 326
Defibrillator interrogation 23
Deficit fluid correction 250
Dehydration, degrees of 250*t*
Dental disorders 243
Depression 317
Dermal clues 305
Dexamethasone 290, 325
Dextran 172, 273-275
    formula 272
Dextrose 196, 290
Diabetes 193
    insipidus 180
    management 196, 297
    mellitus
        type 1 194
        type 2 194
Diabetic ketoacidosis 97, 139, 187, 187*f*, 188
    initial assessment of 189*b*
    management of 189
    pathophysiology of 188*fc*
    treatment of 189
Dialysis 170
    membrane 168
Diaphoresis 30
Diaspirin cross-linked hemoglobin 274
Diazepam 107, 326
Diclofenac 132
Dicyclomine 325
Diffusion-weighted imaging image 112*f*
Digital gangrene 259*f*
Digoxin 290, 324
Diltiazem 290
Diphenhydramine 290
Disability 13, 14, 248
    migraine-associated 132
Disaster
    emergencies 292
    management 298
Ditans 132
Diuretics 38, 165
Diverticulitis 140
Dobutamine 290, 324
Dopamine 165, 290, 324
Doxapram 325
Drinking and driving 215*f*
Drowning 51, 329
    emergency management of 328
    freshwater 328
    near 328
    nonfatal 329
    onset of 329
    saltwater 328
    secondary 328
Dry drowning 328
Dumping syndrome 193
Dupuytren contracture 143
Dysmenorrhea, severe 326
Dyspnea 30, 59
Dysthymias, ventricular 329

E

Eagle's syndrome 244
Earring stuck 237*f*
Echocardiogram, transesophageal 67
Echocardiography 22, 42
    role of 78
    transthoracic 68
Eclampsia 203
Edema 281*f*
    acute pulmonary 29
    cardiogenic pulmonary 276
    pulmonary 297
Elbow injury 219, 219*f*
Electrocardiogram 11, 30, 36, 42, 205, 208
    abnormalities 22
Electroconvulsive therapy 109
Electroencephalography 106, 109
Electrolytes 151, 177
    imbalance 165, 177
    metabolism 188
    serum 138
Eletriptan 132
Embolectomy, surgical 81
Embolism, acute pulmonary 29, 77, 79
Emergency
    airway management 49, 51
    anesthesia 299
    cardiovascular events 293
    classification of 257
    management 52, 98, 102, 184, 215
Emphysema 87
Empyema 118
Encephalitis 104, 123
    acute 123
    antibody mediated 125*t*
    autoimmune 126, 127
    radiologic features of 126*t*
    viral 127
Encephalopathy 123*t*
    hepatic 97
Endobronchial bleeding tumor 75*f*
Endobronchial medical therapy 74
Endobronchial stents 74
Endocrine emergencies 292, 297
Endometrioma, ruptured 209*f*
Endometriosis 208
End-organ function 247
Endoscopy 144
Endotracheal tube culture 150
Endovascular thrombectomy treatment 113
Enophthalmos 233
Enoxaparin 326
Enterocutaneous fistula 281
Epilepsia partialis continua 105
Epilepsy, focal 18
Epinephrine 74, 290
Epstein-Barr virus 150
Erect carotid sinus massage 24
Erythema multiforme 260*f*
Esmolol 323
Esophageal obturator airway 53
Esophageal tracheal combitube 53
Esophagus, upper 237*f*
Estimated glomerular filtration rate 157
Ewart's sign 42
Ewing's sarcoma 178

Exacerbation
   management of 61
      mild 85
      moderate 85
      severe 85
Exercise
   intolerance 85
   pulmonary 284
Expiratory positive airway pressure 60
Extracorporeal membrane oxygenation 91
Extracorporeal renal replacement therapy 168
Extraperitoneal anastomosis 280
Eye
   infection, treatment of 231t
   injuries 232

F

Fatigue 87
Febrile status 252
Fecal peritonitis 281f
Feeding 151
Fenoldopam 165
Fetor hepaticus 97
Fibroid red degeneration 203
Fine-needle aspiration 148
First aid 267
   care 271
Fish bones stuck 238
Fistula, pancreatic 280f
Fluid 147, 191, 268
   attenuated inversion recovery image 112f
   choices 273t
   intravenous 291
   management 87, 270fc
   removal, complications of 44
   requirements 250t
   resuscitation formulae 272t
   therapy 165, 249, 272
Flumazenil 326
Food allergens 317
Foot injury 220
Forced expiratory volume 88
Foscarnet 172
Fosphenytoin 108
Free fatty acid 188
Fresh frozen plasma 115, 272, 273, 313
Frovatriptan 132
Fungal infections 70
Furosemide 290, 325
Furunculosis 243
Fusobacterium 121

G

Gallstone disease 139
Gangrene 310f
Gastric antral vascular ectasia 143
Gastroenteritis 140f
Gastroesophageal reflux disease 87, 143
Gastrointestinal bleeding 142
   initial assessment of 142
   management of 142
   overt 142
   severe 142
   upper 142, 144fc
Gastrointestinal emergencies 262
Gastrointestinal endoscopy, upper 142
Gastrointestinal tract 178, 316
   carcinoma of 178
Gelatin 275

Geneva Clinical Prediction Rule for Pulmonary Embolism, revised 78t
Geneva scores 79
Genital examination 138
Gepants 132
Glasgow coma scale 26, 97t, 99, 106, 248, 329
Glipizide 252
Global Initiative for Asthma Guidelines 85
Glomerular filtration rate 158, 158f, 161, 163f
Glottic obstruction 53
Glucagon response, loss of 196
Glucocorticoids 260
Glycemic control 166
Glyceryl trinitrate 324
Golfer's elbow 218
Gouty arthritis, acute 258
Granulomatosis, eosinophilic 87
Gynecological disease 147
Gynecological emergencies 203, 207t
Haemophilus influenzae 118, 243

H

Hamptons sign 78f
Head
   injury 96, 218
   laceration 218
   tilt-chin lift maneuver 5f, 50f
Headache 129, 322
   chronic 130t
   disorders 130, 131, 131t
   improvement of 134
   thunderclap 98
Head-up tilt testing 23
Hearing loss 26
Heart
   disease 22b, 35
      ischemic 317
   failure 34, 87
      acute 34, 35t-37t
      chronic 37
      congestive 13, 31, 64
   rate 11, 270
Heimlich maneuver 51, 51f
Hematemesis 142
Hematochezia 142
Hematogenous seeding 119
Hematoma
   intra-abdominal 279
   subdural 119, 244
Hemodialysis 168, 171
Hemodynamics, invasive 43
Hemofiltration 168
Hemolytic uremic syndrome-thrombotic thrombocytopenic purpura 160
Hemoptysis 71
   etiology of 71t
   massive 70
   severity of 71
Hemorrhage 278
   acute gastrointestinal 142
   intracerebral 111, 115f
   intracranial 31, 113
   secondary 278f
   severe 274
   subarachnoid 119
   subconjunctival 232f
   supratentorial 116
Hemorrhoidal bleeding 143

Hemostasis 115
Hepatic dysfunction 280
Hepatic failure, acute 150
Hepatitis
   autoimmune 150
   B core antigen 150
   viral 150
Hepatosplenomegaly 261f
Herpes simplex
   encephalitis 123
   virus 150
Herpes zoster 243
   ophthalmicus 232
High blood pressure 112
   management of 115
High-flow oxygen therapy 90
High-molecular weight dextran 317
Hip injury 219, 219f
Holliday and Segar formula 249t
Holter monitoring 22
Hormone
   antidiuretic 74
   deficiency 193
Hot joint, acute 257
Human chorionic gonadotropin 207
Human herpesvirus 6 126
Human immunodeficiency virus 124, 131
Hyaluronate-carboxymethyl cellulose 279
Hydration 284
   aggressive 147
   level of 226
Hydrocephalus 116
Hydrocortisone 249, 290, 325
Hydrofluoric acid 268
Hypercapnia 57, 87
Hyperemesis gravidarum 203
Hyperglycemia, posthypoglycemic 195
Hyperglycemic emergencies, acute metabolic 187f
Hyperinsulinemia, peripheral 196
Hyperkalemia 177, 183
   etiologies of 184t
   management strategies of 184t
   medical management of 184
   severity of 183t
   treatment of 185t
Hypernatremia 177, 179
   etiologies of 180fc
Hyperosmolar hyperglycemic state 187t, 190
   management of 191
   pathophysiology of 191fc
   sick day rules for 191
Hypersensitivity reaction, mechanism of 318f
Hypertension 296
   portal 144
   pulmonary 19
Hypertensive crisis 29
Hypertensive vascular disease 317
Hyperthermia, malignant 292, 298
Hypertonic saline 116, 273, 274
   formulae 272
Hypertonic solutions 274
Hyperventilation, moderate 114
Hyphema 233, 233f
Hypoglycemia 189, 193, 194, 194fc, 198
   acute complications of 196t
   associated autonomic failure 196, 197fc
   chronic complications of 196t
   complications of 196

defective defense against 194*fc*
defense against 196*f*
diagnosis of 193
effects of 197*fc*
management of 196
nocturnal 195
posthypoglycemic 195
unawareness 195
Hypokalemia 177, 181, 189
  electrocardiography findings of 182*f*
  etiologies of 182*t*
  management 183*t*
  mild 183
  severe 183
  severity of 181*t*
  surgery for 183
Hypokalemic periodic paralysis 181
Hyponatremia 177
  etiology of 177*t*
  management 179*fc*
Hypophosphatemia 87
Hypotension 72, 79, 276, 295, 317
  orthostatic 18, 19*b*
Hypotensive states, acute 324
Hypothermia 109
Hypoventilation 87
Hypoxemia 57, 87
  causes of 58*f*
  degree of 329
  prompt correction of 329
Hypoxia 296
  degree of 35

I

Ibuprofen 132
Ictal paresis 105
Idarucizumab 116
Idiopathic pulmonary arterial hypertension 87
Ileus 278
Immersion 328
Immunoglobulin
  A 162
  M antibody 150
Immunotherapy 317
Infectious Diseases Society of America 66
Infliximab 317
Infratemporal fossa 243
Inhalation injury 87, 269*f*
In-hospital cardiac arrest, prevention of 5
Injuries, penetrating 233
Inspired oxygen, fraction of 90
Insulin
  subcutaneous 190
  therapy 191
Insulinoma 193, 278*f*
Intensive care unit 66, 86, 89, 90, 142, 148
Intensive glycemic control 193
Interferon-gamma 65
Interleukin-18 163*f*
Intermittent pneumatic compression 276
International Classification of Headache Disorders 129
International Headache Society 129
International League against Epilepsy Classification 104
International Normalized Ratio 150, 152

International Study Group of Rectal Cancer 279
Interstitial lung disease 317
Intestinal obstruction 138, 147, 183, 279*f*
Intra-abdominal severe infection 279
Intracerebral hemorrhage 111, 115*f*
  acute 114
  score 115*t*
Intracranial pressure 119
  control 115
  monitoring 116
Intrarenal acute renal failure 160
Intrathoracic blood volume 270
Intravascular injection 292, 299
Intravenous alteplase 113
  exclusion criteria for 113
Intubation, difficult 292
Invasive mechanical ventilation, indications of 62
Ipratropium bromide 249
Iritis 232
Iron 252
Ischemia 112*f*
  intestinal 139
Isoprenaline 323
Isotonic crystalloid solution 147

J

Japanese encephalitis 126
Jaw-thrust maneuver 50
Jugular venous pressure 58, 178

K

Keratitis 232
  adenoviral 232
Ketamine 108, 109
Ketoacidosis, diabetic 97, 139, 187, 187*f*, 188
Ketogenic diet 109
Ketone bodies 188
Ketonemia 188
Ketosis 188
Kidney 168
  biopsy 163
  disease 158*t*
    end-stage 158*f*
  injury
    acute 157, 158, 158*f*, 158*t*, 161, 162, 162*t*, 163*f*, 164*f*, 172*t*
    molecule 163*f*
  test 150
King's College Criteria 152
  for Paracetamol Overdose and Nonparacetamol Acute Liver Failure 152*t*
Knee
  injury 219
  pain 219
Krait bite 313

L

Labetalol 290, 323
Lacosamide 108
Lactate dehydrogenase 64, 208
Laryngeal mask airway 52, 53
  placement of 54*f*
Laryngoscopy, difficult 292
Laryngospasm 296

Lasmiditan 132, 133
Leptospira 40, 160
Leukemia, basophilic 318
Leukotriene 318
  B4 318
  modifiers 91
Levetiracetam 108
Ligate 310
Lipoprotein, low-density 32
Liver 150
  assist devices 152
  biochemistry 138
  dysfunction 142
  failure, acute 150, 151, 151*t*
  transplant 152
Local anesthetic systemic toxicity 298
Low pressure cardiac tamponade 41
Lower airway obstruction 248
Lower gastrointestinal bleeding 145*fc*
Lower respiratory tract 316
Lower segment cesarean section 205
Low-molecular weight heparin 69, 69*t*, 113, 276, 326
Lumbar puncture, technique of 120
Lung
  diseases, immunologic 71
  scintigraphy 79
Lupus, acute flare of 261*f*
Lymphoma 178

M

Macrolide 243
Macronutrient abnormalities 188
Macrophage activation syndrome 261, 261*f*, 261*t*
Magnesium 109
  sulfate 87, 91, 290
Magnetic resonance imaging 42, 126
Malignancy 119, 243
Malignant diseases 178
Mannitol 116, 172, 290
Mask ventilation, difficult 292
Massive hemoptysis 70
  management of 73*fc*
Mast cell activation syndrome 317
Mastocytosis 317, 318
Mean arterial pressure 151
Mechanical circulatory support 37
Medication, theophylline group of 87
Melena 142
Meninges, inflammation of 118
Meningitis 118
  acute 118
  anaerobic bacterial 121
  bacterial 119
  healthcare-associated 118
Menstrual bleeding, heavy 208
Mental
  disorders 224*b*
  function, higher 86
  illness 223
Mephentermine 324
Metabolic emergencies 177, 292, 297
Metabolic hyperglycemic emergencies 187
Methylenedioxymethamphetamine 178
Methylprednisolone 249, 290
Meticulous surgical techniques 284
Metoprolol 290

Midazolam 107, 108, 109, 290
Middle cerebral artery 112*f*
    segment 114
Migraine 25, 129*t*, 132, 133
    acute 129
        treatment of 132*t*, 133*fc*
    basilar-type 25
    clinical features of 130*t*
Mineralocorticoid receptor antagonists 38
Miscarriage 206
    types of 207*f*
Monoamine oxidase inhibitors 317
Monocled cobra 310*f*
Monomorphic ventricular tachycardia 295*f*
Monosodium glutamate 318
Morbilliform rashes 316
Morphine 147, 326
Motor examination 110
Motorbike
    accident 216*f*
    ambulance 310*f*
Mouth-to-mouth
    breathing 5*f*
    respiration 329*f*
Movement disorders 124
Multiple endocrine neoplasia syndromes 193
Multiple myeloma 161
Mushroom poisoning 323
Mycobacterium tuberculosis 40
Myeloperoxidase 160
Myocardial infarction 29, 30, 35, 36, 139, 276, 318, 324
Myocardial injury 277
Myocardial necrosis 35
Myocardial rupture 44
Myoma, pedunculated 209

N

Naproxen 132, 134, 290
Naratriptan 132
Nasal endoscopy 72
Nasal septum 238*f*
Nasogastric tube 143
Nasopharyngeal airway 54*f*
Nasopharyngeal tube 53, 217
National Institute of Health Stroke Scale 111
National Poison Information Centre 305
Natriuretic peptide 35, 165
Nausea, postoperative 278
Nebulization 90
Nebulized salbutamol 248
Neck stiffness 98
Necrotizing vasculitis 259*f*
Neisseria meningitidis 118
Neoplasms 243
Neoplastic disease 258
Neostigmine 313*f*
Nephrotoxic medications, discontinuation of 166
Nerve, trigeminal 243
Nervous system, disorders of 178
Neuralgia 244
    trigeminal 244
Neuroimaging 101, 111
Neurological emergency 292, 297
Neurosurgery, role of 116
Neurosurgical emergency 292, 297
Neuroviral diagnostic tests 126

Neutrophil gelatinase-associated lipocalin 163*f*
Nicotinic toxidrome 306
Nipah virus 126
Nitroglycerin 290
Noninvasive mechanical ventilator 61
Noninvasive positive pressure ventilation 35, 36
Noninvasive ventilation 59, 59*t*, 60*b*, 90
Nonprotein colloid solutions 274
Non-ST-elevation myocardial infarction 29, 30
Nonsteroidal anti-inflammatory
    agent 323
    drugs 85, 132, 133, 257, 260, 316
Noradrenaline 290
Norepinephrine 74
N-terminal pro brain natriuretic peptide 37, 65
Nutrition 147
    enternal 270

O

Obstetric emergencies 205*t*, 292, 297
Obstructive sleep apnea 277
Obtundation 95
Ocular emergencies 261
Oculocephalic responses 100*t*
Oculovestibular responses 100
Odours 97*t*
Odynophagia 317
Oligemia, benign 111
Ondansetron 326
Ophthalmic emergencies 231
Opioids 252
    toxidrome 306
Optic fundus examination 99
Oral activated charcoal 115
Oral anticoagulants 115
Oral hypoglycemic agents 257
Orbital injuries 233
Organophosphorus 97
    poisoning 323
Oropharyngeal airway 53, 53*f*
Oropharyngeal malignancy 243
Oropharyngeal tube 217
Oropharynx 329
Orthostatic hypotension 18, 19*b*
    causes of 18*b*
Orthostatic intolerance 21
Osteoporosis 259
    fracture 258
Otalgia 242
    causes of 242
    referred 243, 244*f*
    types of 242*fc*
Otitis externa
    acute 242
    malignant 243
Otitis media, acute 243
Otomycosis 242
Otorhinolaryngological emergencies 237
Outflow tract obstruction 157
Out-of-hospital cardiac arrest, prevention of 5
Ovarian cyst
    ruptured 209
    torsion of 209, 209*f*
Ovarian neoplasm, rupture of 204
Over speeding 215*f*

Oxygen
    monitoring 87
    saturation 62, 90, 270
    therapy 36, 87
Oxygenation 61

P

Paget disease 258
Pain
    abdominal 137, 139*fc*, 146, 326
    duration of 140
    features of 140
    intensity 132
    parietal 137
    patterns of 140*f*
    progressive 140*f*
    types of 140
    visceral 137
Palmar erythema gynecomastia 143
Pancreas, head of 278*f*
Pancreatitis 139, 146, 258, 280
Pandora's box 137
Paracetamol 132, 252
Paralysis 52, 73
Paraovarian cyst 209
Parenchymal blush 75*f*
Parenteral nutritional support 270
Paroxysmal atrial fibrillation 277
Paroxysmal supraventricular tachycardia 323, 325
Partial heart block 323
Peak expiratory flow 62, 89
Pedal edema 178
Pediatric cardiac arrest algorithm 12*fc*
Pediatric emergencies 247, 292, 297
Pelvic
    endometriosis 204
    examination 138
    ultrasonography of 206
Penicillinase-resistant penicillin 243
Pentamidine 172
Pentobarbital 109
Percutaneous coronary intervention 31, 32, 36, 41
Pericardial effusion 40
Pericardial fluid 41*f*
    drainage 44
Pericardial injury syndromes 41
Pericarditis, effusive-constrictive 40
Pericardium, volume curve of 41*f*
Perichondritis 242
Perineum 267
Periorbital hematinic proptosis 233
Peritonitis 280
Perivascular injection 292, 299
Pheniramine 290
Phenytoin 108, 290
Pheochromocytoma 318
Phosphorus 268
Physical trauma, types of 218*fc*
Plasma glucose concentration 195
Platelet-activating factor 318
Pleocytosis, polymorphonuclear 125
Plethoric inferior vena cava 42
Pleural effusion 61, 63, 64*fc*, 277*f*
Pleural fluid cytology 65*fc*
Pneumonia 34, 61, 63, 277, 139
    community-acquired 248*t*
Pneumothorax 34, 61, 63, 64*fc*

Poisons 252, 306
    household 251*t*
    hypnotic 325
    type of 305
    unabsorbed 307
Pollen-food syndrome 318
Polyangiitis 87
Polymorphic ventricular tachycardia 295*f*
Polyp, endometrial 210*f*
Positive end-expiratory pressure 330
Positive pressure ventilation 59
Positron emission tomography 127
Postresuscitation 144
    care 291
Potassium 87
    chloride 183
    excess intake of 183
    excretion 181
    levels 189
    loss 183
    replenishment of 183
Pott's spine 258
Prednisolone 249
Pre-embolization digital subtraction angiographic image 75*f*
Pregnancy 150, 203, 204*fc*, 209*f*
    ectopic 139, 203-205, 206*f*
    types of 205*f*
Premature ventricular contraction 31, 294*f*
Pressurized metered dose inhaler 62, 88
Procainamide 290
Promethazine 327
Propofol 108, 109
Prostaglandin D2 318
Protein binding 173
Prothrombin
    complex concentrate 115
    time 152
Proton pump inhibitors 143
Pseudohemoptysis 72
Pseudohypoglycemia 195
Pseudomonas 243
    aeruginosa 242
Pseudosyncope 26
    psychogenic 18, 21
Psychiatric disorders 224
Psychiatric emergencies 224
Psychogenic nonepileptic
    seizures 18
    syndrome 21
Psychosis 224
Psychotic disorders 317
Ptosis 313*f*
Pulmonary artery
    sling 87
    wedge pressure 270
Pulmonary disease 119
Pulmonary disorders 178
Pulmonary embolism 19, 34, 61, 67, 67*fc*, 68, 77, 78*f*, 80*fc*, 81*fc*, 82, 276, 277, 296, 318, 326
    differential diagnosis of 79
    early diagnosis of 78
    management protocol of 68*fc*
    severity index 82, 82*t*
Pulseless electrical activity 7, 12
Pulseless ventricular tachycardia 7, 12
Pulsus paradoxus 42

Pupils 98
    examination 99
Purulent discharge 283*f*
Pyridoxine 109

R

Radiotherapy, extrathoracic 74
Raised intracranial pressure 116
Rankin scale score, prestroke modified 114
Rapid airway management position 52, 53*f*
Rapid tranquilization medication 226*fc*
Rash driving 215*f*
Rasmussen's aneurysm 71*f*
Recombinant tissue plasminogen activator 69
Rectal examination 138
Red blood cell 142
Red eye 231
Reflex 100
    syncope 18
        diagnosis of 25
Refractory hypoxemic acute respiratory failure 59*f*
Rehabilitation 272
Renal artery stenosis 183
Renal calculi 138
Renal disease 147
    end-stage 168, 170
Renal emergencies 262
Renal failure
    acute 157, 158, 158*f*
    indices 162
Renal function tests 138
Renal infarction 157
Renal insufficiency 168
Renal replacement therapy 166
Renal syndromes, pulmonary 262
Renal trauma 157
Respiration, abnormal patterns of 97*t*
Respiratory arrest 59*f*
Respiratory complications 277
Respiratory distress, sudden onset 79
Respiratory emergencies 61, 262, 292, 296
Respiratory failure 57, 58*fc*, 59
Resuscitation 6, 143
    cardiopulmonary 3, 6, 7, 9-12, 67, 330
    fluid 249, 270*b*
    neonatal 297
Reteplase 31
Retrograde intubation 54
Revascularization 31
Reversible cerebral vasoconstriction syndrome 131
Rheumatoid
    arthritis 41, 263*f*, 323
    vasculitis 259*f*
Rheumatological emergencies 257
Rheumatology 257, 260*t*
Rhinocerebral mucormycosis 189
Rifle criteria 157, 158*f*
Ringer's solution 147, 273, 274
Rituximab infusion 259*f*
Rizatriptan 132
Road traffic accidents 215
Rotator cuff pain 218
Rule of nine 257, 268*f*
Russell's viper 309*f*, 311
Ryles tube 147

S

Salbutamol 87
Salicylates 193
Salt intoxication 179
Sarcoidosis 41
Saw-scaled viper 309*f*
Scar ectopic pregnancy 203
Schizophrenia 224
Scleroderma renal crisis 260
Screening tests 98, 98*t*, 102
Scrub encephalitis 125
Sea snakes 309
Seizures 21*t*, 25*t*, 114, 116, 125, 252
    disorder 259
    refractory 259*f*
    repeated focal motor 105
    types of 253*t*
Sepsis 279
Serum ceruloplasmin 150
Serum creatinine 158
    concentration 158*f*
Serum protein electrophoresis 161
Severe acute asthma treatment 90*fc*
Sexual assault 207
    and rape 210
Sgarbossa criteria 30, 30*f*
Shock 276, 318, 325
    anaphylactic 322
    cardiogenic 322, 324
    lung syndrome 328
    resuscitation fluid for 249
Shoulder injury 219, 219*f*
Sick day rules 190, 191
Sickle cell anemia 118
Silver sulfadiazine 272
Simplified pulmonary embolism severity index 82
Simultaneous argon plasma coagulation therapy 74*f*
Sjögren syndrome 41
Skin
    excoriation 281*f*
    failure, acute severe 258
    flap necrosis 283*f*
Small pulmonary artery branch 71*f*
Snakebite 309
    management 311, 312*fc*
        syndromic approach of 312
    treatment 311
Sodium 178, 184, 273
    bicarbonate 290
    glucose cotransporter 38
    valproate 108
Somogyi effect 195
Spectacled cobra 309*f*
Spinal fractures 259
Spontaneous circulation, return of 8, 10
Spontaneous eye
    examination 99*t*
    movements 99
Spontaneous pneumothorax
    primary 63
    secondary 63
Spot urine
    potassium 182
    sodium 182
Standard cerebrospinal fluid test, analysis of 120

Staphylococcus aureus 242
    methicillin-resistant 66
Status asthmaticus 325
Status epilepticus 104, 106, 109*fc*
    classification of 104, 105*b*
    convulsive 105
    emergency treatment of 104*t*
    etiology of 105*b*
    evaluation of 105
    general management of 105
    management of 106*fc*
    nonconvulsive 105, 106, 109
    refractory 107, 108*t*
Status migrainosus 133
ST-elevation myocardial infarction 8, 29, 32, 36
Sterile suturing set 291
Steven-Johnson syndrome 260*f*
Stomal prolapse 281*f*
Stomal retraction 281*f*
Streptococcus pneumoniae 118
Streptokinase 31
Stridor 317
Stroke 104, 111
    acute ischemic 111, 112
    ischemic 118
Stupor 96
Stylohyoid
    ligament 244
    syndrome 244
Subglottic obstruction 53
Succinate dehydrogenase 208
Sudden cardiac death 5, 29
Suicides 328
Sulfasalazine treatment 260*f*
Sulfite additive allergy 318
Sumatriptan 132
Super-refractory status epilepticus 108, 109*t*
Supine carotid sinus massage 24
Supportive therapies 166
Supraglottic obstruction 53
Surgery
    laparoscopic 277
    noncardiac 277
Surgical bleeding, trauma related 322
Surgical site infections 282
Syncope 17, 19, 21*t*, 25*t*, 27*b*
    arrhythmic 22*b*
    cardiac cause of 22
    cardiopulmonary 22*b*
    cardiovascular 19
    classification of 18, 18*b*
    clinical manifestations of 20
    development of 20*fc*
    diagnostic evaluation of 20
    differential diagnosis of 25
    epidemiology of 19
    pathophysiology of 20
    prodromal phase of 20*b*
    vasovagal 18
Syndrome of inappropriate antidiuretic hormone secretion 178
    etiologies of 178*t*
Synkope 17
Systemic inflammatory response syndrome 146
Systemic lupus erythematosus 41, 259*f*
Systemic venous return 40

T

Tachycardia 7, 21, 79, 293, 293*f*
    adult 13*fc*
    supraventricular 13, 322
Tachypnea 72, 79
Tacrolimus 172
Telangiectasia, hemorrhagic 143
Temporomandibular joint 243
Tendonitis 218
Tenecteplase 31
Tennis elbow 218
Tenofovir 172
Tension
    headache 129, 130*t*
    pneumothorax 29
Testis, torsion of 139
Thallium 97
Thiopental 108, 109
Thrombocytopenia 261*f*
Thromboembolic disorders 324
Thromboembolism 276
Thrombolysis 30
Thrombolytic
    intravenous 113
    regimens 68, 69*t*
    therapy 31
        prehospital initiation of 32*t*
    thrombocytopenic purpura-hemolytic uremic syndrome 159
Thymoma 178
Thyroglobulin 148
Thyroid
    function tests 178
    stimulating hormone 37
    storm 325
Thyrotoxic periodic paralysis 181
Tibial shaft fracture 219
Ticagrelor 31
Tilt table test 21, 24
    indications for 23
Tonsillitis 243
Total parenteral nutrition 148
Toxic epidermal necrolysis 259, 259*f*
Toxic vital signs 305
Toxidromes 305, 306, 306*t*
Toxins 150
Tracheostomy 240
    preoperative management of 240
Tramadol 147
Transcranial magnetic stimulation 109
Transient ischemic attack 111
Transtubular potassium gradient 182, 184
Transvaginal scan 204, 205
Trauma 292, 298
Triage system, level of 298*f*
Tricuspid insufficiency 36
Tricyclic antidepressants 317
Triptans 132, 134
Troponins 35
Tubercular meningitis 121
Tuberculoma, multiple 259*f*
Tuberculosis 64, 70
Tubular necrosis, acute 161, 171
Twenty-four hours urine potassium 182
Twenty-minute whole blood clotting test 313*f*

U

Ultrasonography 138, 204, 205, 207, 208

Unconsciousness 99*t*
    evaluation 101*fc*
Upper airway obstruction 248, 248*t*
Upper respiratory tract 316
Ureteric calculus 139
Urine
    analysis 138
    osmolality 163, 182
    output 157, 158, 158*f*, 270, 272
    potassium 184
    protein electrophoresis 161
Urokinase 31
Uterine bleeding, massive 210

V

Vagal nerve stimulation 109
Vancomycin flushing syndrome 318
Varicella zoster 118
    virus 126, 150
Vascular disease, peripheral 324
Vasculitis
    systemic 41
    urticarial 259, 318
Vasopressors 165, 319
Veillonella 121
Venom detection testing kit 311
Venous thromboembolism 67, 276
Venous thrombosis 190
Ventilation, technique of difficult 53
Ventricular ectopic beats 294
Ventricular fibrillation 7, 12, 295, 295*f*
Ventricular tachycardia 7, 294, 322, 323
Vertebral body compression fracture 219
Vertigo 98
Villous adenoma 183
Violence 223
    etiological explanations of 223
Vital signs 306
    abnormalities in 306*t*
Vocal cord
    dysfunction 87
    edematous 269*f*
Vomiting, postoperative 278

W

Water metabolism 188
Wells scores 79
Whipple's procedure 280*f*
Whipple's triad, modified 193
World Allergy Organization 317*b*
Wound 268
    complications 282
    dehiscence 280*f*, 282*f*
    surgical-site infections 282*f*
Wrist injury 218, 218*f*

X

X-ray 138
Xylocaine 290
Xylocard 290

Z

Zero order kinetics 108
Zoledronate 172
Zolmitriptan 132

EU GSPR Authorised Reprsentative
Logos Europe, 9 rue Nicolas Poussin
1700, La Rochelle, France
Phone: +33 (0) 6 67 93 73 78
E-mail: contact@logoseurope.eu

www.ingramcontent.com/pod-product-compliance
Ingram Content Group UK Ltd.
Pitfield, Milton Keynes, MK11 3LW, UK
UKHW050430150426
5217IPUK00019B/1330